Foundations of Dental Technology: Anatomy and Physiology

Foundations of Dental Technology
Anatomy and Physiology

Arnold Hohmann

Retired Instructor of Dental Technology
Carl-Severing Vocational College
Bielefeld, Germany

Werner Hielscher

Medical Illustrator
Bad Salzuflen, Germany

Former Head of Design Department
Carl-Severing Vocational College
Bielefeld, Germany

Quintessence Publishing Co, Inc
Chicago, Berlin, Tokyo, London, Paris, Milan, Barcelona, Beijing, Istanbul,
Moscow, New Delhi, Prague, São Paulo, Seoul, Singapore, and Warsaw

This book was originally published in German under the title *Lehrbuch der Zahntechnik, Band 1: Anatomie, Kieferorthopädie.*

Library of Congress Cataloging-in-Publication Data

Hohmann, Arnold, author.
  [Lehrbuch der Zahntechnik. Band 1, Anatomie, Kieferorthopädie. English]
  Foundations of dental technology. Anatomy and physiology / Arnold Hohmann and Werner Hielscher.
      p. ; cm.
  Anatomy and physiology
  Includes index.
  ISBN 978-0-86715-611-9 (softcover)
  I. Hielscher, Werner, author. II. Title. III. Title: Anatomy and physiology.
  [DNLM: 1. Stomatognathic System--anatomy & histology. 2. Orthopedic Procedures. 3. Technology, Dental. WU 101]
  QP146
  612.3'1--dc23
                                    2014017755

5 4 3 2 1

© 2014 Quintessence Publishing Co Inc

Quintessence Publishing Co Inc
4350 Chandler Drive
Hanover Park, IL 60133
www.quintpub.com

Editor: Leah Huffman
Design: Ted Pereda
Production: Sue Robinson

Printed in the USA

Contents

Introduction *vi*

1 Fundamental Concepts of Dental Technology *1*

2 Cells and Tissues *25*

3 Dental Tissues *41*

4 Morphology of Teeth *71*

5 Morphology of the Dentition *115*

6 Cranial Anatomy *151*

7 Physiology of Mandibular Movement *201*

8 Articulators *245*

9 Pathology of the Orofacial System *275*

10 Orthodontics *295*

11 Splint Therapy *357*

Index *381*

Introduction

Trainee dental technicians are introduced to working in a health care profession by being taught the nomenclature of dentistry and dental technology and being given wide-ranging basic medical knowledge. However, students often have difficulty relating this basic knowledge to the job-specific tasks in dental technology. An understanding of the functional interrelationships of anatomical form not only makes it easier but actually makes it possible to comprehend the whole purpose of dental technology work. Therefore, this book focuses on the relationship between anatomical form and function in dental technology, providing the high-level technical knowledge necessary to develop profession-specific competence and innovation in dental technology.

The close cooperative relationship between dentist and dental technician is a process of doing preparatory work for each other in a series of established working steps. Depending on the particular nature of the prosthetic replacement, these steps can vary in their internal structure, but they nevertheless reflect the principle of providing a specific medical service and division of work. Only when dental technicians understand how to relate form to function can they succeed in providing excellent restorations and laboratory work to their collaborating dentists.

Fundamental Concepts of Dental Technology

Specialization

The purpose of any professional training is to become fully capable of performing a specific job. Successful specialists should be able to undertake professional tasks, perfect and appraise their work, and also show a willingness to be innovative and open to alternative solutions while reflecting on their own work. Sound technical skills are also necessary, and these skills rely on in-depth technical expertise as well as craftsmanship. For dental technicians, the goals of specialist training are the following:

- To acquire a detailed understanding of:
  - The anatomical principles of the masticatory system
  - The physiologic effects of the materials used for dental prostheses
  - The esthetic principles of oral rehabilitation
- To acquire practical knowledge regarding the interdependence of the form and the function of tissues, organs, and organ systems
- To work out criteria and construction conditions for producing dentures

Form and Function

Skilled dental technicians should have a fundamental medical knowledge, which will enable them to produce functional dental prostheses. In dentistry, prosthetic work is objectively assessed using criteria based on the form and function of anatomical tissue structures. Anatomy is therefore a primary discipline for dental technicians.

Anatomy is the study of the structure and form of the human body as well as animal and plant bodies (Fig 1-1). The word *anatomy* is derived from Greek and means "to dissect or dismember." When the human body is dissected and examined, the position, shape, and composition of the organs and organ systems can be defined. *Macroscopic anatomy* involves describing the form and structure of what is visible to the naked eye; *microscopic anatomy*, on the other hand, involves examination of the structure of organs and tissues that can only be seen under the microscope. Focus directed specifically to the positions of the organs and the relations of the organs and tissues to each other is known as *topographical anatomy* (ie, describing position). However, focus directed to the tissues themselves and their constituents is known as *histology* (ie, the study of tissues). *Cytology* (ie, the study of cells) is a specific branch of histology.

The study of form and organization (ie, the study of interactions), mutual influences, and interdependence of organs and organ systems is carried out using techniques that involve studying the processes of life; this discipline is known as *physiology*. All normal processes in the human body and any normal demands on organs and tissues are therefore considered physiologic. For example, chewing hard foods, which puts strain on the teeth because they are embedded in the jaw, is a physiologic process (and a physiologic stress) because the tissues involved were created for this very purpose and designed to withstand this type of strain. Meanwhile, the discipline of *pathology* focuses on the abnormal changes in the body as well as the causes of diseases and their courses; changes due to disease are therefore known as *pathologic disorders*.

While medical practitioners draw on their experiences of anatomy, physiology, and pathology in their daily practice of treating patients, dental technicians do not interact with patients directly but rather base their restorations on physical reproductions (models) of the patients' teeth. Therefore, a sound knowledge of anatomy, physiology, and pathology is essential for any dental technician. The goal of any artificial replacement, whether it be for the teeth, parts of the alveolar ridge, or mucous membrane, is to integrate this prosthesis with the living structures; not only is the form being replaced, but function is also being restored. In other words, the dental prosthesis should not only replace the tissue but should also function in the same way as the original tissue.

Law of form and function

There is a close link between the unique form of a tissue (eg, of teeth) and the function it is intended to carry out. This relationship has led to the establishment of the *law of form and function*, which states that a tissue developed for a specific purpose takes on a specific form for that purpose. This law also states that when the function of the tissue changes, its form alters to the same extent and vice versa.

Disuse atrophy is a particular aspect of the law of form and function, and it may explain the association between the form and the function of a tissue. If a leg is immobilized in a plaster cast after a fracture, the muscles begin to waste away and weaken because they are not being used; their form or shape therefore changes. However, this process is reversible. If the leg is used again after the fracture has healed, the muscles return to their original form. *Atrophy* is the wasting away of tissue caused by lack of nutrition, while *disuse atrophy* is specifically a shrinking of tissue caused by reduced blood flow when there is a lack of use.

Once this association between form and function is established, it becomes clear that a denture, like any other component in the body, must have the correct anatomical form in order to function reliably. An artificial prosthesis that does not have the correct form cannot fulfill the original function of the tissue.

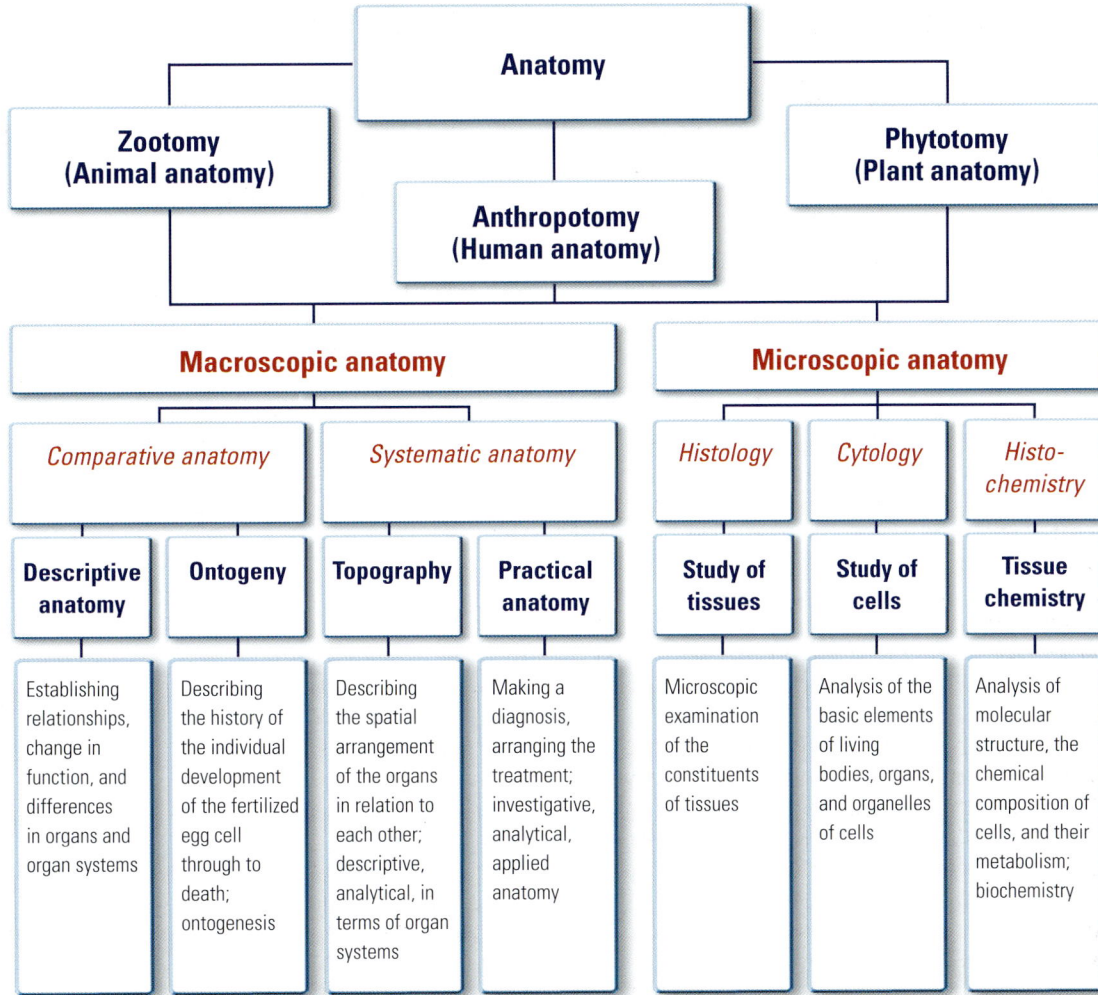

Fig 1-1 Subdivisions of anatomy.

Structure of the Human Body

The human body can be divided into two portions: *(1)* the trunk, head, and neck and *(2)* the extremities (Fig 1-2).

Trunk, head, and neck

The **trunk** *(truncus)* comprises the chest, abdomen, and pelvis. The posterior region of the trunk is known as the *back (dorsum)*. The upper region of the trunk, the *chest (thorax)*, is formed from the bony rib cage, which protects the lungs. The *chest cavity (cavitas thoracis)* is separated from the abdominal cavity below by the diaphragm. The *abdomen* describes the area between the thorax and the pelvis, its bony structure being formed by the lumbar spine. The *abdominal cavity (cavitas abdominalis)* contains the abdominal viscera, which are bordered by the peritoneum. The lower part of the trunk, the *pelvis*, contains the pelvic organs and connects the trunk to the lower extremities.

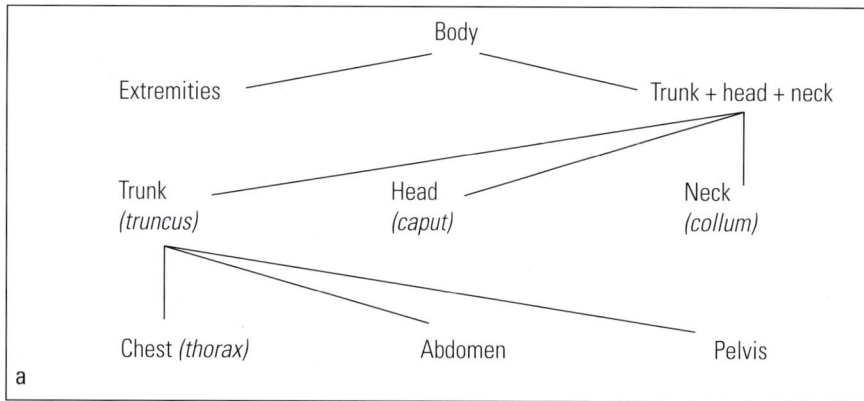

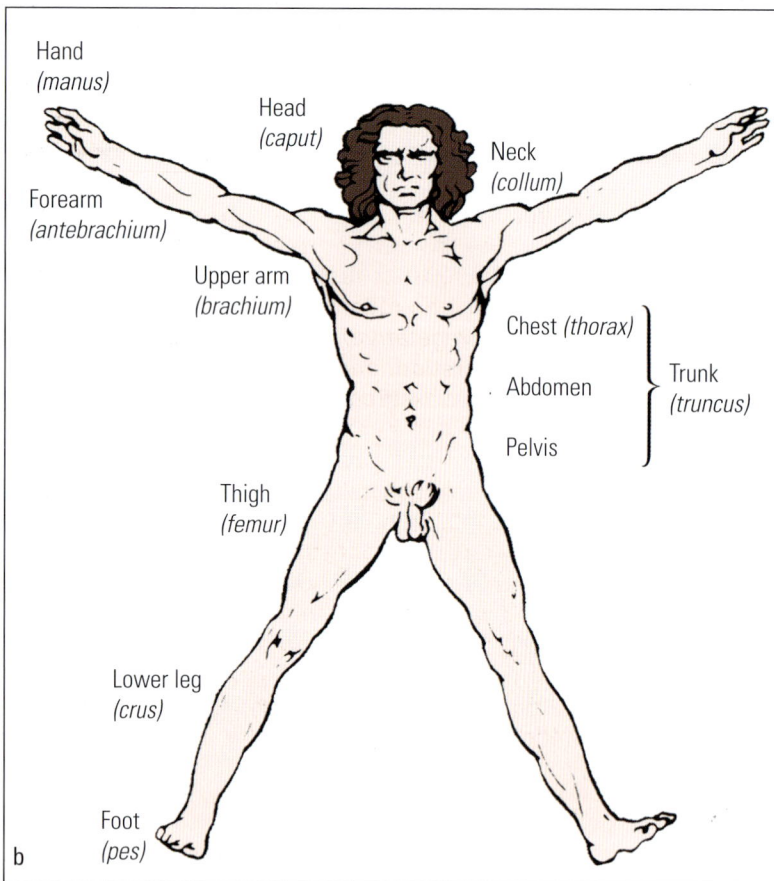

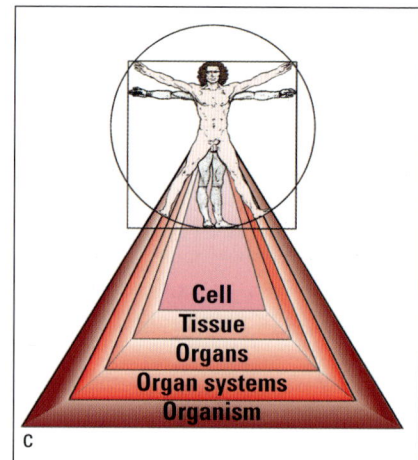

Fig 1-2 *(a)* Structural diagram of the human body. *(b)* Illustration of the locations of the major structures of the human body. *(c)* Diagram depicting the increasing complexity of human body structures.

The **head** *(caput)* includes the cavities that house the brain and the sensory organs. The head also includes the mouth and nose, responsible for food and air intake, respectively. The basic bony structure of the head is the skull (cranium), the tooth-bearing parts of which are formed by the skeletal tissue of the jaw. The crown (vertex) forms the highest point of the vault of the cranium. The front half of the head is known as the *sinciput*, the posterior area is known as the *occiput*, and the side regions are known as the *temples (tempus)*. The front surface of the head is known as the *face (facies)*, in which the eyes *(oculi)*, nose *(nasus)*, and mouth *(os)* are located. The ears *(auris)* are positioned on the sides of the head.

The **neck** *(collum)* connects the head to the chest. Its basic bony structure is the cervical spine, in front of which lie the windpipe and the gullet as well as the nerves and vessels supplying the head. The back of the neck is known as the *nape (nucha)*.

Extremities

The four **limbs** (ie, arms and legs) are connected to the top of the trunk by the shoulder girdle and to the bottom of the trunk by the pelvic girdle. The arm is subdivided into the upper arm *(brachium)*, lower arm or forearm *(antebrachium)*, and hand *(manus)*, which includes the fingers *(digiti)*. The leg is composed of the thigh *(femur)*, lower leg *(crus)*, and foot *(pes)*.

Complexity of the human body

There is a scale of increasing complexity within the structure of the human body, ranging from a single cell—the smallest unit of life—to a complete organism (see Fig 1-2c). Cells make up tissues, the next level of complexity, which then differentiate into organs with characteristic functions. Organ systems, which comprise combinations of several organs, form the next level of complexity, with the unit of highest complexity being the complete organism.

The **cell** is the smallest functional unit of all living creatures that is capable of independent life and reproduction. A cell is able to undertake various metabolic processes including growth, movement, and reaction to stimuli, and it can reproduce by cell division. Cells exist in a diversity of forms and, in multicellular organisms, become specialized to form specific types of tissue.

Tissues are structures composed of cells that have the same structure, function, and intercellular substances. Individual tissues are never independent, but as several tissues combine, they form more complex functional units such as organs and organ systems. Tissues can be classified according to their structure and function as protective, supporting, and connective tissue as well as muscle and nerve tissue.

The **intercellular space** is the gap between cells, and these spaces contain intercellular substances in which nutrients, active substances, and breakdown products are transported from the vessels to the cells. The intercellular substances determine the unique properties of different tissues (eg, the high tensile strength in tendons is due to collagenous fibers, and the strength of the hard tissue in teeth results from the deposition of calcium salts).

Organs are functional units composed of different tissues that are characterized by their specific function and their histologic microstructure. Examples include muscles, lungs, kidneys, etc. *Autonomic (vegetative) organs* are involved in nutrition, excretion, and procreation, while sensory organs are classified as *somatic organs*.

Organ systems are units of organs that work together to perform particular functions. Examples include the respiratory, digestive, excretory, and nervous systems. Interrelationships among organ systems are coordinated and regulated by nervous and hormonal control.

The **organism** is the whole system of organs in a living body. It is made up of various functional units (ie, the organs), which are responsible for the development, maintenance, and procreation of the organism.

Anatomical Nomenclature for Direction and Position

Terms that denote direction and position are standardized in anatomical nomenclature so that all the positional descriptions of areas of the human body can be located by reference to specific planes and directions. In dentistry, these systems

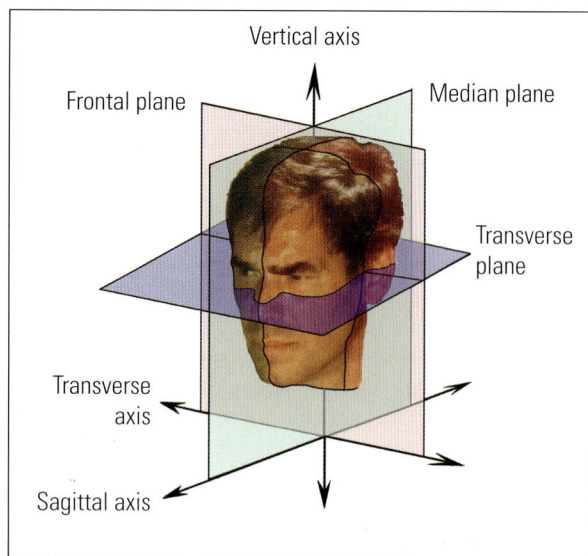

Fig 1-3 Principal planes and axes relating to the head.

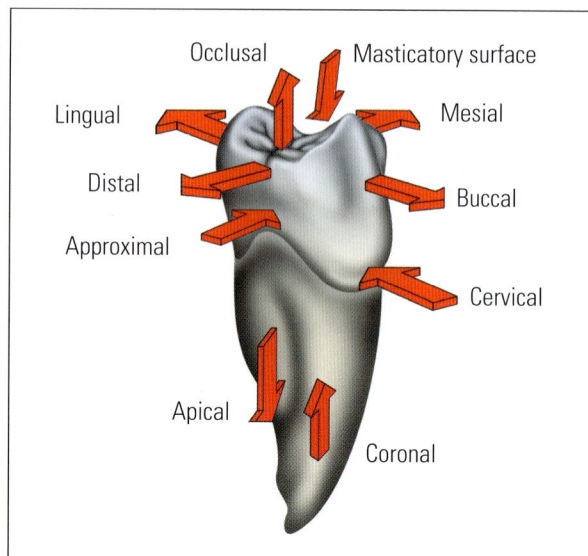

Fig 1-4 Directional terms relating to the tooth.

of reference can be used, for example, to fit a row of teeth into the geometry of the skull. To locate the position of parts of the body or organs, the human body can be divided into four principal planes and three main axes (Fig 1-3).

The **median** or **symmetry plane** divides the body into the right and left halves. The following adjectives are used to distinguish between the two halves of the body: *dexter, dextra, dextrum* = right; *sinister, sinistra, sinistrum* = left. A **sagittal plane** (*sagitta* = arrow), or paramedian plane, is a plane parallel to the median plane through the body. The median plane is therefore unique among the numerous sagittal planes.

The **frontal plane** (*frons* = forehead) is the plane parallel to the forehead and perpendicular to the median plane, which divides the body into the posterior (rear) and anterior (front) regions.

The **transverse plane** is the horizontal plane that is perpendicular to the median and frontal planes and divides the body into the upper and lower regions.

The main axes run as follows:

• **Vertical axis**: from top to bottom
• **Sagittal axis**: from front to back
• **Transverse axis**: from left to right

To locate the position of a tooth, directional names that relate to the anatomy of the tooth are used. For each tooth, a distinction is made between the visible area protruding into the oral cavity, the crown of the tooth *(corona dentis)*, and the root *(radix dentis)*, which is anchored in the jawbone. The transition between the crown and the root is known as the *neck* of the tooth *(collum dentis, cervix dentis)*. The tip of the root *(apex dentis)* is the only part of the tooth that is perforated, and the perforation is known as the *apical foramen (foramen apicis dentis)*.

The location of a particular tooth in relation to the head, the occlusion, and the other teeth is identified using directional terms in addition to other terms that specify a point within the body, head, occlusion, or tooth that lies in the specified direction. Common directional terms used in relation to the teeth and the dental arches include (Figs 1-4 and 1-5):

• **Vestibular**: the area of the vestibule (*vestibulum* = space between cheeks and gingiva/teeth); directed toward the outside of the dental arch
• **Buccal**: the cheek area (*bucca* = cheek); directed outward in the region of the posterior teeth
• **Labial**: the lip area (*labium* = lip); directed outward in the region of the anterior teeth

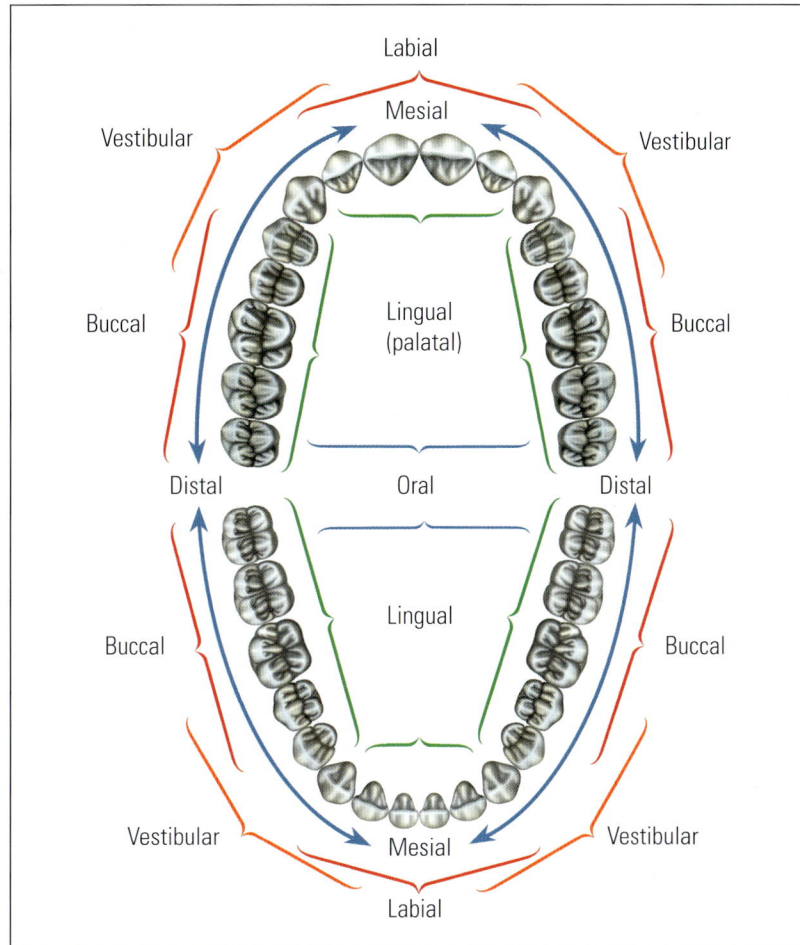

Fig 1-5 Positional and directional terms relating to the dental arch.

- **Oral**: the area in the mouth (*os* = mouth) facing the inside of the dental arch
- **Lingual**: the tongue region (*lingua* = tongue)
- **Palatal**: the palate area (*palatum* = palate)
- **Approximal**: adjacent; toward the contact surface (*ad* = to, *proximus* = nearest)
- **Mesial**: toward the midline of the dental arch (*medium* = middle, *medial* = toward the middle)
- **Distal**: toward the back of the dental arch (*distare* = to be away from)
- **Occlusal**: toward the chewing surface of the tooth (*occludere* = to close)
- **Masticatory**: toward the chewing surface (*masticare* = to chew)
- **Incisal**: toward the cutting surface (*incidere* = to cut into)

- **Apical**: toward the apex of the root (*apex* = tip)
- **Coronal**: toward the crown of the tooth (*corona dentis* = crown)
- **Gingival**: toward the soft tissues (gingiva)
- **Cervical**: toward the neck of the tooth (*cervix* = neck)

General directional terms for the body and head region include:

- **Anterior**: at the front (*ante* = before, in front of)
- **Basal**: toward the base of the skull, downward (*basis* = floor of the skull)
- **Central**: in the middle
- **Dorsal**: toward the back (*dorsum* = back)

- **Frontal**: toward the forehead, forward (*frons* = forehead)
- **Caudal**: downward (*cauda* = tail)
- **Cranial**: in an upward direction (*cranium* = skull)
- **Lateral**: toward the side (*latus* = side)
- **Marginal**: toward the edge (*margo* = margin)
- **Nasal**: toward the nose (*nasus* = nose)
- **Occipital**: toward the back of the head (*occiput* = back of head)
- **Peripheral**: outlying, located in the periphery
- **Posterior**: at the back (*post* = after/behind)
- **Sagittal**: in the plane of the suture between the parietal bones of the skull or in a parallel plane (*sagitta* = arrow)
- **Temporal**: toward the temple (*tempus* = temple)
- **Ventral**: in a forward direction (*venter* = belly)

The Orofacial System

The masticatory system, or orofacial system (system of mouth + face system; in Latin, *os* = mouth, *facies* = face; facial = relating to the face), includes all the different types of tissue that are involved in the chewing process. The *stomatognathic system*, as the masticatory system is also called, is not described as an organ unit according to the biologic descriptive model but as a unit with functionally coordinated tissue structures.

The ***orofacial system*** comprises the following functional components: teeth and their supporting tissues, jaws and their alveolar sections, the temporomandibular (jaw) joints (TMJs), muscles responsible for facial expression, nerve and vessel pathways, mucous membranes, salivary glands, mucous glands, cheeks, lips, and the tongue.

The system forms a functional cycle in which each part has a specific role to play that contributes to the operation of the whole system. Within such a controlled cycle, the functionality of each component is important because the operation of the whole cycle is disrupted if just one component fails.

A functional cycle will work successfully only if all the parts of the system involved are present and functioning in a normal physiologic manner. This is because the individual components mutually influence each other. Because the individual parts of the system have a unique function, they have evolved and developed so that they can meet these requirements. Any changes due to disease in any of the components of the system will influence the entire functional cycle. Furthermore, a defect in one area of the system will not only lead to alterations in the functioning of the whole system but also affect the other components of the system.

The ***biologic functional cycle*** is controlled by the central nervous system and regulates the actions of the system. For example, in the regulation of the degree of force needed to crush food, the jaw muscles first receive a stimulus that activates the teeth to crush the food. The nerves around the teeth and in the jawbone, in addition to the TMJ itself, act as sensors to measure and record the actual force applied so that an optimal pressure can be achieved.

In the orofacial system, a ***normal occlusion*** describes a regular, well-formed, and perfectly functioning masticatory system. It is the didactic descriptive model of an ideal occlusion based on statistical mean measurements. In terms of the form and function of a masticatory system, the normal occlusion is the standard to which all dental technicians work, since the purpose of their work is to produce a well-formed and, most importantly, a properly functioning (artificial) occlusion.

In exceptional cases where a dental prosthesis that differs from the normal occlusion has to be used because the individual conditions do not permit any other solution, the aim is always to provide the best possible compromise between what is available and the ideal occlusion. If there is anything in dentistry to which the term "skillful" can best be applied, it is the ability to produce an individual denture that is close to the ideal normal occlusion.

To achieve an appropriate understanding of the functions of the masticatory system and teeth, they should be regarded as a single system (an integrated whole). Detailed observation of the individual components in isolation is only appropriate where a precise description of form is required. Because form has an effect on the functions of a component, any description of the overall system should include form, function, and the interdependence of the components of the system (Figs 1-6 and 1-7).

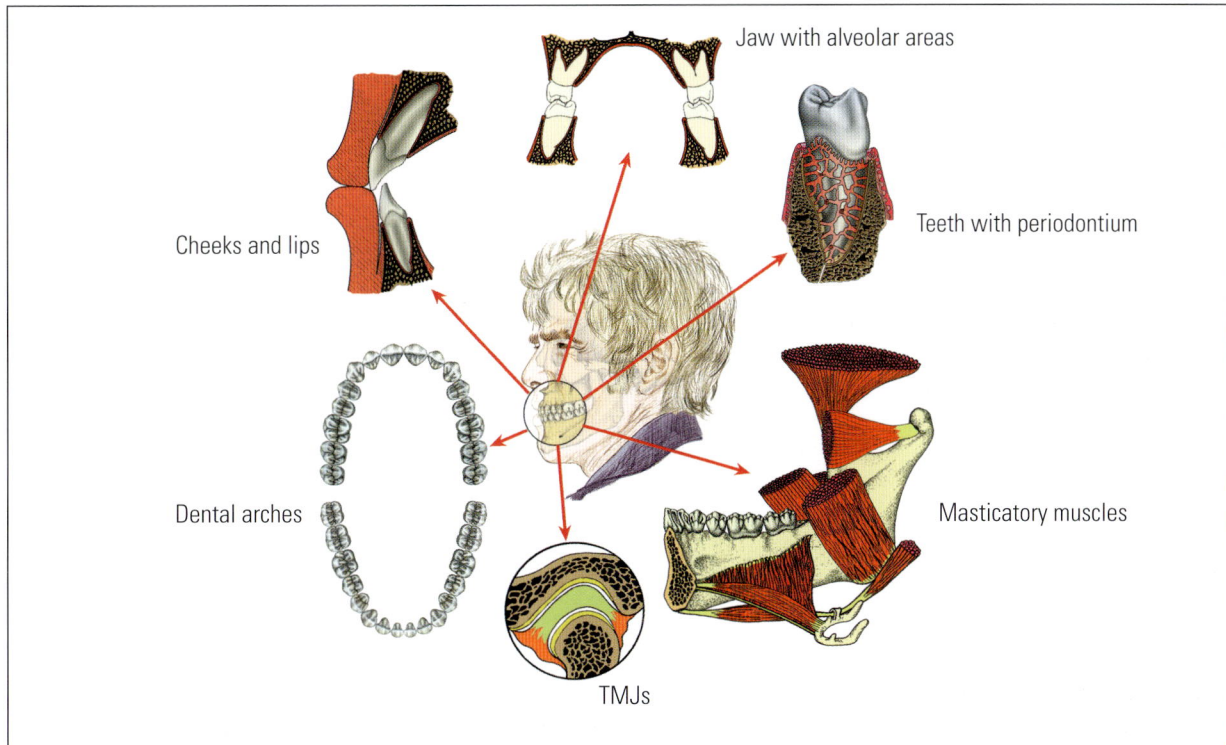

Fig 1-6 Structural elements of the orofacial system.

Functions of the orofacial system include:

- Mechanical preparation of food, biting, and chewing
- Salivation and preparation of food for swallowing
- Identification of tastes
- Preventing the ingestion of harmful substances that may be present in food by identifying them and separating them out
- Formation of speech using the closed rows of teeth and the resonance chamber of the oral cavity
- Providing static support for the facial skeleton
- Giving shape to the face, the esthetics of which will have psychologic effects
- Self-cleaning during chewing through the activity of the tongue

The individual components of the orofacial system are examined in the following sections, starting with the surface topography of the face and head and including the oral cavity with the teeth, jawbone, muscles, nerves, TMJs, and the movement of the mandible.

Features of the face

The **human face** *(facies)* can be divided into three areas by the interpupillary line (a line through the pupils with the eyes looking straight ahead; see Fig 1-10) and a line through the oral aperture:

1. Upper face, from the hairline over the forehead *(frons)* to the eyebrows *(supercilium)*
2. Middle part of the face, including the maxilla, nose, and upper lip
3. Lower face, including the mandible, from the orifice of the mouth *(rima oris)* to the chin *(menton)*

At the sides, the face extends over the temple region *(tempus)* and the external ear *(auricula)* as far as the posterior and inferior edge of the mandible. From the frontal view, cephalometric (or anthropometric) measuring points can be es-

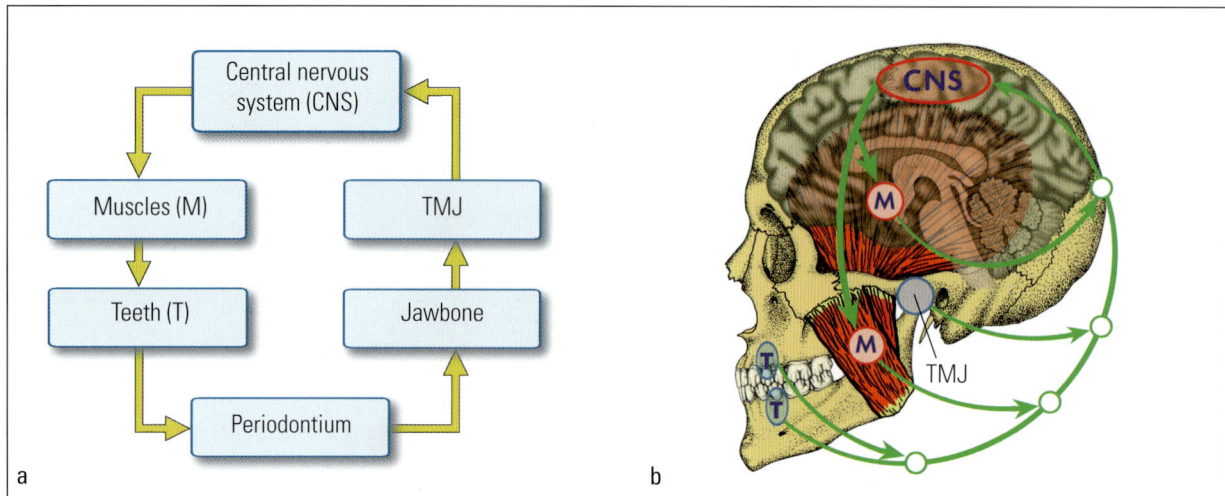

Fig 1-7 *(a)* Simplified diagram of the functional masticatory cycle. The necessary force, eg, the degree of force needed to crush food, is determined by the control mechanism (central nervous system). The impulse is transmitted to the muscles. Nerves in the periodontium, muscles, and TMJ register the actual value. The amount of force required is then adjusted by the central nervous system. Within a control cycle, the functional capacity of all the components is important because the whole cycle is disrupted if one part fails. Each part of the cycle is assigned a specific function, which determines the specific form of that part. *(b)* Illustration showing the controlling factors of the masticatory cycle.

tablished, which are used for analysis of the facial profile. The facial landmarks described in this section are illustrated in Fig 1-8.

The **eyeballs** can be covered by both eyelids *(palpebra superior/inferior)*, the upper and lower edge of the lids forming the palpebral fissure *(rima palpebrarum)*. In the medial angle of the eye at the root of the nose, there is a small mucosal projection, the lacrimal caruncle *(caruncula lacrimalis)*.

The external part of the nose projects from the **midface**. The nose extends from its root *(radix nasi)*, which is located between the eyes, to the bridge *(dorsum nasi)* and finally to the mobile tip *(apex nasi)*, whose sides or wings *(alae nasi)* form the entrance to the nose or the nasal vestibule.

The **orifice of the mouth** *(rima oris)* forms the entrance to the oral cavity, which is enclosed by the upper and lower lips *(labium superius and inferius)*. When the mouth is closed, the orifice forms a curved line.

The **angles of the mouth**, where the upper and lower lips meet, lie level with the maxillary canine teeth. The upper lip is bordered above by the nose and at the sides by the nasolabial sulcus *(sulcus nasolabialis)*. The *philtrum*, a flat furrow, divides

the upper lip into two halves and forms the tubercle *(tuberculum labii superioris)*.

In the middle of the **lower lip**, there is a gentle depression into which the tubercle of the upper lip fits. Below this, the labiomental groove *(sulcus mentolabialis)* delineates the lower lip from the chin area.

The **lips** *(labia oris)* are folds of skin that mainly contain muscles but also glands. Three different types of skin are found in the lip area:

1. The outer skin section *(pars cutanea)* up to the nose or the chin. In men, this may be largely covered with hair and well supplied with sebaceous glands.
2. The transitional area *(pars intermedia)*, which forms the red lip margin and is responsible for the redness of the lips. There are no sebaceous glands or hair in this area.
3. The mucosal area *(pars mucosa)*, the section of the lips up to the oral vestibule that contains the lip glands with outlets into the vestibule.

In the fornix or trough *(fornix vestibuli)*, the lips intersect with the gingiva, which is attached to the jaws. Lip shape and fullness are essentially

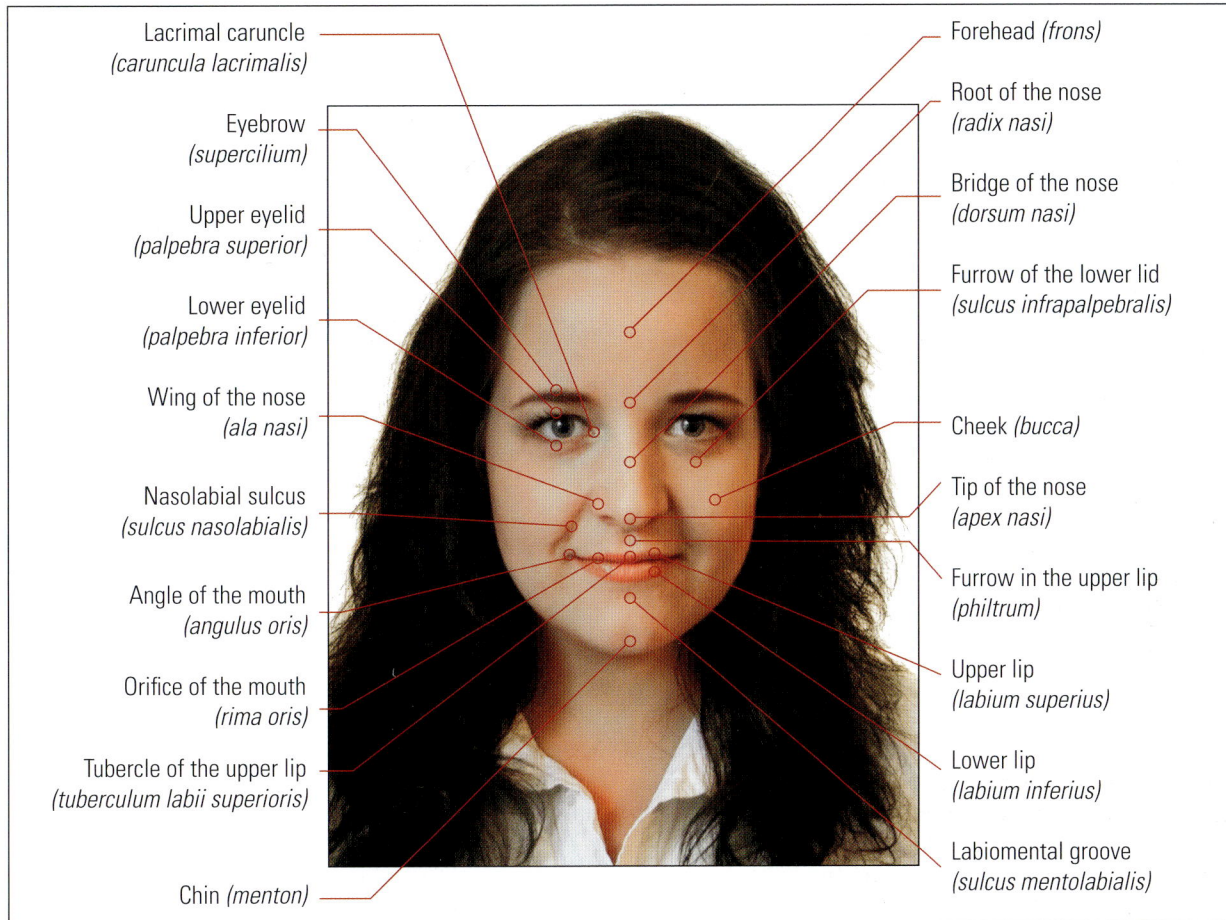

Fig 1-8 Facial landmarks.

achieved by the maxillary anterior teeth. The upper lip lies directly over the labial surfaces, while the lower lip gently bulges outward over the incisal edges of the maxillary anterior teeth. Therefore, the natural and functionally ideal position of the maxillary anterior teeth must be carefully reconstructed during dental treatment for each individual patient.

The *distance between the mouth and the nose* is smaller than that between the mouth and the chin. In many cases, the space between the nose and the mouth is roughly half the distance to the chin. In other cases, the upper lip is even shorter so that the distance from the orifice of the mouth to the chin is three times that to the nose. When a person laughs, the orifice of the mouth widens,

and the angles of the mouth can be drawn back to behind the second premolars, so that the maxillary anterior teeth and gingiva may become visible.

The *lip muscles* make the mouth area one of the most mobile parts of the body. The lips play an important role in the creation of facial expressions; they take on characteristic shapes during speaking, smiling, frowning, and otherwise nonverbally expressing emotion and are also involved in the ingestion of food.

The *cheeks (buccae)* originate from the sides of the face at the nasolabial sulcus *(sulcus nasolabialis)* and, together with the lips, form the external border of the oral vestibule. The cheeks can contain thick pads of fat; the layer of fatty tissue in the faces of women may be twice as thick as in

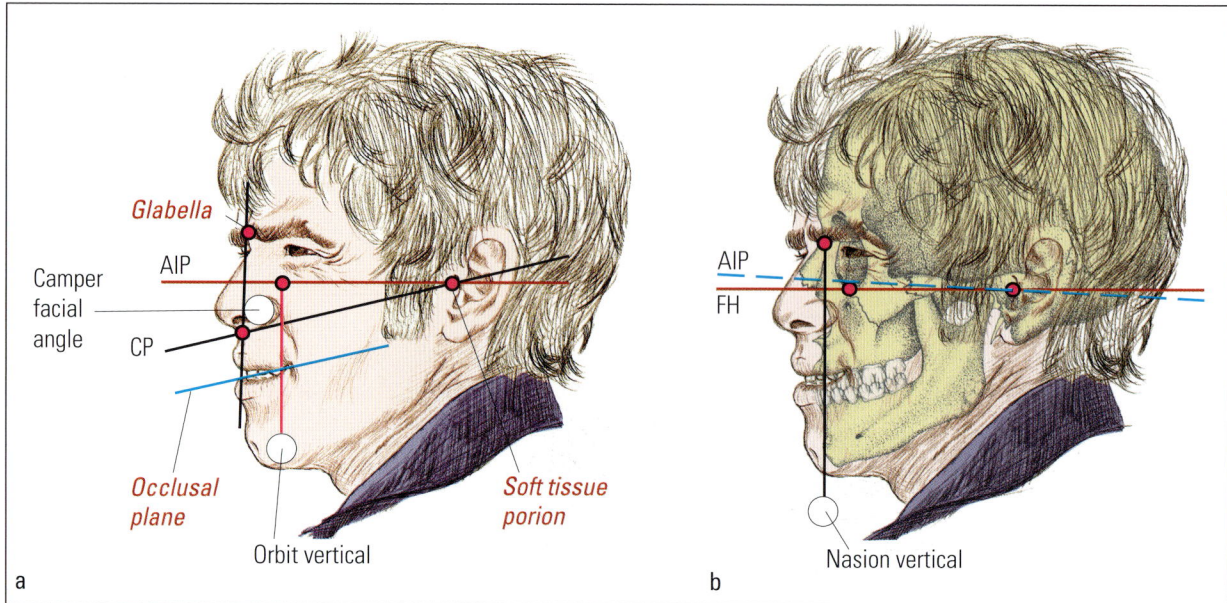

Fig 1-9 *(a and b)* Cephalometric planes of the head. AIP, auriculo-infraorbital plane; CP, Camper plane; FH, Frankfort horizontal plane.

men. The thickness of facial skin varies across the different sections of the face, but it is highly elastic in all areas and has a plentiful supply of blood vessels and nerves.

The **muscular basis of the cheeks** is formed by the buccinator muscle *(musculus buccinator)*, which attaches the cheeks to the molars and premolars. The mucosa of the cheeks, like that of the lips, contains small mixed salivary glands *(glandulae buccales)*. The exit point of the parotid gland in the form of a small mucosal protuberance *(papilla parotidea)* is located close to the second molar, and this is the reason for the tartar deposits that are commonly found on the vestibular surface of the maxillary molars.

The **chin** *(menton)* is a characteristic feature of the human face that developed as the cranium grew larger and the jaw became shorter. Owing to the development of speech, the tongue became larger, and the arch of the mandible widened. This resulted in a significant buildup of bone at the middle fusion line of the two halves of the mandible *(symphysis)* in order to absorb initial transverse stresses. After birth, the chin develops as the primary teeth are shed. The chin may be wide, narrow, long, short, square, oval, or round and, depending on the occlusal relationship, may

either protrude or recede. It also may be indented to a lesser or greater extent by a dimple.

Cephalometric measurement of the head

The proportions of the face and head can be measured cephalometrically. **Cephalometry** is the science of measuring the skull. Cephalometric points and reference lines are used in profile analysis during orthodontic examination. This facilitates analysis of the maxillofacial relationship and determination of the position of the teeth in the jaws and the relationship of the dental arches.

Starting from a reference point or line, the position of other parts of the skull, in this case the teeth, dental arches, mandible, and lips, can be described on the basis of average measurements and values. A selection of cephalometric points and reference lines used in dental technology are described below and illustrated in Figs 1-9 and 1-10.

- The **Camper plane** (CP; tragus-subnasale plane; nasoauricular plane) runs from the superior margin of the external opening of the ear (tragus point; tragion) to the subnasal point (subnasale)

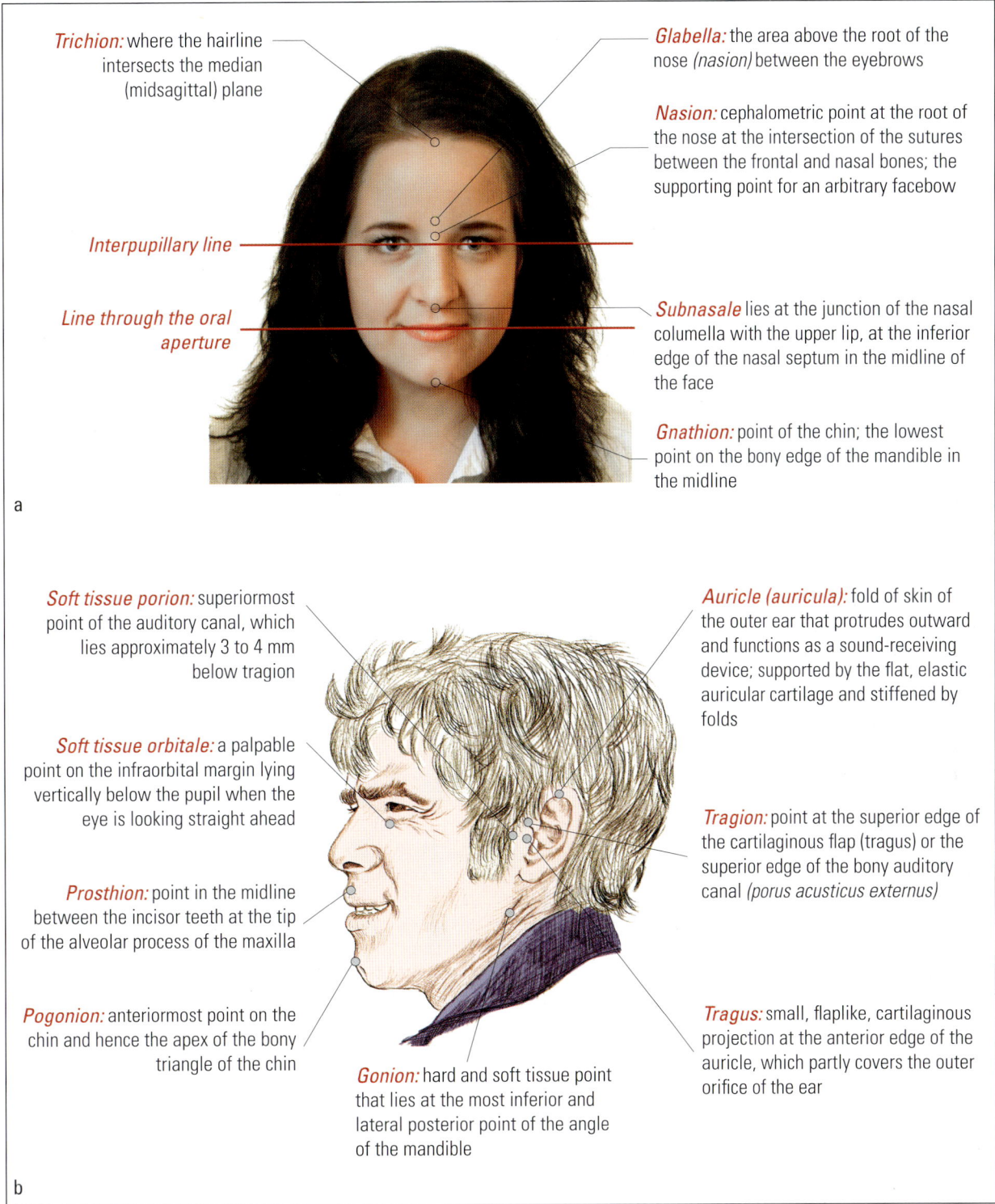

Trichion: where the hairline intersects the median (midsagittal) plane

Glabella: the area above the root of the nose *(nasion)* between the eyebrows

Nasion: cephalometric point at the root of the nose at the intersection of the sutures between the frontal and nasal bones; the supporting point for an arbitrary facebow

Interpupillary line

Line through the oral aperture

Subnasale lies at the junction of the nasal columella with the upper lip, at the inferior edge of the nasal septum in the midline of the face

Gnathion: point of the chin; the lowest point on the bony edge of the mandible in the midline

a

Soft tissue porion: superiormost point of the auditory canal, which lies approximately 3 to 4 mm below tragion

Auricle (auricula): fold of skin of the outer ear that protrudes outward and functions as a sound-receiving device; supported by the flat, elastic auricular cartilage and stiffened by folds

Soft tissue orbitale: a palpable point on the infraorbital margin lying vertically below the pupil when the eye is looking straight ahead

Prosthion: point in the midline between the incisor teeth at the tip of the alveolar process of the maxilla

Tragion: point at the superior edge of the cartilaginous flap (tragus) or the superior edge of the bony auditory canal *(porus acusticus externus)*

Pogonion: anteriormost point on the chin and hence the apex of the bony triangle of the chin

Gonion: hard and soft tissue point that lies at the most inferior and lateral posterior point of the angle of the mandible

Tragus: small, flaplike, cartilaginous projection at the anterior edge of the auricle, which partly covers the outer orifice of the ear

b

Fig 1-10 *(a and b)* Cephalometric points.

(see Fig 1-9a). The occlusal plane runs roughly parallel to this, about 2 cm below and passing through the closed lips. CP lies at an angle of 15 to 20 degrees to the auriculo-infraorbital plane (AIP). The **Camper facial angle** represents the angular relationship between CP and a line starting from glabella and passing through subnasale. The angle is usually between 80 and 90 degrees. Steep vertical lines (eg, the line from glabella to subnasale) pass through prosthion as well as nasion.

- **Frankfort horizontal plane** (FH) is a cephalometric plane established in 1884. It can easily be constructed on the bony skull by drawing a line through the cephalometric points of tragion (uppermost point on the superior edge of the auditory canal) and the orbital point (orbitale; lowest point of the infraorbital margin) (see Fig 1-9b). With the head positioned normally (in natural head position) and the eyes looking straight ahead, it lies horizontally.
- **Glabella vertical** is a vertical line drawn from the glabella to the AIP; it was formerly used for profile analysis but has now been superseded by the nasion vertical.
- **Nasion vertical** (nasal vertical) also runs vertical to the AIP. It starts from the root of the nose (nasion) and touches the upper lip (see Fig 1-9b). It can be used to assess the profile.
- The **auriculo-infraorbital plane** (AIP) is a plane of orientation that runs through the highest points of the superior margins of the two external bony openings of the ears (ear points, poria; soft tissue porion) and the lowest point at the inferior margin of the orbit (orbitale) (see Fig 1-9b). The AIP is not identical to the FH, differing from it by about 2 degrees.
- **Orbital vertical** is a vertical line perpendicular to the AIP, starting from the soft tissue orbital point, running via the apices of the incisors, and meeting the bony tip of the chin (gnathion) (see Fig 1-9a). This relationship can be seen on the skull within the normal range of variation.

Anatomy of the oral cavity

The **oral cavity** is the space between the orifice of the mouth and the isthmus of the fauces (*isthmus faucium*; also called the *oropharyngeal isthmus*) (Fig 1-11). The alveolar processes, which bear the teeth, divide the oral cavity into the oral vestibule (*vestibulum oris*) and the oral cavity proper (*cavitas oris propria*), the mucosa of which is covered by stratified squamous epithelium.

The oral cavity proper is formed by the oval space behind the dental arches and is almost fully occupied by the tongue. The palate, which is like a roof, marks the superior boundary of the oral cavity; the other boundaries are the isthmus of the fauces posteriorly and the floor of the mouth below.

The **floor of the mouth** lies between the parabolic mandibular body and extends as far as the root of the tongue. It is the muscular base of the oral cavity, being formed by some of the suprahyoid muscles of the hyoid bone, mainly by the mylohyoid muscles (*musculus mylohyoidea*; running from the mandibular body transversely to the midline of the skull), on which the tongue rests. Above and below these muscles are the sublingual and submandibular salivary glands. The boundary of the floor of the mouth is shaped laterally by the mylohyoid line and anteriorly by the movable sublingual area. This limited sublingual space is often referred to as the *floor of the mouth*. Sublingual and submandibular salivary glands are found in the floor of the mouth.

The **palate** (*palatum*) is the roof of the oral cavity. It is divided into the hard palate (*palatum durum*) and the soft palate (*palatum molle*), which consists of the movable velum palatinum and ends at the uvula. The hard palate also forms the floor of the nasal cavity and the maxillary antrum.

The bony foundations of the **hard palate** (*palatum osseum*) are the incisive bone (*os incisivum*) anteriorly, the palatine processes of the maxillae (*processus palatinus*), and the horizontal plates of the palatine bones (*lamina horizontalis*). The hard palate is covered with mucosa, which is attached to the periosteum by bands of connective tissue. The firm attachment of the mucosa to the underlying bone means that the tissue is not displaced during mastication.

Over the median palatine suture (*sutura palatina mediana*), the mucosa of the hard palate forms a midline elevation, the palatal raphe (*raphe palati mediana*), which starts behind the incisor teeth at the incisive papilla (*papilla incisiva*) at its tip and may show a protuberance known as the *torus palatinus* in the middle of the palate. The incisive papilla lies over the incisive foramen (*foramen incisivum*) of the bony palate and is

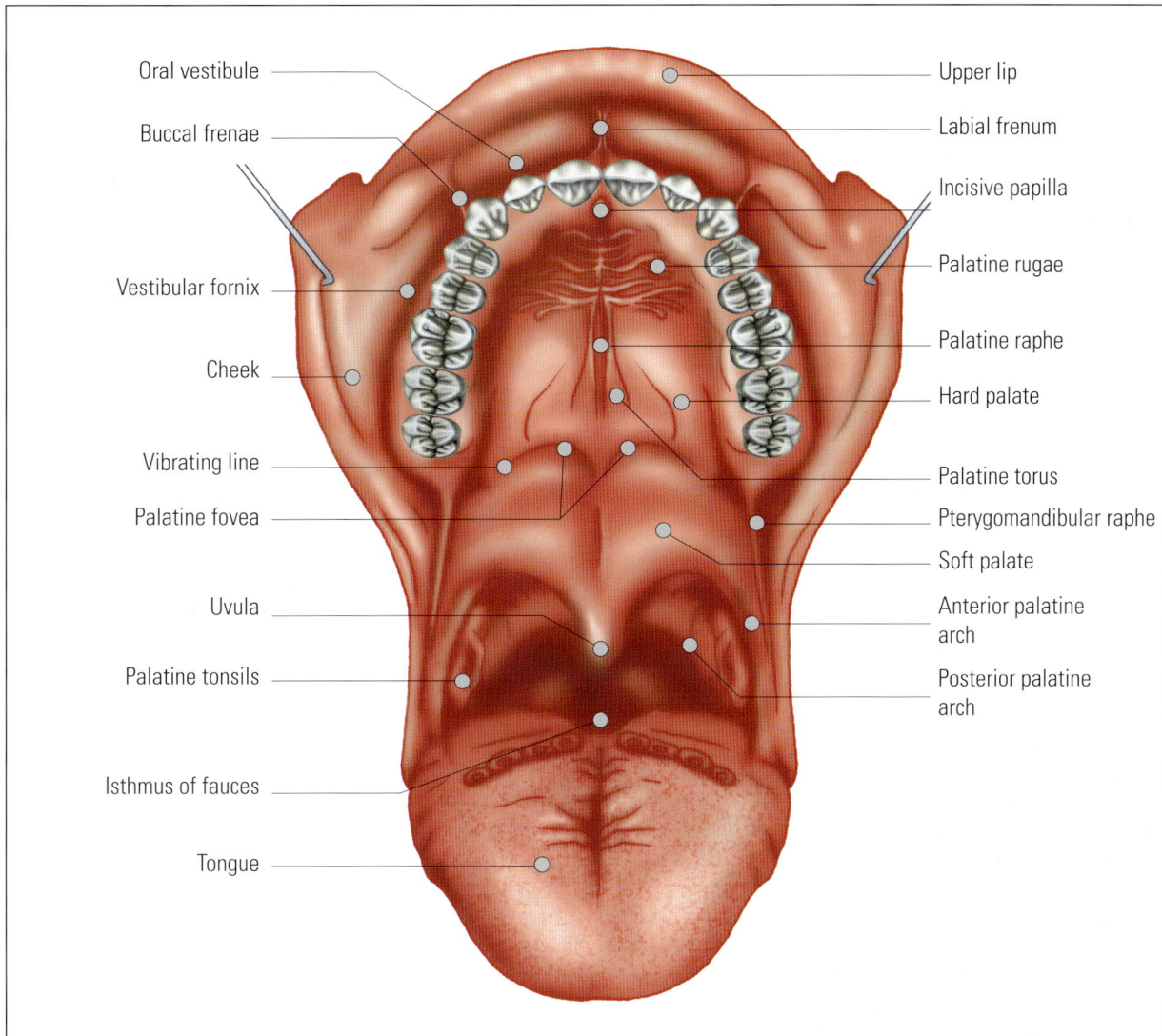

Fig 1-11 Major structures in and near the oral cavity.

protuberant. Below the papilla, blood vessels and nerves emerge from the incisive canal.

In the anterior part of the palate, a few irregular mucosal ridges emanate from the raphe: these are the palatine rugae *(plicae palatinae trans-versae)*. Along with the firmly attached mucosa, they help create **friction** between the palate and the tongue to help in mastication and speech; the moving bolus of food does not displace the mucous membrane, and the tongue is able to turn food over and let the saliva infiltrate it. The rugae are made up of a network of connective tissue fibers and isolated cartilage cells. An accumulation of tactile nerves is found here. So that food can slide along in the rear part of the hard palate during swallowing, this area contains the palatine mucous glands *(glandulae palatinae)* and is padded with fatty tissue. These glands become more numerous toward the soft palate.

The **vibrating line** denotes the transition from the hard palate to the soft palate. It is a line formed into a double arch that runs from one maxillary tuberosity to the other and encloses the posterior nasal spine. To the left and right of this line are the foveae palatinae, which are openings for the palatine glands. The vibrating line can be identified by producing a nose-blowing effect and generally forms the posterior border of a denture. This line is usually etched on the cast to mark the peripheral seal of the denture. Thus, the maxillary denture should end in the area of transition between the hard and soft palates, which results in a peripheral seal and ensures that no air enters between the fitted surface of the denture and the palate; in this way, the denture is kept in place by suction.

The **soft palate**, continuing from the hard palate, is a mucosal fold filled with muscles and a solid connective tissue framework, the superior surface of which forms the posterior floor of the nose. The highly mobile posterior part of the soft palate is known as the *velum palatinum*, and it terminates in the midline as the uvula, which is a continuation of the palatal raphe. The sides become the palatine arches or pillars *(arcus palatini)*.

The muscles of the soft palate are the tensor veli palatini, levator veli palatine, musculus uvulae, palatoglossus, and palatopharyngeus. These muscles are able to pull the velum palatinum posteriorly as far as the root of the tongue so that the oral cavity is sealed posteriorly and airtight. With the mouth closed, the mandible can thus be held in its resting position by the pressure of air; normally it is kept in this position by resting muscle tension *(tonus)*. The palatine glands are found on the inferior surface of the soft palate (toward the oral cavity). These are mucous glands, just as in the hard palate area, which enable the food to slip down smoothly when swallowing. The soft palate, with the palatine arches or pillars at the sides and the root of the tongue, forms the isthmus of the fauces. Between the two palatine arches lie the palatine tonsils *(tonsillae palatina)*. When the soft palate is touched, it can trigger a gag reflex.

Oral vestibule

The structures of the maxilla and mandible discussed in this section are illustrated in Fig 1-12. The **oral vestibule** *(vestibulum oris)* is the space between the cheeks and lips laterally and the teeth, gingiva, and the alveolar region medially. Usually the tissue surfaces lie close together so that the space in between is only potential in nature. An actual space can be produced if the cheeks are puffed out or pressed in when chewing food.

The **vestibular fornices** *(fornix vestibuli superioris and inferioris)* form the superior and inferior margins of the oral vestibule, where the mucosa of the cheeks and lips reflect back onto the alveolar mucosa. The furrow formed by the vestibular fornices is also known as the *vestibular sulcus*. It lies roughly at the level of the apices of the roots of the teeth, which is why surgical removal or treatment of tooth roots can be performed via the vestibule (eg, apicoectomy or root end resection).

The fornices can be pushed tangentially up to the alveolar ridge. However, this area can be extremely sensitive if, for example, it is chronically stressed. The loose submucous connective tissue is capable of storing a lot of fluid. Extensive fluid accumulations can cause severe swelling (creating an appearance of "fat" cheeks).

When the mouth is closed, the vestibule communicates with the oral cavity proper through the retromolar space (posterior to the molars). With the mouth wide open, the pterygomandibular raphe *(raphe pterygomandibularis)* marks the boundary between the oral cavity and the vestibule. The shape of the vestibular sulcus varies from one individual to another, and it is interrupted by various ligamentous attachments and mucosal folds.

The **labial frenula** or **frena** *(frenula labiorum; frenulum labii superioris and inferioris)* are free-edged mucosal folds in the midline that run from the lips to the alveolar mucosa. The vestibule is virtually halved by this frenum, both in the maxilla and in the mandible. A thick superior labial frenum can push apart the two middle incisors to form a median diastema (a gap between the two maxillary central incisors).

The **buccal frena** *(frenula buccales; frenulum buccae superioris and inferioris)* are fibrous bundles covered with buccal mucosa that run laterally in varying numbers as part of the tendons of origin of the buccinator muscle *(musculus buccinator)*. They are usually located in the region of the premolars and run from the alveolar ridge dorsally into the fornix; they prevent excessive

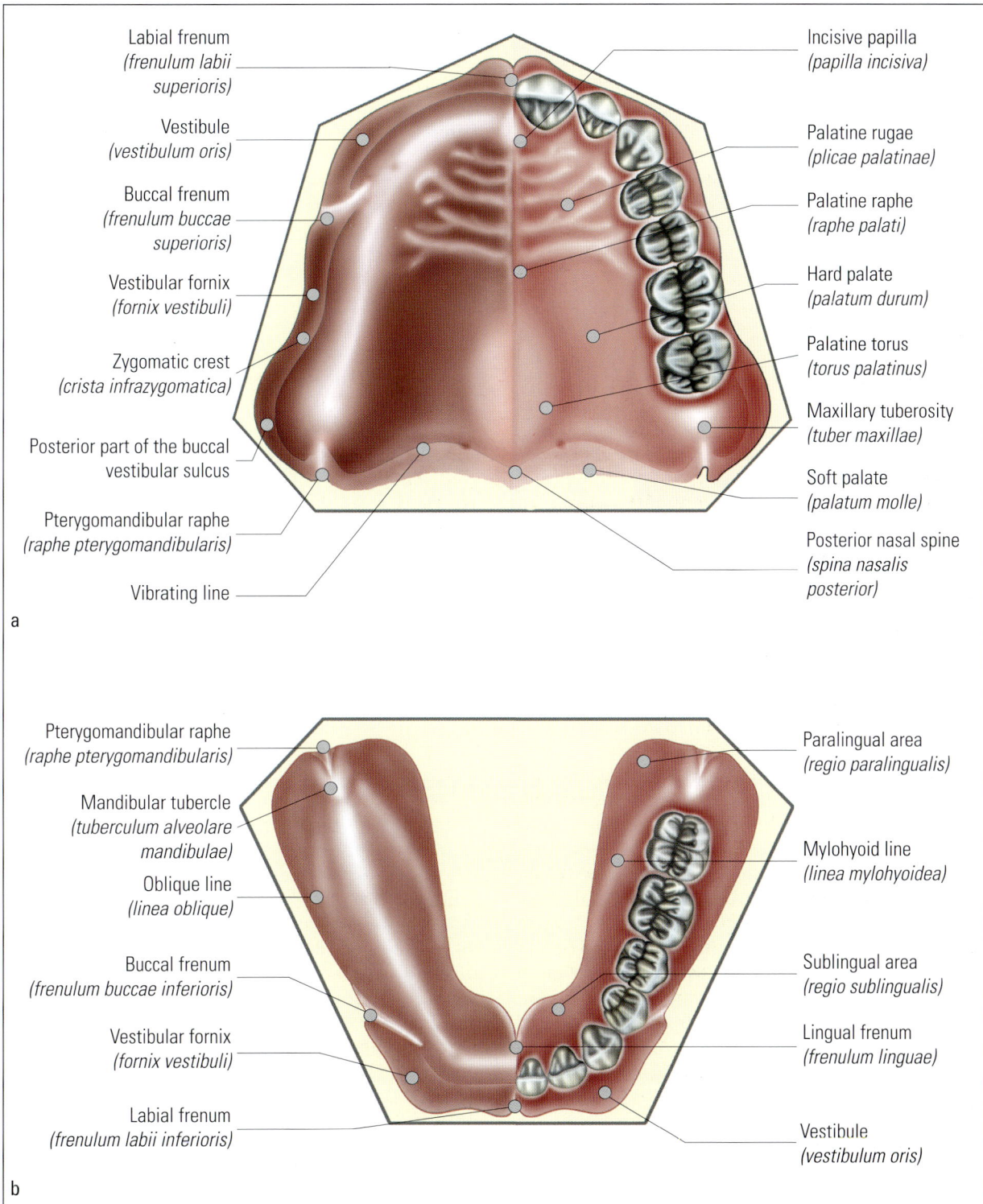

Labial frenum
(frenulum labii superioris)

Vestibule
(vestibulum oris)

Buccal frenum
(frenulum buccae superioris)

Vestibular fornix
(fornix vestibuli)

Zygomatic crest
(crista infrazygomatica)

Posterior part of the buccal vestibular sulcus

Pterygomandibular raphe
(raphe pterygomandibularis)

Vibrating line

Incisive papilla
(papilla incisiva)

Palatine rugae
(plicae palatinae)

Palatine raphe
(raphe palati)

Hard palate
(palatum durum)

Palatine torus
(torus palatinus)

Maxillary tuberosity
(tuber maxillae)

Soft palate
(palatum molle)

Posterior nasal spine
(spina nasalis posterior)

a

Pterygomandibular raphe
(raphe pterygomandibularis)

Mandibular tubercle
(tuberculum alveolare mandibulae)

Oblique line
(linea oblique)

Buccal frenum
(frenulum buccae inferioris)

Vestibular fornix
(fornix vestibuli)

Labial frenum
(frenulum labii inferioris)

Paralingual area
(regio paralingualis)

Mylohyoid line
(linea mylohyoidea)

Sublingual area
(regio sublingualis)

Lingual frenum
(frenulum linguae)

Vestibule
(vestibulum oris)

b

Fig 1-12 Major structures of the maxilla (a) and the mandible (b).

True Teeth

In the animal kingdom, a distinction is made between true teeth and structures that are similar to teeth but are not true teeth. ***True teeth*** are made of enamel, dentin, and cementum as well as pulp. They are called *dentinal teeth* because they are mainly made up of dentin.

Structures that are **not true teeth** do not have any of the hard substances of the true teeth, ie, enamel, dentin, and cementum. They are mainly the horny teeth found, for example, in the pharynx and esophagus of leatherback sea turtles.

---

stretching of the vestibule. Additional mucosal folds may also be present, and these must be taken into account when shaping a denture border.

Directly below the fornix, but slightly above the alveolar ridge, there are muscle attachments that, during movements, alter the vestibular sulcus. It can also be constricted during speaking and chewing.

The ***pterygomandibular raphe*** (*raphe pterygo-mandibularis*; suture of the pharyngeal wall; *pterygo* = winglike) is a vertical fold of mucosa that limits the vestibule posterior to the molars. This fold is shaped by a strip of tendon that runs from the hamular (hooklike) process of the sphenoid bone *(hamulus pterygoideus)* to the inside (hylohyoid line) of the mandible.

The ***buccal vestibular sulcus*** is narrowest posteriorly where the coronoid process of the mandible reduces the space considerably during lateral movements. The vestibule is also narrowed here by the activity of the masticatory muscles, which is why a denture flange must not be too thick in this region.

After tooth loss, the alveolar processes of the jaw resorb, causing the folds to lose their original height and in some cases completely level out. It is possible to increase fold depth surgically to compensate for badly shrunken alveolar ridges and to create undercut retention areas for the denture base.

The ***zygomatic crest*** (*crista infrazygomatica*) is a bony process of the cheekbone *(zygoma)* level with the roots of the first molars. Owing to the presence of this crest, the fornix is shallow in this region.

The ***maxillary tuberosity*** (*tuber maxillae*) is a robust bony prominence at the posterior end of

the maxillary dental arch that is not resorbed after tooth loss.

The ***mandibular tubercle*** (*tuberculum alveolare mandibulae)* is a mucosal elevation over the bony retromolar trigone *(trigonum retromolare)*. It can arise from special muscle attachments. The mandibular tubercle is also frequently known as the *retromolar triangle*.

The ***oblique line*** (*linea oblique)* is a bony elevation that runs from the retromolar triangle anteriorly and inferiorly to the premolars and into the vestibular sulcus. The attachment of the buccinators extends to this line.

Teeth

Form, formation, and function

In Latin, the word *teeth* is *dentes* (*dens* = tooth; *dentis* = of the tooth). *Dental* means relating to the tooth. In Greek, *tooth* is *odous* (*odontes* = teeth).

Teeth are hard structures in the oral cavity that, as modified parts of the dermoskeleton, form the dentition. Each tooth is comprised of a basal bony mass, a dentinal crown, and an inner pulp cavity. Food is held, incised, ground, and chewed by the teeth. Figure 1-13 presents comparisons of the forms and arrangements of teeth in different animals. Primitive rootless teeth are found in fish, amphibians, and reptiles and are the basic form of tooth. They can be slightly pointed, conical teeth, which can be angular or serrated (in sharks) and are shaped into so-called pavement teeth in fish and fangs in venomous snakes. These teeth of the same form (haplodont) vary only in size

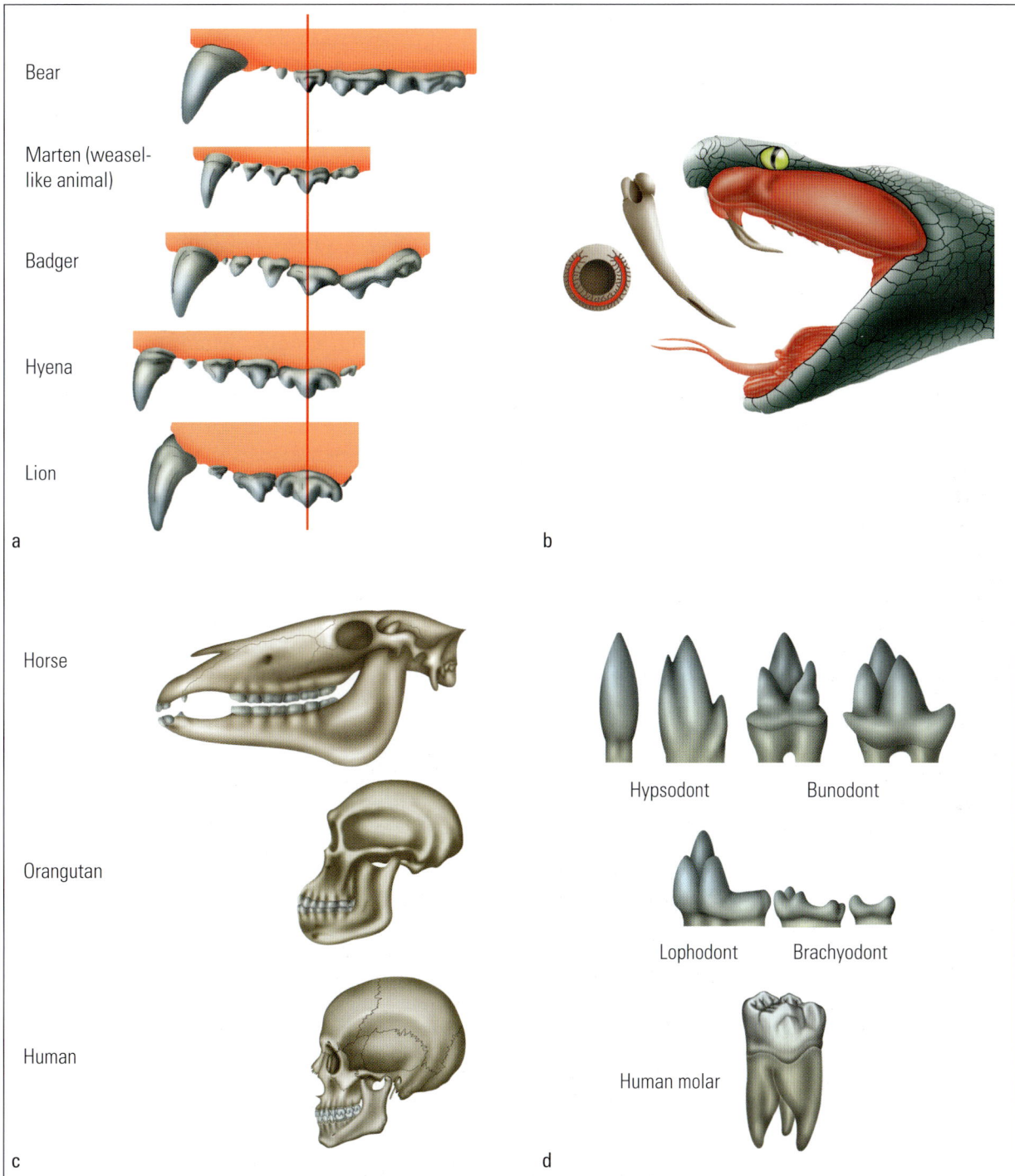

Fig 1-13 *(a)* The red line intersects the maxillary "tearing" teeth of various animals for purposes of comparison. *(b)* The specialization of teeth illustrated by a snake's fang. When the mouth is closed, the fang is tilted inward. The tooth is hollow and has an opening at its tip through which the venom can flow out of the poison gland. *(c)* A comparison of the arrangement of the teeth in different mammals. *(d)* Mammals and humans have dentitions with different types of teeth, the occlusal surfaces of which display a variety of shapes and forms.

and thus create a dentition with just one shape of tooth, ie, a haplodont dentition.

The dentitions of mammals consist of teeth of different shapes (heterodont). The names of the different teeth are incisors, canines, premolars, and molars. Depending on the animal species, molars can take various different forms (see Fig 1-13d): bunodont (with cone-shaped cusps), hypsodont (with a high cylindric crown), brachyodont (with a shallow crown), lophodont (with a broad crown and yoke-like enamel crests), or selenodont (masticatory surfaces with crescent-shaped enamel crests).

The teeth are anchored in the jaw by fibrous structures (*acrodontia*; in Greek, *acros* = highest) in sharks, bony fish, snakes, and some lizards. The teeth of amphibians and reptiles are firmly joined to the underlying bone mass on the inside of the jaw (*pleurodontia*; in Greek, *pleura* = side). In mammals and crocodiles, the root of a tooth lies in a cavity *(alveolus dentalis)* of the jawbone and is firmly and flexibly anchored to the bone with collagenous fibers and a connective tissue periodontium (*thecodontia*; in Greek, *theke* = container).

With a few exceptions, the teeth are shed several times or, in the case of mammals, once. This is known as **exfoliation of the teeth**. The rather smaller teeth of the first dentition are known as *primary* or *deciduous teeth (dentes decidui)*. A distinction is made between vertical and horizontal exfoliation.

In **vertical exfoliation**, the old or erupted tooth is replaced by a new tooth from below (that is, from within the jawbone), with the root of the old tooth being resorbed. In **horizontal exfoliation**, the teeth located in the posterior region of the jaw gradually migrate anteriorly as the anterior teeth are worn out and shed (eg, in elephants, manatees, and kangaroos).

The size of the teeth is hereditary and differs between individuals. Size is inherited independently of the jaw size, which is also hereditary. This is why relatively small teeth can develop in a large jaw with gaps between the teeth, and relatively large teeth can develop in a small jaw with resultant crowding.

Following are the **functions of human teeth**:

- Cutting (biting off) food (by the incisors)
- Preparing food for swallowing (by teeth with grinding surfaces)

- Transmitting masticatory forces via the attachment apparatus to the jawbone
- Protecting the marginal periodontium during chewing
- Allowing unimpeded sliding contacts during mandibular movements
- Preventing overclosure during jaw closing movement
- Detecting foreign bodies in food and thereby performing a protective function (by proprioception)
- Allowing self-cleaning
- Enhancing esthetics
- Orienting the tongue when making sounds (phonation)
- Biomechanical transfer of forces to the other teeth

Anatomy

The roots of teeth are located in sockets *(alveolus dentalis)* of the jawbone, where they are firmly and flexibly anchored with collagenous fibers and a connective tissue periodontium. In addition, there is a special ligamentous apparatus at the gingival margin. Teeth are slightly mobile within the alveolar sockets, rather like a joint. Anatomically, the attachment apparatus includes the gingiva, the root cement (cementum), and the bony alveoli. The tooth is supplied via the blood vessels and nerves that enter the periodontium and the tooth itself.

A tooth is divided into the following parts (Fig 1-14):

- **Crown** *(corona dentis)*: the visible part protruding into the oral cavity with a grinding surface or a cutting edge. The following distinctions are made:
  - **Clinical crown** *(corona clinica)*: the treatable portion of the part visible at that time.
  - **Anatomical crown** *(corona anatomica)*: the part of the tooth covered with enamel. Thus, the clinical crown and root differ in length from the anatomical crown and root, depending on the patient's age or the position of the gingival margin.
- **Root** *(radix dentis)*: the portion attached inside the jaw.
- **Neck** *(collum dentis or cervix dentis)*: the area of transition from crown to root; where the enamel

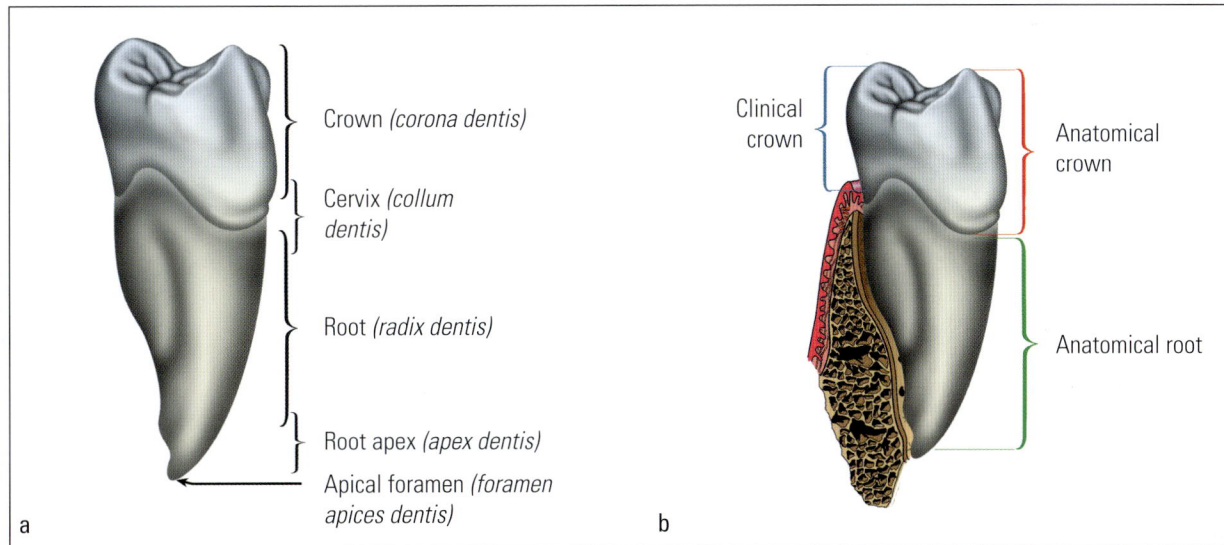

Crown (corona dentis)

Cervix (collum dentis)

Root (radix dentis)

Root apex (apex dentis)

Apical foramen (foramen apices dentis)

Clinical crown

Anatomical crown

Anatomical root

a

b

Fig 1-14 (a) Parts of the tooth. (b) Distinction between the anatomical crown and the clinical crown and depiction of the anatomical root.

of the crown changes into the cementum of the root and the gingival margin is located, which tends to lie above the anatomical neck of the tooth in young people and migrates more apically (toward the root) with increasing age.

• **Root apex** (apex dentis): the only part of the tooth with an opening (the **apical foramen** [foramen apicis dentis], where nerves and blood vessels enter the tooth).

Types of dentitions and teeth

In dentitions that are only shed and replaced once (diphyodontia), the rather smaller teeth of the first dentition are replaced by the larger teeth of the second dentition. In humans, the primary dentition appears first with 20 teeth (dentes decidui). It is replaced and supplemented by the complete, secondary dentition of 32 permanent teeth (dentes permanentes). The primary dentition is also known as the temporary dentition.

The teeth in the primary and permanent dentitions are arranged in superior and inferior dental arches (arcus dentalis superior and inferior). In mammals, and hence in humans, the dentition is heterodont (different kinds of teeth), and the

teeth can be divided into the following functional groups (Fig 1-15).

• **Anterior teeth** (dentes anteriores):
  – **Incisors** (dentes incisivi; dens incisivus; incidire = to cut; pre-canine teeth = teeth in front of the canines)
  – **Canines** (dentes canini; dens caninus; dens angularis; angulus = corner, angle)

• **Posterior teeth** (dentes posteriors):
  – **Premolars** (dentes praemolares; dens praemolaris; dens bicuspidatus = two-cusp or two-point teeth; cuspis = point; dens buccalis minoris = small back tooth)
  – **Molars** (dentes molares; dens molaris; dens multicuspidatus = multi-point teeth; dentes buccales majores = large back teeth)

The dentition is symmetric in both dental arches: The maxilla and mandible each contain the same number of teeth and groups of teeth, and they show mirror symmetry. Each half of either jaw contains a quarter of all the teeth: two incisors, one canine, two premolars, and three molars. The third (last) molar is often called the wisdom tooth (dens serotinus).

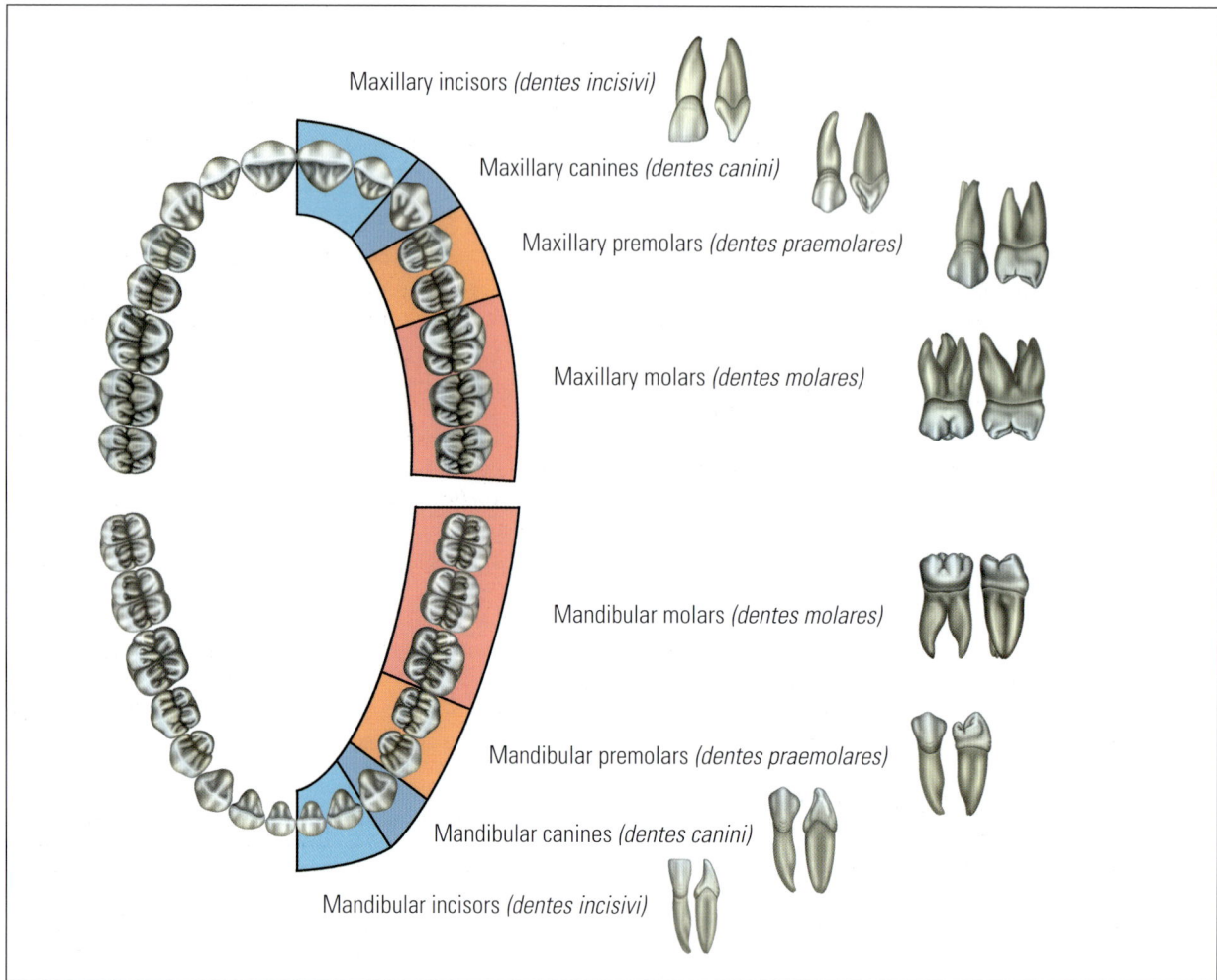

Fig 1-15 Types of teeth.

Below is the typical dental formula for the permanent dentition in humans:

3M	2P	1C	2I	2I	1C	2P	3M
3M	2P	1C	2I	2I	1C	2P	3M

where I = incisor, C = canine, P = premolar, and M = molar.

• The **_permanent dentition_** contains:
  – 12 anterior teeth (8 incisors, 4 canines)
  – 20 posterior teeth (8 premolars, 12 molars)

• The **_primary dentition_** contains:
  – 12 anterior teeth (8 incisors, 4 canines)
  – 8 posterior teeth (all molars)

The primary dentition has no premolars and only two so-called primary molars in each half of each arch.

Notation

In their close collaboration, dentists and dental technicians need to be able to refer to specific teeth clearly. The term *mandibular left second molar* is correct and clear as it stands, but it is far too long-winded. Based on the dental formula, various notations have been developed to allow clear communication when referring to the teeth within each dental arch.

The ***Zsigmondy-Palmer system*** (also called the *Set-Square* or *Chevron system*) names the teeth as the observer sees the dentition from the front. The teeth are numbered consecutively from one to eight starting from the midline to the back, so that the same teeth in the four halves of the jaws (maxilla and mandible, left and right) are given the same numbers. The numbers are arranged in a cross, where the lines of the cross indicate the occlusal plane (horizontal) and the middle of the face (vertical):

Right | 8 7 6 5 4 3 2 1 | 1 2 3 4 5 6 7 8 | Left

Right | 8 7 6 5 4 3 2 1 | 1 2 3 4 5 6 7 8 | Left

The tooth notation is written as one sees the teeth when sitting opposite someone and looking into that person's mouth, ie, the directionals right and left refer to the patient's right and left.

An individual tooth is identified by drawing a section of the dentition cross and writing the number assigned to the tooth in it; for example, a maxillary right first molar is represented as 6| (Fig 1-16a).

For the primary dentition, the notation follows the same pattern as the permanent dentition, but the teeth are named using lowercase letters in the cross:

Right | e d c b a | a b c d e | Left

Right | e d c b a | a b c d e | Left

Thus, the primary mandibular left second molar is designated as e|.

Fédération Dentaire Internationale (FDI) tooth notation is the two-digit system of notation for the permanent and primary teeth that was introduced internationally on January 1, 1971. The maxilla and mandible are divided into four quadrants: maxillary right (1), maxillary left (2), mandibular left (3), and mandibular right (4).

Starting from the midline of the arch and moving distally, the teeth are numbered consecutively from one to eight, and the number of the quadrant is placed in front of the tooth number (Figs 1-16a and 1-16b). Tooth 36 is therefore the mandibular left first molar.

The FDI notation for the primary teeth uses the following consecutive numbers to name the quadrants: maxillary right (5), maxillary left (6), mandibular left (7), and mandibular right (8). The primary teeth are numbered from one to five, starting from the midline of the arch (Fig 1-16c). Thus, the primary mandibular right first molar is designated 84.

The ***Haderup system*** (or European system) is set out like a cross, but the maxillary teeth are denoted with a plus symbol (+) and the mandibular teeth with a minus symbol (–). The position of the symbol denotes which half of the jaw it refers to: in front of the tooth number (ie, to the left) means the left side, and after the number (ie, to the right) means the right side. The maxillary right first premolar is therefore 4+.

Right | | Left
8+ 7+ 6+ 5+ 4+ 3+ 2+ 1+ | +1 +2 +3 +4 +5 +6 +7 +8

8– 7– 6– 5– 4– 3– 2– 1– | –1 –2 –3 –4 –5 –6 –7 –8

In the Haderup system, a zero placed in front of the tooth number indicates a primary tooth; for example, the primary mandibular left second molar is –05. Studies have shown that the permanent dentition appears to be evolving, so that the last molar (wisdom tooth) and the maxillary lateral incisor are gradually reducing in size or are completely absent in some individuals. When a complete replacement of the permanent dentition is carried out, the wisdom teeth are not replaced, which is why such dentures are often known as "28ers" and why the diagrams of the dental arches for prosthetic restorative treatment show only 28 teeth.

Fig 1-16 *(a)* Tooth notation: Zsigmondy-Palmer *(red)* and FDI *(blue)* systems. *(b)* FDI system: permanent teeth. *(c)* FDI system: primary teeth.

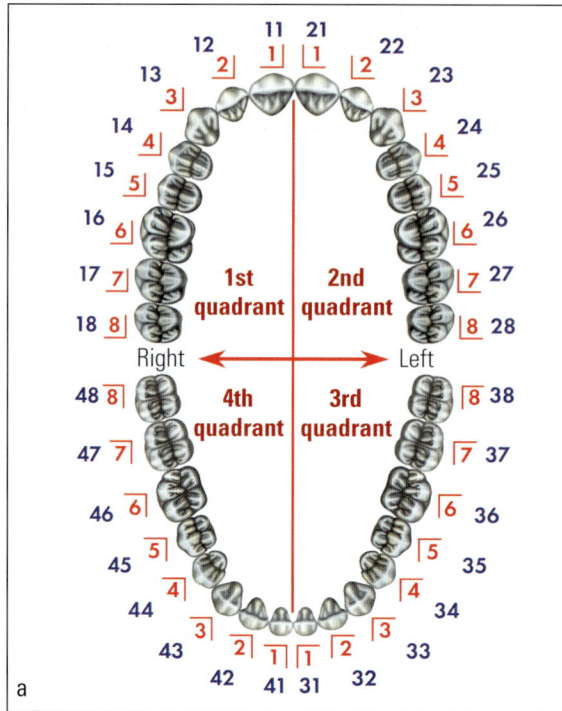

a

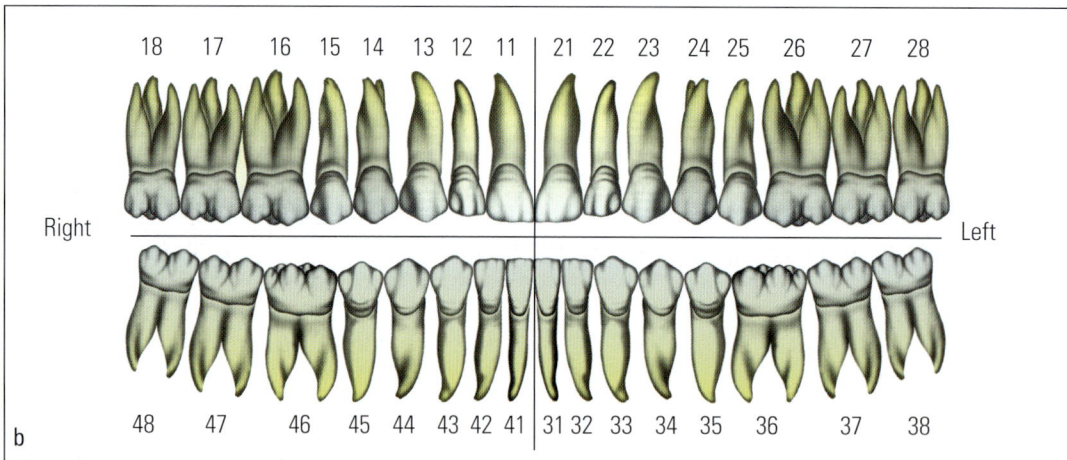

b

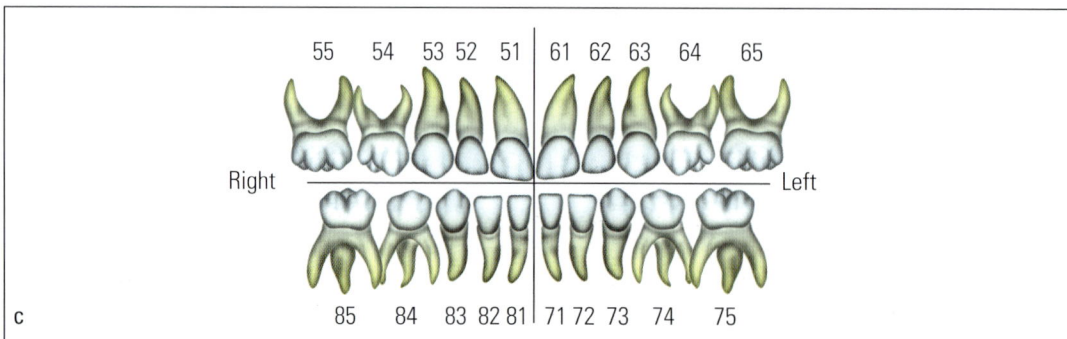

c

2

Cells and Tissues

The Cell as a Functional Unit

Sound knowledge of the structure and functions of the human body starts from the very smallest components, moves through increasingly larger units, and ends with the whole organism. The smallest independent functional unit of any organism is the cell. The structure and function of the cell are described in general cytology (*cytos* = cell, *cellula* = small chamber). The cell as an independent functional unit displays the characteristics of life:

- *Metabolism:* The ability to absorb substances and use them to build up the body's own cell substance and obtain heat. In plant cells, metabolism mainly takes place via photosynthesis, in which carbohydrates are formed from carbon dioxide and hydrogen by the chlorophyll molecules. In animal cells, metabolism mainly takes place with oxygen, in which complex carbohydrate compounds are broken down into the smallest basic building blocks and carbon dioxide is released.
- *Growth:* Enlargement of the cell substance made up of the products of metabolism, where certain protein compounds reduced during catabolism are used for protein synthesis.
- *Reproduction:* In cells, the re-creation of their own cell substance by cell division or some other principle of reproduction. Reproduction means that all the skills, characteristics, and external form of the cell are passed on.
- *Movement:* The ability of certain parts of cells to perform specific motions as a reaction to stimuli.
- *Regulatory ability and reactivity:* Keeping the living conditions inside the cell constant by an exchange of substances with and, to a certain extent, reacting to changes in the external environment.

From simple to complex

The simplest animal life is single cells that perform all the functions of life. One example of such unicellular organisms or protozoa—of which there are about 20,000 species—is the amoeba, which moves by extending and retracting so-called pseudopodia (false feet).

Multicellular organisms without any specialization of individual cells are networks or colonies of cells in which each cell is still capable of living and therefore possesses all the characteristics of life. These colonies of cells are the precursor to true multicellular organisms. Organisms made up of networks of cells, or metazoa, have cells that have specialized in certain functions, so that specialized cells undertake partial functions of the whole organism. In networks of cells, however, not every living cell has all the defined abilities; the cells have given up certain skills for the sake of the network functioning as a whole.

In multicellular living beings, only the cells that have specially developed flagella (whiplike structures) have the ability of independent movement, while cells that have developed an ocellus (eye-spot) take on a function of orientation.

Viruses

Viruses are not cells, but they have the capacity to exploit the reproductive mechanism of other cells to reproduce a viral body. They are made up of a protein envelope for a DNA molecule, which contains the instruction to utilize the reproductive apparatus of a living cell and to prepare the receptacle and the blueprint itself. Viruses are dependent on living cells for all their functional characteristics.

Organs arise from the joining together of similar types of cells geared to a specific function. In the human body, the cells of the various tissues and organs can be classified by form and size:

- Largest cell: egg cell (oocyte)—200 to 252 μm
- Smallest cell: lymphocyte—4 μm
- Average cell size: 10 to 20 μm
- Longest cell: nerve cell (due to the axon)—up to approximately 1 m

Despite the differences in form and function of specialized cells, there is an underlying structural principle: Cells have a cell membrane that encases the cellular fluid and the organelles it contains (Fig 2-1). The nucleus, demarcated by a nuclear membrane, contains the cell's genetic material. The organelles are highly specialized subcellular structures with their own membrane border. They are small, specially structured, separate reaction areas within the cell for the specific function of metabolism.

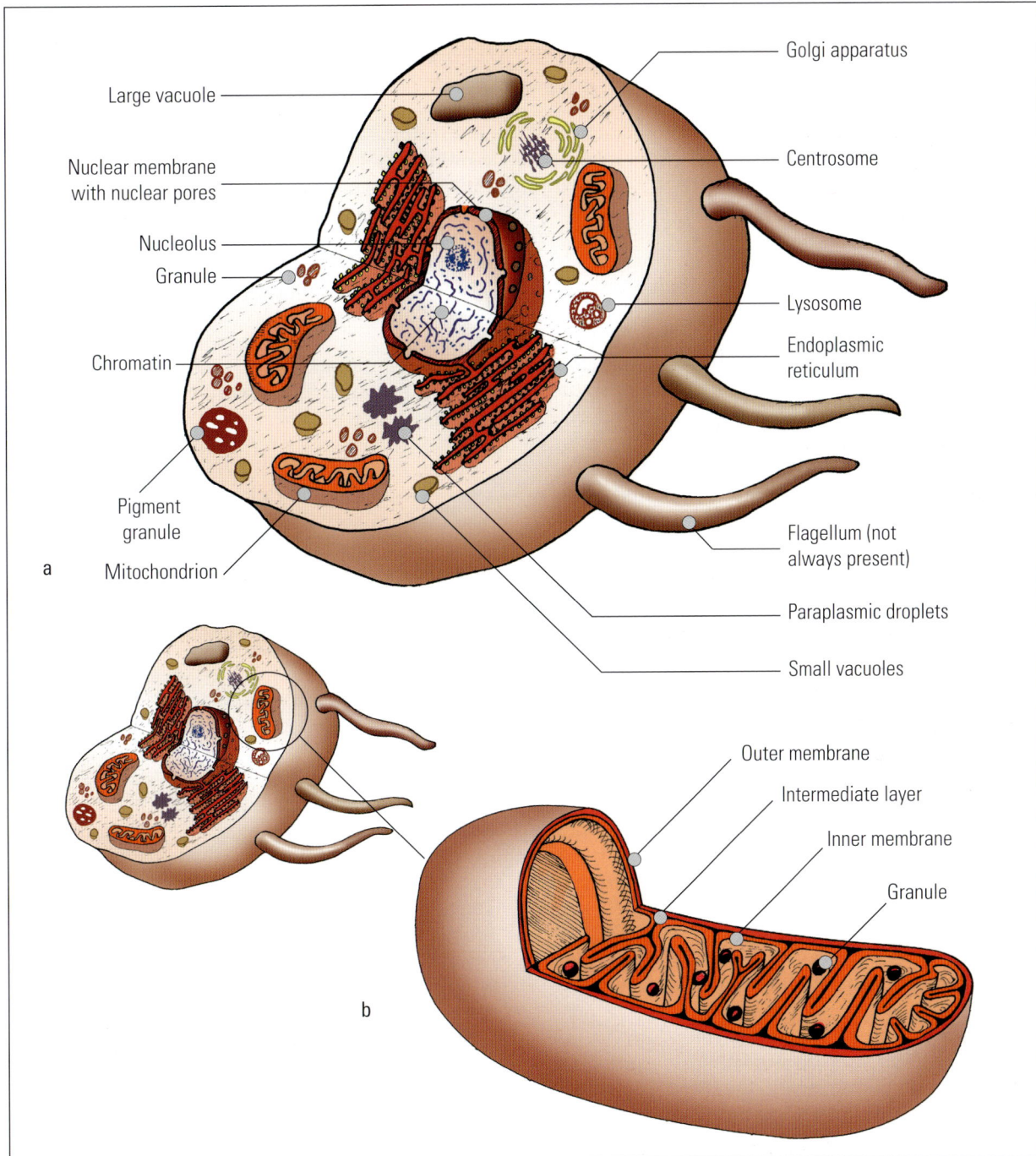

Large vacuole

Nuclear membrane
with nuclear pores

Nucleolus

Granule

Chromatin

Pigment
granule

Mitochondrion

a

Golgi apparatus

Centrosome

Lysosome

Endoplasmic
reticulum

Flagellum (not
always present)

Paraplasmic droplets

Small vacuoles

b

Outer membrane

Intermediate layer

Inner membrane

Granule

Fig 2-1 *(a)* The cell is regarded as the smallest unit capable of life. In the functional unit visible under the microscope, differentiated structures that are separated from the inside of the cell by the cell membrane can be identified. *(b)* The diagram of a typical mitochondrion shows the oval structure with an outer double membrane, which turns inward to form a lamellar system that increases the surface area. This is where the enzymes for organic oxidation are found. These organelles are seen as the energy suppliers of cells.

Microstructures of the Cell

Cytoplasm

The cytoplasm can be divided into four structural units: hyaloplasm, cell organelles, metaplasm, and paraplasm.

Hyaloplasm

Hyaloplasm forms the main substance of the cell body. It is made up of the jelly-like cytoplasm, a protein colloid in which filamentous protein molecules join together to form a spatial lattice, a matrix of protein filaments on which to suspend the cell organelles and other working structures. The hyaloplasm comprises 70% to 80% water, approximately 10% proteins, around 2% nucleic acid (RNA and DNA), and about 1% lipoids (fatlike substances) and fats, as well as organic materials such as sugar and inorganic ions (eg, sodium chloride and calcium). In addition to this matrix, ribosomes and the endoplasmic reticulum are present.

The **endoplasmic reticulum** is a branched system of fissures and cavities; it is a working structure of protein synthesis in which constructive metabolism takes place. Proteins, carbohydrates, and lipids are synthesized here and broken down to produce cell components. Broken-down carbohydrates are stored in oval structures called *cytosomes*. Ribosomes are found on the membrane of the (rough) endoplasmic reticulum.

The **ribosomes** form the working structure of protein synthesis, which means they form the templates for special protein molecules: the RNA molecules. The matrices for identical replication of RNA molecules are found on the surface of the ribosomes.

Ribosomes and endoplasmic reticulum, to put it simply, can be seen as duplicating material for the RNA molecules, while the RNA molecules represent the duplicating material by which the DNA molecules are produced. DNA molecules are the finished protein molecules, in which all the "blueprints and working instructions" for the structure and function of a cell are stored.

Cell organelles

Cell organelles are the small organs of a cell and include:

- The mitochondria, threadlike or oval structures comprising a lamellar system with an outer and inner membrane. They contain active substances (enzymes) for organic oxidation. The respiratory enzymes of the mitochondria can break down amino acids, fats, and glucose with the aid of oxygen while generating heat; therefore, these organelles can be seen as the cell's energy suppliers.
- The **Golgi apparatus**, a vesicular membrane system in which the secretory activities of the cell take place. This is where the cell's secretions are stored, altered, and if required, released as a functioning secretion. The Golgi apparatus is mainly found in glandular cells.
- The centrosome (centrosphere, centriole), which only becomes active upon cell division, when it produces protein threads, with which it arranges, divides, and attracts the chromosome threads to itself.
- Lysosomes, which contain enzymes to break down molecules that are then further broken down by the special enzymes of the mitochondria.

Metaplasm

Metaplasm is made up of specific fibrous structures with functional tasks:

- Tonofibrils: give the cell special resistance to tensile stress
- Myofibrils: can contract like muscle cells
- Neurofibrils: conduct nerve impulses

Paraplasm

Paraplasm is made up of dead cell inclusions, which have either been absorbed from outside or developed as degradation products from the breakdown of nutrients. However, so-called reserve carbohydrates can also be found as paraplasm, and these are still of use for cell metabolism.

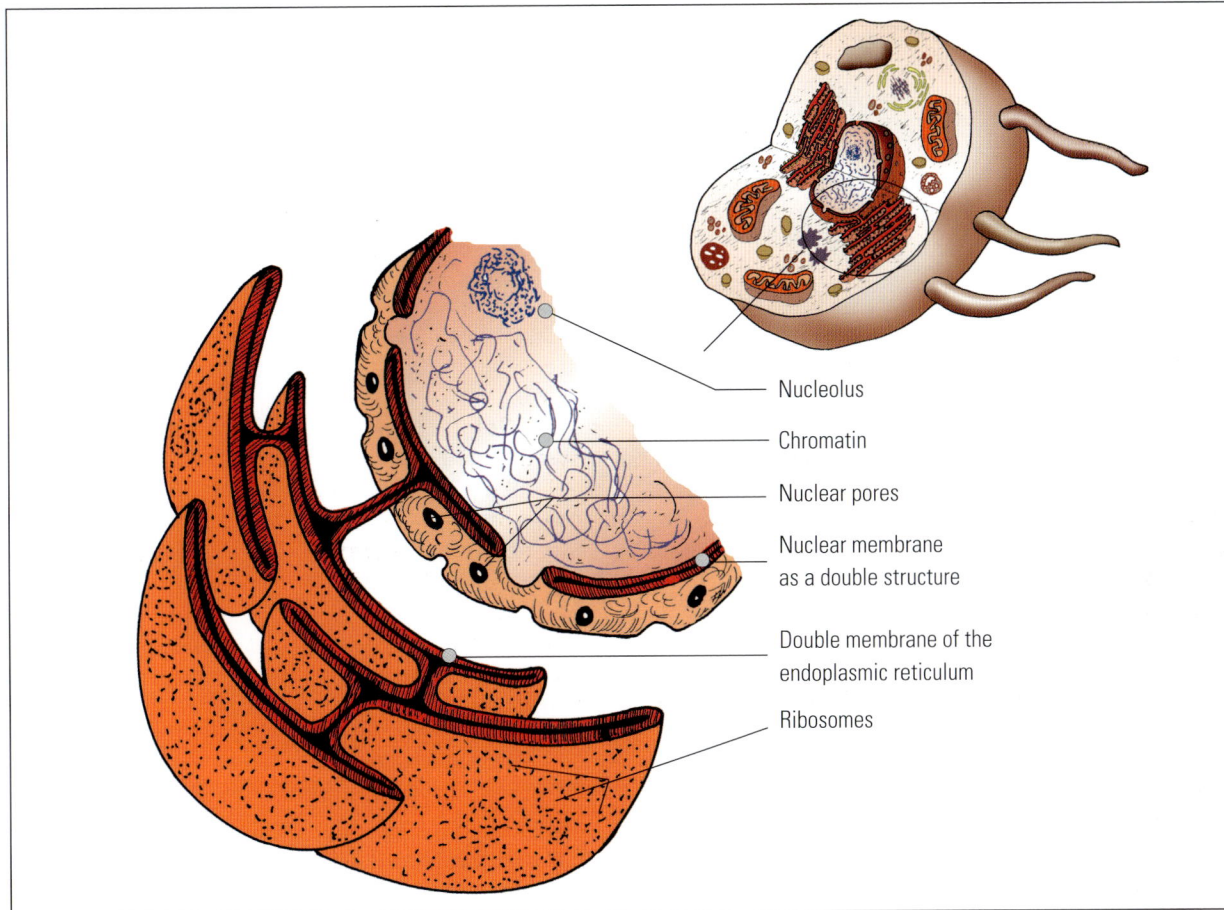

Fig 2-2 Normally every cell contains a cell nucleus, which can be seen in the living cell. It is separated from the cytoplasm by a double-walled membrane and contains the chromatin, the carrier of genetic information.

Nucleus

The cell nucleus is separated from the hyaloplasm by a nuclear membrane. It is the cell's control center and contains the chromosomes, which carry the genetic information. The cell nucleus is part of each and every cell. The most important exceptions are the red blood cells, which only live for about 100 days because they lack a nucleus.

The functions of the cell nucleus are to ensure control of protein synthesis by the formation of transfer RNA, to take over control of species-specific cellular reproduction by the formation of special RNA molecules, and to store the chromosomes.

The cell nucleus comprises the following constituents (Fig 2-2):

- The **nuclear membrane**, which is an inner membrane, a lipoid layer through which exchange of materials between nuclear contents and hyaloplasm is possible. The outer membrane is part of the endoplasmic reticulum; it forms a narrow gap with the inner membrane, the perinuclear space, which is connected to the channel system of the reticulum.
- The **nucleolus**, part of an active chromosome; transfer RNA, with which protein synthesis is regulated, is formed in the nucleolus.

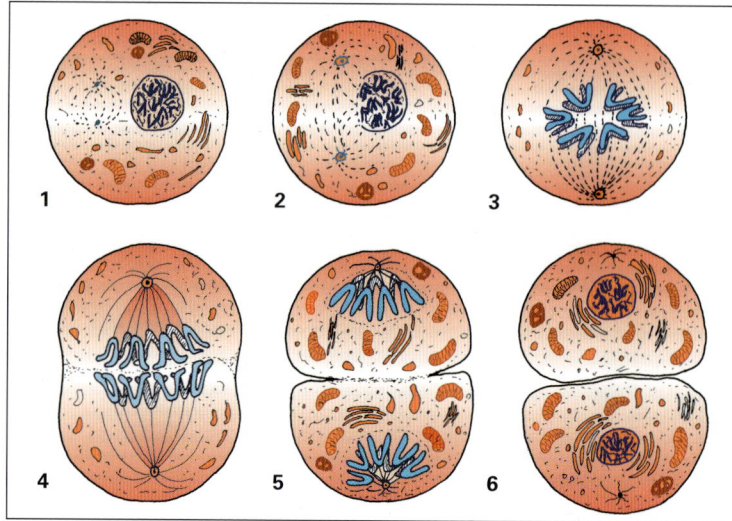

Fig 2-3 A living cell has the capacity for reproduction, a characteristic of life. This means duplication by division of the cellular substance and the genetic factors. By this form of reproduction, identical genetic factors are passed on to the daughter cells. There are different types of cell division. The five phases of mitosis—the normal form of cell division—are shown here: 1 and 2, prophase; 3, metaphase; 4, anaphase; 5, telophase; 6, reconstruction phase.

• *Chromatin*, which consists of largely unwound chromosomes from the resting or interphase nucleus. The chromosomes are long spiral threads of DNA molecules. They are always found in pairs. In humans, a diploid set of chromosomes comprises 23 pairs of chromosomes, ie, a total of 46 chromosomes. The DNA molecules carry the genetic information (genes); this is where the functions, structure, and timing for coordinating living processes are stored.

Cell Division

The reproduction of cells involves the division of existing cells. This process of cell division is known as *mitosis*. This means the equal distribution of the genetic information stored in the cell nucleus and division of the cytoplasm. This process of cell division takes between 20 minutes and 4 hours and can be broken down into five different phases, each of which smoothly transitions into the next (Fig 2-3):

1. *Prophase* (*pro* = before): The nucleus absorbs water and swells up while the chromosomes from the chromatin framework develop into fine threads. This differentiation is also known as *spiralization*. During prophase, the nuclear membrane breaks down, and the centriole divides and migrates to the poles of the cell.
2. *Metaphase* (*meta* = after): The chromosome threads become short and thick and split into two chromatids each. These chromatids come to lie on the equatorial plate.
3. *Anaphase* (*ana* = onto): The halved chromosomes (chromatids) migrate to the poles, being pulled by the spindle fibers of the centriole. The so-called stem fibers (protein threads) between the chromatids also push them to the poles.
4. *Telophase* (*telos* = target): The cytoplasm starts to narrow while migration of the chromatids to the poles is completed. A chromatin structure re-forms. The spindle and stem fibers break up so that a new nuclear membrane forms around each chromatin structure.

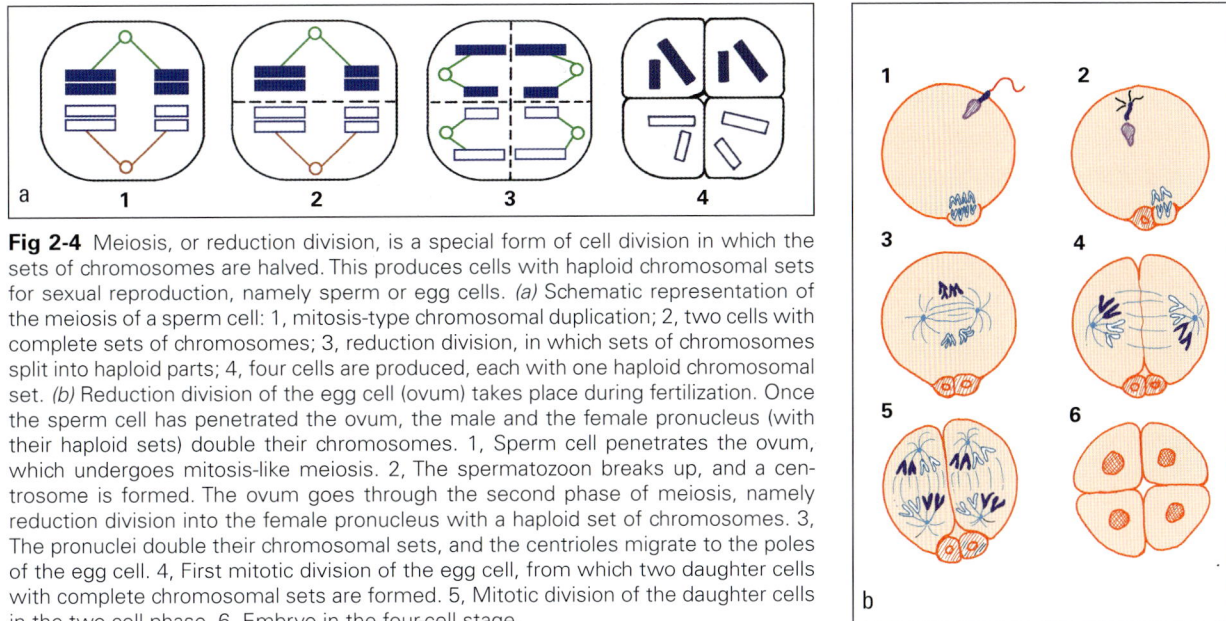

Fig 2-4 Meiosis, or reduction division, is a special form of cell division in which the sets of chromosomes are halved. This produces cells with haploid chromosomal sets for sexual reproduction, namely sperm or egg cells. *(a)* Schematic representation of the meiosis of a sperm cell: 1, mitosis-type chromosomal duplication; 2, two cells with complete sets of chromosomes; 3, reduction division, in which sets of chromosomes split into haploid parts; 4, four cells are produced, each with one haploid chromosomal set. *(b)* Reduction division of the egg cell (ovum) takes place during fertilization. Once the sperm cell has penetrated the ovum, the male and the female pronucleus (with their haploid sets) double their chromosomes. 1, Sperm cell penetrates the ovum, which undergoes mitosis-like meiosis. 2, The spermatozoon breaks up, and a centrosome is formed. The ovum goes through the second phase of meiosis, namely reduction division into the female pronucleus with a haploid set of chromosomes. 3, The pronuclei double their chromosomal sets, and the centrioles migrate to the poles of the egg cell. 4, First mitotic division of the egg cell, from which two daughter cells with complete chromosomal sets are formed. 5, Mitotic division of the daughter cells in the two-cell phase. 6, Embryo in the four-cell stage.

5. ***Reconstruction phase***: The identically structured daughter cells thus formed develop working nuclei; ie, the cell nuclei take on their typical form and start their working functions. Constriction of the cytoplasm continues until complete separation. What is known as the *interphase* (resting phase) now begins. For most of their lives, the cells are in the interphase, ie, in a working state with their defined functions.

There are various forms of cell division. *Mitosis* means the equal distribution of the genetic stock between the daughter cells. *Endomitosis* denotes division of the chromosomes without the nuclear membrane breaking down or the cell body dividing. This gives rise to cells with nuclei that have multiple sets of chromosomes.

Amitosis means division of the cell nucleus without ordered, equal distribution of the chromosomes. If the cytoplasm also divides, this produces daughter cells whose nuclei have different proportions of genetic material. This type of cell division happens in:

• Striated muscle cells
• Osteoclasts (cells that break down bone tissue)
• Diseased cells (eg, tuberculosis cells)

Meiosis (in Greek: reduction) is a special form of nuclear division that occurs in living creatures that procreate sexually. Mitosis is an asexual form of reproduction, whereas meiosis is a prerequisite for sexual reproduction.

In meiosis, sperm cells and egg cells with half sets of chromosomes are produced so that when an egg cell (ovum) is fertilized by a sperm cell, another complete set of chromosomes can arise. Meiosis therefore ensures that sexual reproduction does not lead to a linear increase in the number of chromosomes from generation to generation.

Meiosis always involves two different processes of division (Fig 2-4). First the sexual germ cell divides as in mitosis with doubling of the chromosomes. This means it divides normally, as described above, to give two daughter cells. This is followed by nuclear division, in which the sets of chromosomes are halved. This second process is known as *reduction division*. As a result of the process of meiosis, four sperm or egg cells, each with half of a set of chromosomes, are therefore produced from one sexual germ cell (gamete).

On fertilization, the half chromosomal sets lead to the normal genetic stock in the next generation. Thus, any linear increase in the number of chromosomes from generation to generation is prevented.

As the fertilized egg cell divides again and again, the cells differentiate to form tissues during human embryo development. As this development continues, cell differentiation results in cells of different formations determined by their functional specialization.

Tissue

In a multicellular living being, work is divided among uniquely differentiated cells. Each of the 60 billion cells in the human body exhibits a typical form, which is determined by the function of the particular complex of cells where the cell is located. This indicates a universal characteristic of living cells, namely to react flexibly to particular functional requirements. In the human body, a large number of different cells with differing functions can be identified.

Classification of tissue

Organic tissue is made up of a complex of cells that are differentiated in the same way and form the building blocks of the whole body; they have the same or similar functional tasks or responsibility for partial functions. Depending on their specific functions, four types of tissue or matrix can be distinguished. In the organs and organ systems, different tissues are always mixed up together to form one functional unit.

The four matrices are:

1. *Epithelial tissue* or *covering tissue* refers to closed colonies of cells that cover external and internal surfaces.
2. *Connective* or *supporting tissue* is a fibrous or tendinous tissue that joins together tissues and organs of the body. This includes fatty tissue, which acts as a fuel store, padding, and heat protection. Supporting tissues are cartilage and bone in the passive locomotor system. Supporting tissues give groups of tissues elasticity and stability while at the same time helping to protect the internal organs.
3. *Muscle tissue* makes up the active locomotor system or allows body cavities to contract, eg, the heart, blood vessels, and digestive tract.
4. *Nerve tissue* has the task of receiving, transmitting, and processing stimuli. It is part of the body's control system.

Epithelial tissue

The word *epithelial* is of Greek origin (*epi* = upon; *thele* = nipple). The epithelium covers or lines surfaces: the outer skin (epidermis), mucous membranes, gastrointestinal tract, urinary tracts, and inner linings of the blood vessels.

Epithelial tissue takes on various functions:

- General protection (eg, in the outer skin and mucous membranes)
- Respiration (eg, in the ciliated epithelium of the airways)
- Absorption (ie, absorbing substances in the epithelium of the intestinal villi)
- Secretion (ie, releasing substances from the glands; special groups of epithelial cells are designed to secrete fluids; Fig 2-5)
- Receiving stimuli (ie, sensory function, eg, in the retina of the eye)

Depending on the partial functions undertaken, epithelial tissue can be classified as surface or tegumentary epithelium, glandular epithelium, or sensory or neuroepithelium (Fig 2-6).

Distinguishing features of *surface epithelium* are that it is divided from other tissues by a basement membrane, it contains no blood vessels, and it is found as a flat collection of cells on the inner and outer surfaces of the body. The cells of the surface epithelium can be classified according to their form as follows (Fig 2-7):

- Squamous (flat): in the lungs, the blood and lymphatic vessels, and the inner surfaces of the joint capsules
- Cuboidal: such as the epithelium of the eye lens and the retinal pigment epithelium
- Columnar: such as the mucous membrane lining the digestive tract; often also as ciliated epithelium

Fig 2-5 The glandular epithelium forms organs from specialized epithelial cells, which are distinguished by their structure and mode of secretion. 1, The goblet cell of the intestinal mucosa is a unicellular gland. 2, Multicellular glands made up of goblet cells in the nasal mucosa open outward. 3, Glands with apocrine secretion collect their secretory material at the apex of the cell and expel it with a piece of cytoplasm. 4, Glands with holocrine secretion on a thick basement membrane form daughter cells. 5, Glands with merocrine secretion expel their fine granules in droplet form at the cell surface.

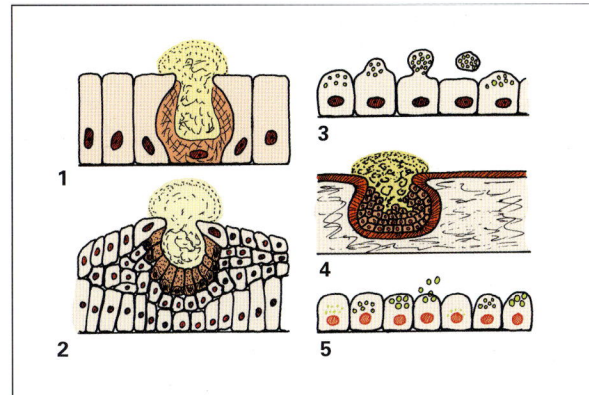

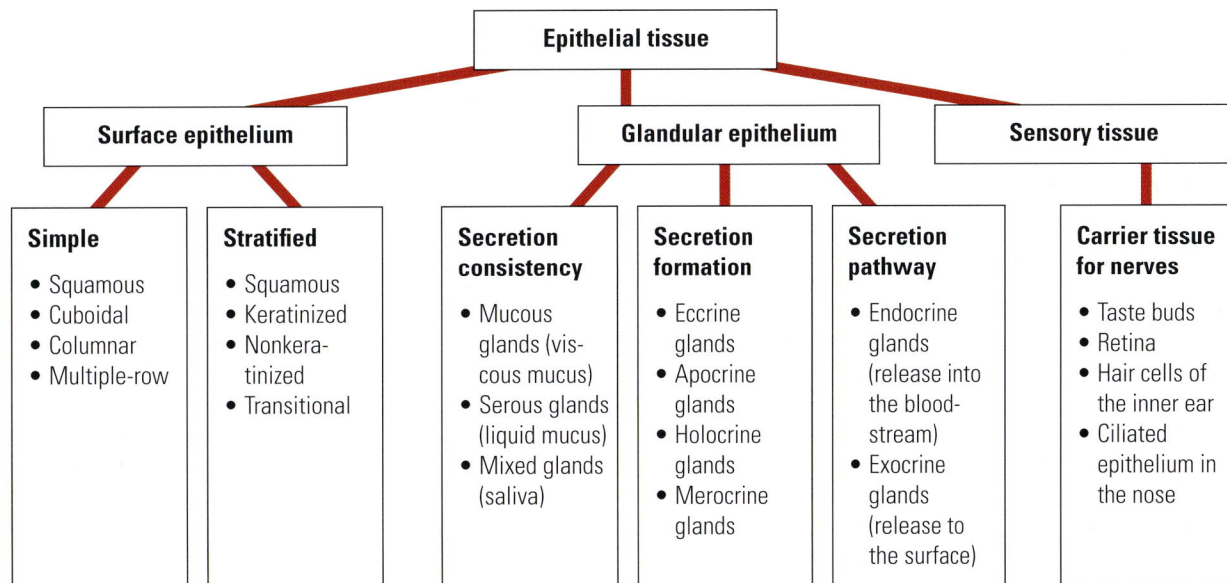

Epithelial tissue

Surface epithelium | **Glandular epithelium** | **Sensory tissue**

Simple
• Squamous
• Cuboidal
• Columnar
• Multiple-row

Stratified
• Squamous
• Keratinized
• Nonkeratinized
• Transitional

Secretion consistency
• Mucous glands (viscous mucus)
• Serous glands (liquid mucus)
• Mixed glands (saliva)

Secretion formation
• Eccrine glands
• Apocrine glands
• Holocrine glands
• Merocrine glands

Secretion pathway
• Endocrine glands (release into the bloodstream)
• Exocrine glands (release to the surface)

Carrier tissue for nerves
• Taste buds
• Retina
• Hair cells of the inner ear
• Ciliated epithelium in the nose

Fig 2-6 Classification of epithelial tissue.

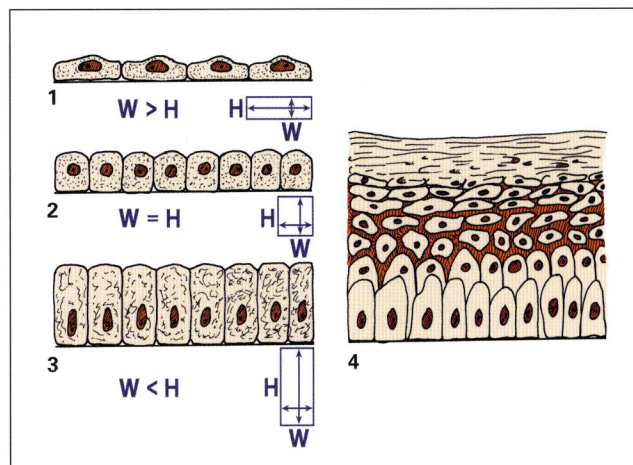

Fig 2-7 The epithelial cells sit on a basement membrane and form the typical cells of the various basic forms. 1, Simple (single-layer) squamous epithelium; cell width (W) is greater than cell height (H). 2, Cuboidal epithelium; cells are of the same height and width. 3, Columnar epithelium; cells are taller than they are wide. 4, Stratified, keratinized squamous epithelium.

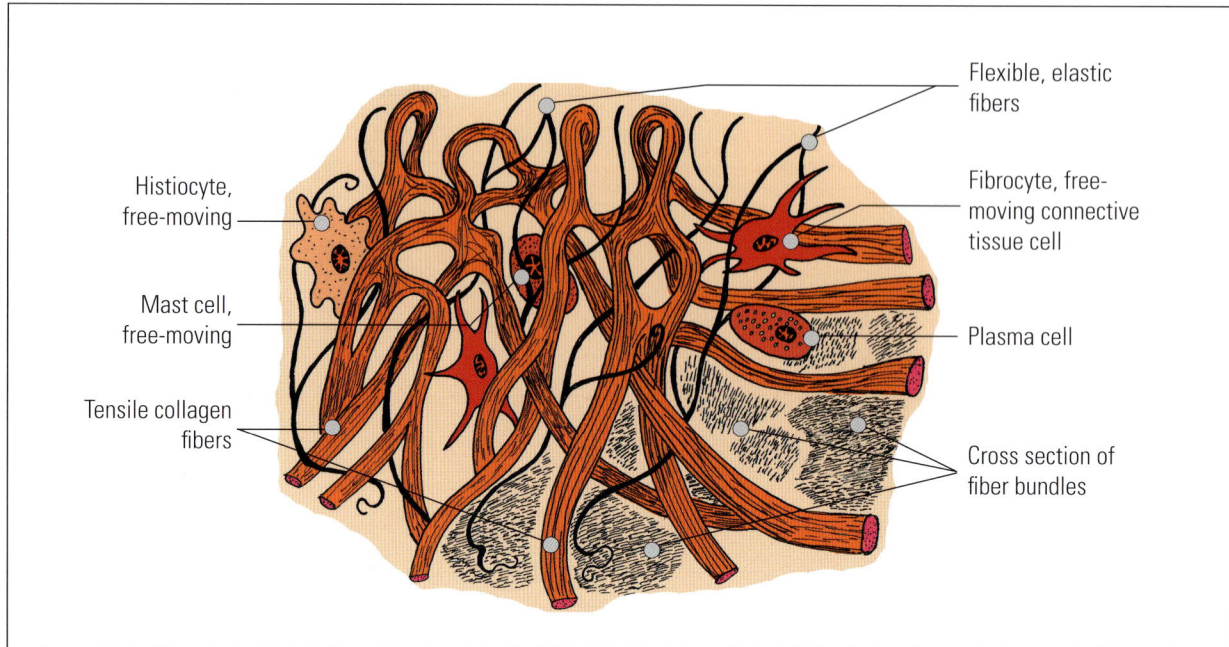

Fig 2-8 Schematic diagram of connective tissue structures.

Labels (clockwise from top right):
Flexible, elastic fibers
Fibrocyte, free-moving connective tissue cell
Plasma cell
Cross section of fiber bundles
Tensile collagen fibers
Mast cell, free-moving
Histiocyte, free-moving

The epithelial cells can be found in various arrangements:

• Single-layer (simple) epithelium: in the digestive tract
• Multilayered (stratified) epithelium: for example, on the outer skin as horny or keratinized squamous epithelium or on the mucous membrane as nonkeratinized squamous epithelium
• Transitional epithelium: for organ coverings where there are great fluctuations in volume (eg, urinary bladder)

The horny layers of keratinized squamous epithelia are made up of dead, hardened epithelial cells.

Connective and supporting tissue

This tissue group includes many different cell complexes, which, apart from their histologic origin, still have a few similarities of form that relate to the main mechanical function of that tissue. For instance, it is noticeable in connective tissue cells that the intercellular substance (ie, connecting substance between the cells) is highly developed.

In connective tissue, a distinction can be made between the actual connective tissue cells (fixed cells), which make up intercellular substance, and the free cells, which as accompanying cells move around freely in the gaps in the connective tissue (not in supporting tissue) (Fig 2-8). This distinction suggests that the free connective tissue cells and blood should be viewed in conjunction because the main purpose of these free connective tissue cells is to supply the other cells of the body and to defend against toxins, foreign matter, and bacteria. Lymphocytes, for example, are typical free connective tissue cells. Granulocytes, also free connective tissue cells, have their own ameoba-like mobility and phagocytize, which means they can engulf bacteria and ingest them so that the bacteria can be dissolved with the aid of special enzymes.

Connective and supporting tissue can be classified according to the amount and structure of the intercellular substance (Fig 2-9):

Cell-rich connective tissue
– Embryonic connective tissue (mesenchyme)
– Reticular (netlike) connective tissue
– Fatty tissue

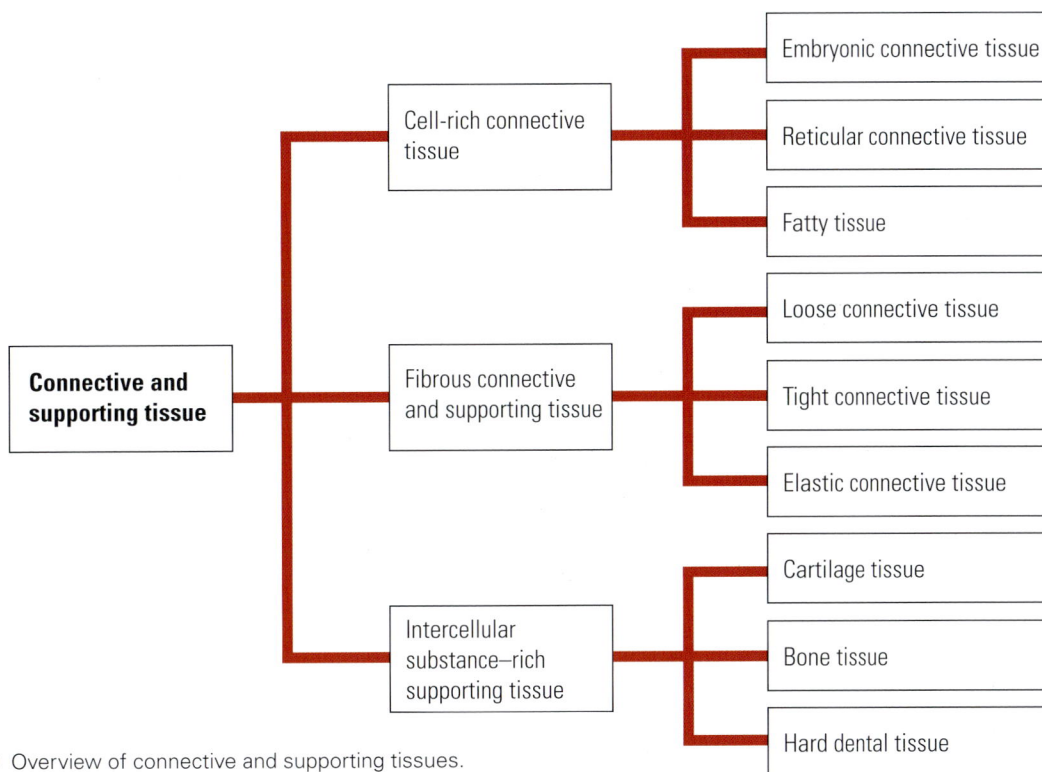

Fig 2-9 Overview of connective and supporting tissues.

Fibrous connective and supporting tissue
- Loose connective tissue
- Tight connective tissue
- Elastic connective tissue

Intercellular substance–rich supporting tissue
- Cartilage tissue
- Bone tissue
- Hard dental substances

The first two categories of tissue are discussed briefly here; subsequently bone and cartilage tissue are addressed in greater detail in dedicated sections, and hard dental substances are covered in chapter 3.

Cell-rich connective tissue

Embryonic connective tissue is a loose, filling, and elementary tissue in the embryo. The star-shaped cells form a loose mesh in which tissue fluid is still deposited instead of intercellular substance.

Reticular connective tissue is also structured as a three-dimensional lattice that holds a fluid ground substance (the lymph) in which numerous lymphocytes are suspended. The reticular connective tissue forms the basic framework of the lymphatic organs (spleen, tonsils, lymph nodes, and bone marrow). Reticulum cells can kill foreign bodies and absorb toxins. The free connective tissue cells are produced in the reticular tissue.

Fatty tissue is a type of reticular connective tissue with a high level of paraplasmic substance, namely fat, which is stored there instead of the fluid ground substance. It is important as an elastic pad, a reserve for calorie-rich fat, a store to maintain the water balance (fat:water = 1:7), and heat protection against sudden cooling.

Fibrous connective and supporting tissue

Loose connective tissue acts as filling tissue because it is found between organs, vessels, and nerves and thus provides cohesion. It is also described as interstitial connective tissue because it fills up the spaces in between. Bundles of tensile, inelastic (collagenous) fibers permeate the loose connective tissue in all directions and provide

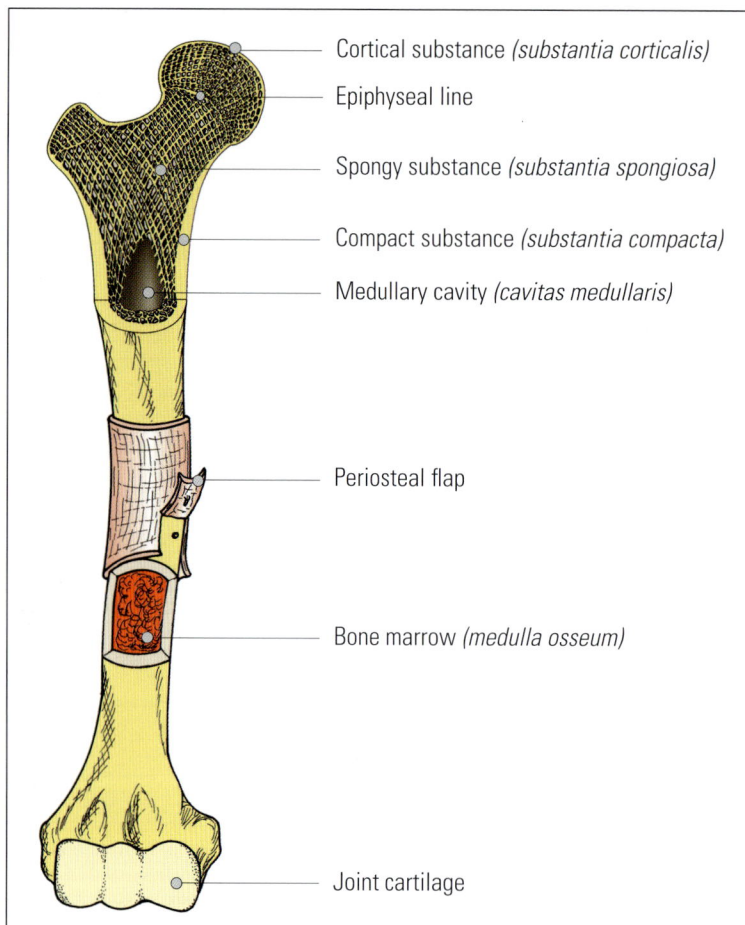

Cortical substance (*substantia corticalis*)

Epiphyseal line

Spongy substance (*substantia spongiosa*)

Compact substance (*substantia compacta*)

Medullary cavity (*cavitas medullaris*)

Periosteal flap

Bone marrow (*medulla osseum*)

Joint cartilage

Fig 2-10 Diagram of bone structure.

resistance and stability. However, elastic fibers (elastin) are also found there, so that the tissue has a high level of mobility and returns to its original position after pressure has been placed upon it. Loose connective tissue is a filling and displacement tissue that serves as a water store (eg, in subcutaneous connective tissue).

Tight connective tissue is mainly interspersed with many tensile, inelastic, collagenous fibers to give a highly tensile, not very elastic tissue. It is found as shiny white tissue in the form of a muscular coat (fascia) and as tendinous tissue.

Elastic connective tissue largely comprises elastic fibers (elastin), which make it a highly stretchy tissue that is nevertheless very dimensionally stable. It is found in the walls of blood vessels, as vocal cords in the larynx, and as connecting ligaments attached to the spine.

Bone tissue

The **basic substance of bone tissue** is two-thirds inorganic mineral salts and one-third organic substances (living cells). The collagenous connective tissue fibers are responsible for the high bending strength of bone, while the mineral salts create the enormous compressive strength (15 kPa/mm²). The mineral salts are mainly calcium phosphate in the form of hydroxyapatite crystals. Apatites are crystallized molecules that were once easily confused with other crystals, hence the name (*apatan* = they deceive).

Bone develops in two ways: embryonic connective tissue is converted directly into bone substance by the deposition of bone-forming cells (osteoblasts), or cartilage tissue forms first as a precursor that later develops into bone tis-

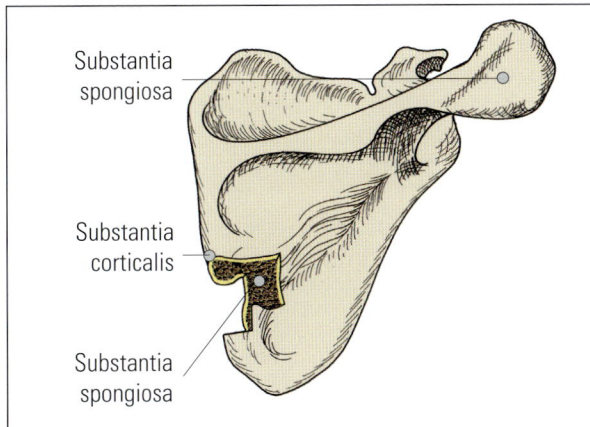

Fig 2-11 Bone structure in the shoulder blade.

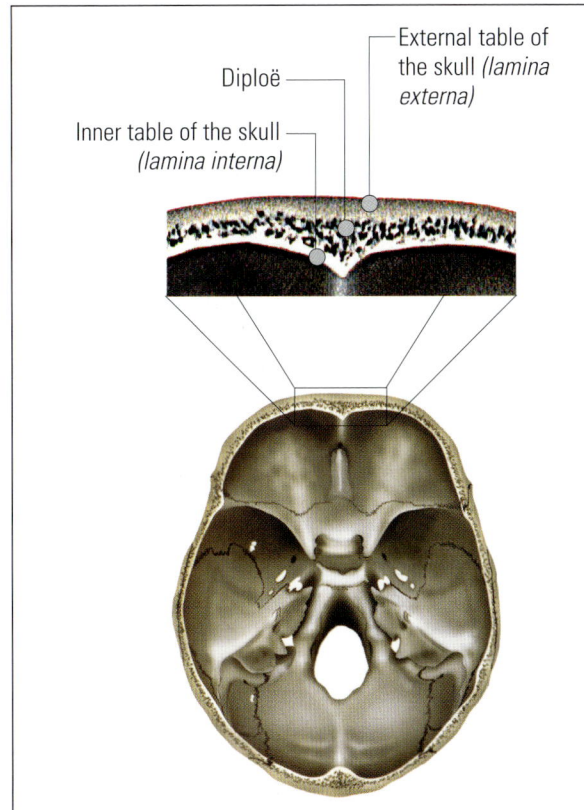

Fig 2-12 Diagram of bone structure in cranial bone.

Isolating organic and inorganic components of bone

The organic substance can be removed from the bone by heating until red hot, which renders the bone noticeably brittle. The calcium salts can be removed from the bone by acid treatment, which leaves only the flexible substances. In response to both treatments, the bone retains its original form, but the mechanical properties are exactly reversed; whereas the organic part of the bone is so rubbery and elastic that it can be coiled into a knot, the inorganic part of the bone remains brittle and hard.

sue through calcification. The first type is known as *membrane* or *dermal bone* and the second as *replacing* or *cartilage bone*.

Constituents of bone

In bone, a distinction is made between three constituents that together form a functional unit: periosteum, bony substance, and bone marrow (Figs 2-10 to 2-12).

Periosteum

Periosteum is a tight envelope of connective tissue that completely encases the bone, except at the joints. It contains blood vessels and nerves and is made up of an outer fibrous layer and an inner germ layer of bone-forming cells, the osteoblasts. The periosteum nourishes the bone and bone marrow. In mature bone, the osteoblasts are in a resting state; they become active and regenerate the bone if there is a fracture.

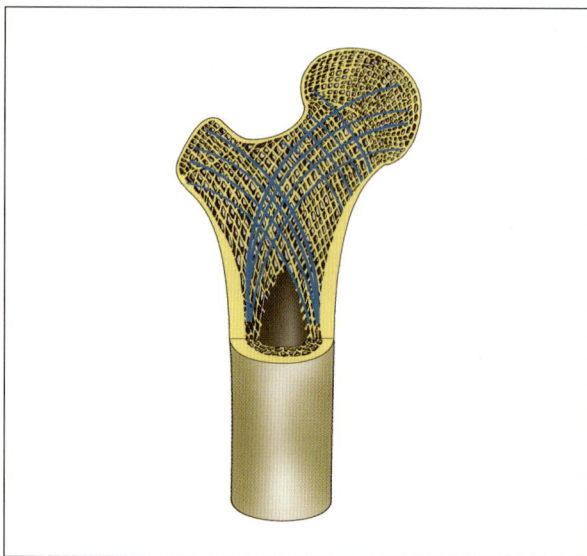

Fig 2-13 The osseous lamellae of the spongy substance of bone are arranged along the lines of force in a bone.

Bony substance

Bony substance comprises two differentiated structures: the outer compact cortical layer and the inner spongy material (lamellar or cancellous bone).

The **compact cortical layer** (substantia compacta, corticalis) forms a layer of thickened bone material at the surface of the bone, which is particularly thick in the middle part of a tubular bone and thinner at the joints. At the surface of the cortical layer, there are small openings to the Volkmann and Haversian canals, in which blood vessels and nerves run from the periosteum through the bone into the bone marrow.

The **spongy material** (substantia spongiosa) forms a framework of fine trabeculae, whose holes are filled with soft bone marrow. There are no trabeculae in the middle section of a long or tubular bone, so that a uniform bone cavity is produced (cavum medullare). The fine trabeculae (spongy trabeculae) are arranged according to lines of pressure and traction (Fig 2-13) with two guiding principles: (1) the minimum and maximum rule, whereby the greatest work is achieved with the least effort; and (2) the form and function rule, according to which the function determines the form and form influences function. Bone mass is only built up at points where mechanical stresses are exerted. Where there is no mechanical strain, this substance is absent. Owing to the special arrangement of the spongy trabeculae along the lines of mechanical force, the bone becomes pliable in a specific way and equally resistant to bending. This is because a bone only bends in response to stress as much as the spongy trabeculae will allow, and this provides the stimulus to strengthening the spongy trabeculae in their particular form.

Bone marrow

Bone marrow (medulla osseum) is a soft, jellylike substance that is found both in the gaps between the spongy trabeculae and in the bone cavity of long bones. A distinction is made between red and yellow bone marrow. The red, blood-forming marrow in adults is only found in the gaps between the spongy trabeculae of flat bones (eg, ribs, cranial bones, sternum, vertebral bodies, and wrist bones). Yellow bone marrow is mainly found in the medullary cavity of the long bones. The bone marrow and bony substance are nourished via blood vessels. These vessels run from the periosteum through to the bone cavity via a system of Volkmann canals, which in turn branch into Haversian canals.

Form and function of bone

Bone has the following functions:

- To support the soft tissues
- To form attachments for the active locomotor system (the muscles)
- To protect sensitive organs such as the heart, lungs, and brain
- To produce red blood cells (as the blood-forming center)

The passive locomotor system comprises bones and their joint cartilages. The bones are connected to each other via joints.

The form of bone is determined by its specific function (Figs 2-14 and 2-15). This means that pressure loading from vessels, nerves, or muscles can cause the formation of, for example, depressions, grooves, and cavities, while tensile strain may result in the formation of processes, spurs, or tubercles on the relevant bones.

Skull *(cranium cerebrale)*
Facial part of the skull *(cranium viscerale)*
Spinal column *(columna vertebralis)*
Shoulder blade *(scapula)*
Upper arm *(humerus)*
Radius
Ulna

Collarbone *(clavicula)*
Breastbone *(sternum)*
Ribs *(costae)*

Upper extremity

Lower extremity

Hip bone *(os coxae)*
Thigh bone *(femur)*
Knee cap *(patella)*
Shin bone *(tibia)*
Calf bone *(fibula)*

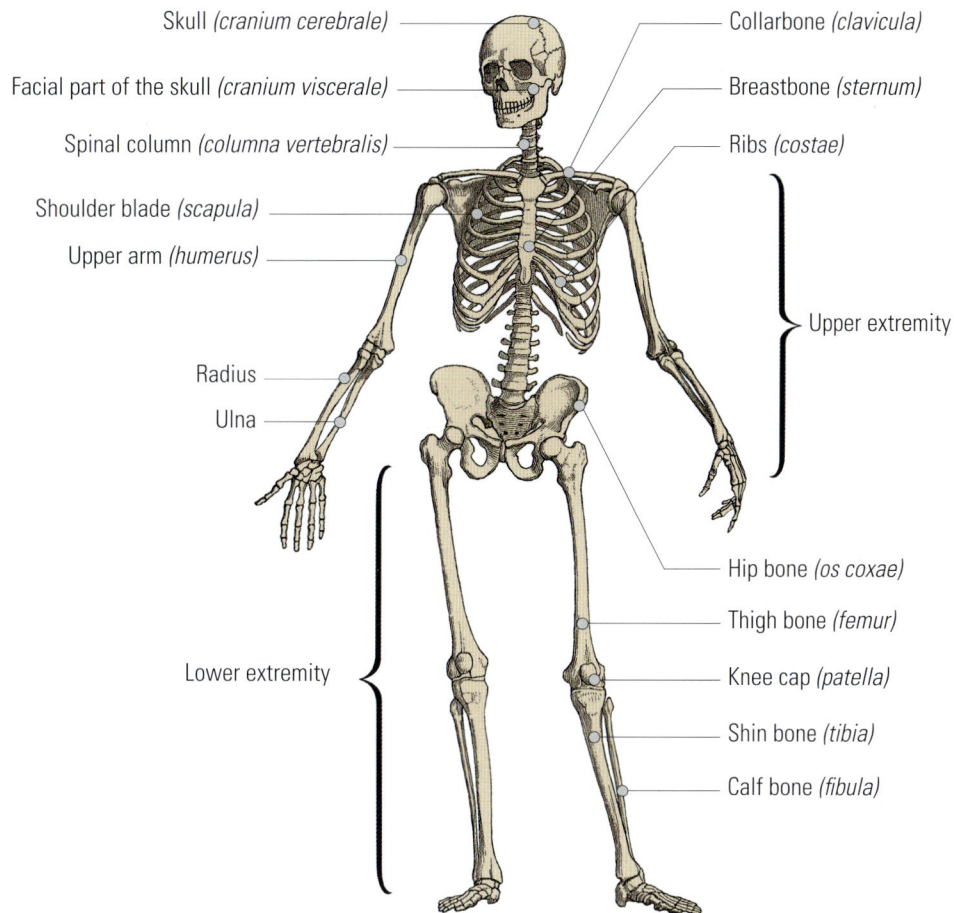

Fig 2-14 The human skeleton.

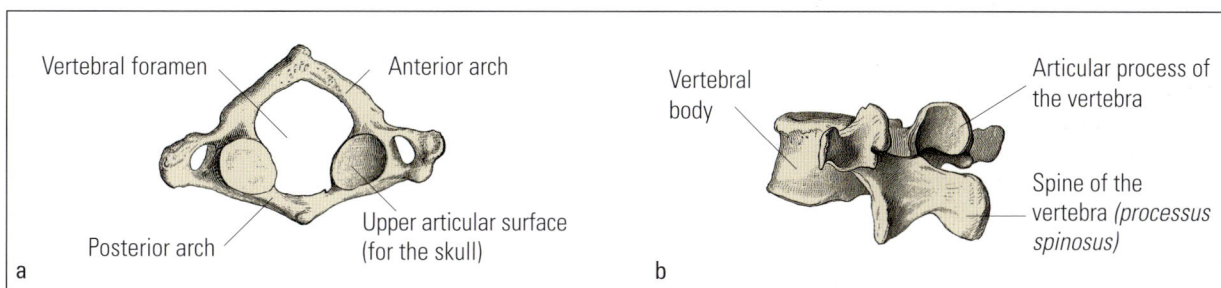

Vertebral foramen   Anterior arch
Vertebral
body
Articular process of
the vertebra

Posterior arch   Upper articular surface
(for the skull)
Spine of the
vertebra *(processus
spinosus)*

a   b

Fig 2-15 *(a)* First cervical vertebra (atlas) seen from above. *(b)* Lumbar vertebra seen from the side.

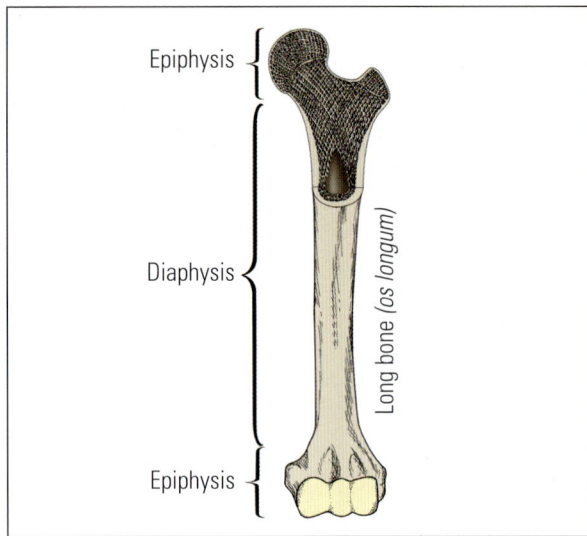

Fig 2-16 Structure of a long bone.

A distinction is made between the following forms of bone:

- **Long tubular bones** *(ossa longa)* (Fig 2-16) or supporting bones are the long bones of the extremities, which are made up of a tubular middle section (diaphysis) and the two thickened ends covered with joint cartilage (epiphyses). There is a region of lengthwise growth (metaphysis) between the diaphysis and the epiphyses. The diaphysis ossifies, unlike the two ends, which remain cartilaginous at first. Tubular long bones have a medullary cavity in their middle section, which is filled with red, blood-forming bone marrow in young people and with yellow (fat) marrow in older people.
- **Flat bones** *(ossa plana)* comprise two layers of compact bone with spongy material lying between the layers. The skull bones, hip bones, and shoulder blades are typical flat bones, which surround the cavities to protect sensitive organs and are therefore also known as *protective bones.*
- **Short bones** *(ossa brevia)* are the carpal and tarsal bones of the hands and feet, which mainly consist of spongy bone and are surrounded by a thin cortical layer.
- **Irregular bones containing air** perform protective, supportive, and locomotor functions, as shown by the example of the craniofacial bones.

The cavities of spongy bones, epiphyses, and long bones as well as short and flat bones contain red, blood-forming bone marrow in which the red blood cells, granulocytes, and platelets are formed.

If the bone marrow has to be clinically examined, a biopsy is taken from the sternum, and the bone marrow specimen obtained is stained.

Cartilage tissue

Cartilage tissue, like bone tissue, is classified as intercellular substance–rich connective and supporting tissue. Supporting tissues give the body its form because of their strength; they surround important organs and create stable protective spaces. The intercellular substance in supporting tissue is formed not by fibers but by the ground substance. This ground substance comprises 75% water, 5% protein, 15% collagenous substance, and 5% mucopolysaccharides as a strengthening material (put simply, these are macromolecules of amino sugars and one sulfuric acid residue). The cartilage-forming cells are called *chondroblasts*.

Cartilage usually does not contain blood vessels. It is nourished by diffusion. In metabolic disorders, the cartilage may calcify because the chondroblasts are also being transformed into cartilage substance.

Three forms of cartilage tissue are identified, based on their differing composition, which is due to different mechanical stresses: glassy or hyaline cartilage, elastic cartilage, and fibrous cartilage.

Hyaline cartilage is glassy, transparent, and permeated by collagen fibers. It is very smooth and ideally suited to withstanding compressive stresses. It is mainly found as a covering of joint surfaces, as part of the nasal septum, and as costal (rib) cartilage.

Elastic cartilage consists of the same ground substance, but it is permeated by a large number of elastic fibers, making this cartilage highly resistant to bending. It forms the cartilage of the outer ear.

Fibrocartilage is also known as *cartilaginous connective tissue* because it is very densely permeated by parallel collagen fibers. It is therefore highly resistant to mechanical strain. The meniscus in the knee, the intervertebral discs, and the articular disc of the mandibular joint are made up of fibrocartilage.

Dental Tissues

The individual tooth is composed of five different tissue layers, which can be seen without magnification in a cross section of a tooth (Figs 3-1 and 3-2). These tissues can be divided into soft and hard substances:

- Hard substances
  - Enamel *(enamelum)*
  - Dentin *(dentinum)*
  - Cementum
- Soft substances
  - Dental pulp *(pulpa dentis)*
  - Periodontal ligament *(desmodontium)*

The whole tooth with its root is fixed in a bony socket in the jaw, the alveolus. Because the periodontal ligament is connected to both the cementum of the root and the alveolar bone, a cross section reveals the junction between the alveolar bone and the periodontal ligament; the junction between the tooth and the gingival tissue is also evident.

Development of Dental Tissues

The development of dental tissue starts in the fifth week of embryonic life and is not complete until the twentieth year of life, with the formation of the third molars. The developmental processes are genetically controlled and are the same for all teeth. The development of dental tissue is known as **odontogeny** and starts when the embryo is roughly 9 mm in size. The side swellings for the nose and the primary palate are already

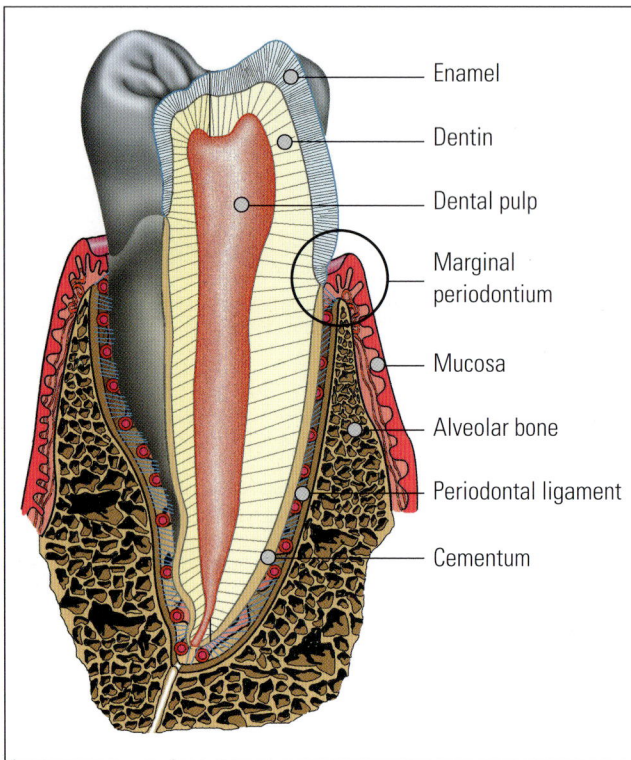

Fig 3-1 The dental tissues.

Enamel
Dentin
Dental pulp
Marginal periodontium
Mucosa
Alveolar bone
Periodontal ligament
Cementum

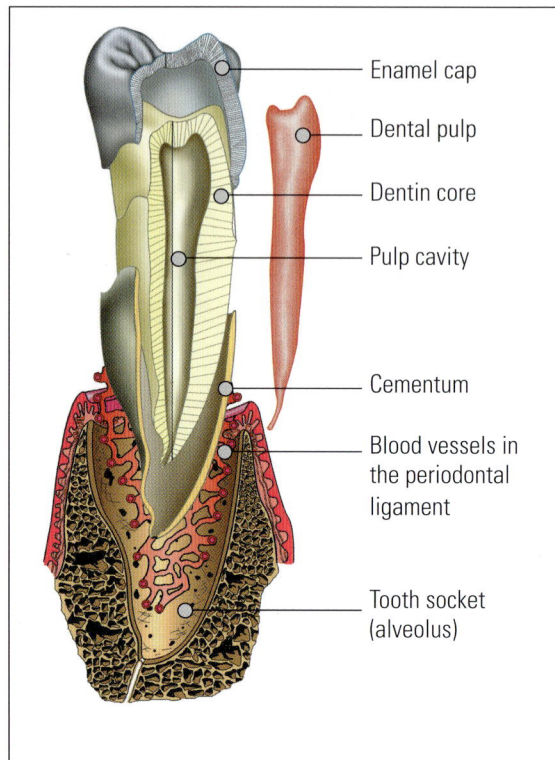

Fig 3-2 Teaching model showing the different dental tissues.

Enamel cap
Dental pulp
Dentin core
Pulp cavity
Cementum
Blood vessels in the periodontal ligament
Tooth socket (alveolus)

identifiable, while there is still a shared nasal and oral cavity. The germ cells for the primary teeth are present in the swellings in the jaw.

The ***tooth germ cells*** arise from proliferation of the epithelial cells in the primary jaws and cells from the neural crest in the jaw swellings during weeks 8 to 17 of gestation. During this period, the proliferation of epithelial cells first gives rise to a dental bud and then a cap, and finally, as a result of the high rate of cell division, the tooth caps enlarge into a bell shape, which has roughly the same form as the eventual tooth. In this stage of development, the cells differentiate into the enamel, dental papilla, and follicle (Fig 3-3).

The ***germ cells of the primary teeth*** reach the bell stage in week 17 of embryonic life. The permanent first molars reach this developmental stage by week 24, and the permanent second molars reach the bell stage at 6 months after birth. The third molars do not reach the bell stage until 6 years after birth. The bell stage also sees

the start of dentin and enamel formation for the primary and accessional germ teeth. The successional germ teeth develop from the fifth month of pregnancy through to the third year of life.

The ***successional germ teeth*** are located lingual to the primary teeth in the bell stage, and then they move to below the roots of the primary teeth when these erupt. This means the anterior germs lie exactly below the tips of the roots, and the premolars are between the splayed roots of the primary molars.

The ***enamel organ*** forms the bell with four functionally distinct layers: the external and internal enamel epithelium, the stellate reticulum, and the stratum intermedium.

The ***enamel epithelium*** covers the whole surface of the enamel organ (Fig 3-4). The external enamel epithelium forms the outer limit of the enamel organ and, with the cervical loop, is continuous with the internal enamel epithelium at the edge of the bell. The cells of the stellate re-

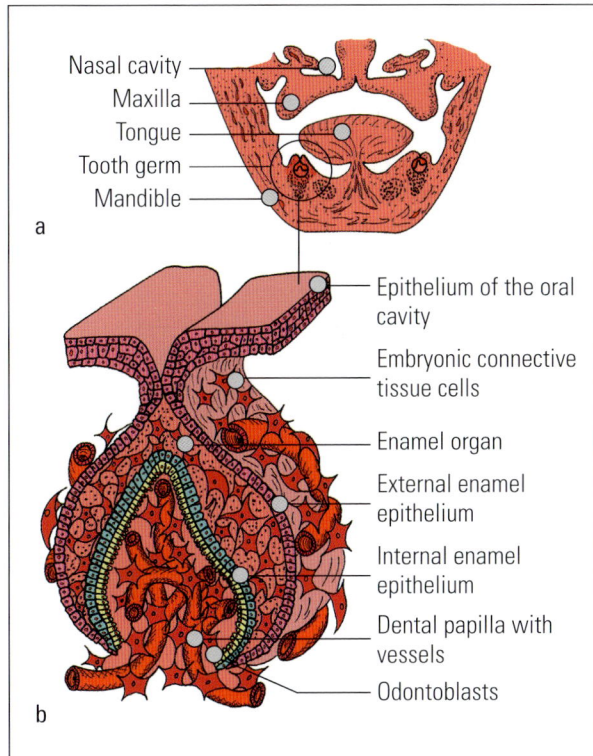

Fig 3-3 *(a)* A frontal section through the skull of a 3-month-old fetus shows the germ teeth. *(b)* Magnification of a tooth germ shows the bell and the enamel organ.

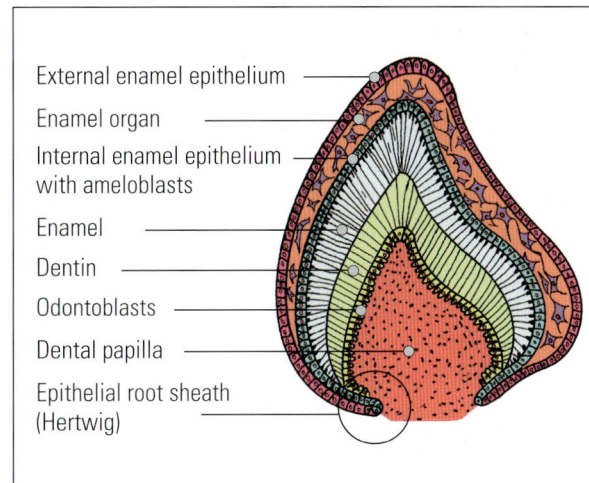

Fig 3-4 Schematic diagram of an anterior tooth germ.

ticulum make up the inner part of the organ; the cells of the stratum intermedium overlie the internal epithelium as a thin layer. The internal enamel epithelium is the inner layer of the bell and marks the separation from the cells of the dental papilla.

The **dental papilla** is an accumulation of cells arising from embryonic connective tissue and migrated nerve fibers, which is enclosed by the epithelial bell. A thin layer of connective tissue known as the *follicle* surrounds the dental papilla and enamel organ.

The **cells of the dental papilla** control formation of the root and the tooth shape. The enamel-forming cells differentiate from the cells of the internal enamel epithelium, while the dentin-forming cells are differentiated from the peripheral cells of the dental papilla.

The odontoblasts secrete the dentin matrix toward the interface with the internal enamel epithelium and thereby stimulate the enamel-forming cells to produce enamel. The formation of dentin transforms the organic shape of the bell into a stable molded shape, against which the dental enamel is deposited.

Dental Enamel

The **crown of the tooth** is covered with a very hard layer of enamel. The enamel is thinnest at the neck of the tooth and increases in thickness up to the incisal or occlusal surface of the tooth. On the occlusal surface, the enamel layer is up to 2 mm thick.

In healthy teeth, the enamel is virtually colorless; it has a slight bluish tinge, making it appear translucent. Therefore, the particular coloring of a tooth is not determined solely by the inherent color of the enamel but by the shade of the underlying dentin. The yellowish dentin is more visible through the thin layer of enamel at the neck of

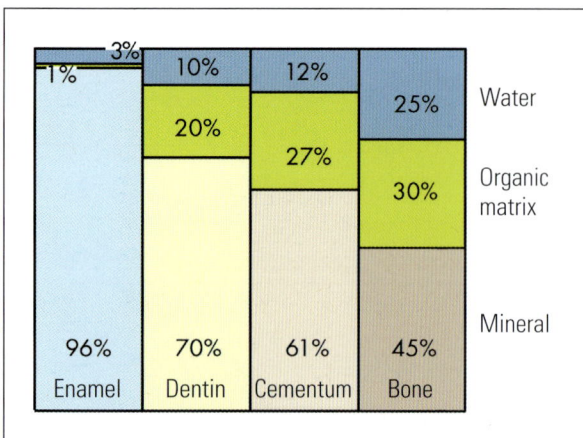

Fig 3-5 Mineral constituents, organic matrix, and water content in percentage by *weight* for enamel, dentin, cementum, and bone.

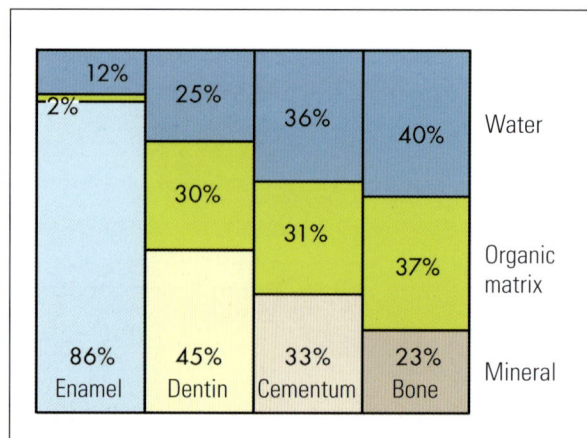

Fig 3-6 Mineral constituents, organic matrix, and water content in percentage by *volume* for enamel, dentin, cementum, and bone.

the tooth. This is why the neck looks darker, while at the incisal edge the tooth appears to have a lighter, almost transparent consistency.

Enamel is the hardest substance in the human body and extremely resistant to mechanical stresses and strains. Being composed of inorganic substances gives enamel very high resistance to chemical influences. However, this hardest dental substance is also the most brittle in the human body and, in line with its mineral density, is harder and more brittle at the surface than in the deeper layers.

Mature enamel differs in its composition and characteristics from the other hard substances of the teeth and bones. It contains 98% inorganic and only 2% organic materials. The crystalline part of enamel is made up of hydroxyapatites of calcium phosphate. It may also contain carbonates such as manganese carbonate, sodium carbonate, calcium carbonate, and fluoride carbonate.

Hydroxyapatite has the chemical formula $Ca_{10}(PO_4)_6(OH)_2$, although the hydroxyl groups can often be substituted by fluoride and chlorine. The fluoride content hardens the dental enamel and varies widely. The fluoride concentration is far greater (20 times) at the surface than in the lower layers and fluctuates further depending on the amount of fluoride consumed in the diet, drinking water, and toothpaste. In its immature state, dental enamel has 50% water content, but

this rapidly decreases as the enamel matures, leaving a residue of only 4% by weight, which accounts for 14% of its volume (Figs 3-5 and 3-6). A quarter of this residual water is found in the organic substance of enamel and makes up about 1% of its weight (2% of its volume). The other residual water is bound to the apatite crystals in the form of hydroxyl groups.

The *organic substance* of enamel comprises proteins, carbohydrates, and lipid compounds. The enamel layer determines the outer shape of the crown of the tooth. However, these shapes are not random but determined by the natural laws of form and function. Every enamel crest, cusp, or fissure therefore has a very specific task. When tooth substance is formed during growth, the *ameloblasts* (enamel-forming cells; adamantoblasts) are the building blocks for enamel, and these give the specific shape to the teeth during development. Shortly after eruption, there is a very thin membrane (1 mm) on the enamel surface. This is known as the *enamel cuticle (cuticula dentis)*. This membrane is very resistant but is soon worn away; the enamel cuticle remains longer at the neck of the tooth. No new enamel is formed once the tooth has erupted. The enamel layer, once developed, has to last for the lifetime of the tooth (ie, the durability of the enamel largely determines the durability of the tooth).

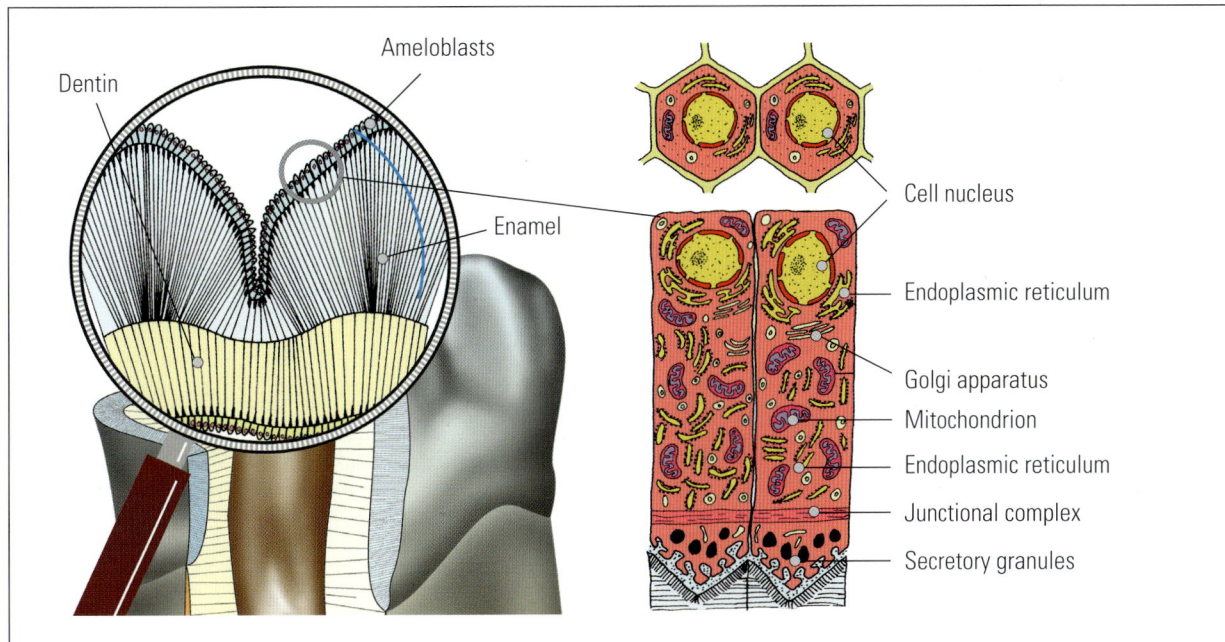

Fig 3-7 Structural diagram of an ameloblast.

The **enamel layer** has several functions. It protects the dentin core of the tooth against thermal and chemical influences. The purpose of its specific hardness is to resist mechanical stresses during chewing, although older teeth will show a certain amount of wear at the incisal and occlusal surfaces (abrasion). The protective effect of enamel also extends to bacterial influences.

Despite its density, **enamel is permeable** to liquids. This means that pigments, water, and alcohol can flow relatively freely through enamel (water penetrates enamel to a depth of about 4 mm within 24 hours). This is why chemical changes that help to maintain or alter the composition of the enamel can be initiated in enamel.

Formation of enamel (amelogenesis)

Dental enamel is a complex product of differentiated cell activities of ameloblasts (Fig 3-7). It arises during three processes taking place in the cells

simultaneously, namely the formation of enamel matrix, mineralization of the matrix, and maturation of the crystalline structure. Enamel is the mature crystalline framework of prisms (Fig 3-8) and the hardest substance in the human body.

The **formation of enamel** starts with the secretion of enamel matrix. This secretory process is similar to that of an eccrine glandular cell: In the distinctly enlarged endoplasmic reticulum of the ameloblasts, the proteins of the enamel matrix are synthesized and secreted in an extracellular direction at the distal pole of the cell. The slightly granulated enamel matrix is secreted drop by drop and proliferates. It is made up of protein, carbohydrates, and lipids.

Needle-shaped crystallization seeds of apatite crystals rapidly form in the secreted matrix. The crystallization seeds develop in orderly rows and with gaps, perpendicular to the cell poles of the ameloblasts. The cells control the formation, arrangement, and orientation of the apatite crystals. Enamel prisms develop and lie almost parallel to each other, reflecting the path of ame-

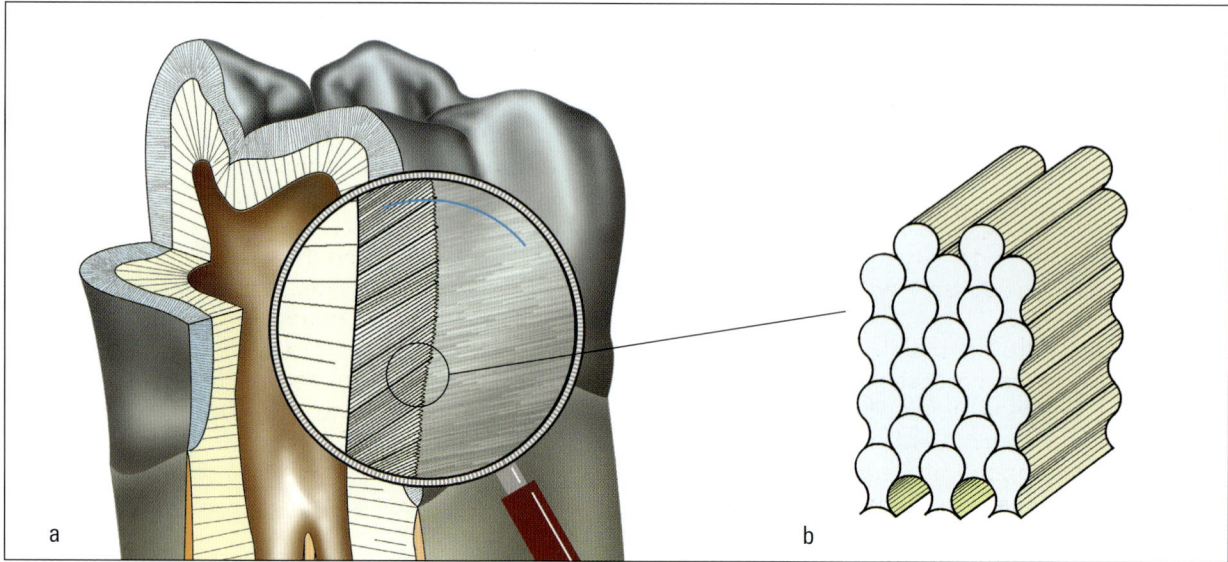

Fig 3-8 *(a)* Perikymata denote a wave-shaped pattern of grooves on the enamel surface, which is visible under the microscope and is formed by regularly arranged enamel prisms. *(b)* A simplified representation of the arrangement of enamel prisms, showing the keyhole type in cross section. Here the head of the keyhole is 5 mm in diameter, and the tail is 9 mm long. In each prism, the apatite crystals are arranged so that crystals overlap adjacent prisms. The apatite crystals therefore interlock at the prism boundaries, which increases the strength of enamel.

loblast movement. During the ongoing synthesis of enamel matrix and its mineralization, the ameloblasts move from the dentinoenamel junction outward just as the enamel prisms lengthen and the enamel thickens. This movement is not linear and centrifugal but happens in growth spurts, as shown by the patterns of lines, the *perikymata*, visible in the mature enamel.

The ***mineralization process*** represents a selective change in the composition of the enamel matrix; when water is removed, the organic parts of the matrix shrink, and calcium phosphate salts are laid down. These rebuilding processes are the cellular activities of the ameloblasts. The preeruptive maturation of enamel denotes the processes in which the mineralized enamel matrix becomes the crystalline structure of enamel. The mineralized enamel matrix initially contains about 25% crystalline components, whereas crystals account for 86% of the volume in mature enamel (see Fig 3-6).

The ***prisms*** in mature enamel are made up of apatite crystals of calcium phosphate in the form of hexagonal rods about 0.016 mm long. An organic matrix is stored in the crystals, occupying

about 2% of the volume (see Fig 3-6). The interfaces between individual prisms can be seen because the crystals with different growth directions collide with each other. No interprismatic filler material that differs from prisms in its chemical composition can be detected. The number of prisms per square millimeter varies from around 20,000 to 30,000 from the crown to the root, while the number of ameloblasts remains equally high. The enamel prisms stop immediately before the enamel surface; the top layer itself is prism-free. The enamel layer regularly found in unerupted teeth is harder, chemically more resistant, and withstands caries far longer than the rest of the enamel. Large amounts of fluoride are stored in this layer.

The ***formation of hard substance*** starts at the tips of the cusps or incisally at the cutting edges and spreads in a labiolingual and mesiodistal direction throughout the crown of the tooth. In the process, the ameloblast layer of the enamel organ moves outward, and the odontoblast layer shifts inward, narrowing the dental papilla on the one hand and the stellate reticulum on the other.

For multicusped teeth, the formation of enamel starts at the various tips of the cusps simultaneously. Once these enamel caps join up, a valley is formed between the enamel ridges. Ameloblasts become compressed in the bottom of this valley so that the valley walls move closer and closer together. This produces the fissures found in teeth with grinding surfaces. Fissure depth and width as well as the density of enamel under the fissures differ considerably within the individual teeth.

After **eruption**, the enamel substance then undergoes changes, a process referred to as *post-eruptive enamel maturation*. During this process, the enamel loses more and more water and organic matrix components. The crystalline structure becomes denser and changes its chemical composition mainly through substitution of hydroxide (OH) groups with fluoride. The enamel becomes even harder and more chemically resistant but more brittle and less permeable. Now the enamel is also more susceptible to fracture, and microcracks appear. When filled with saliva, these microcracks cause discoloration in the form of enamel crack lines. The surface of the enamel also changes as a result of abrasion during chewing and cleaning of the teeth. The enamel layer may be entirely worn away in places, resulting in exposure of the dentin. The dentin layer thus brought to the surface becomes more mineralized by the ongoing activity of the dentin-forming cells (odontoblasts) and is then denser and harder than normal dentin.

As a result of the **aging processes**, enamel changes from transparent to a gray base color. Ingredients of medicines can lodge in the crystals of enamel, forming solid calcium compounds and staining the tooth a brownish or yellowish color.

Topical fluoridation of the enamel, as a caries-preventive measure, builds up a high concentration of fluoride at the enamel surface. Fluoride solutions are applied so that fluoride ions diffuse into the surface, achieving through substitution of the OH groups a stable, crystalline fluoride compound with the apatites, which protects the enamel against attack from caries. Acidic inorganic fluorides (eg, sodium fluoride, phosphate fluoride) are water-soluble and are washed out within a short time. Organic aminofluorides are not washed out and are better suited to fluoridation of the enamel surface.

During eruption, the ameloblasts are resorbed, transform into squamous epithelium, and lose their ability to divide. They migrate to the gingival sulcus and sustain the enamel-mucosa epithelial attachment during eruption, after which they are shed. Whether the enamel cuticle is made up of transformed ameloblasts cannot be said with certainty. The highly resistant enamel surface is the prism-free layer of enamel. Dentin and enamel are formed layer by layer, as shown clearly by the growth lines (including perikymata).

The **root** develops from what is known as the *Hertwig epithelial root sheath*. This is the area of the cervical loop where the internal and external enamel epithelia cross each other. When enamel growth has reached the future cementoenamel junction, the cervical loop lengthens considerably. Hertwig epithelial root sheath determines the ultimate shape, size, and number of roots. The roots differentiate during eruption; while the crown is raised up from the jaw by the primary fibers of the periodontal ligament, the roots grow down in the same way and mechanically support the eruption of the teeth by exerting growth pressure.

Dentin

The enamel and cementum layer together surround the dentin core, which makes up the principal mass of the tooth. Dentin *(dentinum, substantia eburnea)* forms a layer up to 3 mm thick. This layer encloses a hollow cavity in the tooth, the pulp cavity *(cavum dentis; cavitas dentis; cavum pulpae)*, and the root canal *(cavum radicis dentis)*. The dental pulp *(pulpa dentis)* lies inside this cavity.

The **dentin-forming cells** (odontoblasts) produce dentin, a hard bonelike substance that is different than enamel. Between 70% and 80% of the mineralized part of dentin is made up of inorganic hydroxyapatite crystals of calcium phosphate without prismatic alignment, and 20% to 30% is organic substances (see Figs 3-5 and 3-6). The mineral content is relatively uniform, but the fluoride content gradually increases with age. Dentin has an inherent yellow color, is not as hard as enamel, and is highly elastic and hence deformable. Dentin can also be strongly stained

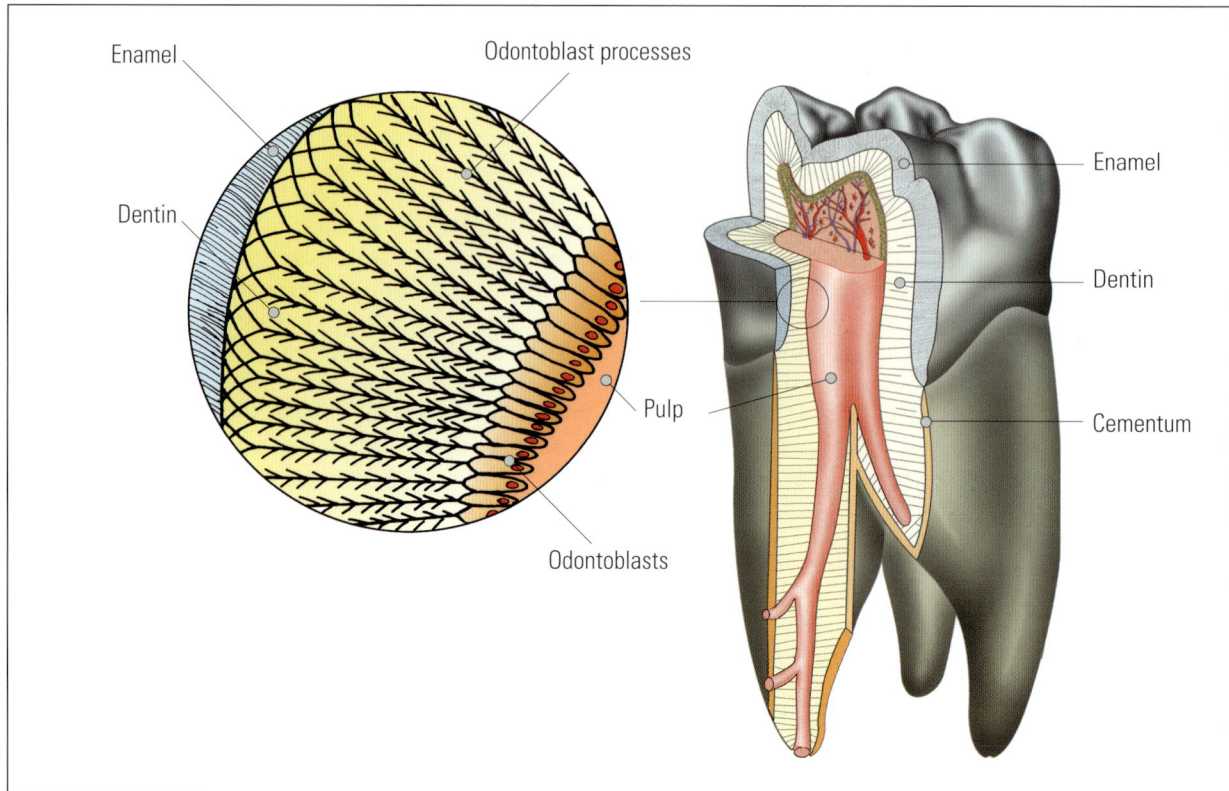

Fig 3-9 The odontoblast processes run from the pulp to the dentinoenamel junction. The dentinal tubules crowd together more densely toward the pulp cavity.

by residues of medicines and by the infiltration of blood pigments.

The ***odontoblast processes*** are the cell processes of odontoblasts, which run from the boundary layer with the pulp cavity through the dentinal tubules to the dentinoenamel junction (Fig 3-9). The odontoblasts probably originate from cells of the neural crest and have the ability to pass on stimuli via their processes. The transmission of stimuli involves the movement of fluid within the processes. The odontoblasts bordering on the pulp are in synaptic contact with nerve fibers. This is why dentin is particularly sensitive to touch, temperature differences, and chemical influences and accounts for painful dentinal sensitivity.

The odontoblast processes can form new dentin throughout the lifetime of a tooth. Dentin is able to keep growing as long as the pulp is healthy. As a result, the originally large pulp cavity becomes increasingly narrow with advancing age due to

dentin growth. In places where the enamel is damaged (eg, by abrasion), new dentin will also form; this is called *secondary dentin*.

Despite this ability to produce new dentin, however, it is rare for an area affected by caries to become fully sealed with secondary dentin. Generally, dentin is not nearly as resistant to caries as enamel. A caries lesion usually results in a small depression in the enamel; this caries then spreads through the enamel to the underlying dentin, where it hollows out the tooth down to the pulp cavity. Once the pulp is affected, this produces the familiar swollen cheek appearance. By this stage, the tooth is very difficult to salvage.

In summary, the ***odontoblast processes*** are responsible for:

• Warning about pain
• The formation of secondary dentin
• Making the dentin permeable to water

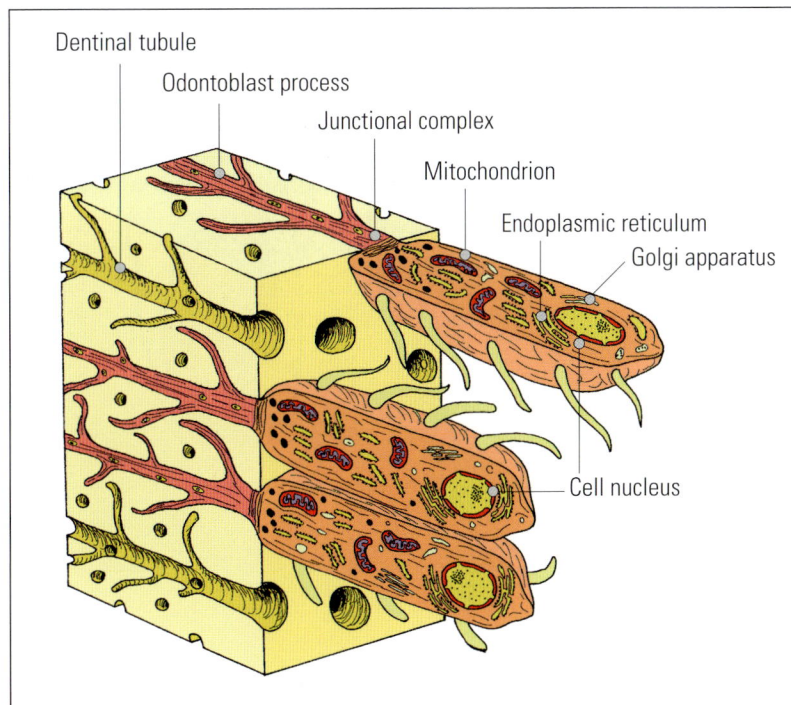

Fig 3-10 Sectional diagram illustrating the spatial relationships of the odontoblasts and their processes to the dentinal tubules. The dentin is tightly covered with the processes of odontoblasts so that the supply of dentin is guaranteed. The odontoblasts retain their function throughout life. Dentin therefore remains vital, elastic, tough, and capable of regeneration to a limited extent.

Dentinal tubule
Odontoblast process
Junctional complex
Mitochondrion
Endoplasmic reticulum
Golgi apparatus
Cell nucleus

The ***dentinal tubules*** with the odontoblast processes run in a wavelike pattern through the dentin and crowd together more closely in the area near the pulp (Fig 3-10). This means the odontoblast processes are densely packed in the dentin close to the pulp; preparing a cavity in this area produces a large wound.

With ***teeth prepared for a crown***, the wound area can be as large as 12 mm²; by comparison, pulp removal only produces a wound measuring 3 mm². On average, up to 40,000 odontoblast processes per square millimeter can be damaged when preparing the base of a normal filling, whereas around 15,000 tubules per square millimeter are opened up in the outer layers of dentin during crown preparation. It is therefore reasonable to call this a "dentin wound."

The continual formation of new dentin is a physiologic aging process by which dentinal tubules can even be fully blocked. However, it does offer a possible means for remedying a caries lesion. This ability of odontoblasts to react to physiologic and pathologic stimuli by forming secondary dentin is a remarkable testimony to the vitality of dentin. This is because odontoblasts still supply dentin even after the mineralization phase, and they can strengthen it by secondary buildup.

Formation of dentin (dentinogenesis)

Dentin is the largest mass in the tooth and is formed and later supplied by the odontoblasts. In the bell stage of tooth germs, the odontoblasts differentiate from the cells of the dental papilla. These cells come from the embryonic connective tissue and the neural crest. The differentiation into odontoblasts can be seen from the increase in cell volume and the cell organelles contained therein. The initially star-shaped (stellate) cells become narrow and columnar, and a thick cytoplasmic process develops, which protrudes from the outer end of the cell. The odontoblasts thus formed lose their ability to divide and become highly specialized secretory cells.

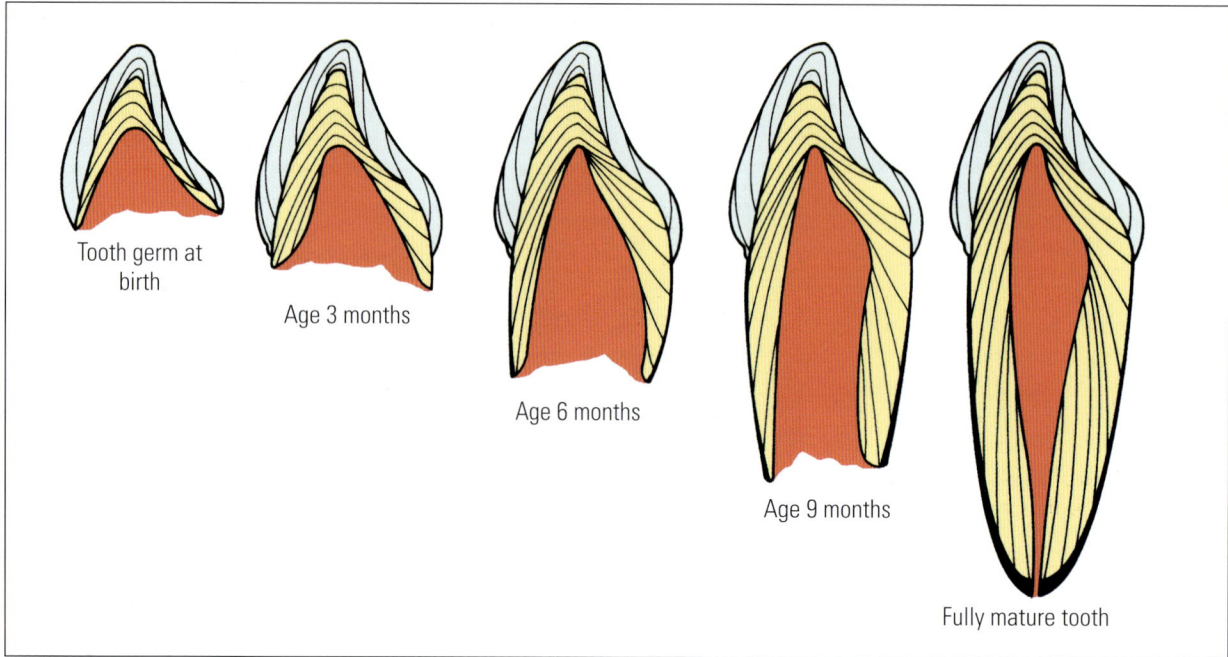

Fig 3-11 The pattern of growth lines in this example of a primary anterior tooth illustrates the growth pattern from the incisal edge to crown formation to root growth. The root does not differentiate until the eruption stage.

Tooth germ at birth

Age 3 months

Age 6 months

Age 9 months

Fully mature tooth

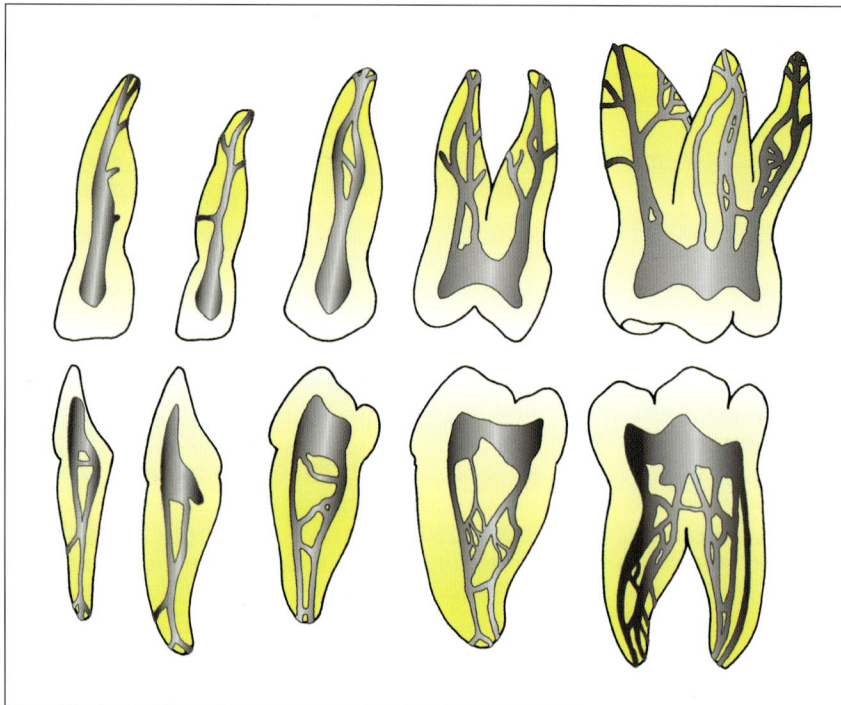

Fig 3-12 During dentin growth, complex root canal formations can develop. In fact, smooth, simple root canals in pulp cavities are rather rare. Shown are a few complex yet typical forms of root canal with several accessory side canals *(from left to right)*: *(top row)* maxillary incisors, canine, premolar, and molar; *(bottom row)* mandibular incisor, canine, premolar, and molars.

The thick **odontoblast process** contains mitochondria, secretory granules, and long microtubules as its typical structural characteristics. It constantly lengthens and gives off short cytoplasmic side branches that can join with each other. Pro-collagen building blocks and mucopolysaccharides are synthesized in the odontoblasts, migrate through the odontoblast process, and are secreted as predentin at the stem of the process. The pro-collagen building blocks polymerize into collagen fibrils, while the mucopolysaccharides form an organic ground substance. Dentin formation therefore goes through an organic precursor phase, namely predentin, followed by mineralization of the dentin.

The **odontoblasts** differentiate at the interface with the internal enamel epithelium, where the dentinoenamel junction later develops. The differentiation of odontoblasts and the formation of predentin start first in the incisal edges and tips of the cusps and gradually move cervically as the dentin layer gets thicker coronally. The first, outer layer of dentin is known as *mantle dentin* and differs from the main mass of dentin in its structure and characteristics. Mantle dentin contains numerous collagen fibers that are distributed with irregular density. This is why mineralization of the mantle layer is not as great as in the rest of the dentin.

The **mass of dentin** between the mantle and the pulp cavity is known as *circumpulpal dentin*. Unlike mantle dentin, the main mass contains no von Korff fibers and has only minimal branching of odontoblast processes. The circumpulpal dentin develops after the mantle dentin as the odontoblasts increasingly withdraw to the dental papilla. Mineralization of the circumpulpal dentin, unlike that of enamel, only starts at some distance from the odontoblasts. It is not until there is a certain thickness (about 20 μm) to the cell layer, due to the secretion of predentin, that the odontoblasts initiate the mineralization process by secreting granules with high levels of phosphates and calcium; ie, the odontoblasts (like the ameloblasts) actively organize the mineralization. Dentin is mineralized layer by layer, with a nonmineralized layer of predentin always being retained between odontoblasts and the mineralization front.

The **formation of dentin** does not take place continuously but periodically in mineralization and resting phases. As the thickness of the dentin layer increases, the pulpal cavity gets narrower, and the border between pulp and dentin becomes smaller (Figs 3-11 and 3-12). The odontoblasts crowd together increasingly closely, but they do not die; they retain their ability to produce new dentin throughout their lives.

However, space for the odontoblast processes and their branches is always left clear during dentin formation so that narrow dentinal tubules develop. The tubule walls are made of far more highly mineralized dentin; this is also produced throughout life, and therefore its thickness also increases. The odontoblast processes and branches become very narrow as well.

The **odontoblasts** lie on the inner surface of the dentin and form the boundary layer with the pulp. The odontoblast processes permeate the dentin as far as the enamel layer, which means that a process can be as long as 5 mm. Cross-linkages are formed with branches from neighboring processes. The quantity of odontoblast processes and branches accounts for 10 times as much mass as the volume of pulp tissue. The volume of the dentinal tubules and branches is 250 mm^3 for the mandibular molars, while the volume of the pulp is only 70 mm^3; in the canines, the ratio of pulp volume to dentinal tubules is 9:90 mm^3.

Cementum

The outer surface of the **tooth root** is covered with mineralized connective tissue, which is known as the **cementum** *(substantia ossea dentis)* and extends from the margin of the dental crown to the apex of the root (Fig 3-13). The cementum is very thin around the neck of the tooth (approximately 0.015 mm) and slightly thicker at the apex of the root (approximately 0.4 mm). Cementum is similar to bone tissue in structure and composition.

The fibers of the tooth attachment apparatus (periodontium) are anchored in the cementum, ensuring that teeth are firmly fixed in the bony alveoli. The cementum overlies the dentin; it can extend into the root canal and even cover parts of the enamel. It is similar to bone tissue but is not permeated with blood vessels. Cementum develops during the formation of the tooth root before and during eruption. It continues to form throughout life, provided there is still a functioning peri-

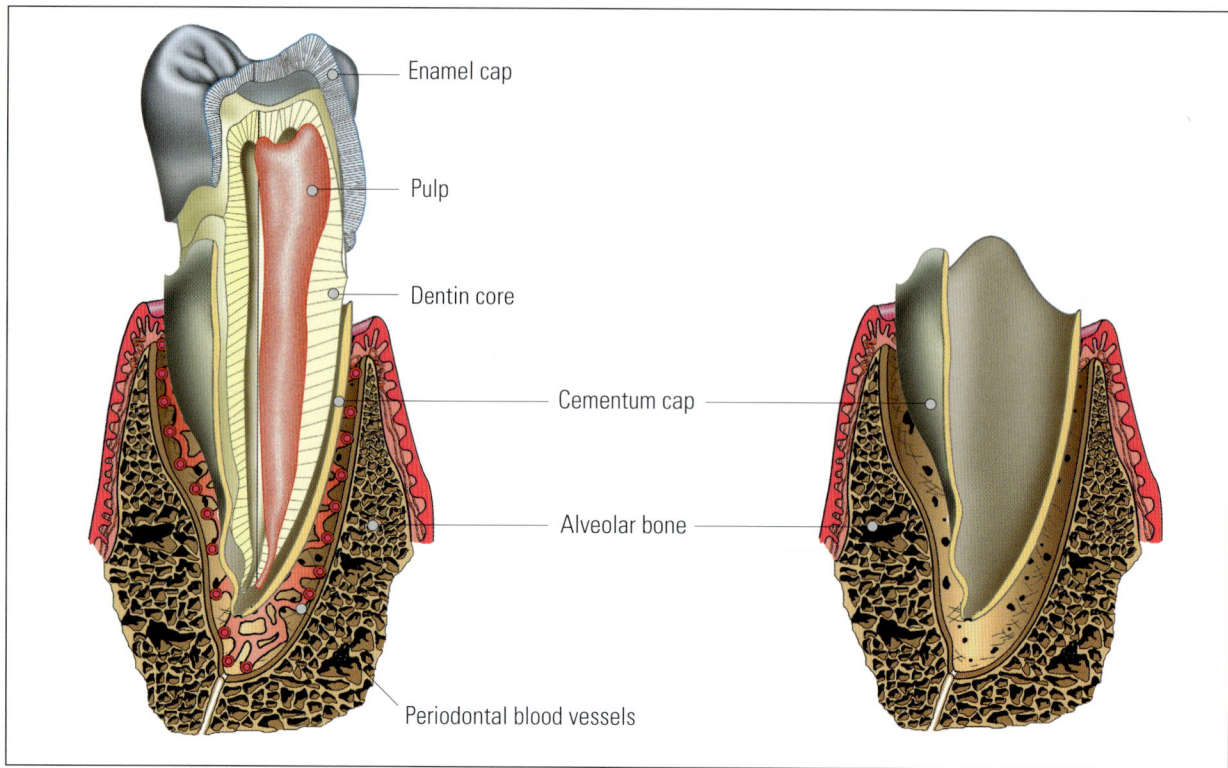

Fig 3-13 Teaching model showing the cementum in relation to the hard tooth substances and surrounding tissues.

Enamel cap

Pulp

Dentin core

Cementum cap

Alveolar bone

Periodontal blood vessels

odontal ligament (desmodontium). It forms a single functional unit with the periodontal ligament and the alveolar bone.

The *cementoblasts* are the cementum-forming cells, which originate from the cells of the dental follicle before eruption; after eruption, cementoblasts can be activated from connective tissue cells. They resemble odontoblasts; they can have several cytoplasmic processes and synthesize a tightly meshed ground substance and collagen fibrils. This then gives rise to cementum, which can be divided into three different types (Fig 3-14):

1. *Acellular-afibrillar cementum*: without any cementoblasts or collagen fibers; overlies the enamel; covers parts of the dental crown
2. *Acellular-fibrillar cementum*: without cementoblasts but with collagen fibers; directly overlies the dentin; is spread over the entire root
3. *Cellular-fibrillar cementum*: with cementoblasts and collagen fibrils; often only deposited over the apex of the root

Cell-poor cementum has a fibrous structure perpendicular to the dentin surface, which is produced by the Sharpey fibers running in the cementum. These fibers exit the cementum in a straight line.

The *organic component* of cementum is collagen, which accounts for about 30% of the whole mass by volume. The cementum mineral accounts for only one-third of the cementum volume and is made up of hydroxyapatites of calcium phosphate. Fluoride is regularly found as a trace element. Water content exceeds one-third of total volume. Cementum is slightly yellowish in color and softer than dentin but as hard as bone. It is permeable, and liquid mainly enters along the Sharpey fibers.

Cementum is counted as part of the tooth because it directly overlies the dentin. However, because it can embed new fibrous parts of the periodontal ligament throughout life, it can also be classified functionally and morphologically as part of the attachment apparatus. The bundles

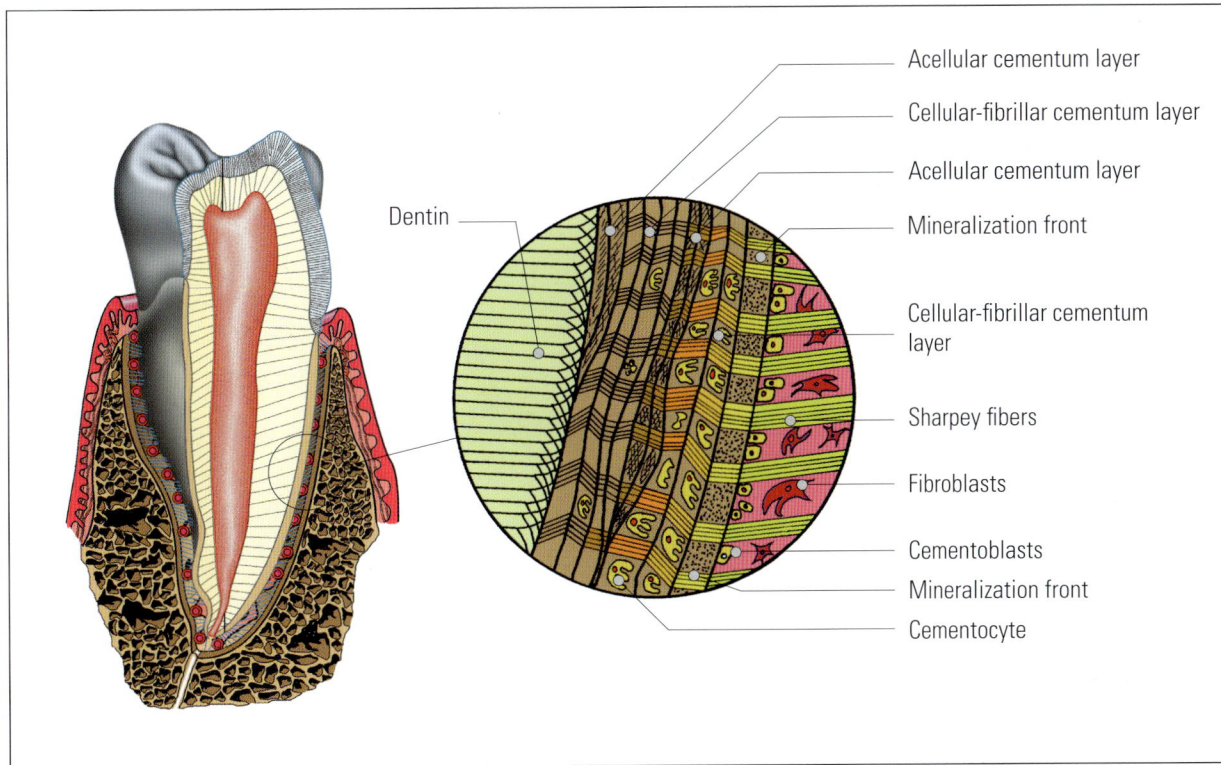

Fig 3-14 Schematic diagram of the structural elements of cementum showing the apposition lines of different cementum layers.

Labels in figure:
- Acellular cementum layer
- Cellular-fibrillar cementum layer
- Acellular cementum layer
- Mineralization front
- Cellular-fibrillar cementum layer
- Sharpey fibers
- Fibroblasts
- Cementoblasts
- Mineralization front
- Cementocyte
- Dentin

of collagen fibers are joined both in the alveolar bone and in the cementum.

The **function of the cementum** is not merely to fix the Sharpey fibers; it can also absorb and displace fibers as a reaction to changing functional demands. For instance, in response to physiologic tooth movements or orthodontic procedures, the cementum can enlarge the periodontal gap by means of resorption or narrow the gap by increasing in size.

If the tooth root tears or breaks as a result of impact, the cementoblasts in conjunction with the odontoblasts are able to heal the wound by producing new hard dental tissue. In doing so, the cementoblasts take on a function similar to that of the osteoblasts of the periosteum in bone fractures by closing the fracture site with bone-type hard substance.

Despite their hardness, the **hard substances** of teeth display a certain elasticity, which means they will deform to a small extent. Hence a tooth can bend without snapping off in response to strong mechanical loading. This remarkable property is displayed particularly by dentin. This is worth noting because such deformability of the dentin core produces a kind of buffer effect when two teeth are linked by a rigid partial denture framework, for example.

Dental Pulp

The **dental pulp** *(pulpa dentis)* lies in the pulp cavity and in the dentinal root canals inside the tooth. This cavity is very large in young people but later becomes progressively narrower as dentin production continues. The pulp is made up of jelly-type connective tissue that contains blood vessels, lymph, and nerve endings. The pulp is generally referred to as the "nerve" of the tooth.

The **pulp cavity** is the chamber that is filled with pulp (Fig 3-15). It is subdivided into the coronal cavity and root canals. The pulp cavity of the

Enamel

Dentin

Capillary plexus of
arterial vessels

Capillary plexus of
venous vessels

Odontoblasts

Coronal pulp

Root pulp

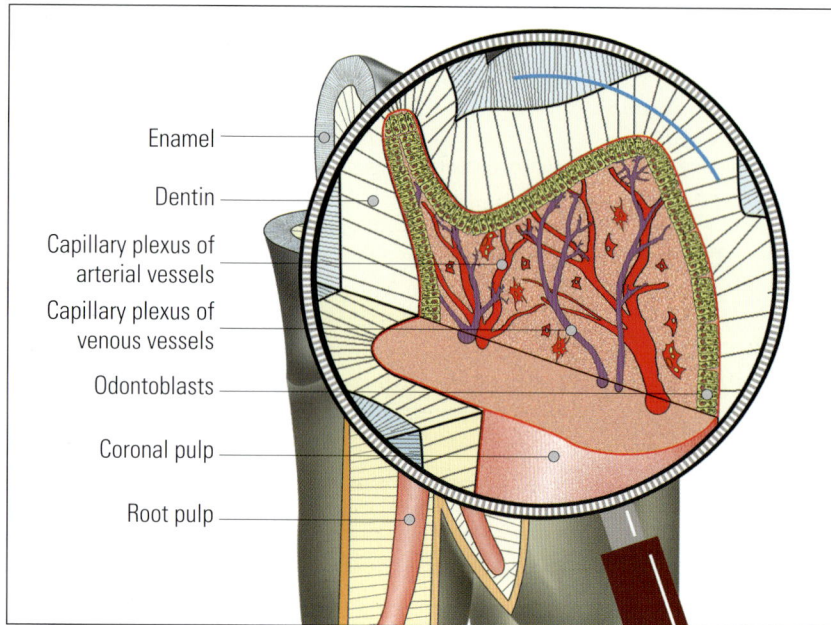

Fig 3-15 The pulp completely fills the pulp cavity. It is made up of differentiated structural elements that perform a diversity of functions.

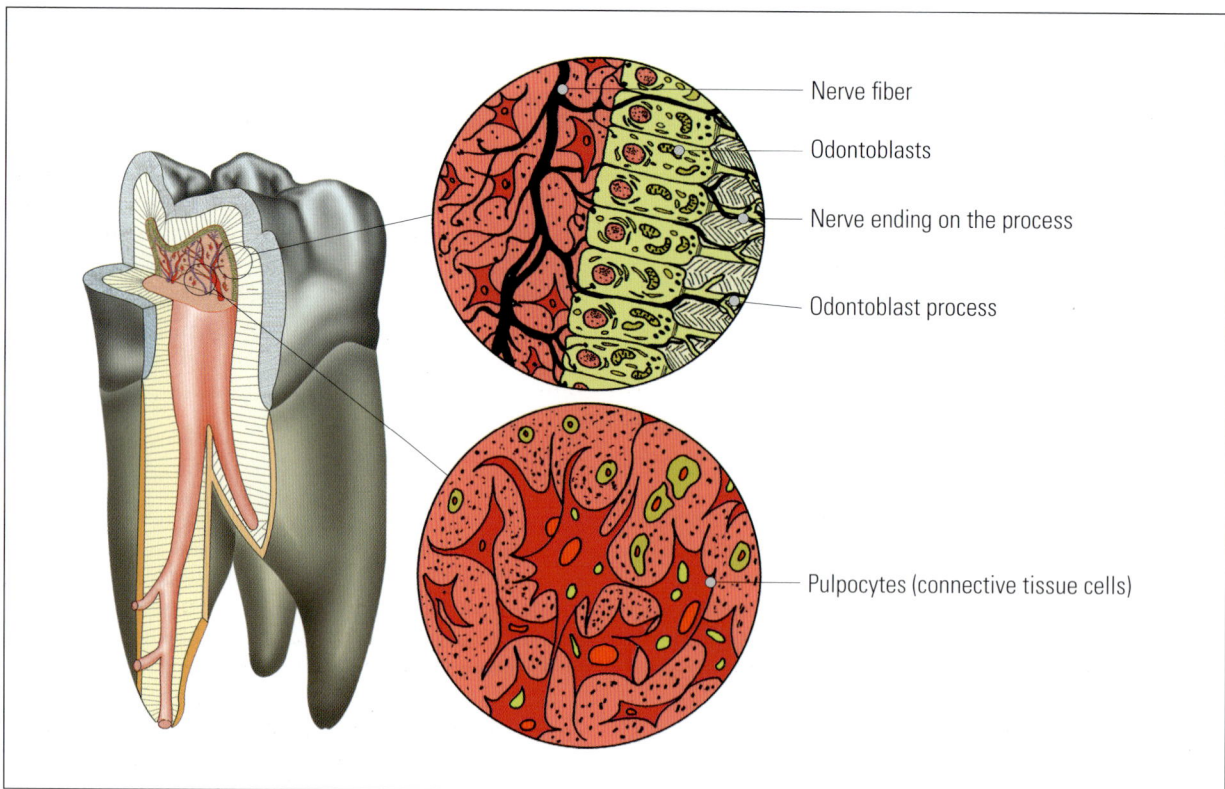

Nerve fiber

Odontoblasts

Nerve ending on the process

Odontoblast process

Pulpocytes (connective tissue cells)

Fig 3-16 Histologic elements of pulp.

crown follows the shape of the tooth in such a way that the pulpal horns lie under the incisal edges and tips of the cusps. The root canals generally end in an apical foramen, but they often have several canals and holes in the apical area and open into the periodontal gap. The pulp cavity and root canals become increasingly narrow as dentin synthesis progresses; the pulp gets progressively smaller, and some root canals may even grow to the point of closure.

The *pulp* is surrounded by a layer of odontoblasts whose processes extend into the dentin and pulp (Fig 3-16). The pulp is packed with blood and lymph vessels that enter through the apical foramina and form a dense network of vessels. Looped branches extend into the odontoblast layer. Nerve fibers also enter the pulp cavities with these vessels through the foramina. The nerve fibers pass into the coronal pulp almost without branching, where they fan out broadly. They are mostly involved in efferent nerve conduction to register pain. Terminal branches reach the odontoblasts and from there enter the dentinal tubules. Impulses that reach the odontoblast processes are thus transmitted to the free nerve endings.

Pulp tissue comprises 25% organic constituents and 75% water and performs its functions under high tissue pressure. It is a loose connective tissue that is packed with fibrils, nerves, and vessels. It develops from the dental papilla. During the formation of dentin, blood vessels from the alveolar arteries grow into the papilla, and the papilla cells are transformed into pulp tissue. The cells are distinguished on the basis of their form and function: the odontoblast layer, fibroblasts, replacement cells, and defensive cells.

The main cell mass is made up of fibroblasts, while the peripheral boundary is occupied by odontoblasts. In addition, there are free-moving cells—lymphocytes, monocytes, and histiocytes—that act as defensive cells of normal connective tissue. The fibers and fibrils of the pulp tissue are connected in orderly states to the fibers of the periodontal ligament (desmodontium) at the apical root pulp.

The *functions of pulp* are to:

- Nourish the odontoblasts
- Replace destroyed odontoblasts
- Be indirectly involved in dentin formation

- Give warning of pain in response to mechanical, thermal, and chemical irritation
- Act as a defensive function via phagocyte systems

Pulp functions are performed better by young pulp tissue than by aging tissue. Functional capacity declines as the pulp cavity narrows, the vessel density decreases, and collagen fibers are embedded. Mineral deposits (pulp stones or denticles) and calcifications, chronic disease processes (eg, caries, infections), as well as careless, damaging dental procedures further limit this functional capacity.

The pulp can sustain reversible or even irreversible damage during preparation of crown stumps or cavities. Pulp irritation can arise, depending on the abrasive pressure applied, heat generated by grinding, or the use of chemical cleaning and filling materials. The best-case scenario is merely short-term, reversible damage to the odontoblast function, combined with inflammatory processes in the pulp that act as a stimulus to the synthesis of secondary dentin. This is exploited for therapeutic purposes to subsequently reach greater preparation depths (eg, for ceramic or composite resin crowns for young teeth).

Temperature increases due to abrasion heat of more than 8°C above 37°C will produce irreversible cell and tissue damage as a result of precipitation of protein. If impression material is too hot, there may be temperature peaks of 53°C in the pulp, which are enough to kill off the odontoblast layer, cause chronic inflammation, and devitalize the tooth. An added problem is that the tooth may remain symptom-free for months or even years after this kind of damage.

Periodontium

The tooth is anchored in the jawbone by a complicated attachment mechanism. Previously it was assumed that the teeth were fused into the bone of the jaw. More detailed analysis of tissue sections, however, revealed a narrow gap between bone and cementum—the periodontal space—in which the tooth is joined to the jawbone by a fibrous apparatus. In descriptive anatomy, this attachment mechanism is called *syndesmosis*.

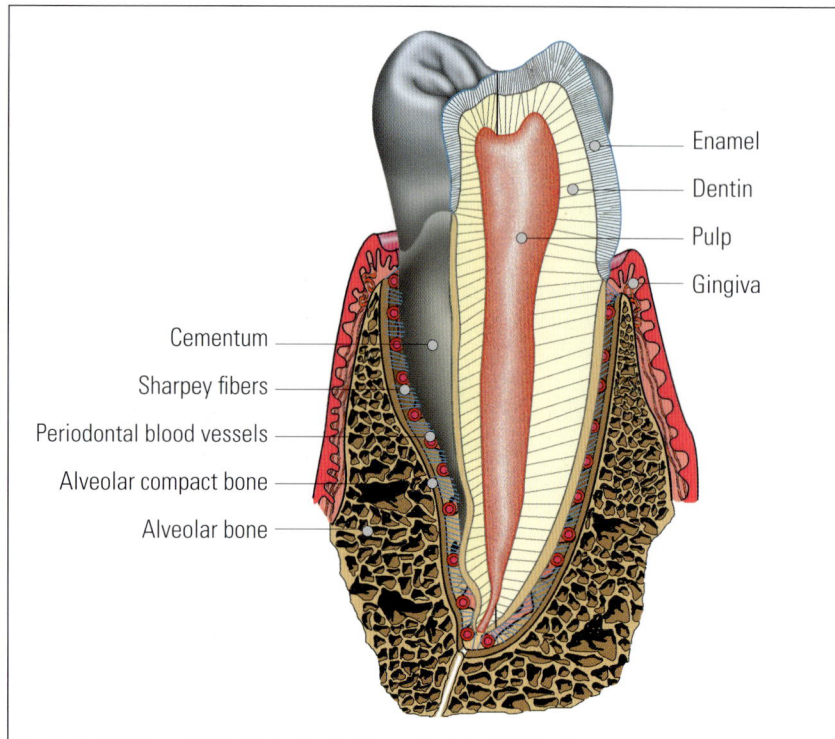

Fig 3-17 Structural elements of the periodontium.

Enamel

Dentin

Pulp

Gingiva

Cementum

Sharpey fibers

Periodontal blood vessels

Alveolar compact bone

Alveolar bone

Syndesmosis means *band attachment*, in which the two bony parts are joined together by ligaments. On closer inspection, some movement of the tooth in its bony anchorage can be detected, so that it could be described as an articulated joint in the sense of a synarthrosis (*arthron* = joint). **Synarthroses** denote articulations uniting bones with extremely limited movement (eg, dentoalveolar articulation).

The **periodontium** comprises all the tissues that anchor the tooth in the bone; ie, it is tooth-supporting tissue (*peri* = around, *odous* = tooth; *paradontal* = near or close to the tooth). This is a functional unit of various supporting tissues. These tissues are seen as a functional unit firstly because they form a single unit once they have developed. Secondly, they belong together in terms of clinical pathology. Thirdly, they form a compact system for the particular task (function) of anchoring the tooth in the jawbone. The bony parts in which the teeth are invested are functionally oriented tissue structures that mature in line with tooth eruption and later can be completely resorbed after tooth loss.

The periodontium includes (Fig 3-17):

• Cementum
• Alveolar bone *(os alveolare)*
• Periodontal ligament (desmodontium)

The **periodontal space** is a gap about 0.1 to 0.2 mm wide (when healthy) between the cementum and the alveolar bone, which is seen as a thin line on radiographs. This is where the periodontal ligament is located. It is mainly made up of connective tissue fibers that join together to form separate bundles of fibers. These are known as *Sharpey fibers*. The periodontal ligament also contains blood vessels and nerves.

Sharpey fibers are fused in the cementum and in the alveolar compact bone tissue, the counterpart of the cementum. The bundles of fibers do not run horizontally from the alveolar bone to the tooth but obliquely down to the root, ie, in an apical direction. A few bundles of fibers also run crosswise from the alveolar bone slightly around the tooth to the root and secure the tooth against twisting. During chewing, the tooth can-

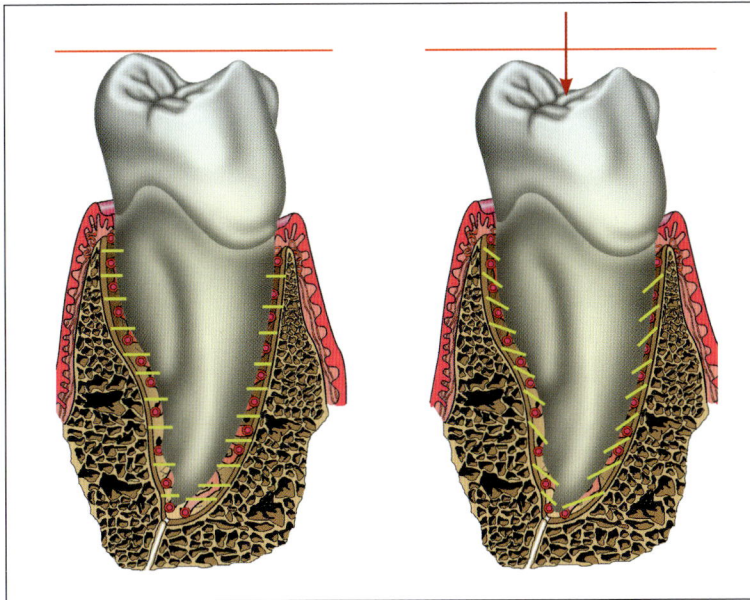

Fig 3-18 The tooth is suspended in the socket by ligaments, which transfer the masticatory pressure loading (arrow) as physiologic tensile stress to the hard tissues (cementum and alveolar compact bone).

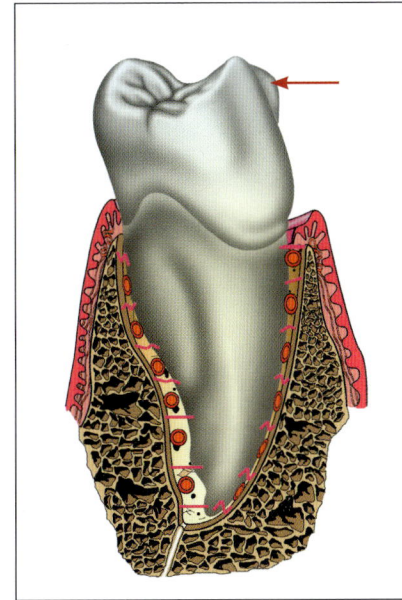

Fig 3-19 Transverse forces (arrow) tip the tooth in the socket and produce one-sided compressive strain and pull in the marginal and apical periodontium.

not be compressed very far into the bone because Sharpey fibers are not elastic.

Masticatory loading presses the tooth into the tooth socket (Fig 3-18). Because Sharpey fibers run apically from the alveolar bone in the direction in which the tooth is being pushed, the fibers are immediately placed under tension. They are not elastic and therefore transfer the tensile stress to their anchorage points in the alveolar bone and cementum. They pull on the hard tissues; ie, the hard tissues are placed under tension during masticatory loading. The ligament apparatus transforms compressive forces into tensile forces. This is an advantage because it is a property of bone tissue to atrophy in response to compressive stress; in response to tensile stress, however, it grows or is strengthened in the direction of pull. The same mechanism applies when the tooth is twisted: the crosswise looped fibers then pull on the hard tissues.

The tooth can also be lifted out of the alveolus to a certain extent; this lifting out is limited by fibers at the apex of the root, which run from the alveolar bone up to the root. The tooth is least secured against tipping movements. A few bundles of fibers do run horizontally and can thereby cushion this movement (Fig 3-19). However, tipping movements can put a strain on the periodontium and damage it because they cause uneven loading. Movements of this kind always occur in connection with masticatory pressure loading where the pivot of the tipping is in the bottom third of the whole tooth. The periodontal ligament is thrust or pulled on one side apically as well as marginally. The physiologic tensile stress has to be cushioned by relatively small areas of the periodontal ligament, which can lead to overloading, while other small surfaces are nonphysiologically compressed. At the same time, a vertical masticatory force has to be absorbed.

Alveolar bone

The bony makeup of the alveolar process (os alveolare) has a typical bone structure (Fig 3-20):

• An extremely dense outer bone plate that is covered with periosteum

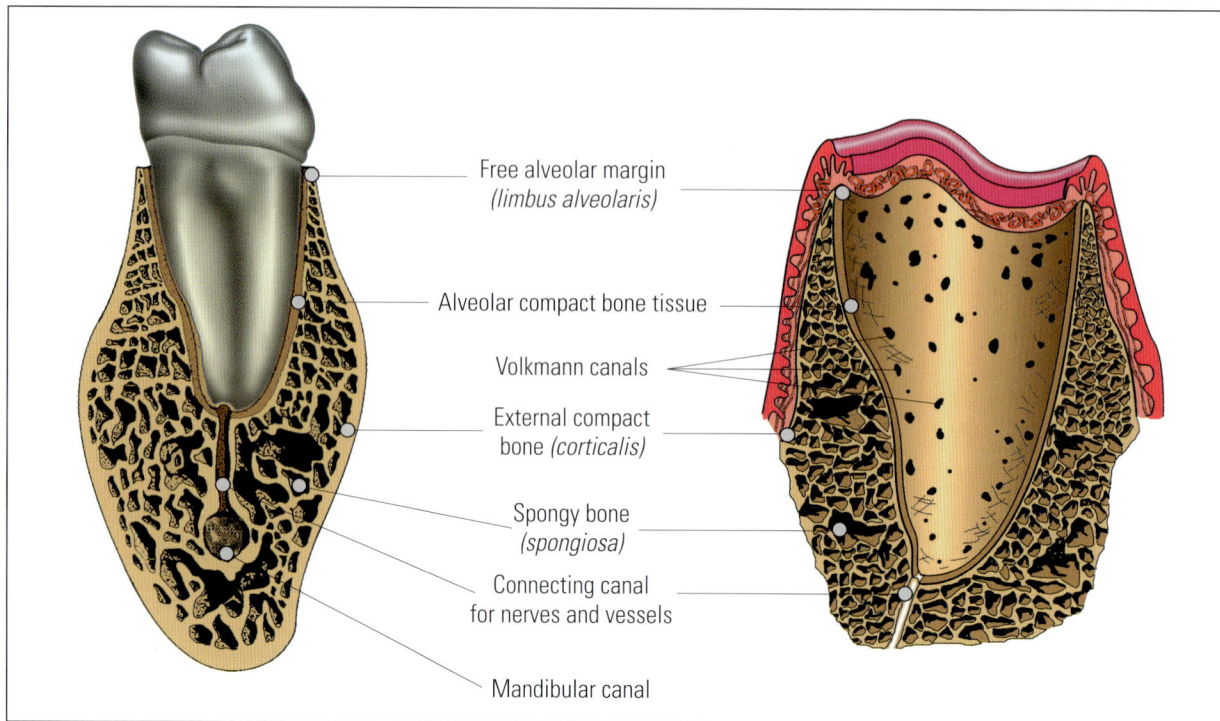

Fig 3-20 Schematic diagram of alveolar bone in the posterior region of the mandible showing the differentiated bone structure and the alveolar shape.

- An inner bony layer lining the tooth sockets that is greatly perforated
- Spongy bone, which lies between the compact layers

Where the compact layers of the outer surface and the tooth sockets merge marks the bony alveolar crest. The outer layer of the alveolar bone is the typical cortical substance (*substantia corticalis*).

The *spongy (cancellous) bone* is composed of thin trabeculae, between which the bone marrow is stored. The bone plate of the jaw contains mainly red, blood-forming bone marrow. The spongy trabeculae illustrate the striking functional orientation corresponding to tension and pressure lines initiated by loading from teeth and muscles. The spongy trabeculae can adapt to altered stresses.

The *internal alveolar wall* to the tooth sockets is a firm, highly perforated cortical layer; it is known as the *cribriform lamina* (or *cribriform plate*). It is particularly perforated in the cervical and apical region. These openings correspond to the Volkmann canals and link the cementum to the bone marrow cavities through which blood and lymph vessels pass. The embedded bundles of Sharpey fibers can be seen in the cortical layer of the tooth socket in the same way as in the cementum.

The *composition* of alveolar bone is the same as that of other bones:

- 45% (by weight) inorganic hydroxyapatite of calcium phosphate
- 30% organic matrix of collagen fibers
- 25% water

The shape and position of the alveolar bone is determined to a great extent by the teeth and their function (Fig 3-21). For instance, all permanent incisors and maxillary canines, premolars, and molars are inclined in a vestibular direction; the mandibular canine stands rather vertically, while the mandibular posterior teeth show a lingual tendency. The bony layer on the roots is noticeably thin in the external (vestibular) alveolar re-

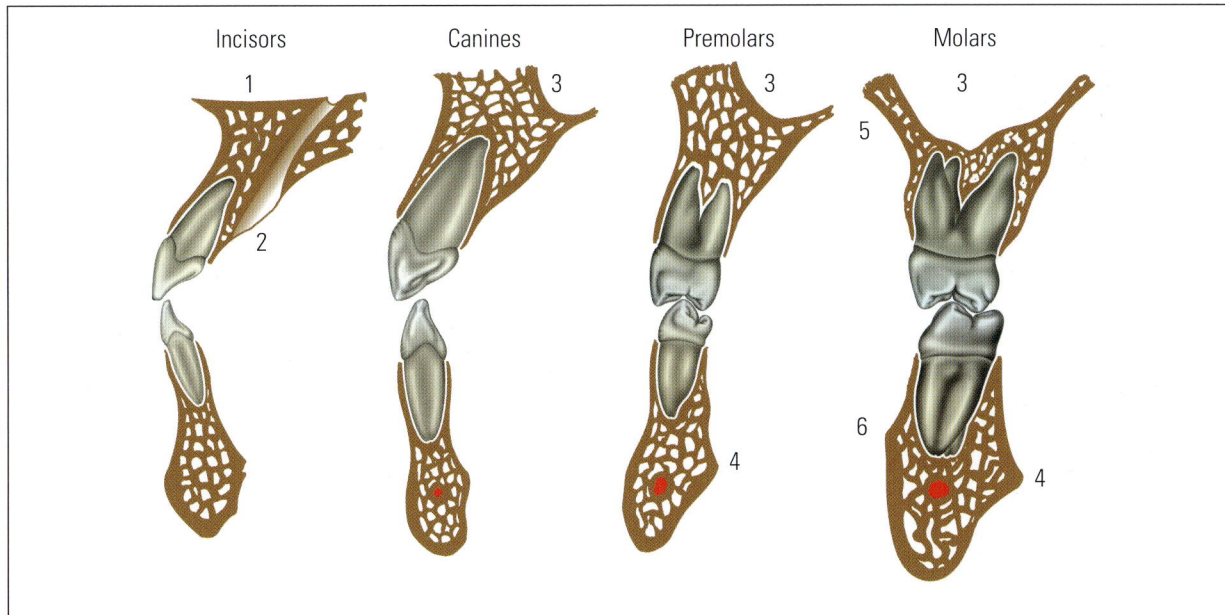

Fig 3-21 The position of the teeth in the alveolar bone and the distribution of the bone tissue in the area of the vestibular and lingual alveolar crest. 1, nasal cavity; 2, incisal canal; 3, maxillary sinus; 4, mylohyoid line; 5, subzygomatic crest; 6, oblique line.

gion of the maxilla, so that the external compact bone and inner cribriform lamina fuse together.

Following **tooth loss**, the bone lamellae of the sockets are resorbed, and the thin, vestibular bone parts are seen to shrink more than the lingual areas. The alveolar crests appear to be shrinking in a direction of incline, which leads to narrowing of the maxillary ridge and widening of the mandibular ridge crest line.

Bone formation of the maxilla and mandible starts in week seven of fetal life from connective tissue cells. The tooth buds are visible at this stage. When the hard tissue is formed from the bell, thin bone lamellae develop and separate the individual tooth germs. These form the separating walls between the alveoli (alveolar septa), which at birth give rise to ten primitive tooth sockets in each jaw for the primary teeth. The permanent first molars are already noticeable in individual tooth sockets.

The **tooth germs** are surrounded by the dental follicles, which are later transformed into the periodontal ligament. During root formation and eruption of the teeth, however, the germs also in-

duce growth of the alveolar processes. At the time of birth, the alveolar bones have grown beyond the occlusal level of the tooth germs. Then, during eruption, they grow in line with lengthening of the roots. At the same time, the fiber systems and the cementum for the periodontium develop.

Alveolar processes and alveolar bone develop as jaw components, dependent on tooth eruption, root growth, and differentiation of the periodontal ligament, and are therefore separate from the growth of the other parts of the jaw. During exfoliation and as the permanent dentition emerges, there are similar growth dependencies leading to a complete change of alveolar parts and alveolar arches to make them suited to the permanent dentition.

Periodontal ligament

The terms *dental periosteum* or *desmodontium* can also be applied to the periodontal ligament (or membrane). This is a firm, fiber-rich connective tissue between the surface of the tooth root and the inside walls of the alveoli with which the

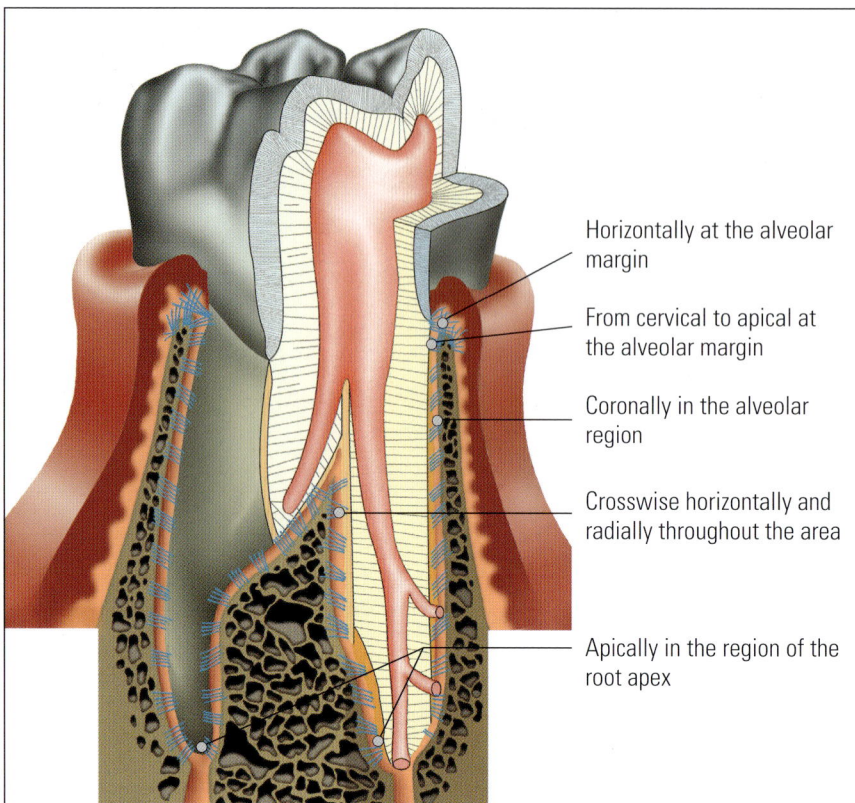

Fig 3-22 Diagram of the paths of fibers in the periodontal cavity, in each case running from the cementum.

Horizontally at the alveolar margin

From cervical to apical at the alveolar margin

Coronally in the alveolar region

Crosswise horizontally and radially throughout the area

Apically in the region of the root apex

tooth is joined to the alveolar bone. The periodontal space is where the tissue structures of the periodontal ligament are found. Its volume varies from single-rooted teeth (30 to 100 mm³) to multi-rooted teeth (65 to 150 mm³) and corresponds to the volume of the particular cementum.

The *tissue elements* of the periodontal ligament are connective tissue fibers, cells, blood vessels, and nerves. The cells undertake a diversity of physiologic processes and are involved in the resorption and remodeling of the cementum and alveolar bone. These cells are cementoblasts, osteoblasts, osteoclasts, and fibroblasts, as well as epithelial cells and leukocytes.

Connective tissue fibers made of collagen form a fiber apparatus that is joined together in bundles and stretched out between the cementum and the alveolar bone. The individual fibers in their mature state are far shorter than the width of the periodontal space so that the bundles of fibers consist of short interwoven fibers. The bun-

dles within the periodontal space can be distinguished by their different functional orientations. If all the fibers are regarded as running from the cementum to the alveolar bone, these cemento-alveolar fibers can be divided into those running (Fig 3-22):

• From cervical to apical at the alveolar margin
• Horizontally at the alveolar margin
• Coronally in the alveolar region
• Apically in the region of the root apex
• Crosswise in a horizontal-radial direction throughout the area

The last of these fiber bundles cross each other and provide anchorage to the root to protect the teeth against twisting (Fig 3-23). The bundles are not stretched in a straight line but follow an undulating path, which means tooth movement is possible because of the difference in length between their coiled and taut states.

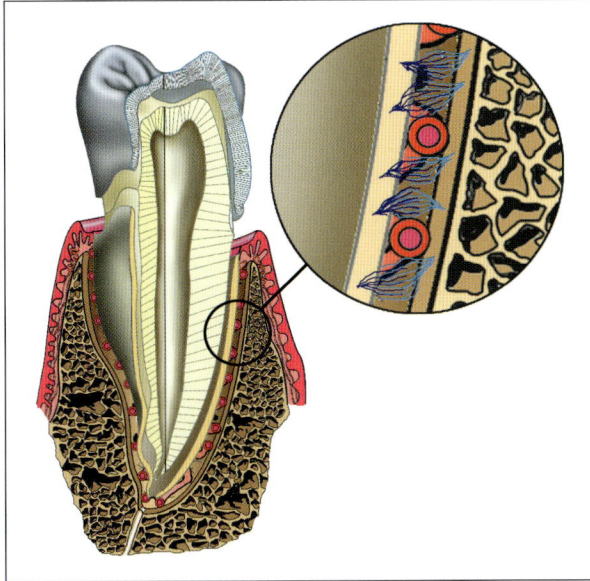

Fig 3-23 The Sharpey fibers of the periodontal space grow as bundles from the cementum and the alveolar bone, bridge the width of the space, and interlock with each other. Forces are transferred via the frictional forces of the interlocked fibers.

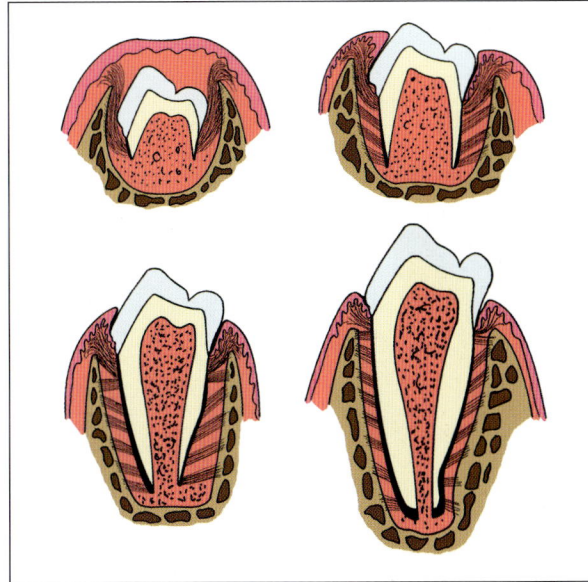

Fig 3-24 The fiber bundles of the periodontal ligament originate during root formation and provide the actual force for tooth eruption. After eruption, the fibers are oriented in their ultimate functional path.

The fibers make up about 75% of the *volume*, the remainder being reserved for vessels, nerves, and free cells. The cementum surface area onto which the fibers can attach is an average of 270 mm^2 for single-rooted anterior teeth and between 400 and 450 mm^2 for multirooted molars. Roughly 28,000 collagen fiber bundles can attach to 1 mm^2 of this root surface. However, because the area of the alveolar compact tissue is about 10% smaller than the corresponding root surface because of the many perforations, the maximum area available for anchorage is 140 to 225 mm^2 for anterior teeth, 170 to 200 mm^2 for premolars, and 300 to 400 mm^2 for molars.

The *functional loading* on the tooth determines the density and thickness of the fiber bundles, just as the width of the periodontal space varies depending on the form of loading. Thus, the space is narrower in the middle of the root and widened cervically and apically; ie, it can take on an hourglass shape.

The *fiber systems of the periodontal ligament* adapt to changing functional demands (Fig 3-24). Active fibroblasts ensure the breakdown of old collagen and the formation of new fibers. The collagen regeneration rate is very high but decreases with age. The formation of new fiber is stimulated by loading caused by masticatory function or by tooth movements controlled for orthodontic purposes. If there is a lack of mechanical stimuli, atrophy of the fiber system ensues, the bundles decrease in density, and the periodontal space can become narrower. This also reduces the functional capacity of the periodontal ligament.

The cells of the periodontal ligament, like those of the cementum and the cribriform lamina, originate from the dental follicle. Before eruption, the dental follicle is mostly transformed into the periodontal ligament as the active fibroblasts of this cell structure start to synthesize collagen fiber bundles. These fibers are embedded in the developing cementum and in the alveolar bone. The fibers run along the cementum, lying parallel to the tooth axis in a coronal direction, with the fibers embedded in the cementum developing first. After that, fiber bundles running in an apical direction and interwoven to form a lattice are also laid down in the alveolar bone (Fig 3-25).

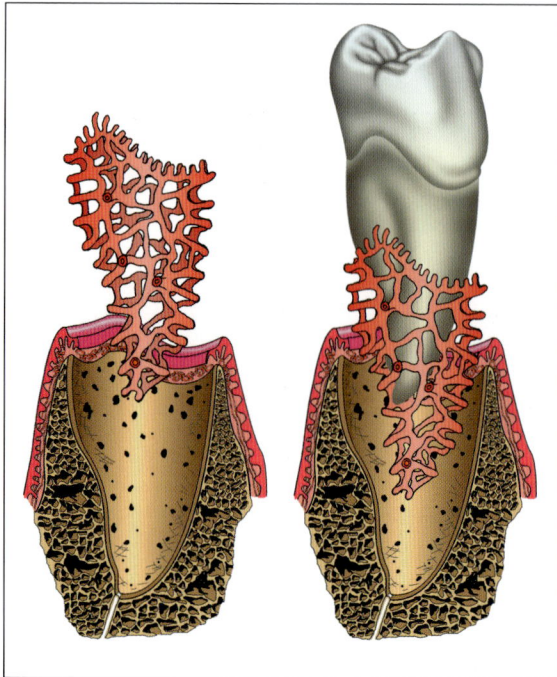

Fig 3-25 The blood vessels form a basket of vessels of varying mesh size, which is narrowed in the marginal region to form the gingival plexus of venules. Here the capillaries are fully grown into convoluted loops of vessels as a reservoir for congested blood.

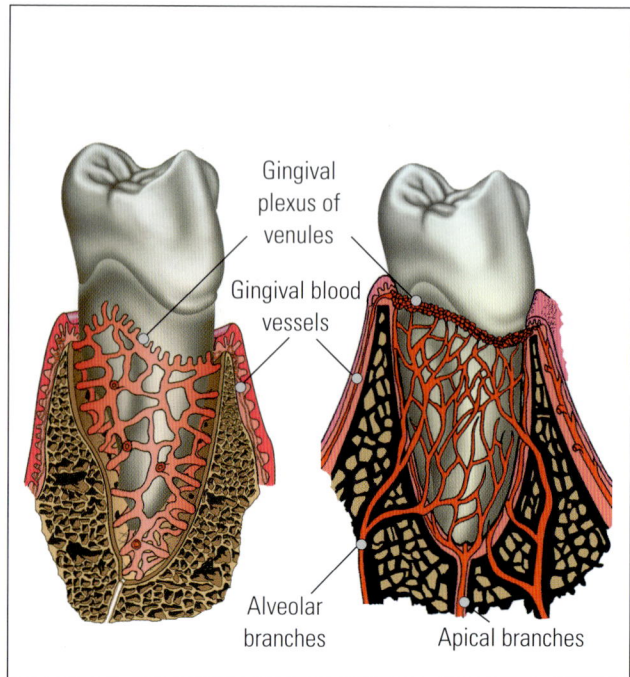

Fig 3-26 The blood supply to the periodontium is fed from three sources: *(1)* branches entering the periodontal ligament apically, *(2)* branches entering within the alveolar spongy bone, and *(3)* branches that feed from the gingiva into the vascular plexus.

The **blood supply** to the periodontal tissue is provided by a dense, basketlike network of vessels that is fed from three main sources (Fig 3-26):

1. Apical inflow from the bloodstream to the pulp
2. Alveolar inflow via the Volkmann canals of the cribriform lamina
3. Cervical inflow via the vestibular and lingual mucosa

The **vessels** are thicker at the root apex than in the marginal area and enter in several places at the root apex and in the alveolar segment. In the marginal area, the vessels are arranged as one-way passages, which causes vascular congestion to build up there. The tightly interwoven vessels of the periodontal space do not have any clear-cut venous outlets, but they follow the arteries. This supports the assumption that there is a pendular blood supply here that is stimulated via a shift in the volume of the vascular network caused by

tooth movement. The tooth is raised out of the alveolus by blood pressure as the blood vessels become engorged with blood. During chewing, the tooth is pressed into the alveolus, and thus the blood is forced out of the vessels. This results in an exchange of blood; ie, the blood supply is set in motion by loading on the tooth.

Lymph is drained via lymph capillaries through the gingival tissue. Otherwise, the system of lymph vessels follows the same kind of basketlike distribution in the periodontal ligament as the system of blood vessels does.

Depending on the state of the blood vessels, the tooth can be found in three different apicocoronal positions in the alveolus (Fig 3-27):

• In the middle position when standing or sitting up
• Coronal when lying down
• Apical when chewing

Fig 3-27 Depending on the state of the blood vessels, the tooth can lie in three different positions in the alveolus.

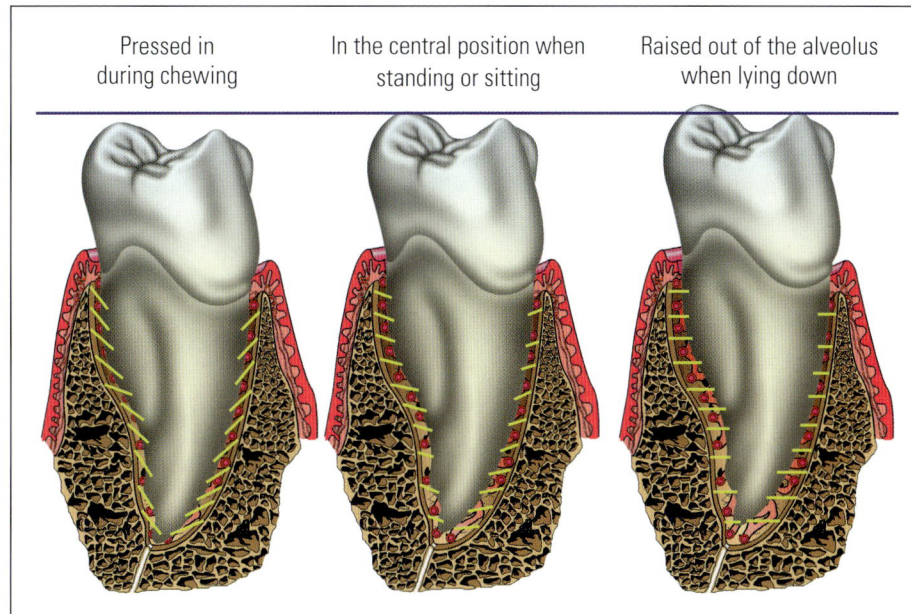

| Pressed in during chewing | In the central position when standing or sitting | Raised out of the alveolus when lying down |

The **nerve supply** in the periodontal ligament is very extensive. This makes the tooth a sensitive, tactile apparatus because it is able to pick up and cushion changes of position and loading and thereby regulate the reflex mechanism with the masticatory musculature.

Two types of nerve fibers run in the periodontal space, namely sensory fibers and fibers of the autonomic nervous system. As branches of the dental nerve, the fibers enter the periodontal ligament apically. The fibers from alveolar entry points also link up with the dense network of nerve fibers. The nerve fibers are either open-ended with tuberous swellings or end in spiral- and ring-shaped receptors. Via the trigeminal nerve, there is a reflex path to the motor end plates of the masticatory muscles as well as to the muscles of the cheeks, lips, and tongue in order to regulate abnormal compressive stresses.

Nerve impulses are picked up in response to pain and pressure. The perception of pressure is so sensitive that the tactile quality can even exceed that of the fingertips. Via a pain message, the nerves indicate when the tooth or the periodontium is being overloaded or when the threshold of mobility is reached. It is clear from this that the periodontal ligament plays a key role in the functioning of the teeth; a tooth with destroyed pulp is more likely to be preserved than a tooth with a defective periodontium. Thus, post crowns, where the pulp has been removed and a post has been placed in the exposed pulp cavity of the root, are a popular option in dental restoration. However, if the periodontal ligament is removed, the link between tooth and alveolar bone ossifies, and the tooth is no longer as capable of bearing stress. This is what happens when a tooth is extracted for root treatment and, after treatment is completed, reimplanted in the cleansed socket. This clinical treatment option is only adopted in very particular circumstances.

Functions of the periodontium include the following:

- A buffer effect is achieved by the fiber apparatus and by the network of blood vessels.
- The fiber apparatus transforms masticatory compressive forces into tensile forces because tensile stress is the natural, physiologic stress borne by the hard tissue.
- The arrangement of the fibers in the periodontal space allows minimal tooth mobility, while the nerve supply registers the loading threshold by means of a pain warning.

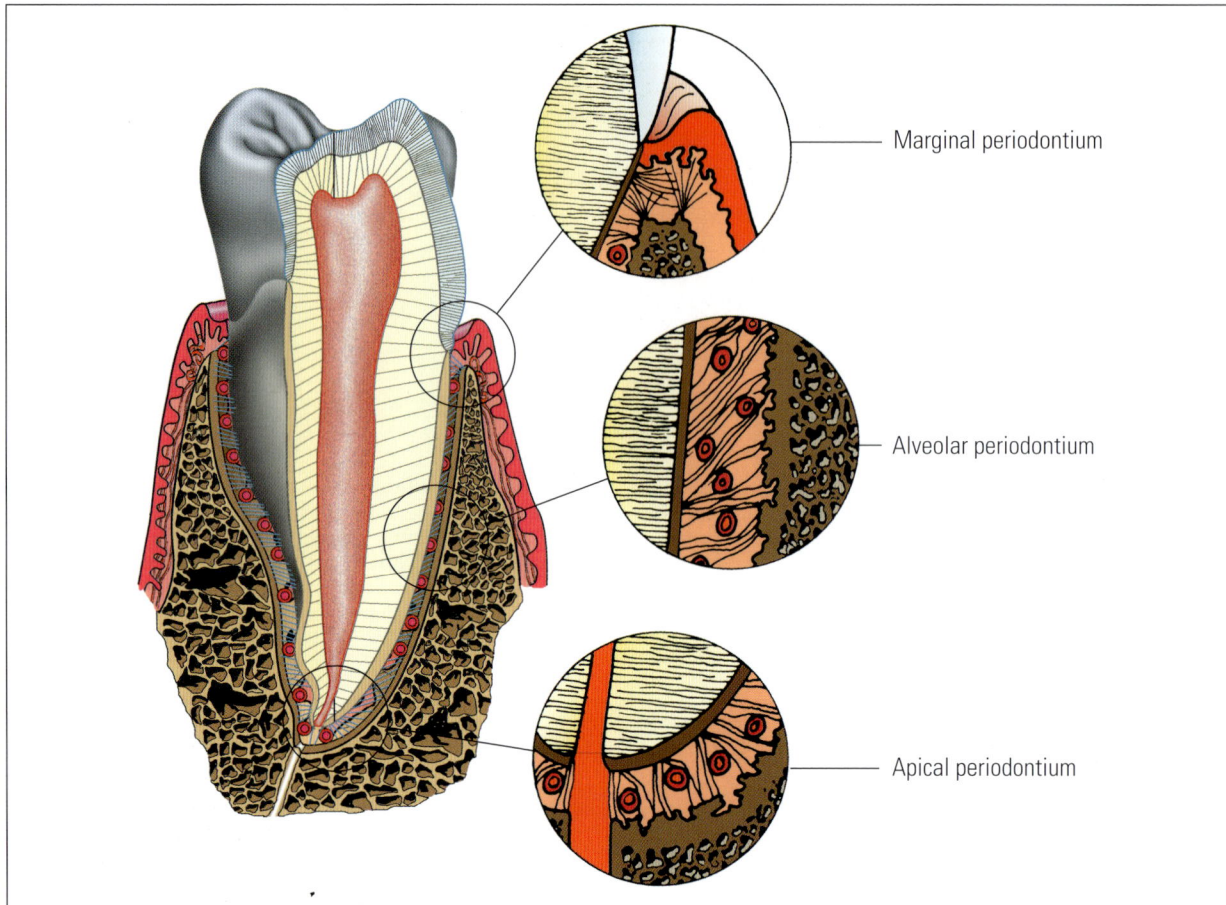

Fig 3-28 Classification of the periodontium.

- The blood supply to the periodontal ligament is ensured by tooth mobility; ie, optimal blood flow in the periodontal ligament is only ever achieved when the tooth is placed under stress. This clearly illustrates how the law of form and function operates: Blood flow in the periodontal ligament is particularly important when the tooth is being loaded, and it is that very loading on the tooth that controls the blood flow.

Classification of the periodontium

The fundamental importance of the periodontium in the functioning of the tooth has already been mentioned. However, this relationship needs to be explained in more detail. Every restoration that is fixed in some way to another tooth and hence puts extraordinary strain on that tooth will also influence the periodontium. This is why a precise understanding of the attachment apparatus is important for every dental technician.

From a topographic point of view, the attachment apparatus is divided into the marginal, alveolar, and apical periodontium (Fig 3-28). As well as differences in structure, differences in forms of loading are found in the various segments. A restoration causes different loading of the natural tooth and hence the various segments of the periodontium. As a result, any damage to the periodontium caused by the prosthetic tooth differs in different segments.

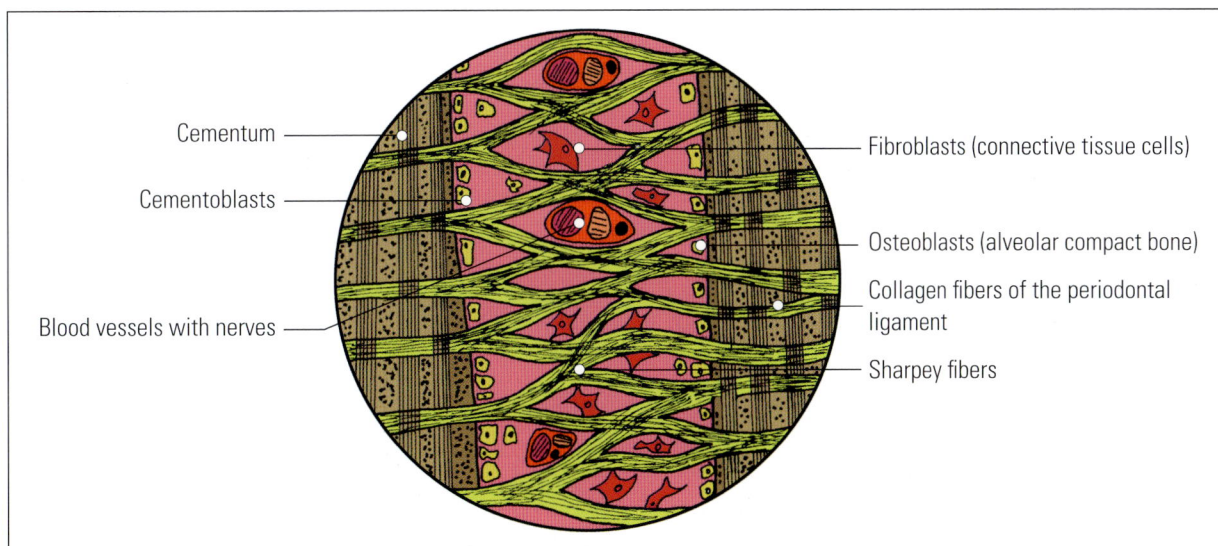

Fig 3-29 The bundles of fibers in the alveolar periodontal space form a network of collagen fibers that cross over, are joined to each other, and are anchored in the cementum and the alveolar bone.

Labels: Cementum — Cementoblasts — Blood vessels with nerves — Fibroblasts (connective tissue cells) — Osteoblasts (alveolar compact bone) — Collagen fibers of the periodontal ligament — Sharpey fibers

Alveolar periodontium

The structure of the alveolar periodontium is the same as the structure already described (Fig 3-29). In response to masticatory loading, the masticatory pressure is transformed into tensile stress on the hard tissue by the Sharpey fibers. In their resting state, the fibers are rather sinuous and thus permit a certain mobility of the tooth until, when stressed in their taut state, they transfer tensile forces directly.

The load-bearing capacity of the alveolar periodontium is in direct relation to the quantity of fibers. The number of fibers in turn depends on the size of the root surface. Hence those teeth that have to absorb very large masticatory forces in the dentition also have larger or even several roots in order to provide a greater surface area to which the fibers attach.

It has also been discovered that increased functional loading in the periodontium leads to an increase in fibers as well as strengthening of the alveolar bone mass and the cementum. The result is that when a tooth is fitted with a crown for a partial denture and more masticatory force has to be absorbed, the periodontium will adapt to this additional loading to a certain extent.

Apical and marginal widening of the **periodontal space** reflects tooth mobility. The space is narrowest around the pivotal point. The average force that the alveolar periodontium has to absorb during chewing is approximately 150 to 300 N (in extreme cases, up to 800 N). This force, however, can best be absorbed if it follows the direction of the vertical tooth axis, because this means the largest area of the tooth root is being loaded. Horizontal forces only put a strain on individual segments of the periodontium.

Tipping movements exert pressures in the marginal and apical periodontium, but these are not noticeable in the central area. In order to avoid compression, the periodontal space is widened marginally and apically. Damage to the alveolar periodontium occurs if the tooth is overloaded as an abutment or clasp tooth.

Apical periodontium

The path of fibers in the apical area differs from that in the alveolar region. The functional orientation of the fibers is intended to counteract any tipping and lifting out of the tooth. The fibers therefore run from the alveolar bone coronally and horizontally to the tooth. Damage to the apical

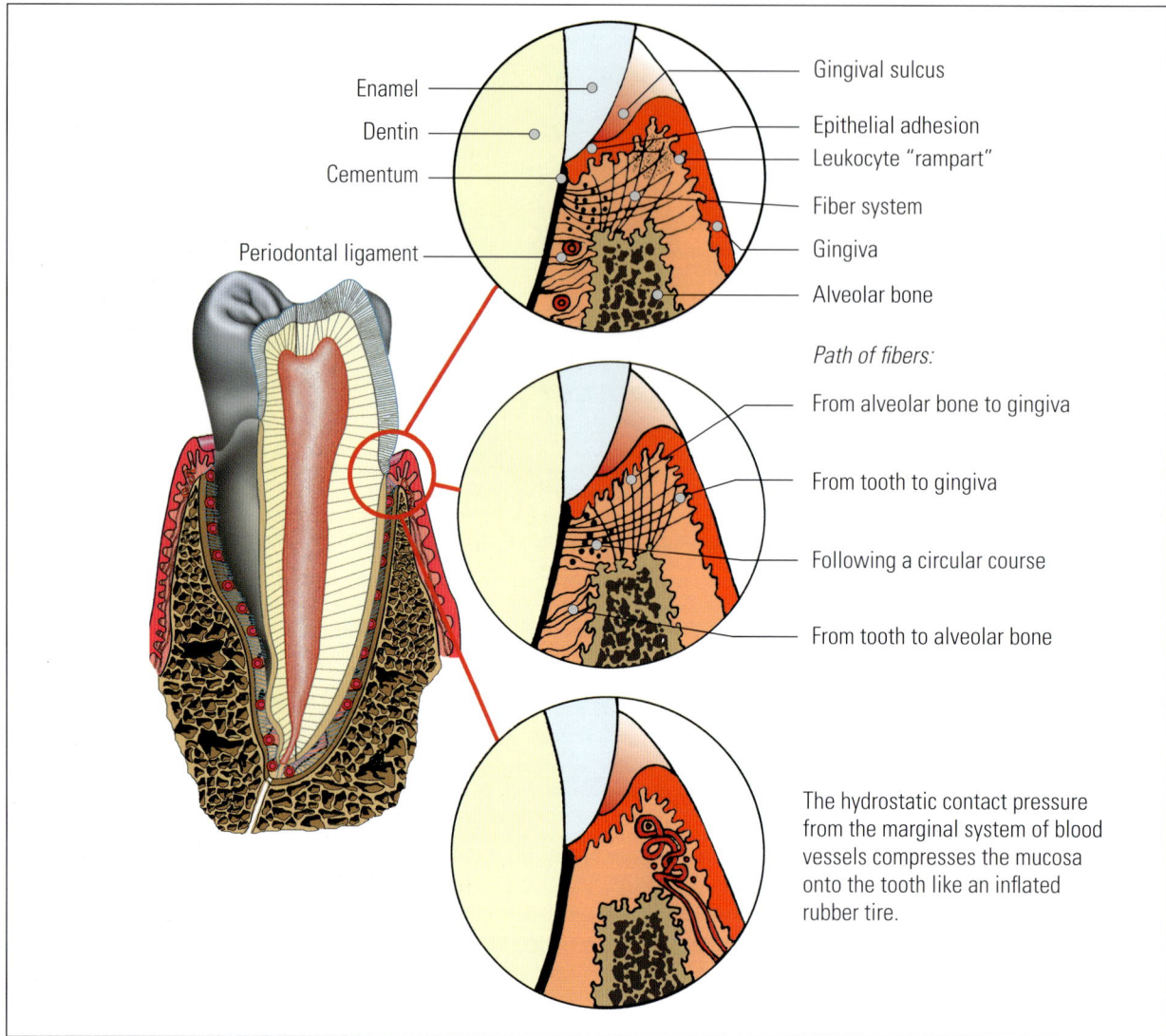

Enamel
Dentin
Cementum
Periodontal ligament

Gingival sulcus
Epithelial adhesion
Leukocyte "rampart"
Fiber system
Gingiva
Alveolar bone

Path of fibers:

From alveolar bone to gingiva

From tooth to gingiva

Following a circular course

From tooth to alveolar bone

The hydrostatic contact pressure from the marginal system of blood vessels compresses the mucosa onto the tooth like an inflated rubber tire.

Fig 3-30 Structural elements of the marginal periodontium.

area occurs if the tooth is tipped too much in the alveolus, ie, if there is incorrect loading caused by a denture.

Marginal periodontium

The peripheral segment of the periodontium, which forms the tissue seal to the oral cavity, is known as the *marginal periodontium*. This tissue segment covers the alveolar margin and the in-terdental spaces. It helps to hold the teeth in the jaws, just as it aids stabilization of the teeth in the closed dentition.

Two fundamentally different tissues are joined together here: hard tooth material and soft mucous membrane. This produces a firm and relatively re-sistant joint and an effective seal that protects against biologic and mechanical intrusion.

Three different mechanisms make this tissue seal possible:

Fig 3-31 Structural elements of the marginal epithelium. The gingival sulcus is a 0.5-mm-deep, groove-type depression of the gingival margin at the tooth surface. The epithelial cells of the gingiva on a basement membrane fit closely to the tooth and form what is called the *junctional epithelium*, which achieves the epithelial adhesion of the gingiva to the tooth.

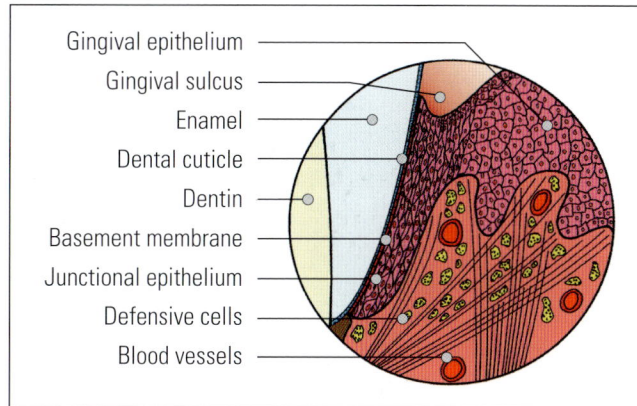

Gingival epithelium
Gingival sulcus
Enamel
Dental cuticle
Dentin
Basement membrane
Junctional epithelium
Defensive cells
Blood vessels

1. Epithelial fusion at the cementoenamel junction
2. Circular, hydrostatic contact pressure from the blood vessels
3. Mechanical constriction by various tissue fibers

The marginal periodontium surrounds the neck of the tooth like an epithelial sleeve (junctional epithelium) that attaches to the tooth surface (epithelial attachment) and is supported by a connective tissue fiber framework. The gingival part of the marginal periodontium can be divided into three distinct topographic areas:

1. Gingival sulcus
2. Free marginal gingiva
3. Attached gingiva

The **gingival sulcus** (*sulcus* = furrow) is a narrow groove about 0.5 mm deep that runs in a circle between the gingiva and the tooth surface. The central wall of the sulcus is formed by dental hard tissue (mainly enamel); the outer wall is the normal mucosal epithelium, while the floor of the sulcus is made up of junctional epithelium, which also forms the epithelial attachment.

The extent of the sulcus can differ from tooth to tooth and widen into periodontal pockets of varying depth as a result of mechanical influences or inflammatory processes and plaque. This formation of pockets then becomes pathologic and can lead to periodontal disease and tooth loss.

The **free gingiva** is the narrow rim of tissue above the bony alveolar margin that follows the scalloped contour of the necks of the teeth or the cementoenamel junction. This rim of tissue is relatively smooth and between 1.1 and 2.1 mm high.

It can be moved along the neck of the tooth but also away from the tooth, while the epithelial attachment to the tooth can be torn.

Attached gingiva is bound immovably to the alveolar bone. This part of the mucous membrane has a different structure from the normal gingiva and varies in height between 1 and 9 mm. It is attached by connective tissue fibers, which start from the periosteum of the alveolar margin and the cementum, marking the course of the topographic borderline. Gingival stippling parallel to the cervical margin often arises from fiber processes.

In the **interdental space**, the vestibular and lingual areas of the gingiva merge and completely fill this space as the interdental papilla when the approximal contact of the teeth is normal. The interdental papillae protrude occlusally in the lingual and vestibular regions, whereas they bend around the teeth in the interdental and apical areas. In normal conditions, the cementoenamel junction of the tooth is covered by the papilla. However, if the approximal contacts are open, the papilla may be displaced, which can result in a significant risk of caries because the cementoenamel junction or the cementum becomes exposed.

The **structural tissue elements** of the marginal periodontium are (Figs 3-30 and 3-31):

• Gingival epithelium
• Junctional epithelium
• Connective tissue fiber structure
• Blood vessels
• Nerves

The tissue seal to the oral cavity between the mucosa and the dental hard tissue is safeguarded by two attachment mechanisms. These are the adhesion of the junctional epithelium (epithelial attachment) and the connective tissue attachment by the fibrous apparatus. Hydrostatic contact pressure caused by the loop-type terminal vascular bed of the blood vessels provides additional support to these attachment mechanisms. All the mechanisms work together in the same way at the level of the cementoenamel junction.

The *gingival epithelium* is similar to the epithelial lining of the whole oral cavity; it is only the specific junctional epithelium in the immediate attachment area that may differ. This tissue forms a ring of epithelium about 2 mm high, which starts at the bottom of the sulcus and provides the epithelial attachment at the cementoenamel junction.

The *junctional epithelium* is a two-layer structure, with a basal layer that is active in cell division and a layer that is inactive in cell division. The intercellular spaces of the two layers differ in width, making this epithelial layer permeable.

Before the teeth erupt, the junctional epithelium develops from reduced adamantoblasts of the enamel epithelium. Conversion from the reduced enamel epithelial cells into the junctional epithelium takes place during and after eruption and ensures the necessary attachment between the epithelium and the enamel. After that, the junctional epithelium is a constantly renewing tissue.

The *epithelial attachment* is based on a biologic principle whereby the junctional epithelial cells stick to the tooth surface by adhesive and cohesive forces. The epithelium is able to stick to the enamel as well as the dentin and cementum. The *junctional epithelial cells* form the *basement membrane* to the dental hard tissues, which renews itself constantly. The junctional epithelial cells with their basement membrane are laid tightly onto the tooth surface so that the molecular forces can take effect. However, it is not the epithelial attachment with its minimal physical binding powers that is crucial to the functioning of this seal; the junctional epithelial cells themselves perform the defensive function. The epithelial and connective tissue structures have enormous powers of regeneration. The shedding of junctional epithelial cells is far greater than that of the normal gingiva. The wound-healing process in the sulcus is fully completed in less than 7 days after total mechanical destruction, after which it cannot be distinguished from the original junctional epithelium. The regeneration rate of the connective tissue parts is also unusually high. This excellent defensive activity allows rapid regeneration after inflammatory and mechanical changes.

The *permeability* of the junctional epithelium in two directions is also a remarkable defense mechanism: firstly, substances that act as antigens penetrate the junctional epithelium and can trigger an antibody reaction; secondly, a flow of various leukocytes directed outward kills the invading bacteria. Around 30,000 neutrophilic granulocytes flow through the junctional epithelium every minute and enter the oral cavity via the floor of the sulcus. The lymph vessels supply the gingiva with numerous populations of leukocytes for defense, so that one could call this a leukocyte "rampart" to the marginal zone (see Fig 3-30).

The *connective tissue fiber structure* of the marginal periodontium is functionally oriented—ie, its path is not purely random—but the fibers run so that they pull the mucosa onto the tooth. The fibers interlink, secure the gingival epithelial layers, and thus form the second attachment mechanism. A distinction is made between several fiber groups that differ in the path they follow (Fig 3-32):

• Tooth to gingiva
• Alveolar margin to gingiva
• Vestibular to lingual papilla
• Forming a circle around the tooth
• Tooth to outer alveolar margin
• Tooth to inner alveolar margin
• Circular fibers to the adjacent tooth
• Cementum to the cement of the adjacent tooth
• External alveolar bone to the gingiva

The *tissue linkage* between the separate teeth is provided by the differentiated paths of the fibers, as a result of which tooth movements are transferred to the closed dentition. The fiber systems of adjacent teeth are so closely interwoven that mutual support between the teeth can take place. If a tooth is tipped buccally, the neighboring teeth are involved as well because of the tis-

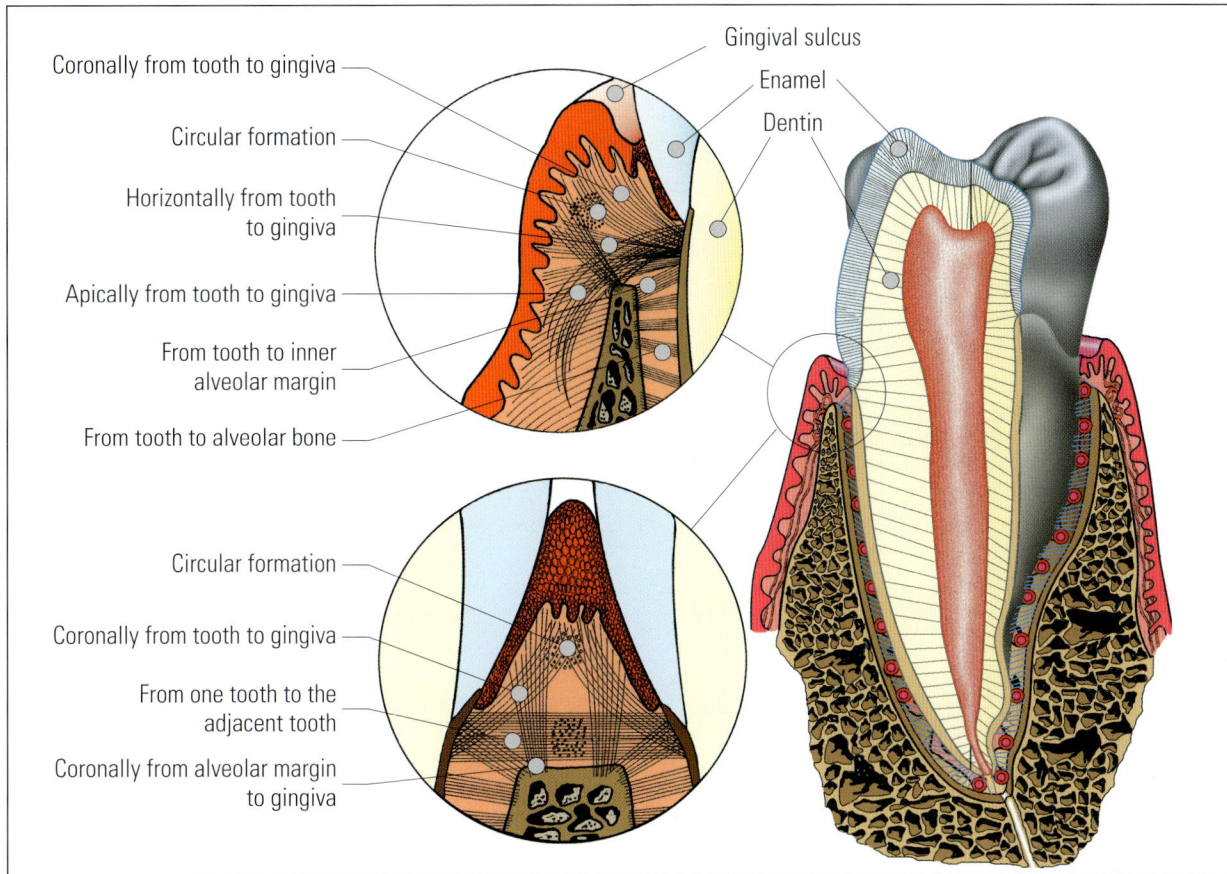

Fig 3-32 Path of fibers at the marginal periodontium. The schematic diagram of the marginal periodontium shows the complex path of fibers with which the gingiva is stabilized onto the tooth and the free alveolar margin. The *top inset* shows the path of fiber bundles in a vestibular direction, while the *bottom inset* shows their path in the interdental papilla between the teeth.

sue linkage, or they prevent excessive tipping of the tooth. This tissue linkage also results in the physiologic mesial migration of the teeth.

Tightening of the gingiva by tear-resistant fiber processes also provides protection against shearing when chewing slippery food. The processes tighten the marginal periodontium against the hydrostatic pressure of the blood vessels and shape the gingiva so that it is compressed onto the epithelial attachment.

The **hydrostatic contact pressure** of the marginal blood vessel system supports the fiber system and the epithelial fusion. The blood vessels of the marginal tissue section are arranged as one-way passages. This leads to congestion of blood as the vessels swell up. They thus transfer the tissue pressure onto the mucosa, which then lies around the tooth like an inflated rubber tire and provides a tight seal. This is why the gingival sulcus must not be displaced; if it is, the epithelial adhesion

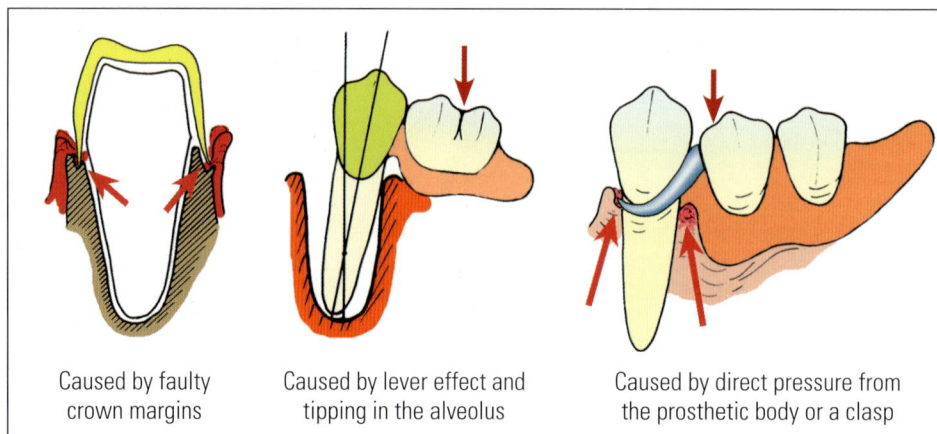

| Caused by faulty crown margins | Caused by lever effect and tipping in the alveolus | Caused by direct pressure from the prosthetic body or a clasp |

Fig 3-33 Prosthetic tooth replacement can cause damage to the marginal periodontium.

might be torn off by the pressure from the blood vessels. Under minimal mechanical stress, this results in gingival bleeding (eg, when cleaning the teeth).

The tissue seal can be damaged by prosthetic work. The following prosthetic errors can cause damage (Fig 3-33):

• Direct compressive stress caused by tight-fitting prosthesis components
• Lever effect on the tooth by anchorage components
• Irritation caused by incorrect crown margins

Morphology of Teeth

Characteristic Features of Tooth Forms

The previous descriptions of dental substances and the tooth attachment apparatus (periodontium) referred to the law of form and function. The connection between form and function also applies when describing the different tooth forms. It explains the extent to which the teeth and the tissue involved form a unit, having developed and grown for their particular functions and hence taken on a particular form. Every characteristic feature of the form of dental tissue therefore indicates a particular significance.

Any replacement tooth will have an influence on the function of the whole masticatory system. Tooth forms should be seen not only as esthetic features but above all as functional forms developed for specific tasks. Dental technicians must be familiar with the tooth forms down to the smallest detail because they are constantly faced with the task of skillfully producing individual teeth for individual dentitions. The dental technician hence needs to recognize anatomical details not only as characteristic features of form but also as functional necessities. The individual teeth are therefore described herein with considerable accuracy, although there are some characteristics of form that are common to all teeth.

Every crown of a tooth has five definable surfaces, which are named after the directions in which they face (Fig 4-1):

1. Occlusal or masticatory surface (*facies occlusalis*; *facies* = surface)
2. Vestibular, buccal, or labial surface (*facies vestibularis*)
3. Lingual surface (*facies lingualis*)
4. Mesial approximal surface (*facies approximalis*)
5. Distal approximal surface

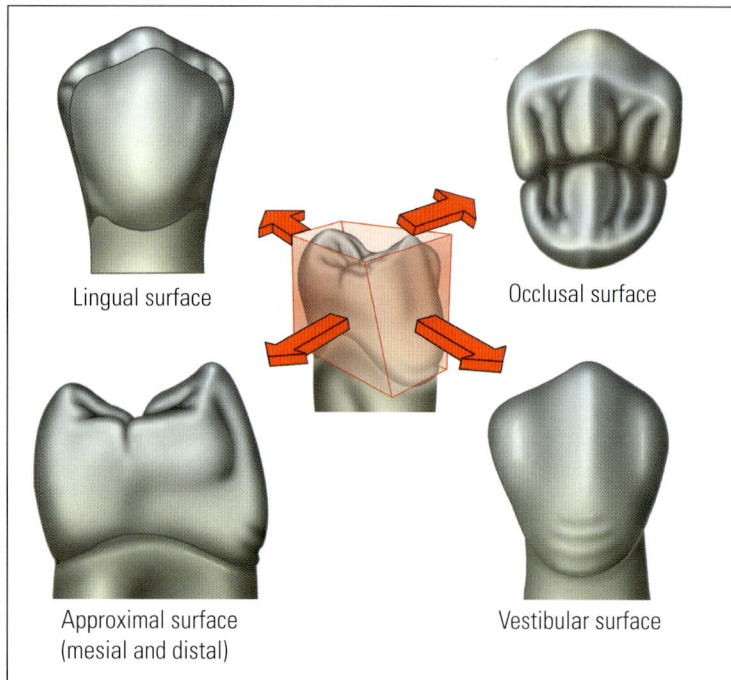

Fig 4-1 Each dental crown comprises five definable surfaces. In principle, the surfaces are trapezoidal, which means a tooth is not cylindric but tapers at the cervix. The shape of the surface is determined by the fact that the teeth form a segment of a circle.

Lingual surface

Occlusal surface

Approximal surface
(mesial and distal)

Vestibular surface

The **occlusal surface** indicates the terminal occlusion or occlusal line in which the teeth rest when biting together. On the posterior teeth this is a true surface, bearing cusps, that fits into the surface of the antagonist (opposing) tooth and is suitable for crushing food (Figs 4-2 and 4-3). It is defined as a true chewing surface and therefore is also known as a *masticatory surface* (*masticare* = to chew). On the anterior teeth, this surface is reduced to a thin edge and is known as the *incisal margin* or cutting edge. The incisal margin of the anterior teeth is suitable for shearing food (Fig 4-4).

The **angle characteristic** denotes the angular transition from the occlusal contour to the approximal surfaces. Looking at the teeth from the vestibular aspect, it can be seen that the occlusal surfaces or incisal margins recede distally; the teeth are higher mesially than distally. Looking at the whole dentition from the vestibular aspect, it is also noticeable that the relative height of the teeth decreases in the distal direction. On an incisor, the transition from the incisal margin to the approximal surfaces mesially is sharp-edged, while the distal transition is rounded and oblique.

Because the pronounced acute angle is always mesial, it is possible to tell from the angles which side of the mouth an anterior tooth belongs to (Fig 4-5).

The **vestibular surface** is the surface that faces the vestibule, ie, is oriented in a buccal or labial direction or facing the outer surface. This surface gets narrower toward the cervical region and wider toward the occlusal surface. Viewed approximally, the vestibular contour bulges outward in a curve at the cervix and is concave occlusally. At the neck of the tooth, this produces an overhanging "belly" that protects the gingival margin. Food is pushed over this bulge away from the margin of the gingiva. Therefore, this bulging form of the vestibular surfaces must be re-created in prosthetic crowns. This curvature is also described as the *vertical curvature characteristic* and is most pronounced in the mandibular teeth.

The **horizontal curvature characteristic** or characteristic of mass denotes the marked transverse convexity of the vestibular surface. The surface contour, when viewed occlusally, is more curved or bulging in the mesial part, while it recedes flatly on the distal side (Fig 4-6). The position of

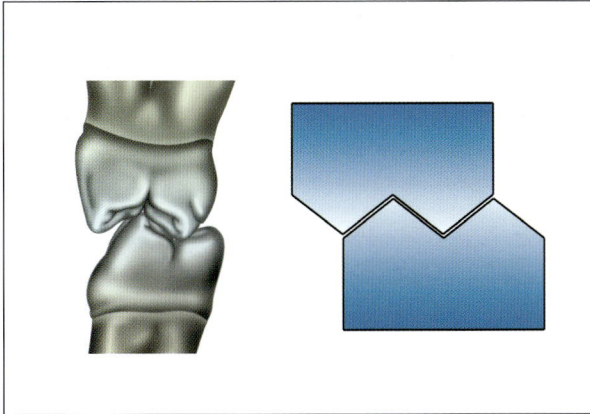

Fig 4-2 The occlusal surfaces of the posterior teeth have cusps and fit into the antagonist occlusal surfaces; they are suitable for crushing food.

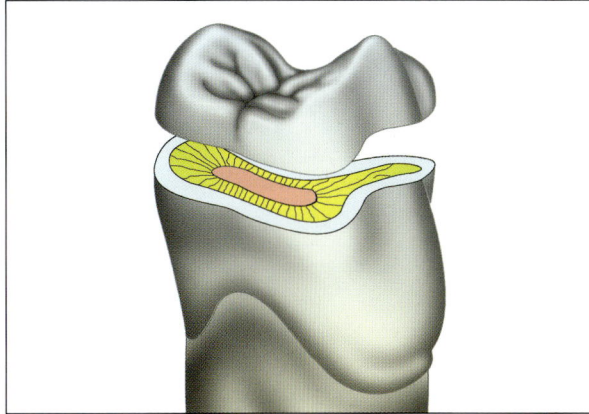

Fig 4-3 Schematic diagram of the occlusal surface of a premolar: The occlusal surface covers the whole occlusal relief from the highest cusp through to the deepest fissure. The occlusal surface has special characteristics that have developed as the best shape for each tooth within the dentition in order to perform specific functions.

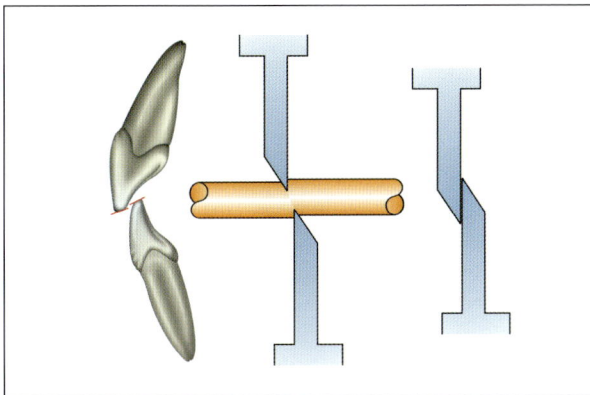

Fig 4-4 The incisal margins of the anterior teeth are ideally suited for cutting food when the mandibular teeth interlock behind the maxillary teeth like a pair of scissors.

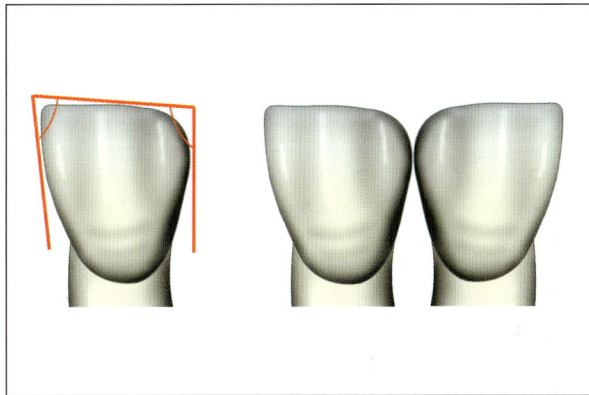

Fig 4-5 When viewed labially, the angle on the anterior teeth between the incisal margins and the approximal surfaces is acute mesially and oblique distally. To illustrate this, the maxillary central incisors have been transposed right to left.

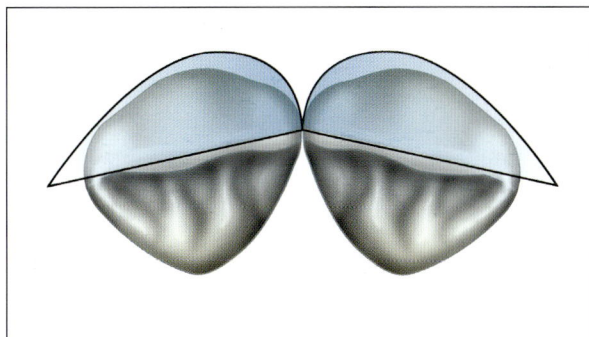

Fig 4-6 The horizontal curvature characteristic is related to the dental arch. When viewed occlusally, the teeth as a segment of the arch are more curved mesially than distally on the vestibular surface.

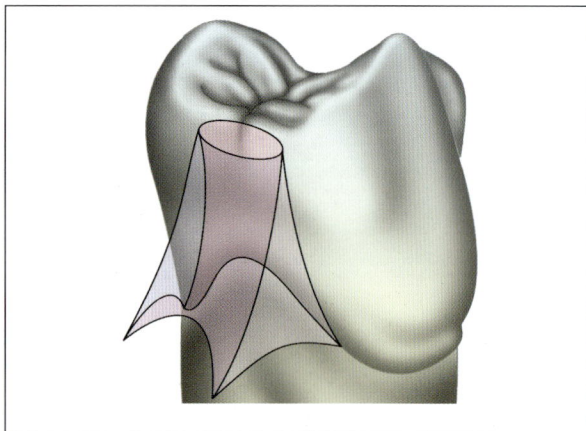

Fig 4-7 The interdental space.

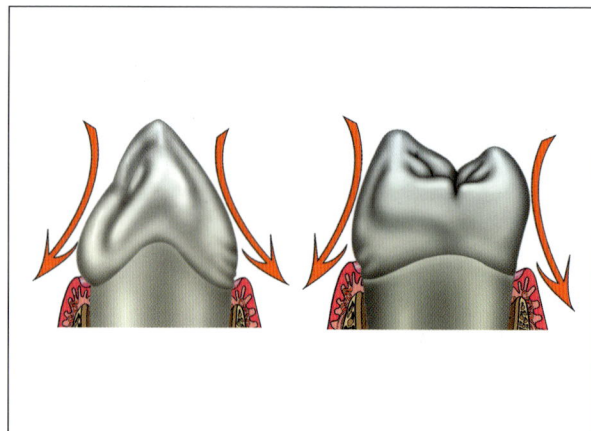

Fig 4-8 The vertical curvatures of the lingual and vestibular surfaces form an overhanging convexity that protects the gingival margin by pushing food away from the gingiva.

the tooth in the dental arch can be classified by this mesiovestibular distribution of mass, which is why it is also referred to as an *arch characteristic*. If it is known whether a tooth is maxillary or mandibular, the side of the mouth to which it belongs can be identified by the curvature characteristic. The curvature and angle characteristics must be reproduced on a prosthetic tooth so that it fits precisely into the existing dentition.

The ***lingual surfaces*** of the teeth face the tongue; in the maxilla, this surface may also be known as the *palatal surface (facies palatina)*. The lingual surfaces are always smaller than the vestibular, which is due to the arrangement of the teeth in the dental arch. When equal slices are cut out of a circular area, the outer surface is bound to be larger than the inner surface.

The lingual surface is also convex, but the widest curvature lies in the middle and is not reduced toward the cervix. The lingual surface always tapers toward the occlusal area, where it becomes the occlusal or masticatory surface.

The ***approximal surfaces*** are the mesial and distal areas of contact with the neighboring teeth; this is where the points of contact with the adjacent teeth lie, which is why these are also known as *contact surfaces (facies contactus)*. Approximal surfaces are basically trapezoidal: The long baseline is at the cervix, while the short line is toward the occlusal surface, and the contour lines of the lingual and vestibular surfaces form the sloping lines. Viewed lingually or vestibularly, the bulg-

ing convexity of the approximal surfaces can be seen to lie directly occlusally or incisally and not at the neck of the tooth. The tooth is thus wider occlusally.

On a tooth, a distinction is made between a mesial and a distal approximal surface. The distal approximal surface is usually smaller than the mesial, but they only differ slightly in their basic form.

Contact points result from the convexity of the approximal surfaces of two adjacent teeth and lie just below the occlusal line. The teeth touch each other above the contact points. As a result, they can support each other (ie, provide reciprocal anchorage) if they are moved sideways or tipped lingually. Then they do not have to bear the sideways pressure alone but can spread the strain to the whole dentition. This is why the contact points are so important and must be re-created in prosthetic crowns. When a tooth is missing, this support mechanism within the dentition is disrupted. Then sideways pressure can very easily lead to excessive strain and damage to the periodontium. This is why even a single tooth within a dentition should be replaced.

Interdental space denotes the space between the teeth that is apical to the contact points and filled with gingival tissue; this is where the interdental papilla lies (*inter* = between) (Fig 4-7). If the teeth are very tightly packed together at the contact points, no food particles can be squeezed between the teeth; the contact points protect the gingival papillae (Fig 4-8). The approximal contact

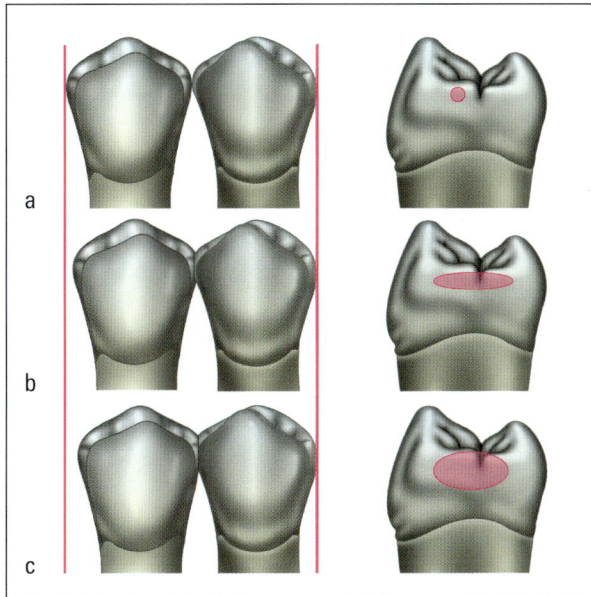

Fig 4-9 The approximal surfaces form the contact surfaces to the neighboring teeth. The contacts are merely points initially *(a)* but become linear *(b)* and then cover a flat area *(c)* with advancing age because of slight tooth mobility. The interdental space forms between the teeth apical to the contact points or lines. The marginal periodontium forms the interdental papilla, which is adapted to this interdental space and is protected by the contact points.

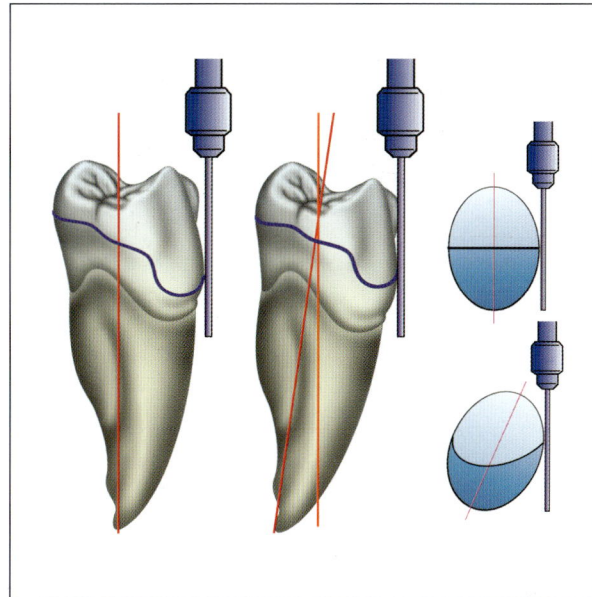

Fig 4-10 A circumference line drawn parallel to the perpendicular changes its course if the tooth (or any oval body) is inclined. When the axis of a natural tooth is parallel to the perpendicular, this gives the anatomical equator; if the path of insertion of a prosthetic tooth lies parallel to the perpendicular, this is the prosthetic equator.

point, which is initially merely a point in young people, becomes linear over time and then is worn away to create a flat area owing to slight tooth mobility with advancing age (Fig 4-9). This makes the teeth crowd closer together in a mesial direction and is referred to as *physiologic mesial migration*. If a tooth is missing, the adjacent teeth lean into the gap.

All the **surfaces of a tooth** put together show that a tooth is not cylindric in shape but concave at the neck, only getting wider coronally and becoming concave again toward the occlusal surface. Therefore, the dental crown is always undercut. This bulging shape serves the purpose of deflecting food or forming the approximal contact.

The **anatomical equator** is the curvature line of the widest circumference of the dental crown. The course of the convexity around the tooth can be traced. Using a black lead pencil to draw a line around the tooth parallel to the vertical dental

crown axis, the anatomical equator or the curvature line can be marked. The course of this equator is not at a single height; approximatly it runs close to the occlusal surface and vestibularly or lingually close to the cervical region.

The **prosthetic equator** denotes the widest circumference line on the prosthetic dental crown, with reference to a freely chosen perpendicular at which the tooth is tipped. If a path of insertion for the denture is fixed during fabrication of partial prostheses, the teeth will be at a different incline to that. The prosthetic equator is obtained by running a black lead pencil parallel to the insertion path around the tooth.

To summarize, the reference line for the anatomical equator is the natural tooth axis; for the prosthetic equator, the reference line is a freely chosen path of insertion that does not necessarily coincide with the tooth axis (Fig 4-10).

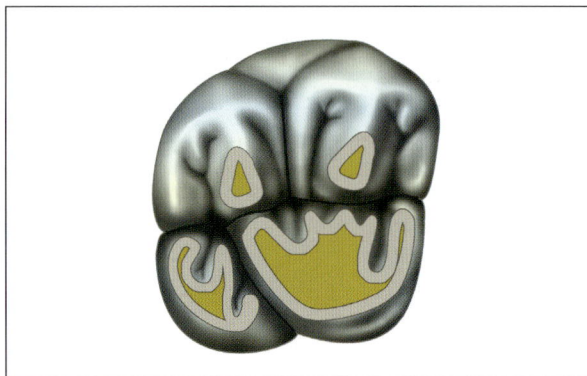

Fig 4-11 The dentin core may be exposed as a result of abrasion, but the pulp chamber is rarely exposed because secondary dentin is constantly being formed.

Description of Tooth Forms

When dental technicians have to fabricate a prosthetic tooth crown, they must be familiar with the normal form (norm) and then individualize it to match the given case. The alternative—knowing all the individual cases and picking out the right one as needed—is simply not feasible. Any description of tooth forms is based on statistical mean values, which are used to work out the normal shape of the tooth concerned, ie, an ideal form.

Individual variations are noticeable when looking at a natural tooth. These variations are mainly deformations of the original form caused by wear. Dental enamel and dentin are subject to mechanical wear known as *dental abrasion (abradere* = to shear off).

Abrasion is the rubbing and erosion of the natural or artificial tooth surfaces by the act of chewing, resulting in the wearing away of incisal margins, occlusal surfaces, and approximal surfaces. The mechanical loss of hard dental substances both occlusally and approximally is known as *horizontal* and *vertical abrasion*. It appears in the form of functional surfaces (ie, incisal margins and occlusal surfaces) being altered by demastication, attrition, and artificial abrasion (defined below).

Normally, abrasion is physiologic wear and can be seen as a functional adaptation: The incisal margins wear each other away like the blades of scissors; the occlusal surfaces lose their high cusps and fit into the abraded surfaces of the opposing teeth (antagonists). If the dentinoenamel junction is reached because enamel (which cannot regenerate) is abraded, dark, yellowish-brown lines and spots appear, and abrasion cavities are formed. The pulp chamber is not generally exposed because secondary dentin is constantly being formed (Fig 4-11).

Demastication is the physiologic wear on teeth as food is crushed, caused by the abrasive force of the food and its impurities. It mainly affects the incisal margins and the occlusal surfaces.

Attrition is the sharply demarcated wear on teeth resulting from friction caused by movements with the empty mouth (ie, parafunctions such as clenching or tooth grinding), so that typical wear facets appear.

Artificial abrasion is the wearing down of hard dental substances as a result of artificial external factors, such as the indentation (erosion) of incisors in pipe smokers.

Generalized abrasion means heavy wear on occlusal surfaces with typical lingual inclination of the occlusal surfaces *(abrasio ad linguam)* in large mandibles, palatal inclination *(abrasio ad palatum)* in the case of a large maxilla, or horizontal inclination where the jaw size is well balanced or there is a reverse articulation.

Interstitial abrasion arises as wear on the approximal contact points caused by natural tooth mobility, so that the mesiodistal tooth diameter shortens, which is compensated for by the physiologic mesial migration of the teeth (Fig 4-12).

Wear facets are the worn areas on natural teeth caused by abrasion. Their typical form and position can be used to identify teeth because very specific wear facets are formed as a result of the position of the antagonists.

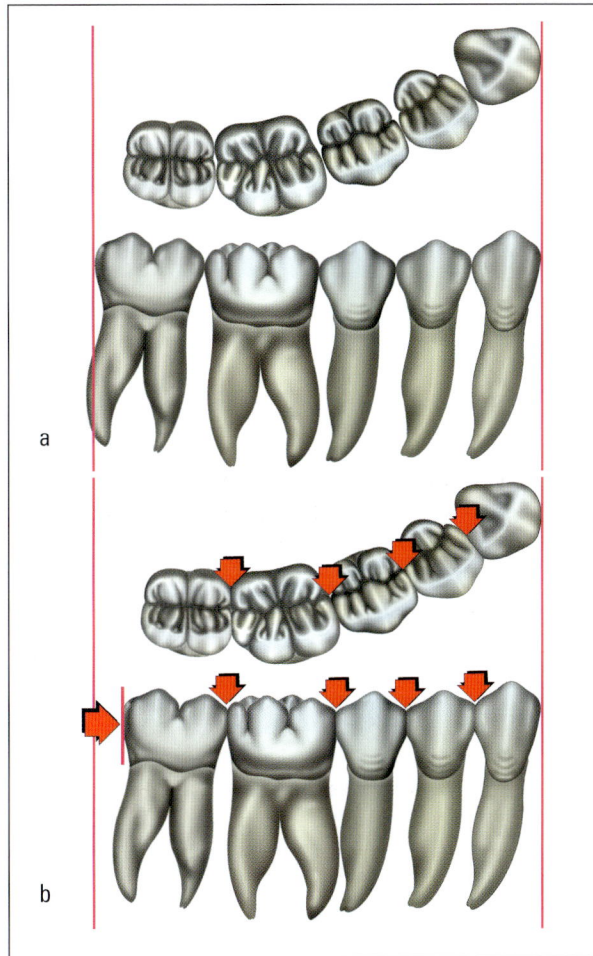

Fig 4-12 *(a)* Before interstitial abrasion. *(b)* After interstitial abrasion. Interstitial abrasion reduces the tooth diameter in the mesiodistal direction; the teeth crowd together more, and the dental arch shortens as a result of physiologic mesial migration.

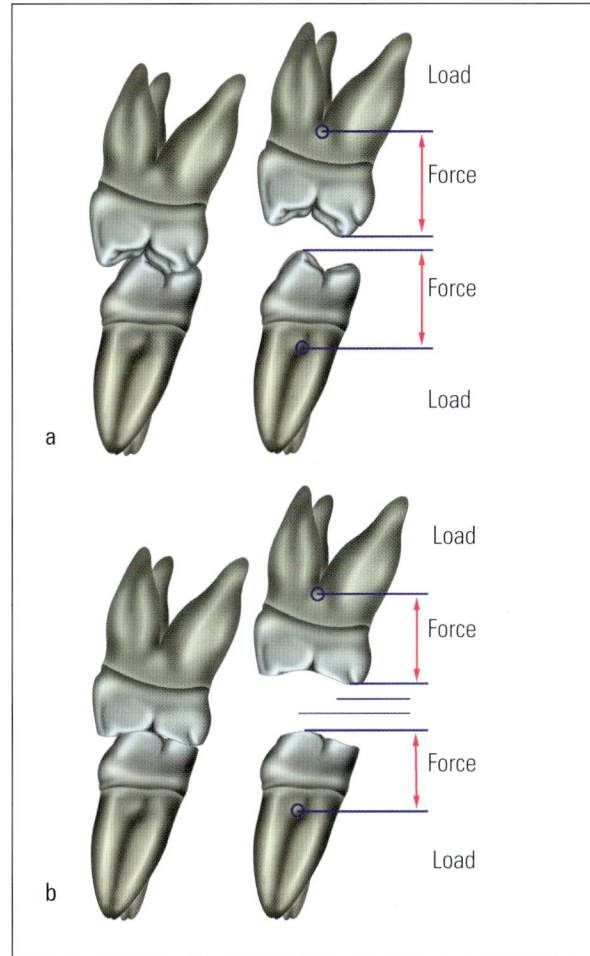

Fig 4-13 *(a)* Before abrasion. *(b)* After abrasion. Abrasion shortens the dental crowns and improves the relationship of load to force. The strain on the periodontium is relieved, the fissures are ground down, and the sites at high risk of caries are reduced.

This raises the question as to why the teeth do not erupt already in a functionally abraded form, but this is based on a false premise. Instead one should ask what is the basic function of highly developed, nonabraded teeth. The answer is that the steep cusps ensure that the teeth find their correct position as they erupt. The emerging teeth are guided by the profile of the occlusal surfaces of their antagonists.

During chewing function, they then wear each other down to their eventual form. This means that the dental crowns are shortened, which im-

proves the relationship of load to force and takes the strain off the periodontium (Fig 4-13). When the fissures are abraded, this also reduces the sites where caries can attack.

A specific system is used to describe the teeth in the following sections: The names and general descriptions are given first, and the functional aspects of the individual teeth are then examined in detail. The actual topographic description emerges from the sequence of surfaces: vestibular, lingual, mesial approximal, and occlusal.

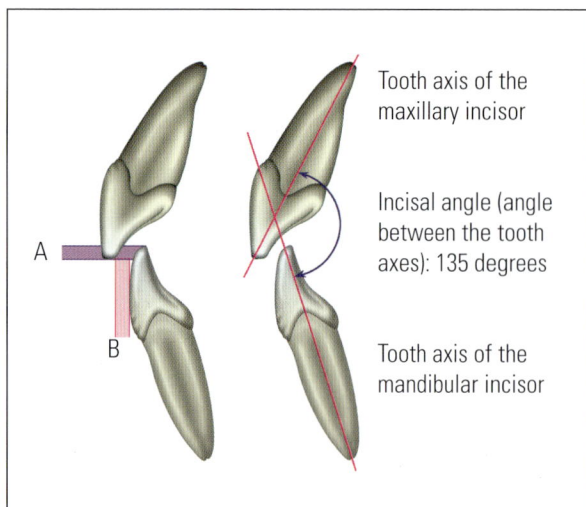

Fig 4-14 Vertical overlap of 2.0 to 3.0 mm (A) and horizontal overlap of 0.1 to 2.0 mm (B).

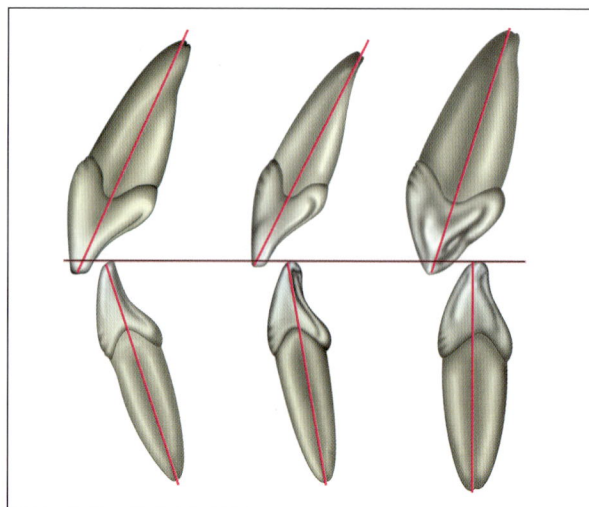

Fig 4-15 Approximal view of the inclination of axes of the anterior teeth in relation to the occlusal line, showing the anterior teeth leaning vestibularly, except the mandibular canine, which stands vertically with its labial contour inclined lingually.

Anterior Teeth

The anterior teeth are the four incisors and two canines in the maxilla and mandible. These 12 teeth form a group of antagonists that produce an interlocking pattern in a normal dentition. When viewed approximally, the maxillary anterior teeth are anterior to and occlude vertically over the mandibular anterior teeth without any contact. The overlap in the horizontal plane is sometimes called the *overjet* and ranges from 0.1 to 2.0 mm; the vertical overlap is sometimes called the *overbite* and can be between 2.0 and 3.0 mm (Fig 4-14).

From the approximal view, the ***interincisal angle*** is the angle of approximately 135 degrees between the axes of the vestibularly inclined maxillary and mandibular anterior teeth (Figs 4-14 and 4-15). The resulting profile view of the dentition looks strongly like a rudimentary snout. The maxillary canine is inclined so far in a vestibular direction that its tip and the cervical margin lie almost vertically on top of each other and, when viewed vestibularly, give the impression that the labial surface is vertical.

Root characteristic refers to the distal bend of the roots (seen from the vestibular view) (Fig 4-16). The incisors have only one root. The inclinations of the axes of the maxillary anterior teeth seen from the vestibular view show a consistent mesial tendency, while the mandibular anterior teeth stand rather vertically (Fig 4-17). The maxillary canines and central incisors are equally long and the lateral incisors rather shorter; the mandibular anterior teeth lie with their incisal margins on a horizontal line.

Incisors have chisel-, paddle-, or shovel-shaped crowns (Fig 4-18a). The labial and lingual surfaces lean incisally toward each other so that a cutting edge is formed. The approximal surfaces thus appear almost triangular, with the apex of the triangle lying at the incisal margin.

Labial surfaces display the vertical curvature that protects the marginal periodontium, while the lingual surfaces form a tubercle toward the cervix that performs the same function. The incisors are ideal for shearing and cutting through food because of their shovel shape and prominent cutting edge. The incisal margins have an oblique abrasion edge, receding palatally in the maxilla and labially in the mandible so that dur-

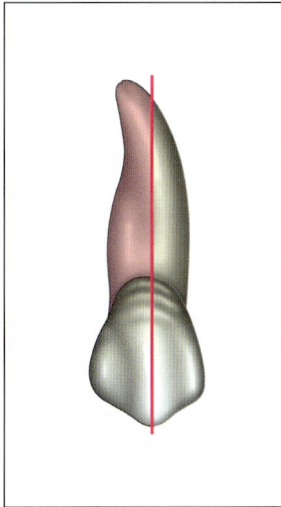

Fig 4-16 Root characteristic: The apical third of the root is curved distally.

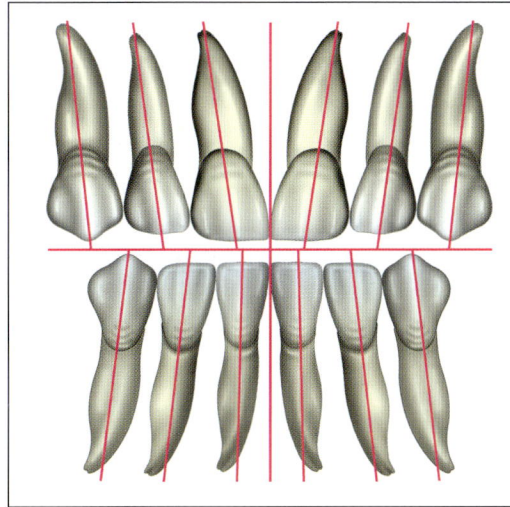

Fig 4-17 Vestibular view showing the mesially inclined maxillary anterior teeth while the mandibular anterior teeth stand rather perpendicular.

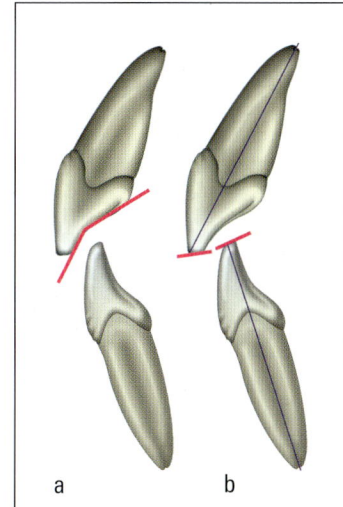

Fig 4-18 *(a)* Shovel-shaped concavity of the lingual surfaces of the maxillary incisors. *(b)* Abrasion edges of the incisal margins. The maxillary incisal margin is chamfered palatally, and the mandibular incisal margin is chamfered labially.

ing anterior movements of the mandible, the incisors slide along on these grinding surfaces (Fig 4-18b).

Mandibular incisors are smaller and narrower than the maxillary incisors; in fact, they are the smallest teeth in the human dentition. The mandibular central incisor, unlike its maxillary counterpart, is smaller than the adjacent lateral incisor. Because they resemble each other very closely, the mandibular central and lateral incisors can be described together. Both teeth have one root, which is significantly flattened in the mesiodistal direction and shows a marked longitudinal groove on the outer surface. They are very weak and short and hence unsuitable for post crowns.

Canines are single-rooted teeth that, unlike the incisors, have a cusp tip and are thus *dentes cuspidati*. They are the strongest single-rooted teeth. The root of the maxillary canine is the longest in the whole dentition. In rare cases, these teeth show stunting or furcation involvement; very rarely the canine is absent.

The canine is an independent tooth form. No animal with a dentition comprising different tooth forms (heterodont dentition) has more than four canines. When the permanent teeth erupt, the canine often shifts, usually being displaced in a lingual or vestibular direction.

The canines form the corners of the dentition: They have an angled incisal margin or masticatory edge, but at the same time they mark the transition between the incisors and teeth with occlusal surfaces, forming a cornerstone between two very different types of teeth. They also form a corner within the row of teeth.

When the ***mouth is closed*** in occlusion, the canines guide the mandibular dentition into the correct hinge position. If the mandible is moved out of the central hinge position laterally or anteriorly, the canines separate the rows of teeth. This phenomenon is known as *canine guidance*. The canines are often referred to as the "anterior joint" of the jaw. The canines can cut food with their mesial cutting edge and crush food with their distal, thickened chewing edge.

Maxillary incisors

The *maxillary central incisor (dens incisivus medialis)* (Figs 4-19 to 4-21) is the largest incisor tooth, having a rectangular to rhomboid, triangular, or oval vestibular surface, which can harmonize with the shape of the face.

Its average dimensions are:

• Crown width (mesiodistal): 8.5 mm
• Crown depth (labiolingual): 7.0 mm
• Crown length: 11.5 mm
• Total apicocoronal length: 25.0 mm

Its *root* forms an elongated cone, is straight from an approximal view, and is slightly bent distally from a labial view (root characteristic). The strong root makes it usable as an abutment tooth or suitable for placement of a post crown.

The *labial surface* (see Fig 4-19a) is almost rectangular and tapers cervically. The mesial edge looks rather straight, whereas the distal edge is curved. The labial surface has a vertical and horizontal curvature characteristic as well as a pronounced angle characteristic. The surface is defined by two marginal ridges and a medial ridge, which are separated by two vertical grooves. When the teeth are freshly erupted, these ridges make the incisal margin appear to have three lobes. This form is lost through abrasion. The distal approximal edge is slightly concave to the cervix and becomes an evenly curved cervical margin. A few slightly pronounced cervical grooves run almost parallel to the cervical margin.

The *lingual surface* (see Fig 4-19b) resembles the labial surface but is smaller and narrower and tapers more sharply, especially in the cervical area. Two marginal ridges run from the incisal edge cervically, then merge in the apical third of the surface to form the dental tubercle. The marginal ridges outline the concave surface like the edges of a shovel. Differently shaped medial ridges emerge from the tubercle. Depending on the concavity of the lingual surface and the number of enamel ridges, the tubercle can be divided into two tubercles, for example, or the margins may form a partially covered canal.

The *mesial approximal surface* (see Fig 4-19c) has a triangular shape, with the apex at the incisal edge and the baseline at the cervix; the functional chisel shape of the incisor can be seen. The cervical line curves considerably in an incisal direction. The surface itself is tapered toward the neck of the tooth. The vertical curvature of the labial surface contour and the prominent dental tubercle, whose curvature is greatest at the neck, can be clearly seen. The mesial approximal surface is larger than the distal surface.

The *incisal view* (see Fig 4-19d) shows the features of the other surfaces described above: The curvature characteristic can be seen, and the distal aspect of the surfaces tapers slightly, while the mesial aspect is prominently curved. The cusplike thickening of the dental tubercle can be clearly seen, as can the marginal ridges and the medial ridge. Figure 4-19d shows both the mesial and the distal contact points as the widest convexity of the approximal surfaces.

The *maxillary lateral incisor (dens incisivus lateralis)* (Figs 4-22 and 4-23) has the same basic shape as the central incisor but is significantly smaller.

Its average dimensions are:

• Crown width (mesiodistal): 6.5 mm
• Crown depth (labiolingual): 6.0 mm
• Crown length: 10.0 mm
• Total apicocoronal length: 23.0 mm

Variations in form and size can be seen with this tooth. It is one of the teeth that is in the process of regression; it may sometimes be entirely absent. It can resemble a primary tooth; even pointed, peg, and pin shapes are possible. The dental tubercle may be developed into a separate lingual tubercle. The lateral incisor is rather shorter than the central incisor, but it is inclined mesially like the central incisor. It has a greater vestibular inclination than the central incisor. The second incisor is single-rooted with a distinctive root characteristic: The root is flattened in the mesiodistal direction and poorly developed with lateral longitudinal fissures, and the root canal is often deformed.

The *labial surface* is the same as that of the central incisor but smaller and more delicate with rounded edges and more pronounced curvature and angle characteristics.

The *lingual surface* has very pronounced marginal ridges and a distinctive tubercle. The surface often appears concave and undercut, especially if

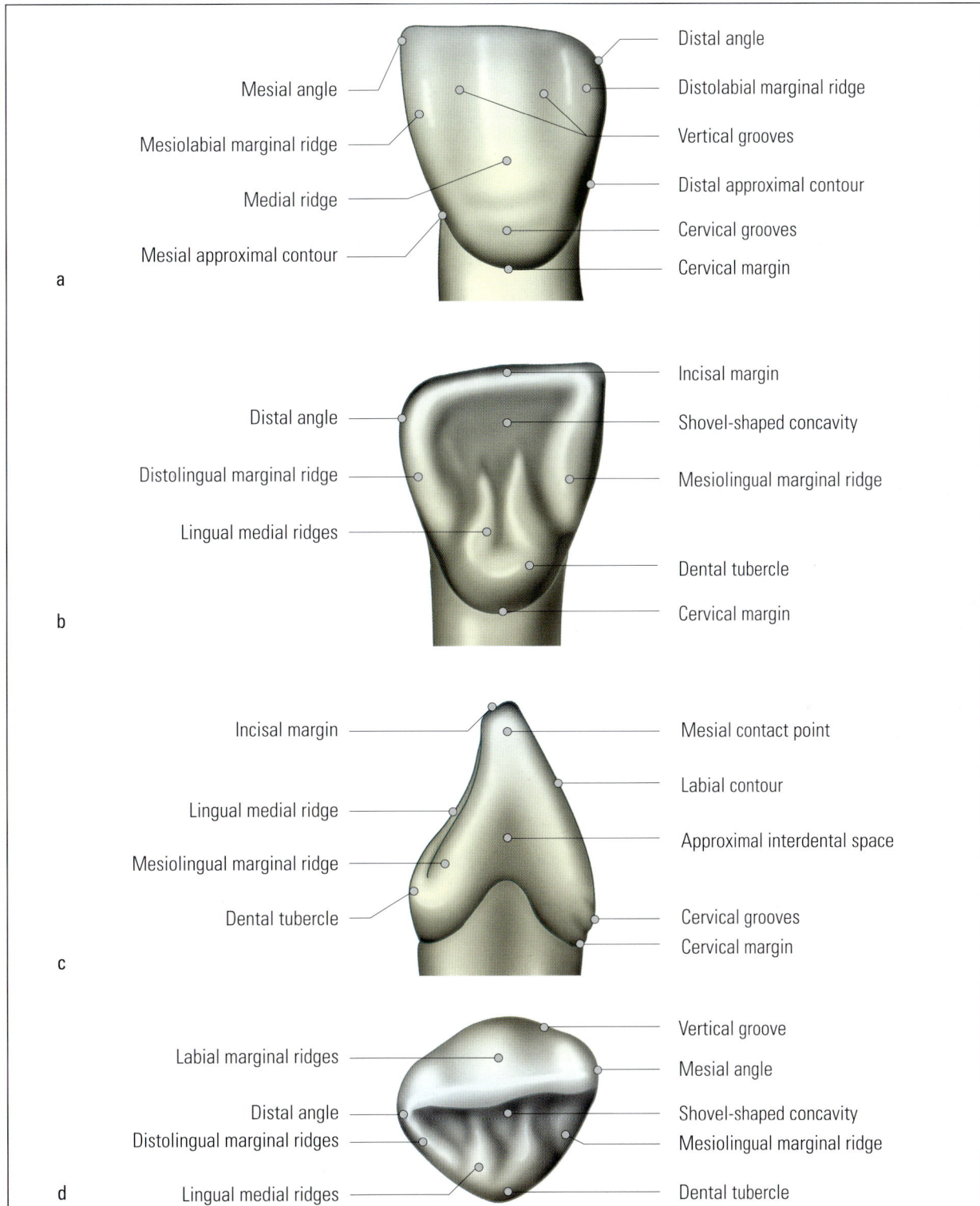

Fig 4-19 Morphology of the maxillary central incisor. *(a)* Labial view. *(b)* Lingual view. *(c)* Mesial approximal view. *(d)* Incisal view.

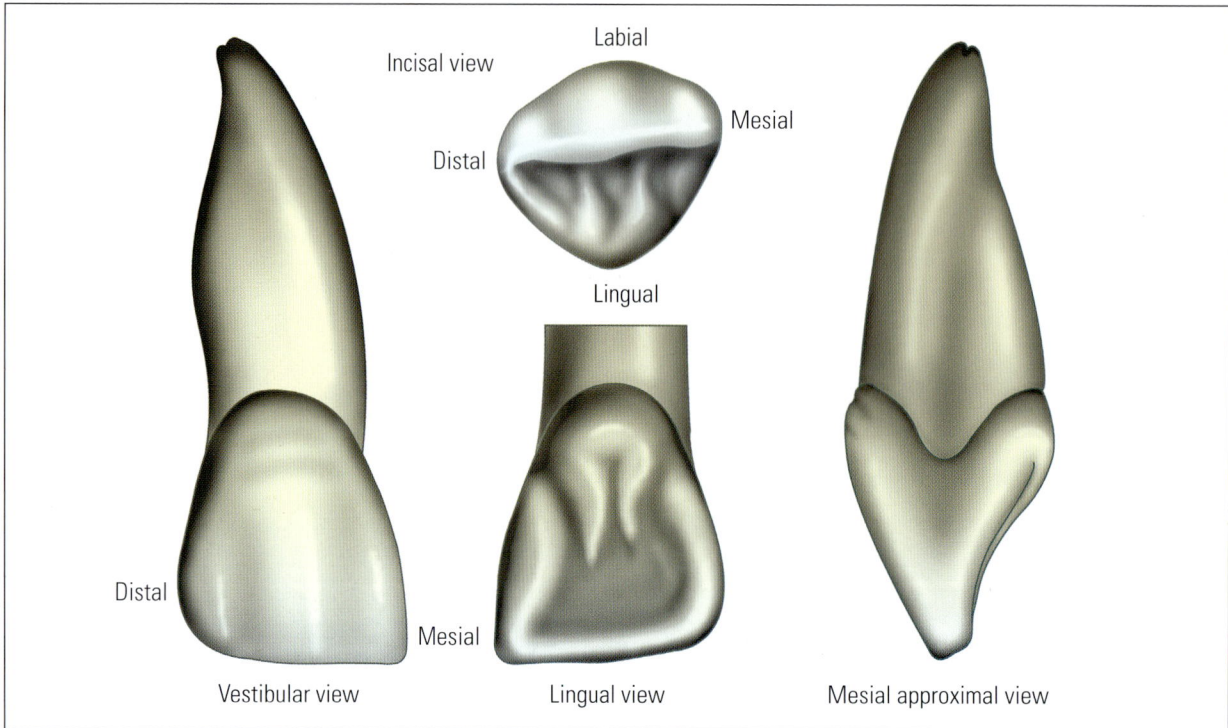

Incisal view
Labial
Distal
Mesial
Lingual

Distal
Mesial

Vestibular view

Lingual view

Mesial approximal view

Fig 4-20 Morphology of the maxillary right central incisor.

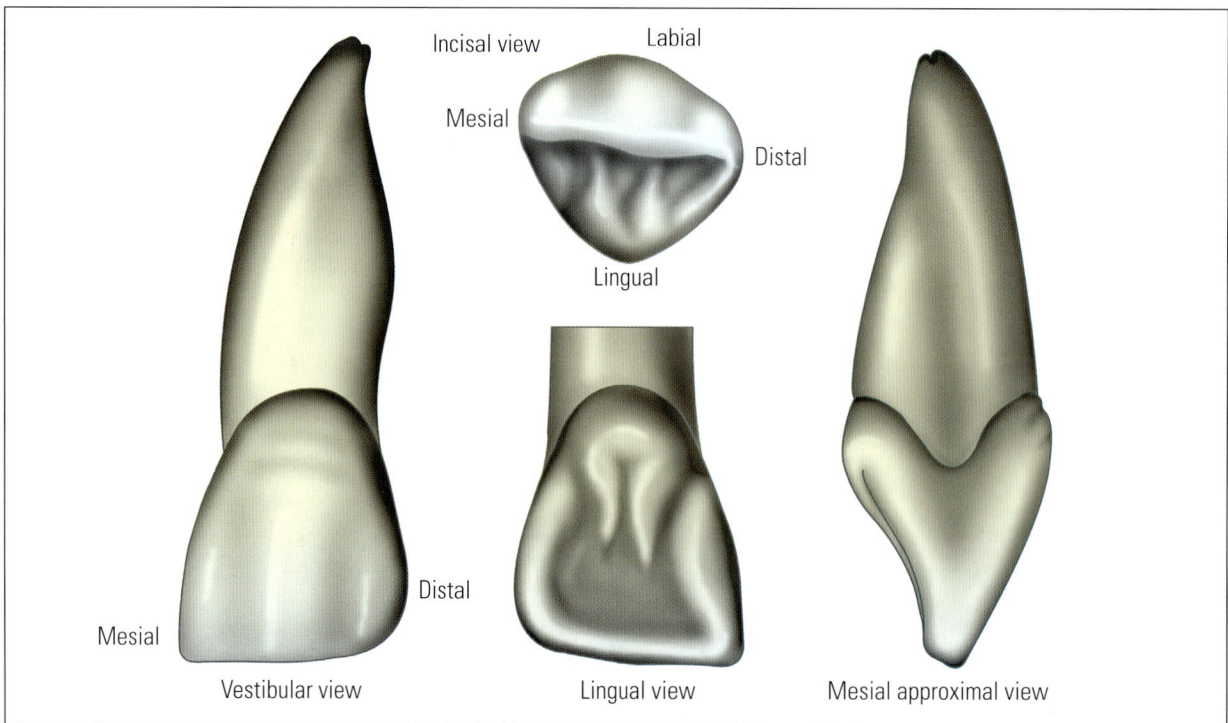

Incisal view
Labial
Mesial
Distal
Lingual

Mesial
Distal

Vestibular view

Lingual view

Mesial approximal view

Fig 4-21 Morphology of the maxillary left central incisor.

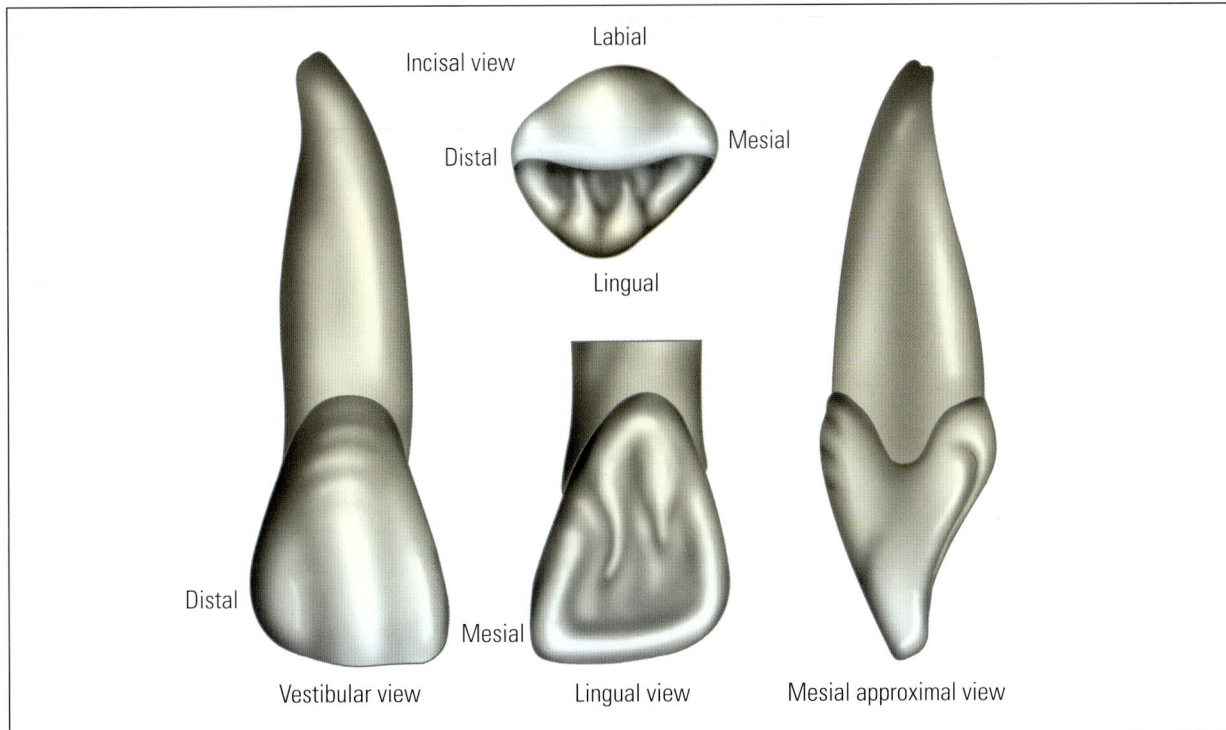

Fig 4-22 Morphology of the maxillary right lateral incisor.

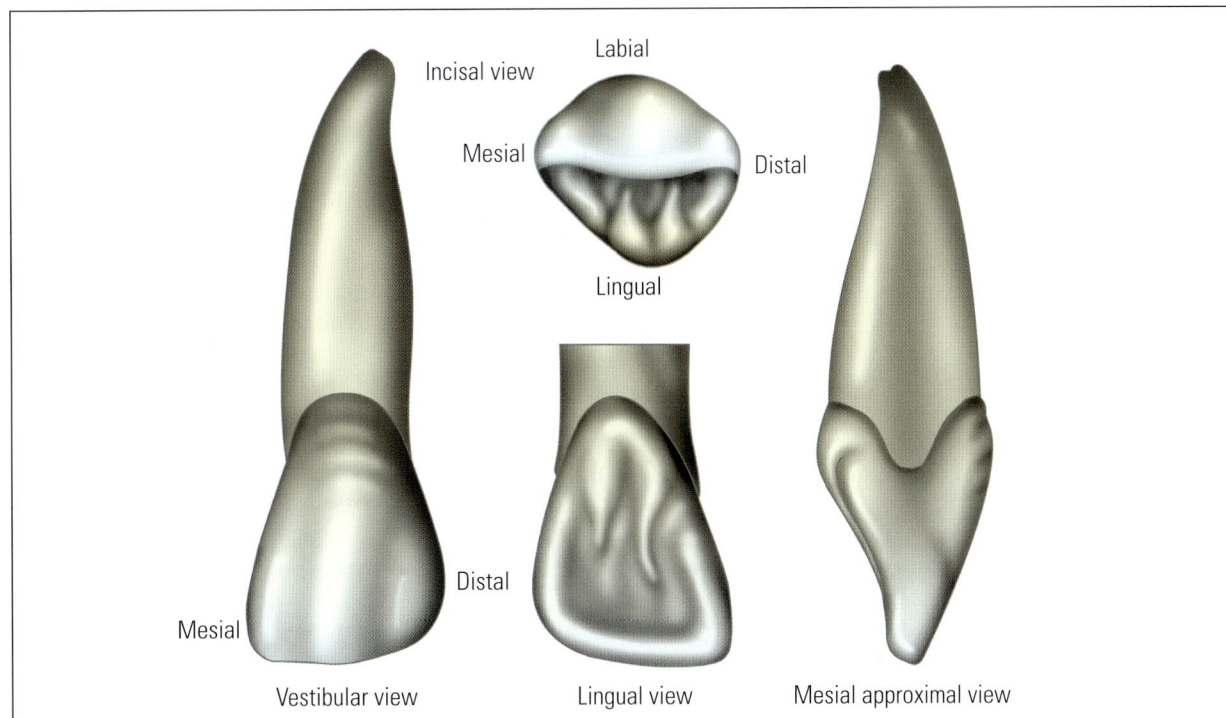

Fig 4-23 Morphology of the maxillary left lateral incisor.

the tubercle is very strongly developed and the surface is rather covered over. This is where caries often develops.

The *approximal surfaces* are markedly concave below the contact points, so that the labial surface appears strikingly triangular. Form variations in the lateral incisors are particularly noticeable in this view.

The *incisal view* shows a very rounded incisal margin, and all the curvatures are clearly visible.

Mandibular incisors

Mandibular incisors differ in size, with the central incisor being smaller than the lateral incisor. The roots of the mandibular incisors are so small and slender that they cannot be used as abutment teeth and should not have crowns placed on them. The size and morphology of these teeth are such that preparation of the tooth may damage the pulp.

The average dimensions of the *mandibular central incisor* are (Figs 4-24 and 4-25):

• Crown width (mesiodistal): 5.2 mm
• Crown depth (labiolingual): 6.0 mm
• Crown length: 9.0 mm
• Total apicocoronal length: 21.0 mm

The average dimensions of the *mandibular lateral incisor* are (Figs 4-26 and 4-27):

• Crown width (mesiodistal): 6.2 mm
• Crown depth (labiolingual): 6.5 mm
• Crown length: 9.5 mm
• Total apicocoronal length: 23.0 mm

In the case of the mandibular incisors, it is difficult to distinguish between left and right because only the lateral incisor has a trace of an angle characteristic. The horizontal curvature characteristic is insufficient on both teeth, but during manual fabrication, it can be constructed in the form of a more pronounced mesial marginal ridge. One possible distinguishing feature is the abrasion of the incisal margin: While the central incisor only has one wear facet, the lateral incisor has two wear facets because it has two antagonists. In addition, the incisal margin of some mandibular incisors is twisted in a distal direction in relation to the base of the crown.

The mandibular incisors need to exhibit a statically optimum chisel shape in order to perform their function because even the sturdy mandibular lateral incisor is generally smaller than the maxillary lateral incisor. This is also why the lingual surfaces are slightly concave. The prominent curvatures and convexities of the individual surfaces are poorly developed in comparison with those of the maxillary teeth.

The incisal margins have minimal mamelons shortly after eruption, similar to the maxillary teeth. These are soon abraded so that the edges are straight and level. This makes it even more difficult to distinguish between right and left. The contact points lie immediately incisally because of the abrasion of the incisal margins.

The *vestibular (labial) surfaces* of both teeth are almost smooth. There are traces of vertical grooves or cervical grooves. The triangular chisel shape of the vestibular surfaces and the straight incisal margin mean that the transition from incisal margin to approximal surface follows an acutely angled course mesially as well as distally. An angle characteristic is only partially present on the lateral incisor. The cervix is narrow and tapers sharply. The distal approximal margin is slightly drawn in compared with the mesial edge.

The *lingual surfaces* have the same basic shape but are slightly narrower. They are rather concave with a trace of marginal and medial ridges. The dental tubercle is less pronounced. The labiolingual diameter at the base of the mandibular incisor crown is greater than the width at the cutting edge.

The *approximal surfaces* are virtually the same size mesially and distally. They are extremely narrow in the incisal area and wider cervically, in keeping with the slender chisel shape. The slight vertical curvature of the labial surfaces and the slight depression in the lingual surfaces over the tubercle can be clearly seen. The cervical lines bend in an incisal direction.

The *incisal views* show the larger labiolingual diameter in contrast to the mesiodistal crown width. The basic incisal shape is oval without any appreciable curvature characteristics. The contact surfaces may be slightly depressed. On the lateral incisor, the cutting edge is twisted in relation to the base of the crown, so that the distal incisal edge lies posterior to the mesial one.

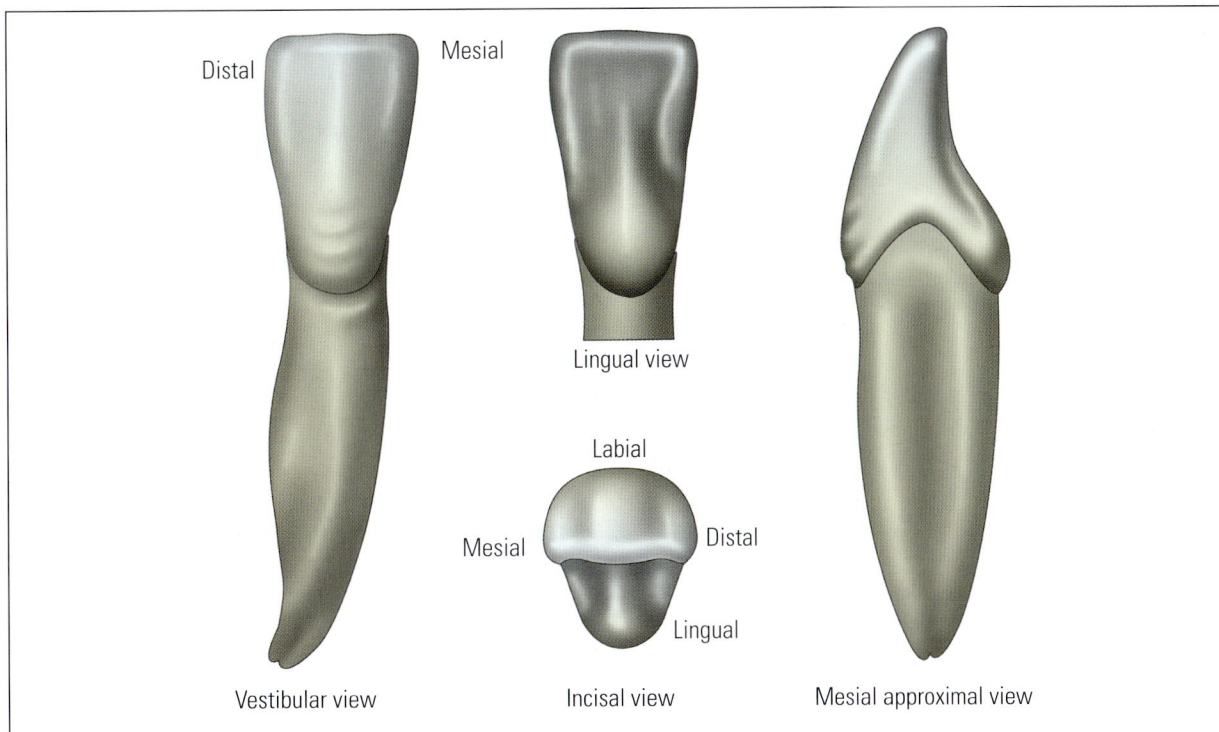

Distal   Mesial

Lingual view

Labial

Mesial   Distal

Lingual

Vestibular view   Incisal view   Mesial approximal view

Fig 4-24 Morphology of the mandibular right central incisor.

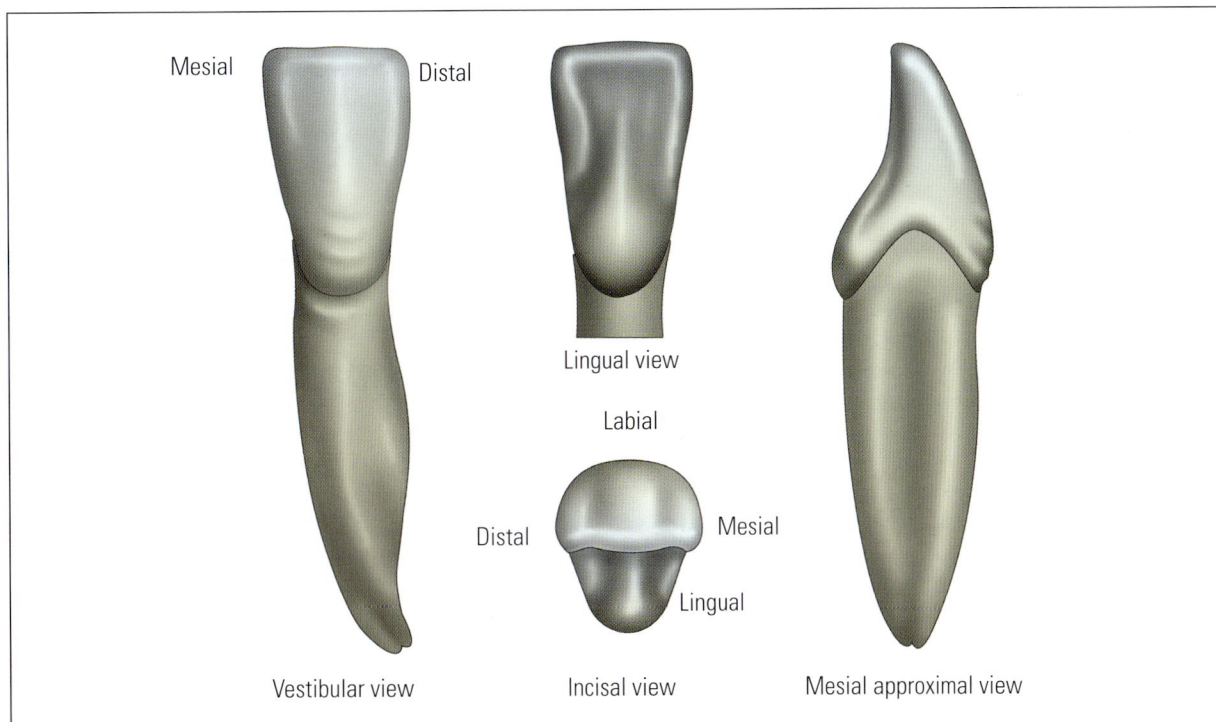

Mesial   Distal

Lingual view

Labial

Distal   Mesial

Lingual

Vestibular view   Incisal view   Mesial approximal view

Fig 4-25 Morphology of the mandibular left central incisor.

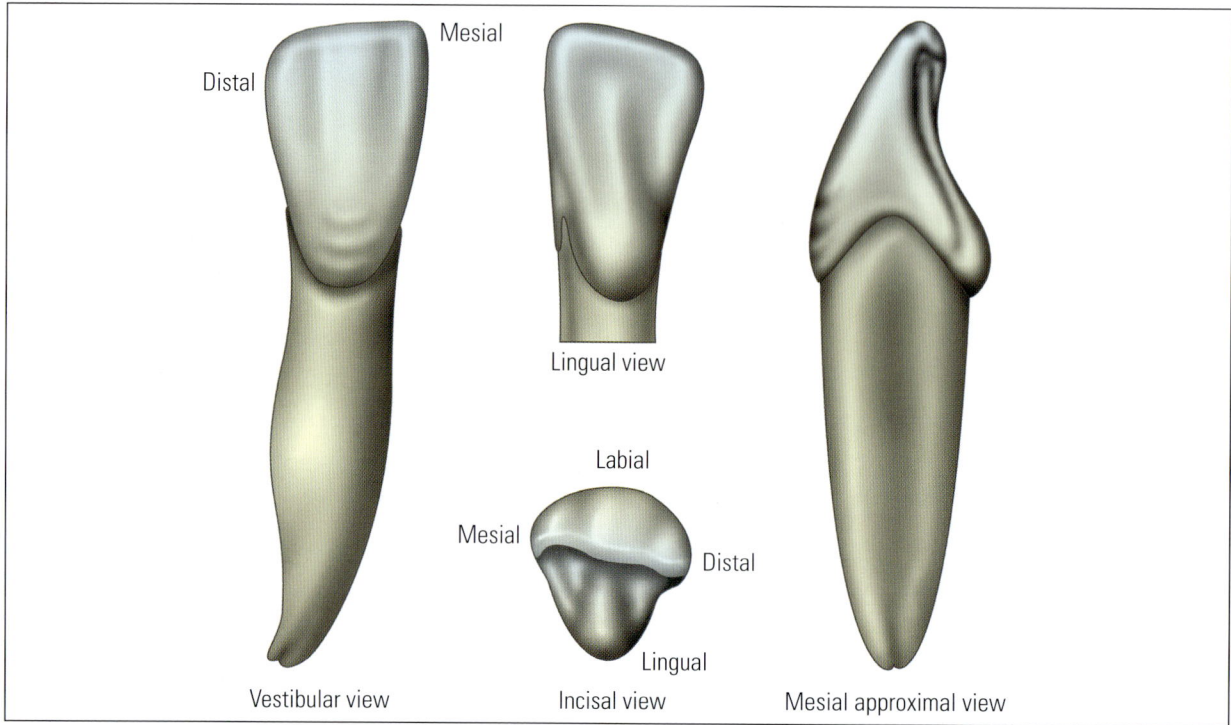

Fig 4-26 Morphology of the mandibular right lateral incisor.

Distal / Mesial — Vestibular view

Lingual view

Labial / Mesial / Distal / Lingual — Incisal view

Mesial approximal view

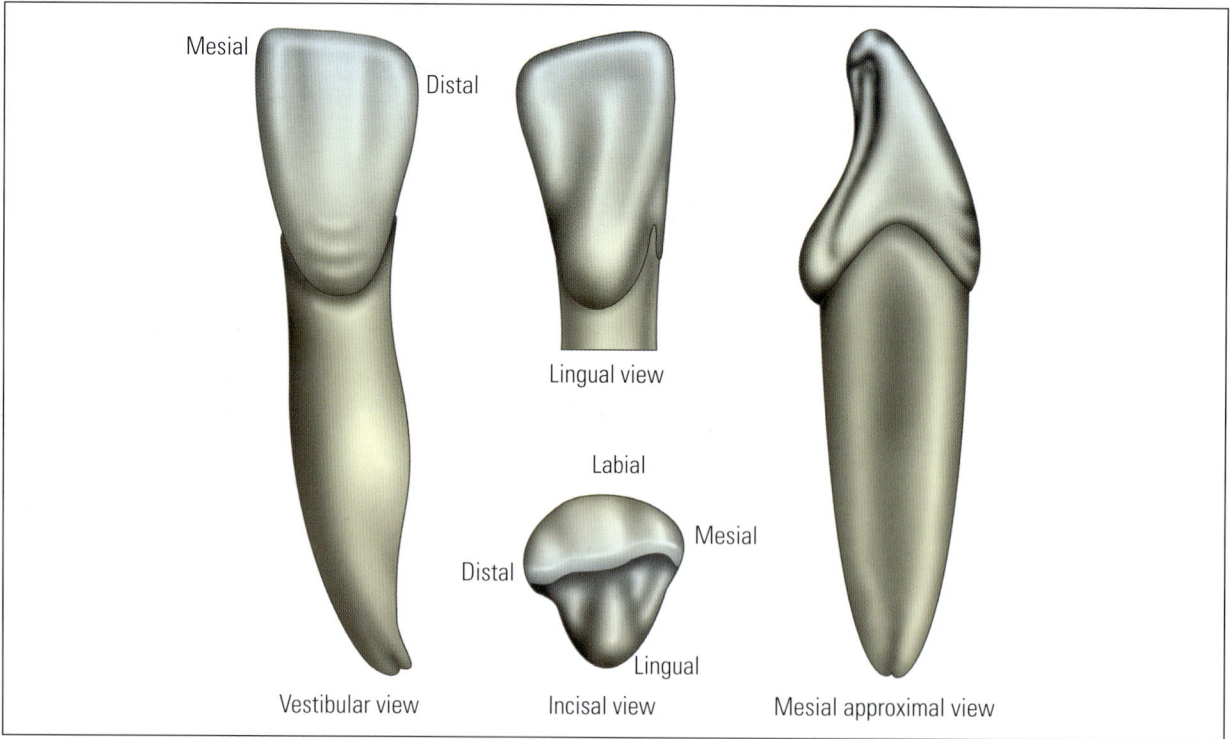

Fig 4-27 Morphology of the mandibular left lateral incisor.

Mesial / Distal — Vestibular view

Lingual view

Labial / Distal / Mesial / Lingual — Incisal view

Mesial approximal view

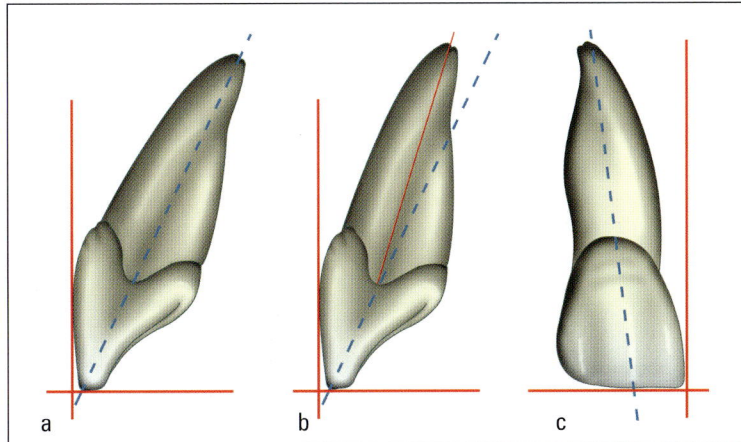

Fig 4-28 *(a)* Crown and root axes are aligned and form the tooth axis; if the crown axis is not in line, adverse lever actions may arise and loosen the tooth in the tooth bed. *(b)* Viewed approximally, the maxillary central incisor is inclined in a vestibular direction; its labial contour stands vertically. *(c)* Viewed labially, the central incisor is inclined in a mesial direction.

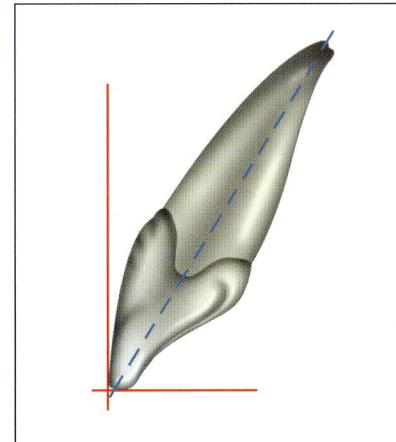

Fig 4-29 The maxillary lateral incisor is slightly more inclined in the vestibular direction than the central incisor; its labial contour does not stand vertically.

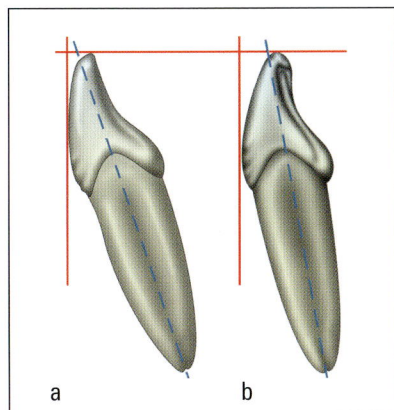

Fig 4-30 Both mandibular incisors lean in a vestibular direction; the labial contour of the central tooth stands vertically *(a)*, while that of the lateral tooth is inclined lingually *(b)*.

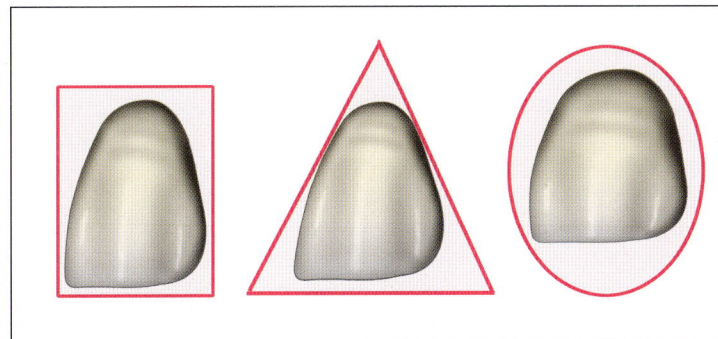

Fig 4-31 The labial surface of the incisors may harmonize with the shape of the face. There are three basic types: rectangular, triangular, and oval.

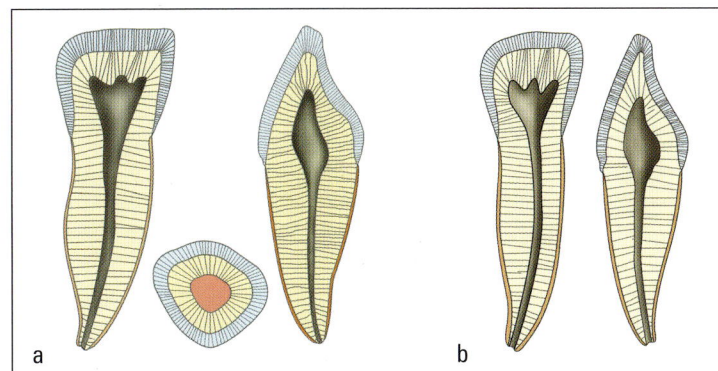

Fig 4-32 *(a)* The maxillary incisors are single-rooted with a pronounced root characteristic; the root bends distally. *(b)* Cross sections of a mandibular incisor. The cross sections show the normal distribution of tooth substance. The pulp cavity is widened in the coronal area.

Figures 4-28 to 4-32 show the inclinations of the tooth axes of both maxillary and mandibular incisors as well as details of their morphology.

Canines

Dens caninus means dog's tooth (*canis* = dog); dens angularis from *angulus* = angle or corner; dens cuspidatus = single-cusp tooth from *cuspis* = cusp, protuberance.

The canine resembles a fang in dogs, which is the origin of its name. The maxillary canine is often popularly known as the "eye tooth" because inflammation affecting the canine root (periapical processes) causes swelling around the eyes.

The **maxillary canine (dens caninus maxillae)** (Figs 4-33 to 4-35) has a long, sturdy root with a stress-resistant periodontium. The root apex is slightly curved distally, reflecting the root characteristic. The pulp cavity widens in the coronal region. Viewed approximally, it is noticeable that the labiopalatal diameter is largest at the cervix. This gives the tooth its statically favorable chisel shape.

The maxillary canine is an excellent abutment and clasp tooth for partial dentures because of its position and its sturdy shape. It should be retained as long as possible. Despite resection of the root apex (apicectomy), ie, the tooth being nonvital, it can still be retained as a load-bearing abutment for a long time (eg, in a partial denture construction). Its periodontium is particularly stress resistant because a large number of fibrous bundles are arranged crosswise and radially, securing the tooth against transverse masticatory forces and torsion. It serves to grasp (and tear) food. The canine is a rudimentary fang that has regressed as a result of functional adaptation; thus, the canine and the premolars are instinctively used to bite tough food.

The average dimensions of the maxillary canine are:

- Incisal crown width (mesiodistal): 7.6 mm
- Cervical crown width (mesiodistal): 6.0 mm
- Crown depth (labiolingual, cervical): 8.0 mm
- Crown length: 11.0 mm
- Total apicocoronal length: 27.0 mm

The **vestibular surface** (see Fig 4-33a) exhibits the striking angular form: The cutting edge is made up of two sides of differing length inclined toward each other. The mesial side is shorter and does not recede as steeply as the longer distal side. The transitions between the cutting edge and the approximal surfaces thus lie at different heights: The mesial edge is shifted incisally, while the distal edge is displaced in a cervical direction; the mesial contact point is displaced more toward the incisal. One angle characteristic can be identified because the distal transition of the incisal margin is clearly rounded, unlike the sharp-edged mesial transition.

From the tip of the incisal edge, the sturdy medial ridge runs cervically as it changes into the prominent transverse convexity of the cervix. Poorly developed cervical grooves are found here. The medial ridge divides the labial surface into a narrow mesial and a broad distal facet. The horizontal curvature of the canine is strongly developed, with both facets receding from the central ridge to the adjacent teeth. Both facets contain a distinct marginal ridge in the vertical direction.

The neck of the tooth is arched and contains the strong vertical curvature to protect the marginal periodontium. The approximal edges run closely together from the contact points in a cervical direction; in the middle, the distal approximal edge is rather concave centrally, whereas the mesial edge runs virtually straight.

The **mesial approximal surface** (see Fig 4-33b) exhibits the pronounced wedge shape of the canine. The mesial incisal edge lies inferior to the tip of the tooth. The vertical convexities of the vestibular and lingual surfaces that protect the marginal periodontium can be seen. While the vestibular convexity runs evenly incisocervically, the lingual surface in the cervical third bends inward and only achieves the outer convexity through the tubercle. The heavy tubercle gives the tooth its bulky appearance. The cervical margin curves in an incisal direction. The tip of the canine lies centrally in relation to the base of the crown. Weak cervical grooves can be seen labially.

The **lingual surface** (see Fig 4-33c) is smaller than the labial surface but with the same basic triangular shape. The tubercle is strongly developed. The marginal ridges are very prominent, as is a central ridge starting from the tubercle. This ridge is described as the *canine guidance ridge* because it is here that a certain guidance of the opposing teeth (antagonists) takes place during mandibular movement. The distal marginal ridge is developed into a strong masticatory edge incisally. The central ridge develops cusplike into the incisal tip, which approximates to a masticatory

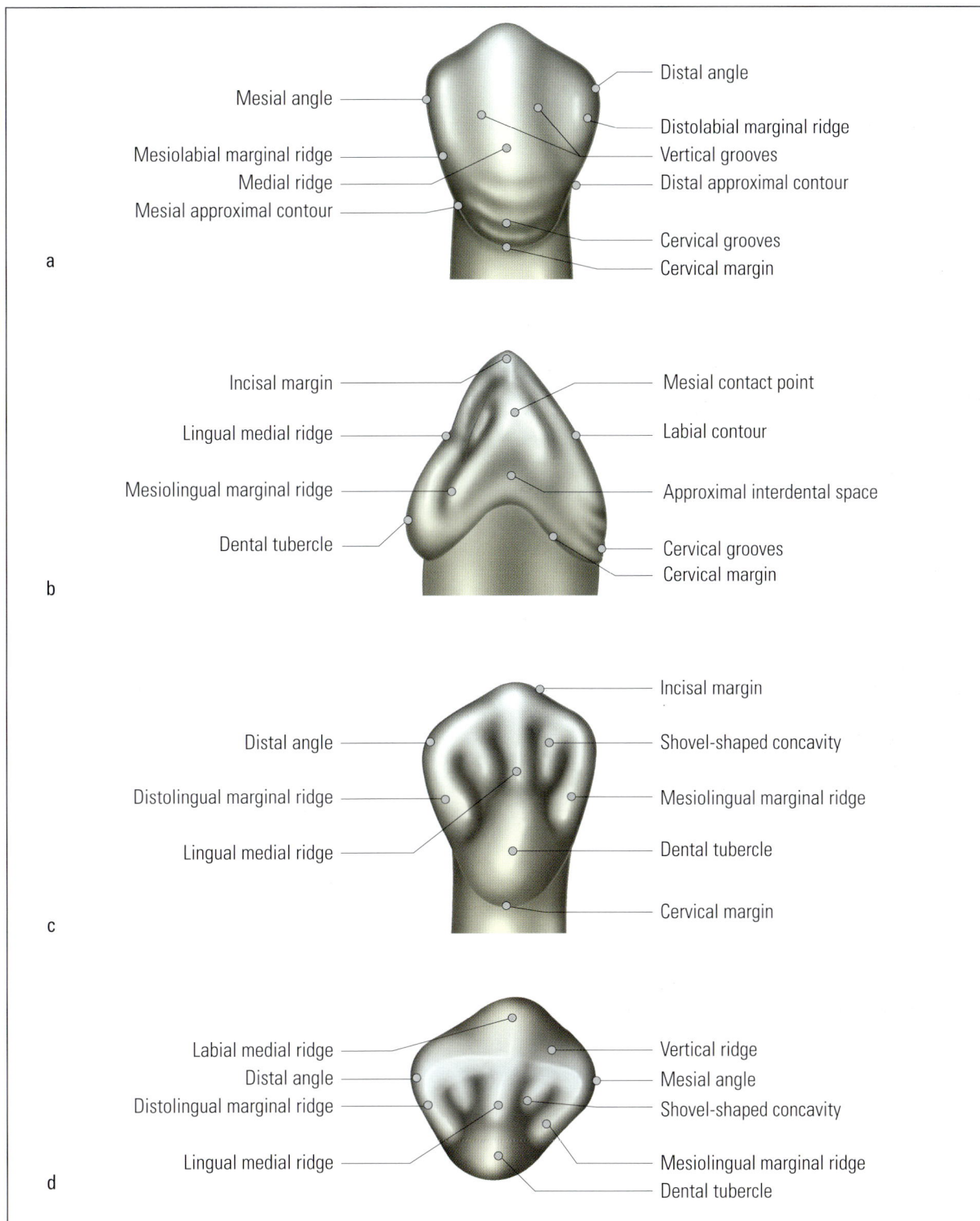

Fig 4-33 Morphology of the maxillary canine. *(a)* Labial view. *(b)* Mesial approximal view. *(c)* Lingual view. *(d)* Incisal view.

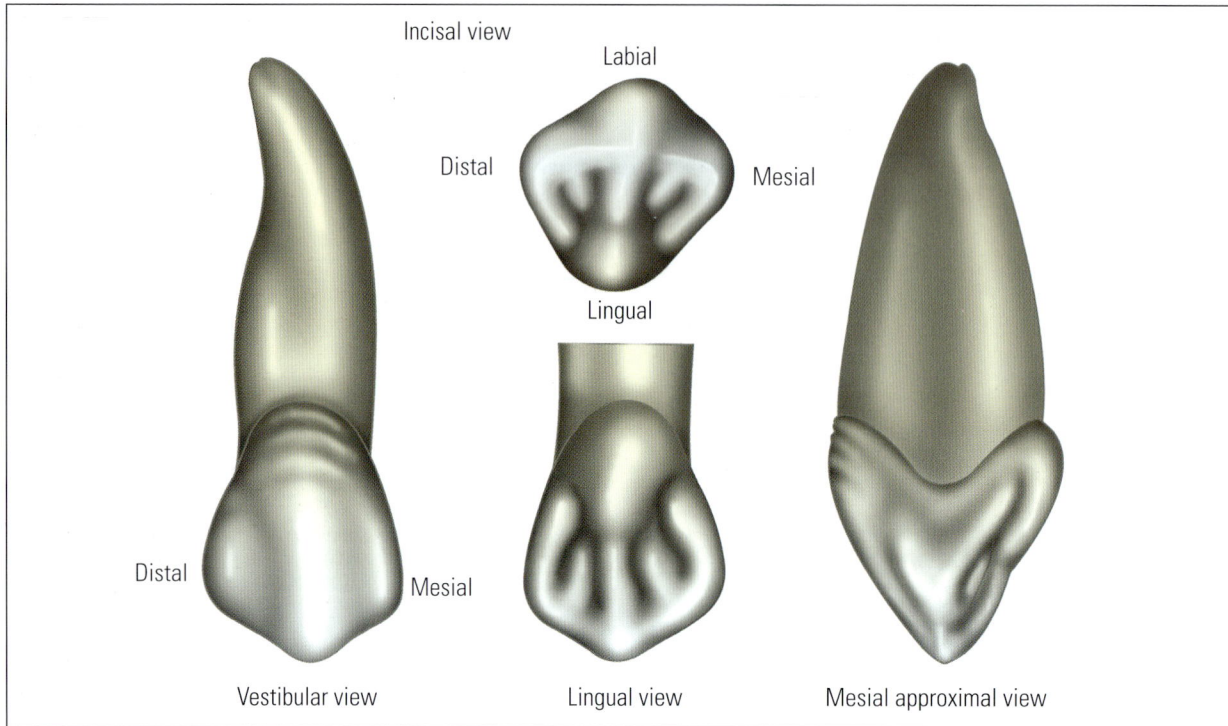

Fig 4-34 Morphology of the maxillary right canine.

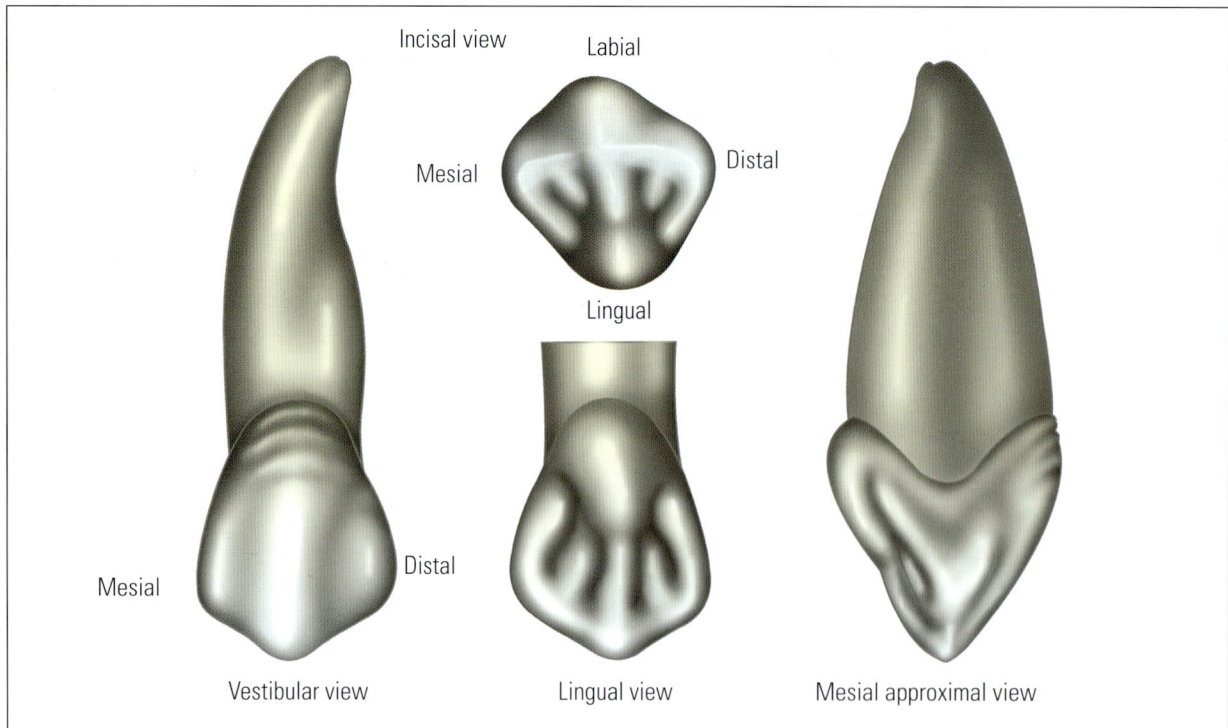

Fig 4-35 Morphology of the maxillary left canine.

surface in the distal portion of the crown. The cervical line is arched, and the tooth bulges out below the line to protect the gingiva.

The *incisal view* of the maxillary canine (see Fig 4-33d) shows the strongly developed curvature characteristic, ie, the mesial facet is narrower than the distal, and both facets recede laterally, following the curvature of the dental arch. The strong medial ridge can be seen labially, and the cusplike tubercle is visible palatally.

The *approximal surfaces* are acutely angled mesially and slightly curved distally. A gentle internal curvature of the distal approximal surface serves as the contact area to the premolar. The incisal margin is curved in line with the curvature characteristic and in the distal portion is wider than the masticatory edge.

The *mandibular canine (dens caninus mandibulae)* (Figs 4-36 and 4-37) resembles the maxillary canine in all characteristics; in terms of form and function, the canines bear the closest resemblance to each other of any teeth. However, the mandibular canine is much more slender and narrower than the maxillary canine, both in the crown and in the root. It has a stronger angle characteristic, with the distal transition from the incisal margin to the approximal surface located more apically than the mesial. Its root is not only much shorter, but in some cases it can be divided: The tooth may even become two-rooted. The stronger horizontal curvature characteristic is also evident; the canine tip generally is in line with the middle of the crown base. The tip of the mandibular canine abrades the tubercle and palatal medial ridge of the maxillary canine, and the teeth show corresponding wear facets.

The average dimensions of the mandibular canine are:

• Crown width (mesiodistal): 6.4 mm
• Crown depth (labiolingual): 7.8 mm
• Crown length: 11.4 mm
• Total apicocoronal length: 25.4 mm

The *vestibular surface* shows the typical canine shape but is narrower at the contact points in comparison with the maxillary canine; the approximal edges do not run parallel. The mesial incisal margin is shorter and higher than the distal margin, which also recedes more sharply than in the maxillary canine. This means that the distal approximal surface is extremely small. The medial ridge, marginal ridges, vertical grooves, and cervical grooves are prominent. The horizontal transverse convexity is more pronounced on the mandibular than on the maxillary canine.

The *lingual surface* is not as strongly developed and is less concave than in the maxillary tooth. There is a weak medial ridge, hardly any marginal ridges, and a very flattened dental tubercle; variations in ridge formation are very rare.

From the *mesial approximal view*, the crown appears to be inclined lingually. However, the tip of the mandibular canine, like that of the corresponding maxillary tooth, is aligned with the midline of the crown base. The appearance of an incline results from the flattened dental tubercle and the vertical curvature of the labial surface.

The *incisal view* shows the stronger horizontal curvature of the labial surface. The lingual surface appears to taper considerably, and the approximal surfaces are depressed. The incisal margin is more strongly angled than in the maxillary canine; ie, the mesial edge faces the anterior teeth, while the distal edge is far more curved toward the posterior teeth. The strong development of the labiolingual diameter at the crown base is noticeable.

Figures 4-38 to 4-40 show the inclinations of the tooth axes of both maxillary and mandibular canines as well as details of their morphology.

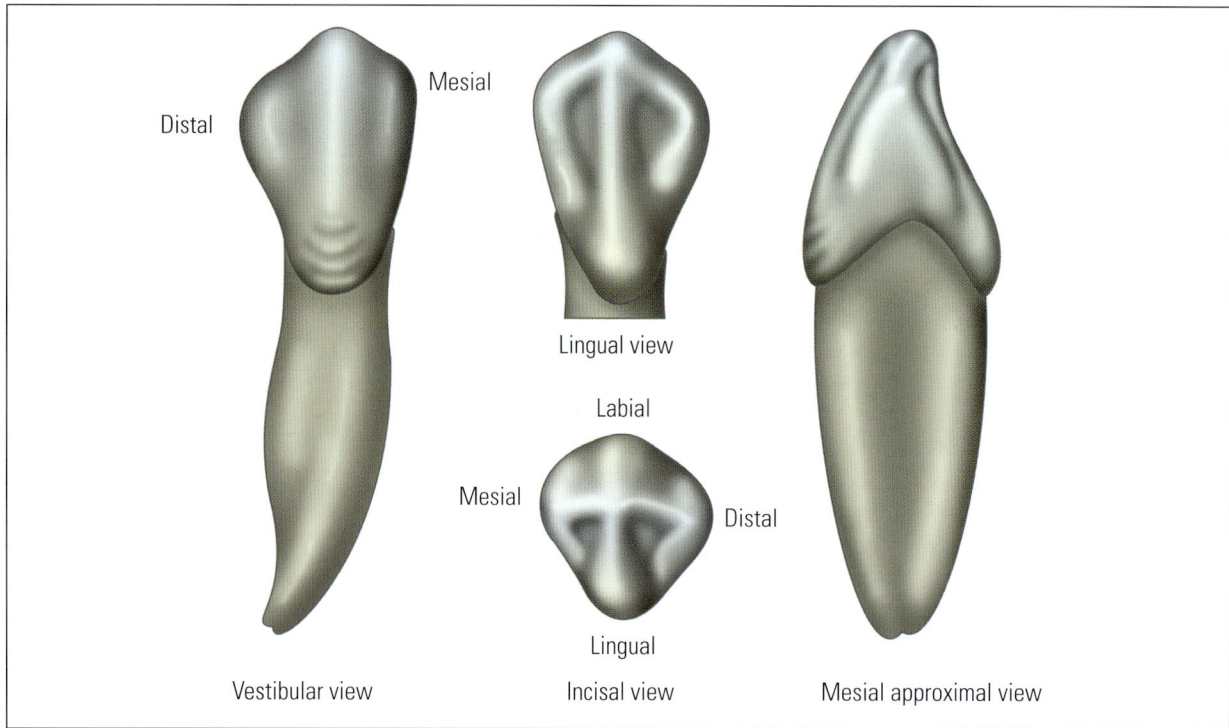

Fig 4-36 Morphology of the mandibular right canine.

Distal / Mesial / Vestibular view

Lingual view

Labial / Mesial / Distal / Lingual / Incisal view

Mesial approximal view

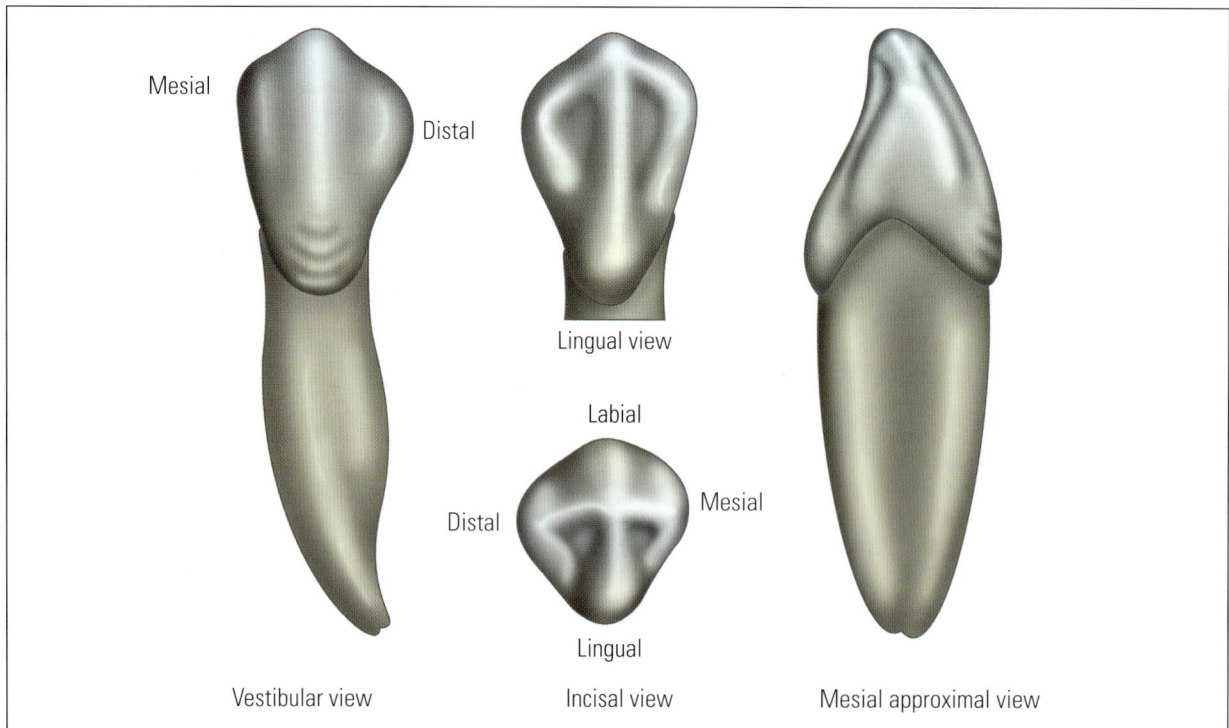

Fig 4-37 Morphology of the mandibular left canine.

Mesial / Distal / Vestibular view

Lingual view

Labial / Distal / Mesial / Lingual / Incisal view

Mesial approximal view

Fig 4-38 The maxillary *(a and b)* and mandibular *(c and d)* canines, viewed labially *(a and c)*, are inclined slightly in the mesial direction; viewed approximally, the mandibular canine *(d)* stands vertically, while the maxillary canine *(b)* is markedly inclined in the vestibular direction; its labial contour is roughly vertical.

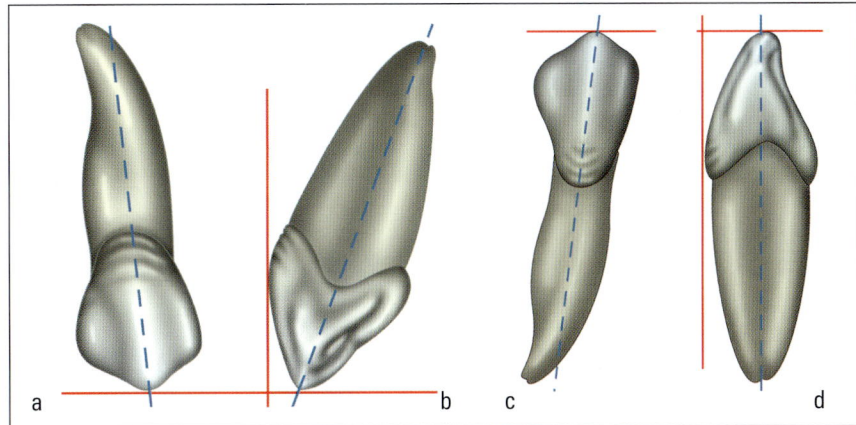

Fig 4-39 The occlusion of the canines, viewed from the vestibular *(a)* and approximal *(b)* aspects, showing the inclinations of the axes. The maxillary canine overlaps the mandibular canine because the former is inclined vestibularly while the latter stands vertically. Both teeth have a slight mesial incline.

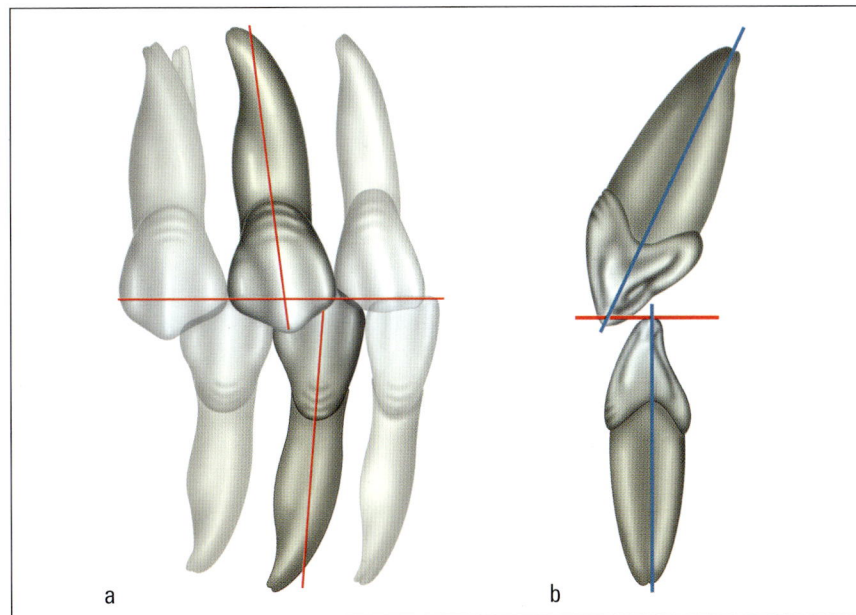

Fig 4-40 *(a)* The maxillary canines are single-rooted and have a pronounced root characteristic. *(b)* The mandibular canines generally are also single-rooted, although the root is often bifurcated. The cross sections show the normal distribution of substance. The pulp cavity of the coronal portion widens into the upper portion of the root.

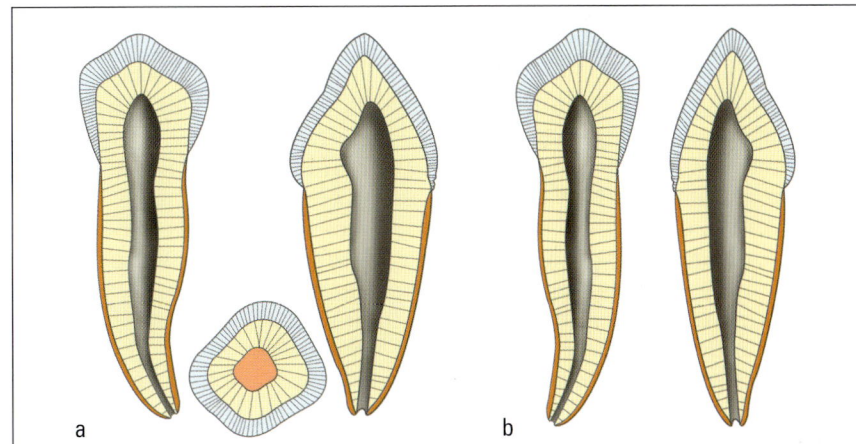

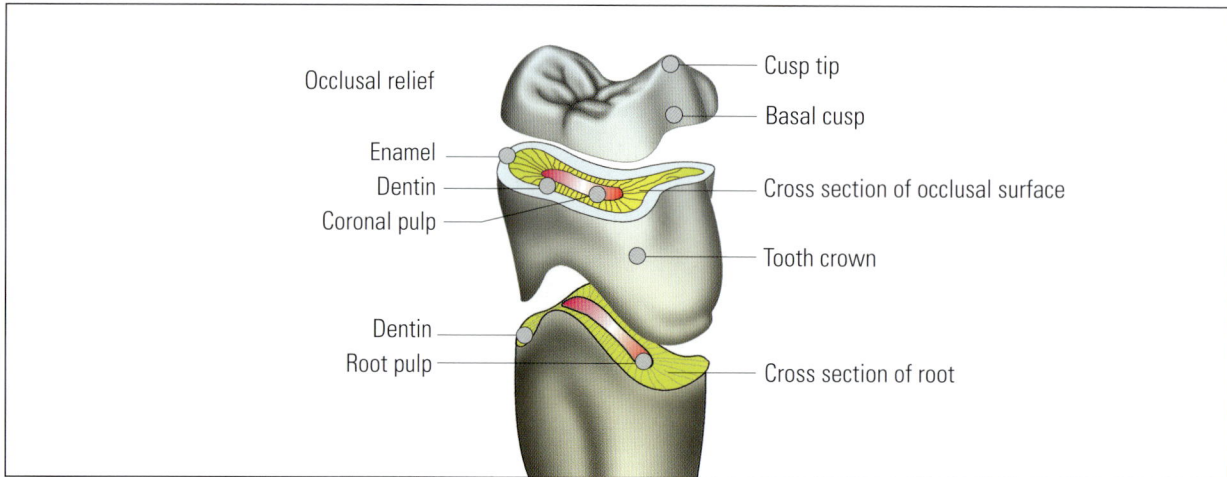

Fig 4-41 Schematic diagram of a premolar divided into horizontal layers.

Posterior Teeth

Occlusal surfaces

Before the individual teeth are described in detail, features common to the posterior teeth are examined.

One common feature is the masticatory or occlusal surfaces *(facies occlusalis)*, ie, the whole occlusal relief with its cusps, grooves, and fossae (Figs 4-41 to 4-43). The specific arrangement, in this case the particular shape of the occlusal surface, develops according to the rule of form and function and should be reproduced in all prosthetic teeth to maximize masticatory function.

Parts of the occlusal surface

Cusps (cuspides dentis) are the elevations on a masticatory surface made up of several surface components; they form the basic structure of the occlusal surface. Their arrangement on the cross section of the crown determines the shape of the tooth. A distinction is made between the basal part and the tip of the cusp. Cusps are classified as crushing or shearing, depending on their function. The crushing cusps of a tooth lie lingually in the maxilla and buccally in the mandible and are referred to as *supporting cusps.* The shearing cusps lie buccally in the maxilla and lingually in

the mandible and are known as *nonsupporting cusps*.

The **cusp tip** forms the contact with the opposing teeth and takes on the actual cusp function of a contact and supporting cusp. There is a varying degree of intercuspation of occluding teeth, depending on the height of the cusp tip. The cusp tips of an occlusal surface are always displaced toward the middle of the occlusal surface, and the masticatory surfaces are always drawn in at the cusp tips. The widest circumference of a tooth with masticatory surfaces is always below the occlusal surface.

The **triangular ridges** are triangle-shaped enamel ridges that run mesially and distally from the cusp tips, along which the cusp tips of the opposing teeth slide during chewing. They are therefore the working surfaces (sliding surfaces) of a cusp for the opposing teeth.

The **cusp crest** or inner cusp slope runs as a ridge of enamel from the cusp tip centrally to the middle of the tooth and divides the triangular ridges.

The **cusp slopes** are ridges of enamel receding in a lingual or buccal direction, which run from the cusp tip to the outer surface of the tooth and thus define the buccal or lingual contour of the tooth. They are the external equivalents of the cusp crests.

The **cusp ridges** are angular enamel ridges that run around the whole occlusal surface from buc-

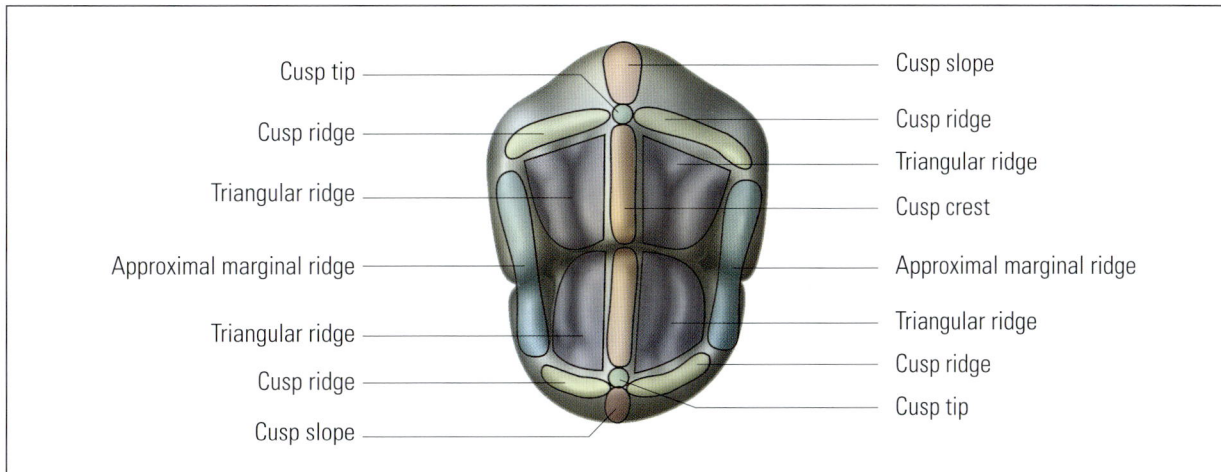

Fig 4-42 Parts of an occlusal surface.

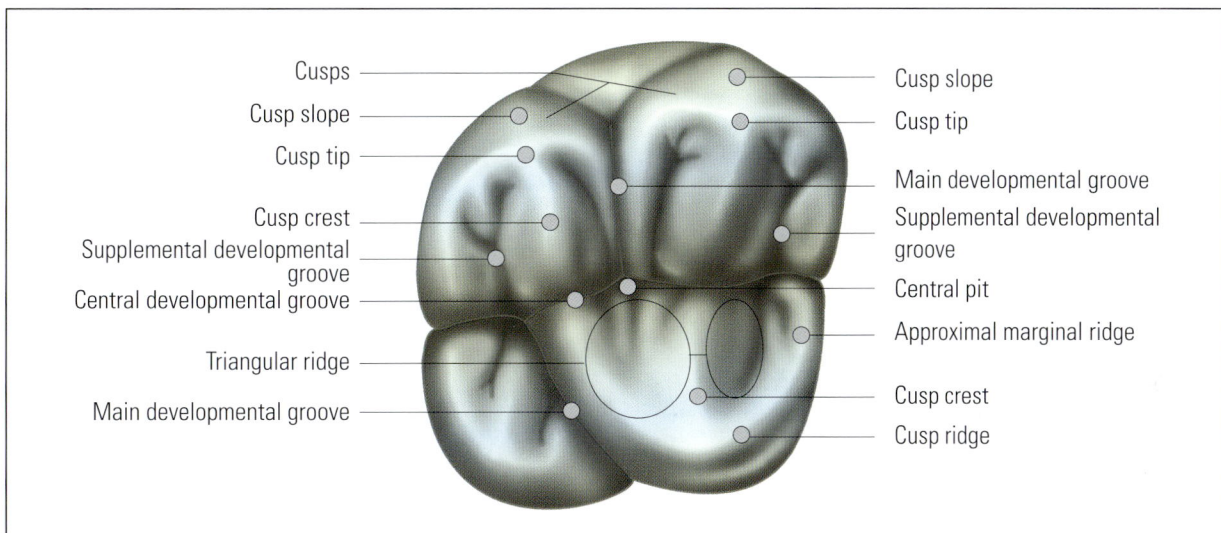

Fig 4-43 Morphology of the maxillary first molar.

cal to lingual and join the cusp tips. In the approximal area, they form the marginal ridges.

The ***approximal marginal ridges*** are the most strongly developed enamel crests of the cusp ridge in the approximal areas. The marginal ridges of adjacent teeth form the interdental embrasure into which the cusp tips of the opposing teeth insert. The approximal marginal ridges thus form the contact with the adjacent tooth but also the functional surface for the opposing teeth.

The ***central developmental groove*** (longitudinal groove; *fissura longitudinalis*) separates the buccal from the lingual cusps. It runs as a deep fissure distomesially, centrally over the occlusal surface, and parallel to the dental arch.

The ***main developmental groove*** (transverse groove; *fissura transversalis*) separates the mesial from the distal cusps in teeth with multiple cusps. It crosses the central groove, running from lingual to buccal or vice versa. Grooves are glide paths for cusps and allow crushed food to flow away.

The **central fossa** or pit *(fovea centralis)* is a deep depression in the middle of the occlusal surface on teeth with multiple cusps, where several cusp crests run together. Central fossae or pits are the preferred sites for the development of caries.

Supplemental or accessory developmental grooves are deep fissures that separate the approximal marginal ridges from the cusps. The central developmental groove branches at the marginal ridges to form distinct supplemental grooves. Deep fossae or pits *(fovea mesialis and distalis)* form in the mesial and distal branching points.

The occlusal surfaces interlock. Reference is made to the cusp-fossa relationship, where a supporting cusp rests in the occlusal fossae of the opposing tooth or on two opposing marginal ridges and where the mandibular posterior teeth are displaced by half a cusp-width.

The cusp surfaces are inclined toward the occlusal plane; this is a theoretical plane in which the occlusal surfaces meet in terminal occlusion. When the occlusal relief is deep and the cusp is steep, this angle of cusp inclination is large; it can vary between 20 and 40 degrees.

Maxillary premolars

Premolars *(dentes praemolaris: prae* = in front of / before, *mola* = mill[stone]; *dentes bicuspidati: bi* = two, *cuspis* = eminence or cusp, bicuspid tooth).

Premolars (and molars) are located in the lateral areas of the dental arch, ie, in the cheek area (bucca), and are known as *posterior, back,* or *lateral teeth.* The premolars have a chewing or masticatory surface instead of a chewing edge. This surface is formed by the pronounced development of the dental tubercle into a genuine cusp. Cusps are referred to as buccal or lingual. Premolars are used to roughly chew food. With tough food, they are instinctively used to hold and bite the food.

The **maxillary first premolar** *(dens praemolaris medialis)* (Fig 4-44) usually has a divided root apex, and in some cases there may be two roots. Very rarely three root apices may be found. A buccal and palatal (lingual) root can be distinguished with independent, very branched root canals, which makes root canal treatment very difficult.

The average dimensions of the maxillary first premolar are:

• Crown width (mesiodistal): 6.5 mm
• Crown depth (buccolingual): 7.8 mm
• Crown length: 8.0 mm
• Total apicocoronal length: 20.5 mm

The **vestibular (buccal) surface** strongly resembles the labial surface of the canine but is slightly smaller. Curvature and angle characteristics are reversed. The medial ridge is displaced distally, the mesiobuccal cusp ridge is longer than the distal, and the mesial facet is larger than the distal. The cervical margin is curved apically, and cervical grooves are present.

The **lingual surface** is smaller than the vestibular surface and more curved; the horizontal curvature is more pronounced and more rounded. The medial ridge and the lingual cusp are displaced mesially so that the distolingual cusp ridge appears longer. The cervical line is curved buccally.

The **approximal surface** is almost rectangular. The contours of the buccal, lingual, and occlusal surfaces can be seen. The vestibular surface contour displays the vertical curvature characteristic: The greatest curvature is at the cervix in order to protect the marginal periodontium. The lingual surface contour is evenly rounded. The occlusal surface contour shows the higher, more angular buccal cusp and the smaller, rounded lingual cusp. The contact points lie directly below the marginal ridges. The cervical line runs slightly toward the masticatory surface.

The **occlusal surface** (masticatory or chewing surface) has an oval outline and is wider buccally and rounded and narrower palatally. The horizontal curvature characteristic is reversed. The cusps are located on half of the buccal and lingual portions of the masticatory surface. The buccal cusp is larger, higher, and more angular, with prominent triangular ridges, cusp ridges, and crests, whereas the lingual cusp is rounded and looks more delicate. There may be displacement of the tip of the lingual cusp distally and the central developmental groove lingually. The central developmental groove branches before the marginal ridges into two small supplemental developmental grooves running crosswise, giving the whole groove formation the appearance of a broad H. Growth-related fossae are formed in the branch-

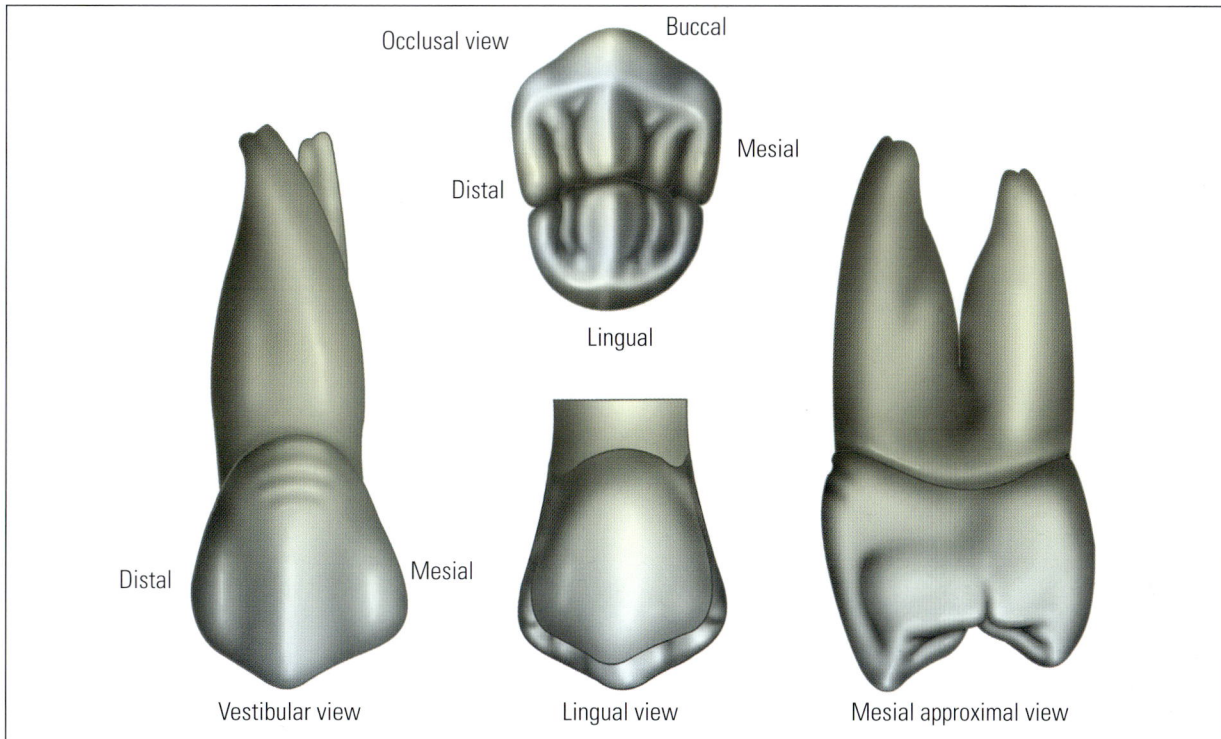

Fig 4-44 Morphology of the maxillary right first premolar.

ing points of the central developmental groove; these are the deepest parts of the occlusal surface.

The mesial approximal marginal ridge is concave for contact with the canine, whereas the distal ridge is convexly shaped. Growth-related depressions form on the triangular ridges, which can sometimes reach the same depth as a supplemental developmental groove.

The *maxillary second premolar (dens praemolaris lateralis)* (Fig 4-45) is smaller, more compact, and more symmetric than the first premolar; the cusps are almost of the same height and virtually the same size, and the central developmental groove lies in the middle. The second premolar is a rudimentary tooth. It has only a single developed root.

The average dimensions of the maxillary second premolar are:

• Crown width (mesiodistal): 6.3 mm
• Crown depth (buccolingual): 8.3 mm
• Crown length: 7.5 mm
• Total apicocoronal length: 20.0 mm

The *vestibular (buccal) surface* is similar to that of the first premolar but smaller and without pronounced angle and curvature characteristics. It contains two identical facets that are separated by a slightly prominent medial ridge.

The *lingual surface* is also similar to that of the first premolar, although the middle ridge lies centrally.

The *approximal surface* shows cusps of unequal height, the buccal cusp being more angular than the rounded lingual cusp. The central developmental groove lies in the middle and is very deep, which indicates a risk of caries. Buccal and lingual curvatures are normal.

The *occlusal surface* is more symmetric than on the first premolar but with the same characteristics: prominent buccal and rounded lingual cusps. The central development groove lies in the middle of the occlusal surface.

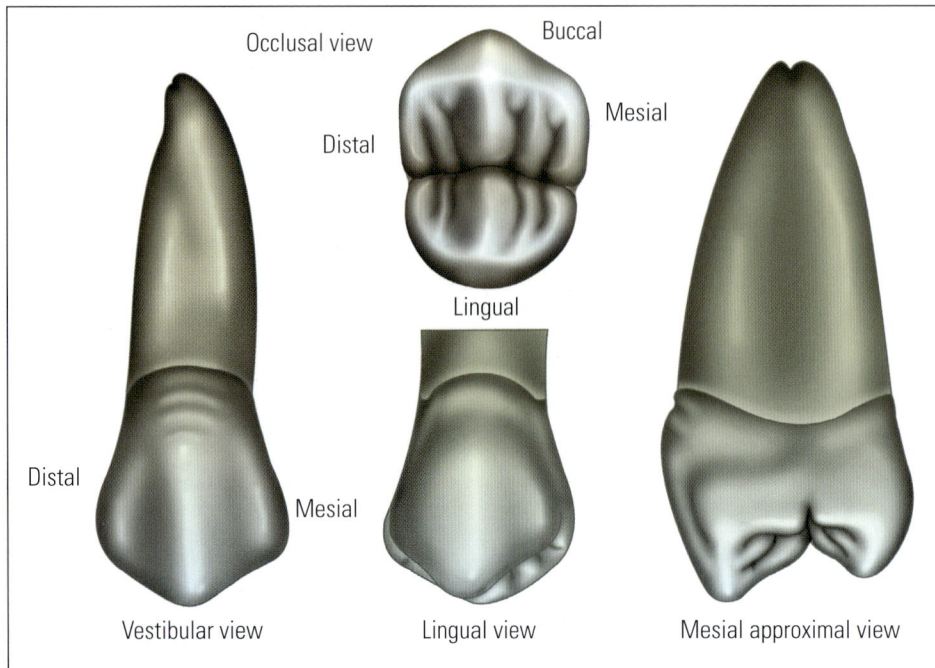

Fig 4-45 Morphology of the maxillary right second premolar.

Mandibular premolars

The main difference between the mandibular and maxillary premolars is that the mandibular ones have an almost circular crown outline. Furthermore, they are always single-rooted. Unlike the maxillary premolars, the mandibular first and second premolars differ considerably from each other.

The **mandibular first premolar** (Figs 4-46 and 4-47) is similar to a mandibular canine, except that the dental tubercle is developed into a very small, independent cusp. As the secondary antagonist of the maxillary canine, the buccal cusp of the mandibular first premolar is most strongly developed. Particularly tough food is often chewed by the maxillary canines and their opposing teeth (the mandibular canine and first premolar).

The average dimensions of the mandibular first premolar are:

- Crown width (mesiodistal): 6.8 mm
- Crown depth (buccolingual): 6.8 mm
- Crown length: 8.4 mm
- Total apicocoronal length: 22.0 mm

The **collum angle** or crown-root angulation (Fig 4-48a) on the mandibular premolars is an angle between the tooth axis and the crown axis. If an axis is drawn through the tooth from the root apex to the tip of the buccal cusp, and another is drawn from the base of the crown to the central developmental groove, there is a striking difference between the paths of these axes. The bend in the root in the crown-root angulation means that the crushing buccal cusp sits centrally, ie, in a statically favorable position over the base of the crown, and strain is placed axially on the periodontium.

The **tooth inclination** (Fig 4-48b) refers to the distinct lingual incline of the mandibular posterior teeth. The tooth inclination is most pronounced on the first premolar, and the degree of inclination declines distally on the posterior teeth.

The **vestibular (buccal) surface** of the first premolar is very similar to that of the mandibular canine. The first premolar is only slightly more compact, and the contact areas may be rather tapered. Overall the surface is highly convex. The ridge-shaped cusp has a rounded tip, while the mesial cusp ridge is shorter than the distal (angle characteristic). One prominent central ridge divides the buccal surface again into two unequally sized facets with vertical depressions. The mesial contact area lies higher than the distal. In the cervical

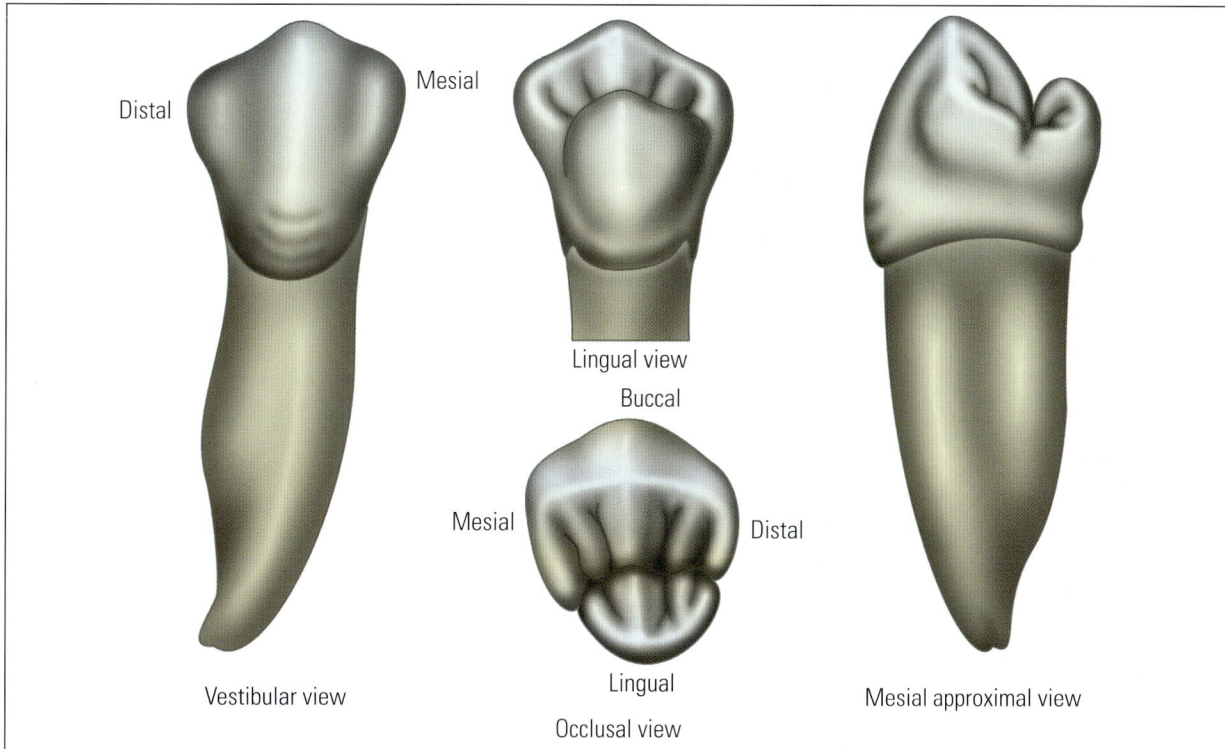

Distal
Mesial

Lingual view

Buccal

Mesial
Distal

Lingual

Vestibular view

Occlusal view

Mesial approximal view

Fig 4-46 Morphology of the mandibular right first premolar.

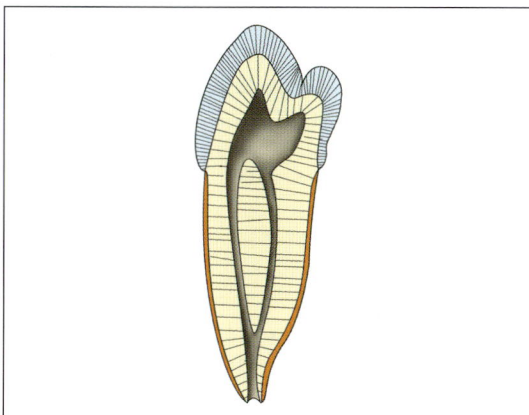

Fig 4-47 The distribution of tooth substances is normal in the mandibular first premolar; the pulp horn may be divided into two root canals in the root area.

Fig 4-48 *(a)* In the mandibular first premolar, the crown and root axes are not in line but produce the so-called collum angle or crown-root angulation; the crown axis is bent lingually in comparison with the root axis. *(b)* Seen approximally, the mandibular first premolar is inclined lingually so that its crown displays what is known as *tooth inclination*.

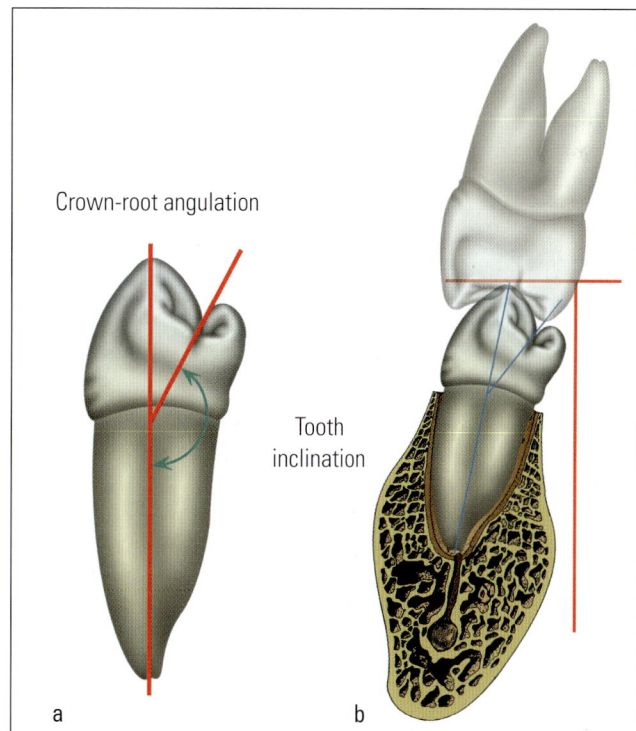

Crown-root angulation

Tooth inclination

a

b

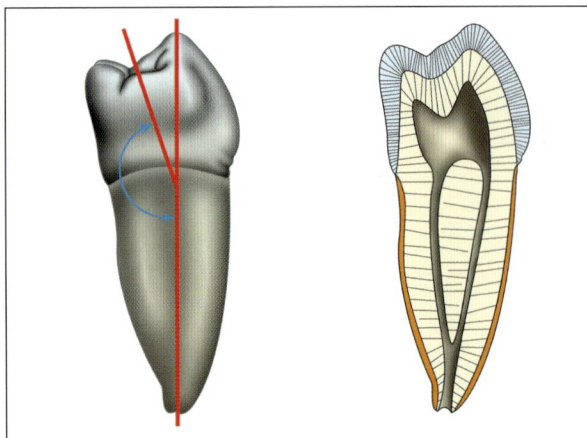

Fig 4-49 The root of the mandibular second premolar is sturdier and has a larger surface area than that of the first premolar. It is therefore capable of absorbing more force. This tooth also has a pronounced crown-root angulation. In this tooth, the pulp horn may be bifurcated in the root to form two canals. The distribution of tooth substances is normal.

runs lingually from the buccal cusp; as a result, the central developmental groove is sometimes interrupted. The central developmental groove is markedly displaced lingually.

The approximal marginal ridges are sturdy and recede in a lingual direction. This produces two distinct fossae, with the mesial one being more superior. The distal marginal ridge also lies more inferiorly. There are three variations on the arrangement of the lingual cusp:

- There is a very regular arrangement of the lingual cusp, where the line connecting the two cusps divides the tooth symmetrically.
- The lingual cusp is small and rudimentary like a tubercle; there is only a suggestion of a central developmental groove.
- The lingual cusp is displaced distally so that the crown takes on a triangular shape with the buccal cusp tip displaced mesially.

The *mandibular second premolar* is larger than the first premolar, but the resemblance is not as strong as that seen between the first and second premolar in the maxilla. The occlusal surface is more horizontal; ie, there is only a slight difference in height between buccal and lingual cusps. The tooth assumes two common forms. One has two cusps, and the other has three cusps, with one buccal and two lingual cusps. Very rarely there may be a four-cusp type with one buccal and three lingual cusps. The root of this tooth is roundish and, consistent with the stronger development of the second premolar, is longer and thicker than the root of the first premolar. The root is only bifurcated in rare cases. This tooth is capable of absorbing considerable masticatory forces. The pulp horn undergoes lobelike widening in correspondence with the cusps (Fig 4-49).

The average dimensions of the mandibular second premolar are:

- Crown width (mesiodistal): 7.5 mm
- Crown depth (buccolingual): 9.0 mm
- Crown length: 8.5 mm
- Total apicocoronal length: 24.0 mm

The mandibular second premolar (Figs 4-50 and 4-51) is a tooth with a true masticatory surface in form and function. It also displays tooth inclination and crown-root angulation, although

third, a short transverse and longitudinal convexity can be seen with poorly developed cervical grooves. The arched line of the cervix converges with concave, curved approximal margins. The curvature characteristic, like the angle characteristic, is well developed.

The *lingual surface* is very small and narrow and shows the very slightly developed lingual cusp. It tapers more cervically than buccally. The buccal cusp can be seen from the lingual aspect; only the central developmental groove is concealed by the small lingual cusp. This cusp has no opposing contact. As a result of the tooth inclination, the lingual cusp greatly overhangs the cervix; however, it is highly concave in the incisal third, so that a pronounced vertical curvature is visible.

The *approximal surface* reveals both the large buccal and the small lingual cusps. The lingual bend in the crown axis corresponding to the tooth inclination is most clearly visible approximally, as is the prominent longitudinal convexity—buccally in the cervical area and lingually in the occlusal. The approximal surfaces are prominent at the contact area and concave cervically.

The *occlusal surface* shows the circular outline of the crown. The lingual cusp is much smaller than the buccal and also more truncated. The occlusal surface is therefore markedly inclined toward the floor of the mouth. A sturdy cusp crest

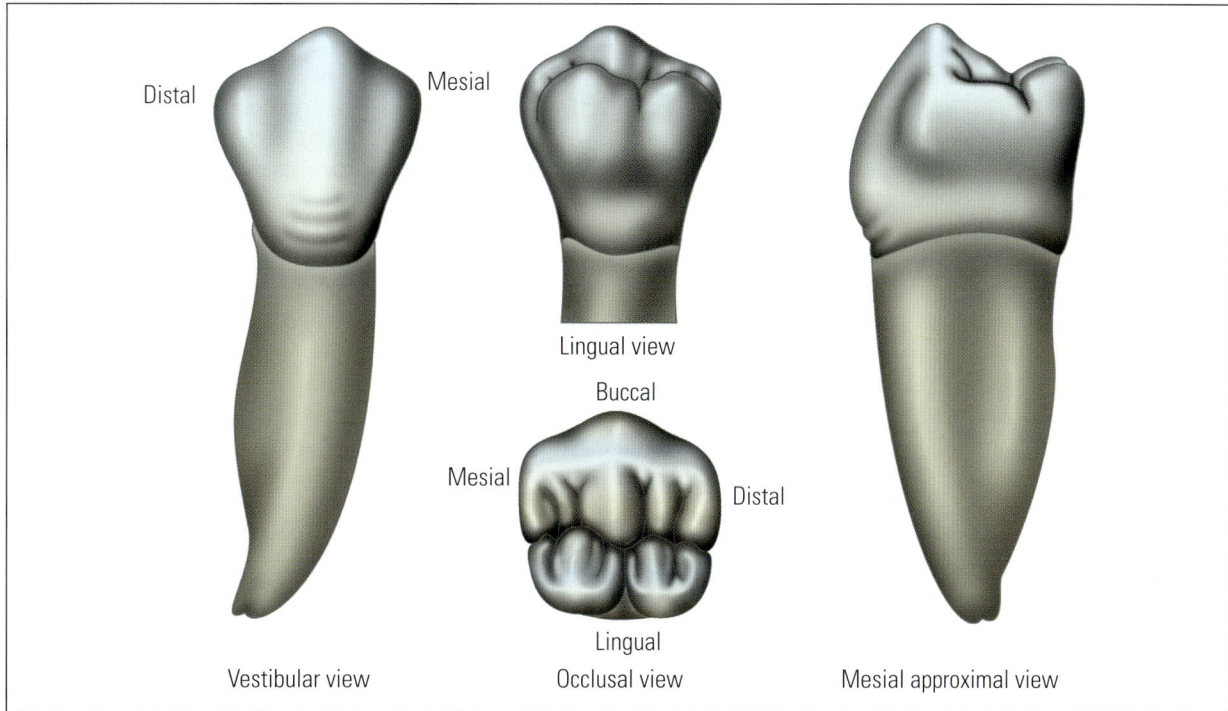

Fig 4-50 Morphology of the mandibular right second premolar.

Distal   Mesial

Lingual view

Buccal

Mesial   Distal

Lingual

Vestibular view   Occlusal view   Mesial approximal view

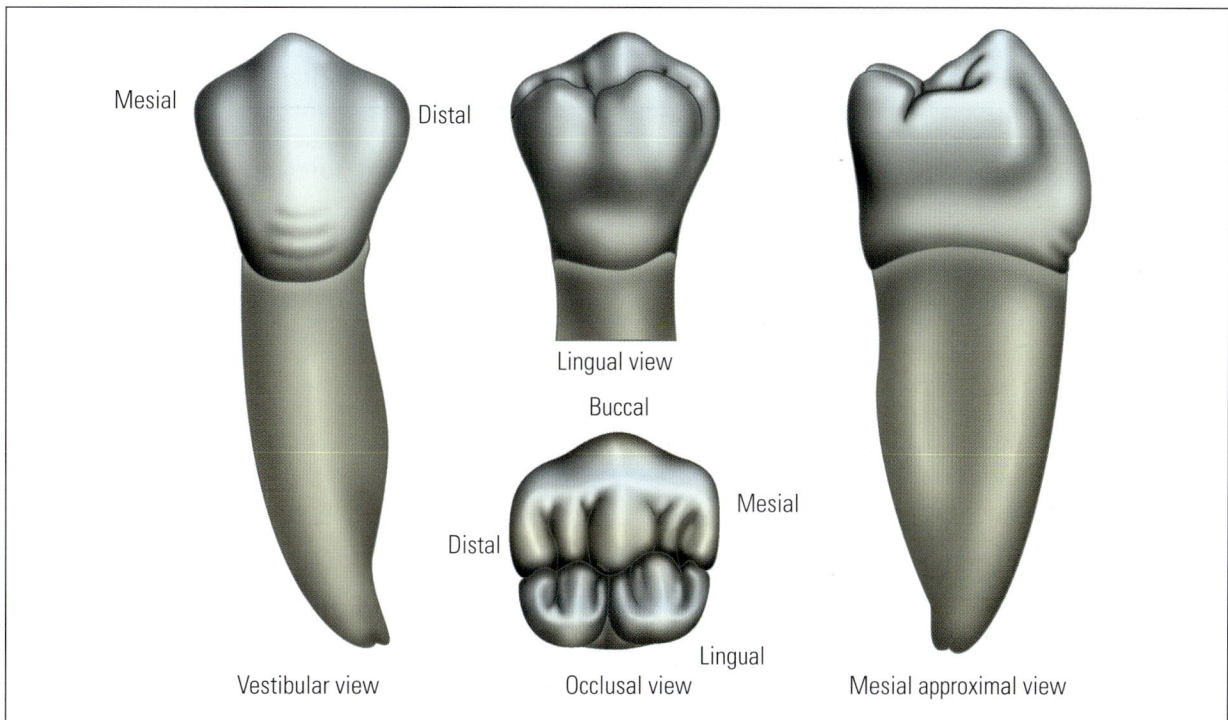

Fig 4-51 Morphology of the mandibular left second premolar.

Mesial   Distal

Lingual view

Buccal

Distal   Mesial

Lingual

Vestibular view   Occlusal view   Mesial approximal view

these are less pronounced than with the first premolar. As a result, the tooth makes full occlusal contact with all of its cusps.

The **vestibular (buccal) surface** resembles a compact, broad canine, with a ridge-shaped cusp ridge and rounded tip. The angle characteristic is pronounced so that the mesial angle lies slightly higher than the distal, as do the contact points. The formation of ridges and depressions is normal, and a curvature characteristic is present. The approximal margins are indented and taper down to the curved cervical margin.

The **lingual surface** is narrower and slightly shorter and has a pronounced transverse convexity. In the three-cusp type, the two lingual cusps are recognizable and make the surface appear divided. It is noticeable that the distolingual cusp is smaller and lower than the mesial. The surface also appears to overhang in the cervical area because of the tooth inclination and the strong vertical convexity. The buccal cusp can be seen in the lingual view because it rises above the lingual cusps.

The **occlusal surface** has all the features of a masticatory surface: cusps, cusp crests and ridges, marginal ridges, and grooves. The two-cusp type resembles the form of the maxillary second premolar. In the three-cusp type, the buccal cusp is the largest, while the linguodistal is the smallest. The three cusps are formed by a large main developmental groove that diverges at a right angle from the central developmental groove: This main groove often originates in the middle or slightly more distally. As a result, the groove formation appears to create a Y shape, which divides the three cusps. A third, very rare form is the four-cusp occlusal surface with three lingual cusps.

The **approximal surface** shows the crown-root angulation, ie, the lingual incline of the crown. In this view, the tooth inclination of the second premolar is also identifiable, but it is less developed than on the mesial neighbor. The vertical curvatures of the buccal and lingual surfaces can also be seen. The lingual contour overhangs in the occlusal area. The occlusal surface is only slightly tilted lingually. The buccal part of the occlusal surface is wider, so that the central developmental groove is displaced slightly lingually. The approximal marginal ridge contains the contact point and tapers so that the approximal surface is concavely indented.

Molars

The **molars (dentes molares)** are ideal for the complete crushing and grinding of solid foods. The occlusal surfaces are capable of withstanding the greatest masticatory pressure. In the maxilla, the lingual cusps have an occlusion-fixing function and are referred to as *crushing cusps*. The buccal cusps have cutting functions and are referred to as *shearing cusps*. In the mandible, the crushing cusps are buccal and the shearing cusps are lingual.

The maxillary posterior teeth show a vestibular inclination. The roots of the maxillary posterior teeth are very characteristically shaped and have a relatively large surface area for a sturdy periodontium. The ratio between the occlusal surface and the surface area of the periodontium is approximately 1:5. At the apices of the roots, there are often small divisions in the root canal, similar to a river delta, which make it difficult to clear the root canal, if necessary. The roots are aligned according to the pattern of forces during mastication, as is the inclination of the teeth to the alveolar crests. The two buccal roots sit almost centrally under the crown, while the distal root is inclined posteriorly and the mesial root anteriorly. This means that central pressures as well as slightly transverse forces that occur within the dental arch can be absorbed. The palatal root is directed palatally and thus absorbs central masticatory pressure and transverse loads.

The mandibular molars have two roots, one distal and one mesial. Both roots have their own canal. These canals can terminate in several outlets at the apex of the root. Development of the pulp horn reflects that of the cusp tips. The prominent roots of the mandibular posterior teeth, like their opposing teeth, have large root surface areas for a robust periodontium. The tooth inclination is not as pronounced on the molars as on the premolars.

Maxillary molars

The **maxillary first molar** (dens molaris medialis) (Figs 4-52 to 4-54) is typical of the maxillary molars. It is the largest of the three large posterior teeth and has all the features characteristic of this form. The occlusal surface contains four cusps, which are separated by developmental grooves.

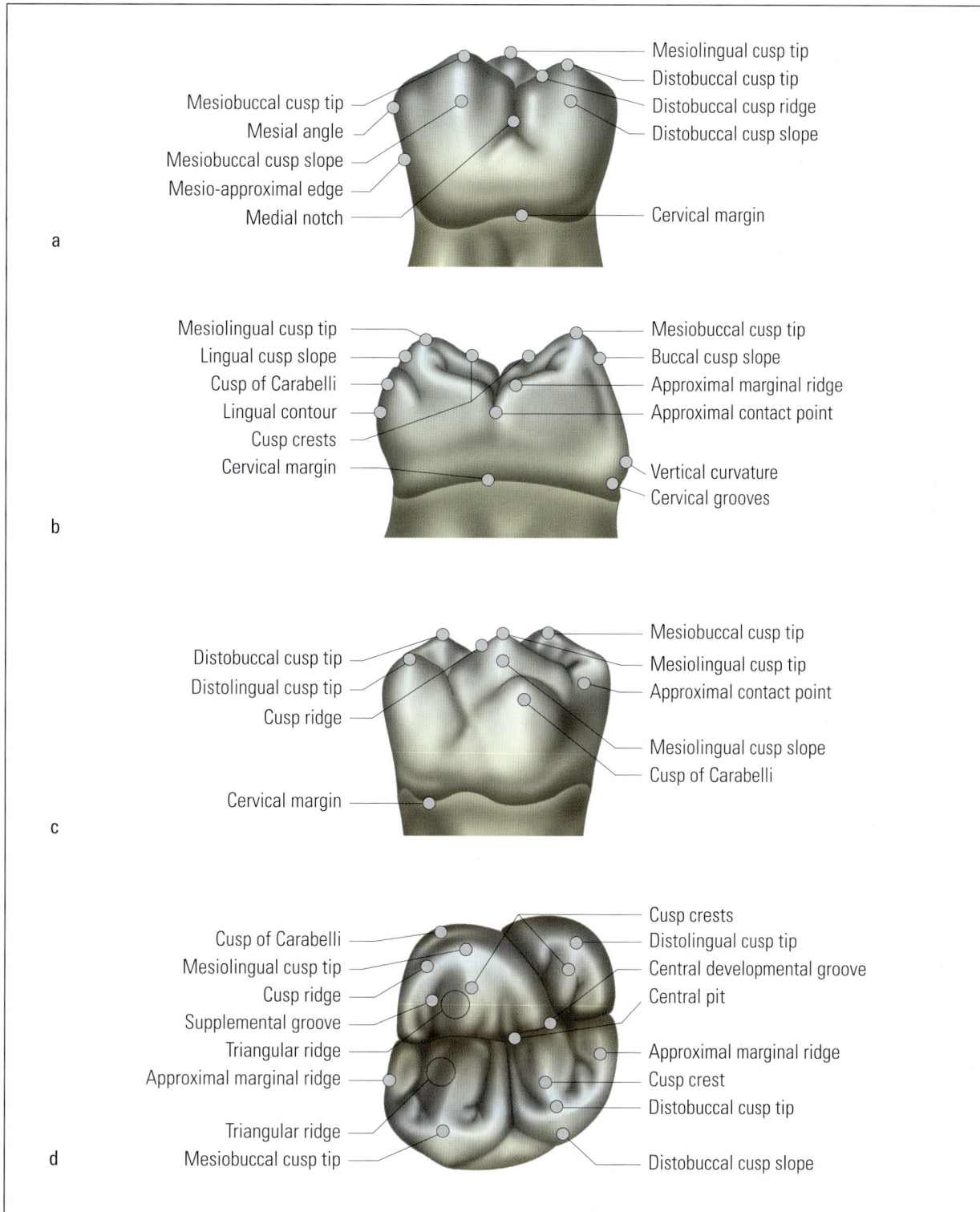

Mesiolingual cusp tip
Distobuccal cusp tip
Distobuccal cusp ridge
Distobuccal cusp slope

Mesiobuccal cusp tip
Mesial angle
Mesiobuccal cusp slope
Mesio-approximal edge
Medial notch

Cervical margin

a

Mesiolingual cusp tip
Lingual cusp slope
Cusp of Carabelli
Lingual contour
Cusp crests
Cervical margin

Mesiobuccal cusp tip
Buccal cusp slope
Approximal marginal ridge
Approximal contact point

Vertical curvature
Cervical grooves

b

Distobuccal cusp tip
Distolingual cusp tip
Cusp ridge

Mesiobuccal cusp tip
Mesiolingual cusp tip
Approximal contact point

Mesiolingual cusp slope
Cusp of Carabelli

Cervical margin

c

Cusp of Carabelli
Mesiolingual cusp tip
Cusp ridge
Supplemental groove
Triangular ridge
Approximal marginal ridge
Triangular ridge
Mesiobuccal cusp tip

Cusp crests
Distolingual cusp tip
Central developmental groove
Central pit

Approximal marginal ridge
Cusp crest
Distobuccal cusp tip
Distobuccal cusp slope

d

Fig 4-52 Morphology of the maxillary first molar. *(a)* Vestibular view. *(b)* Mesial approximal view. *(c)* Lingual view. *(d)* Occlusal view.

The curvature characteristic clearly stands out. The vestibular and lingual surfaces converge distally to create the typical rhomboid shape of the maxillary first molar. The occlusal surface recedes distally. The maxillary first molars have three roots, two buccal and one palatal.

The average dimensions of the maxillary first molar are:

• Crown width (mesiodistal): 10.5 mm
• Crown depth (buccolingual): 12.0 mm
• Crown length: 7.7 mm
• Total apicocoronal length: 23.5 mm

The maxillary first molar is the first accessional tooth in the permanent dentition and is usually the first tooth to be lost during exfoliation. It determines the height of the occlusion and the maxillomandibular relationship. This tooth gives the subsequent teeth their positional orientation at exfoliation. During the transitional phase from primary to permanent dentition, it takes on most of the masticatory work. It is ideally suited as an abutment tooth for partial dentures and should be retained as long as possible.

The *vestibular (buccal) surface* (see Fig 4-52a) gives the impression of being two premolars fused together because it is divided by a distinct longitudinal groove. The mesial and the distal portions of the surface have virtually the same form as a premolar: The occlusal border shows the ridge-shaped cusp form, with the mesial cusp higher and more pronounced than the rounded distal cusp. The medial ridges of the mesial and distal parts of the surface divide each of these into two facets. The mesial part of the surface is more bulging and prominent, while the distal part recedes posteriorly (curvature characteristic). The cervix curves in the middle in an occlusal direction. The cervical grooves are poorly developed.

The *approximal surface* (see Fig 4-52b) has an almost rectangular shape. The typical vertical curvatures of the buccal and lingual surfaces can be seen. The buccal surface has its greatest curvature cervically, whereas occlusally it has a rather sloping and relatively sharp-edged course up to the cusps. The lingual surface bulges considerably so that the lingual cusps appear to be inclined toward the occlusal surface. The cusp tips on this tooth are also about half the tooth width apart. The mesial approximal surface is much larger

(and particularly higher) than the distal; the mesial marginal ridge and hence the contact point are higher. The cervix curves evenly in an occlusal direction.

The *lingual surface* (see Fig 4-52c) is smaller than the buccal surface, in keeping with the constriction caused by the dental arch. There is also some tapering toward the cervix. The longitudinal groove, which separates the two cusps, is displaced distally because the distopalatal cusp is generally only half the size of the mesial. The mesial cusp is again higher, more angular, and more noticeable. Both cusps, however, bulge inward toward the occlusal surface. The occlusal contour recedes distally. The cervical margin curves occlusally, as on the buccal surface.

The *cusp of Carabelli (tuberculum anomale)* is an additional, small, low-lying cusp on the mesial part of the lingual surface of the maxillary first molar.

The *occlusal surface* (see Fig 4-52d) displays typical functional characteristics with four pronounced, differently sized cusps: two buccal shearing cusps and two palatal crushing cusps. Cusps in order of decreasing size are: mesiolingual, mesiobuccal, distobuccal, and distolingual.

The structure of the individual cusps reflects the described features. The buccal cusp ridge and crests are angular, whereas the lingual cusps appear rounded.

The developmental grooves form small pits at their crossover points. Where the central developmental groove comes into contact with the buccal groove, the compact central fossa is formed. The supplemental grooves at the marginal ridges also form pronounced pits at the branching points with the central groove. The shape of the grooves produces a skewed, rather distorted H. The marginal ridges in the approximal area are noticeable, while the mesial approximal edge is rather higher, almost straight, but the distal edge is curved outward. The marginal ridges form the contact points in the transitional area with the approximal surfaces and form the approximal depressions with the adjacent teeth.

The *maxillary second molar (dens molaris laterali)* (Figs 4-55 and 4-56) has the same form as the first molar, with the only difference being that its lingual surface is less developed. The outline of the crown is often modified so that the rhomboid shape appears more acutely angled and the

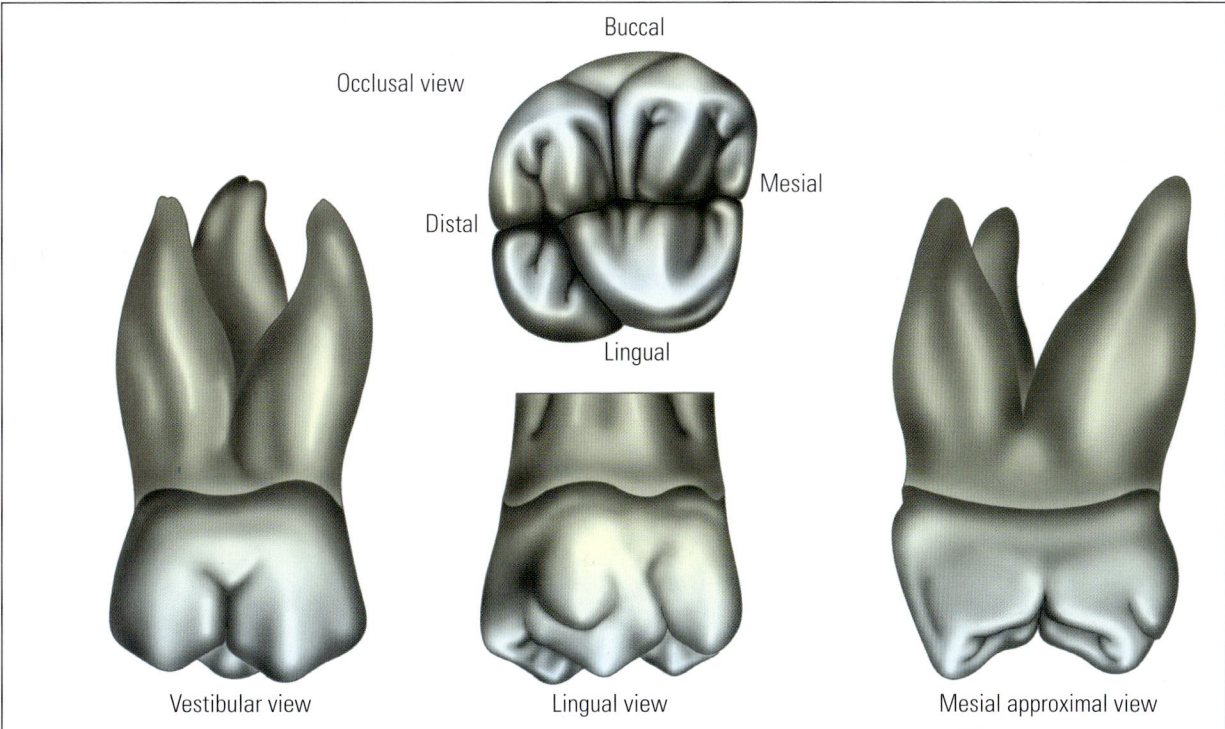

Fig 4-53 Morphology of the maxillary right first molar.

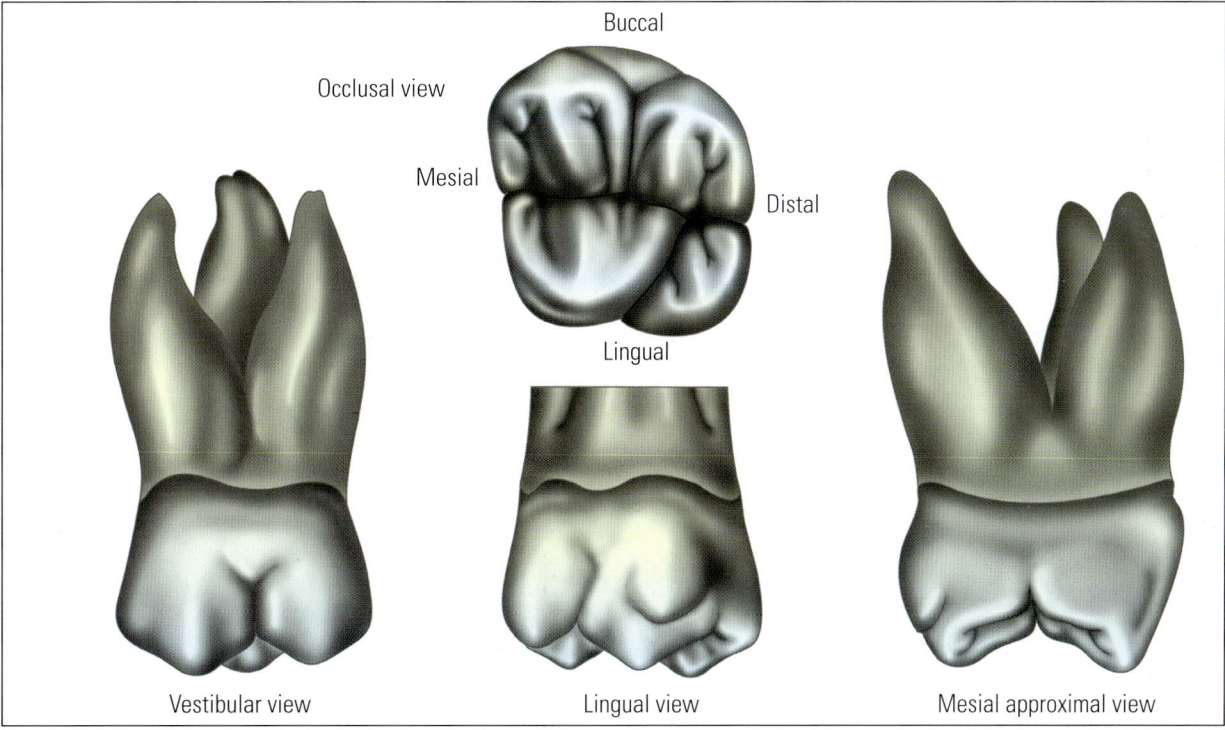

Fig 4-54 Morphology of the maxillary left first molar.

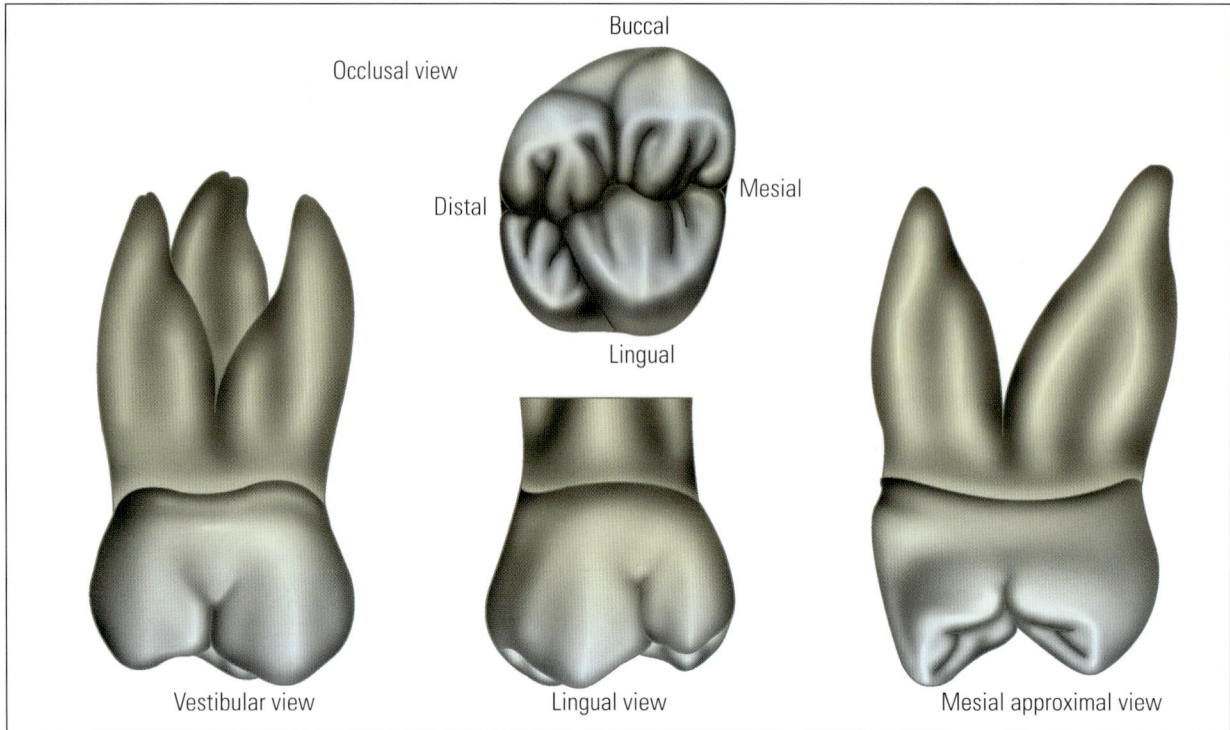

Fig 4-55 Morphology of the maxillary right second molar.

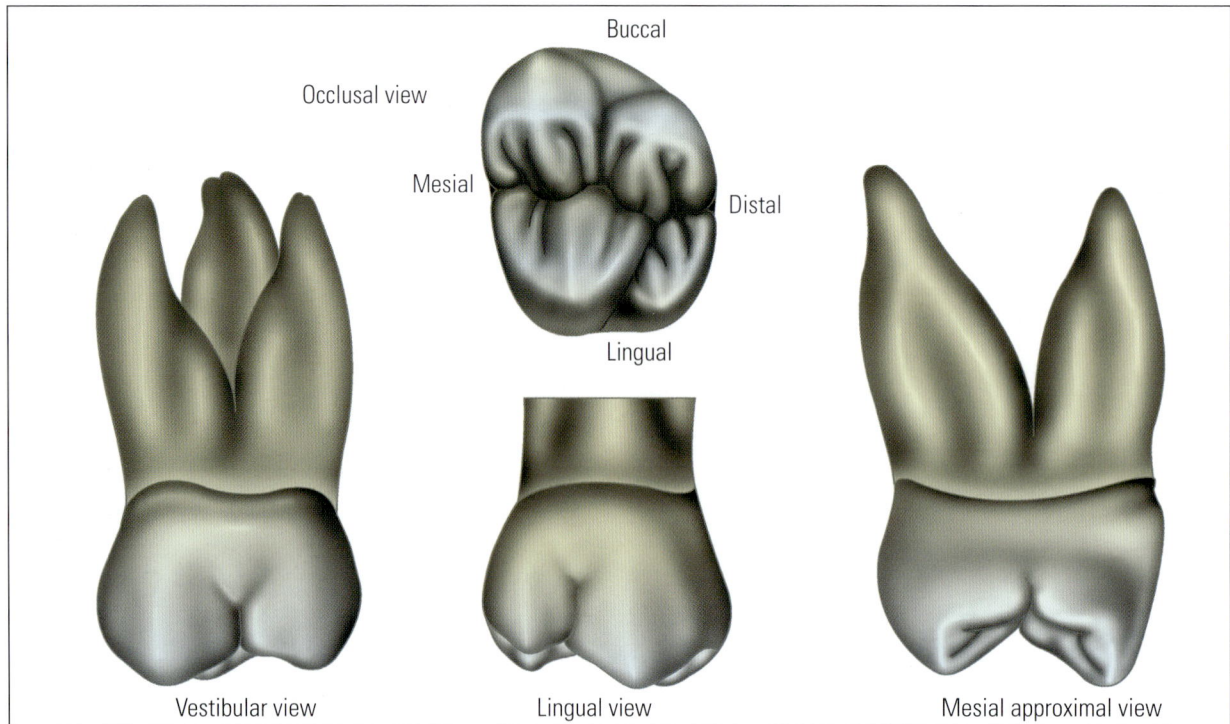

Fig 4-56 Morphology of the maxillary left second molar.

Fig 4-57 The distribution of tooth substance is normal in the maxillary molars. The pulp cavity often develops into several root canals in the root area, and these have several alveolar access points at the root apices; this anatomy makes root canal treatment difficult.

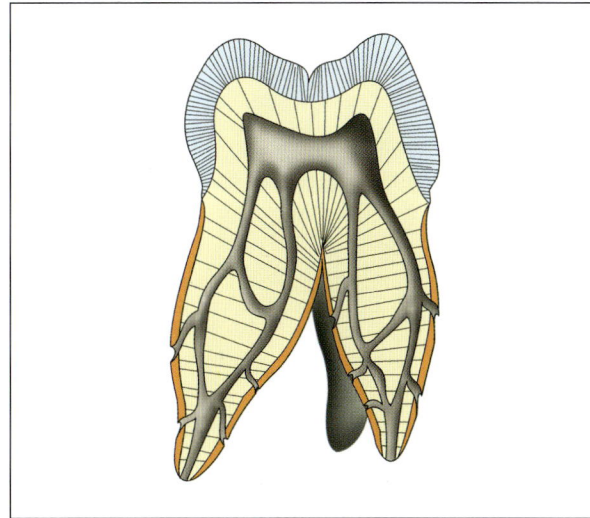

whole crown is far smaller than that of the maxillary first molar.

The cusp of Carabelli is absent, and the distolingual cusp is smaller, sometimes shrunken to a marginal ridge so that the occlusal surface has only three cusps. The three tooth roots are often fused.

The average dimensions of the maxillary second molar are:

• Crown width (mesiodistal): 9.8 mm
• Crown depth (buccolingual): 11.5 mm
• Crown length: 7.7 mm
• Total apicocoronal length: 21.1 mm

The *vestibular (buccal) surface* is divided by a distinct longitudinal depression as in the maxillary first molar. The mesial cusp is higher and more pronounced than the rounded distal cusp, which recedes sharply. The mesial aspect of the surface is much more convex and prominent than the part that recedes distally. The cervical line bends occlusally in the middle. Cervical grooves are only poorly developed.

The *lingual surface* is much smaller than the buccal surface, tapering sharply to the cervix. The distolingual cusp may be rudimentary so that the occlusal contour sharply recedes distally. The mesial cusp is again higher, more sharp-edged, and more developed. There is rarely a cusp of Carabelli present.

The *approximal surface* has an almost rectangular shape. The typical vertical curvatures of the buccal and lingual surfaces can be seen. The mesial approximal surface is also much larger here than the distal surface, with the mesial contact point located much higher. The cervical line bends occlusally.

The *occlusal surface* also displays typical functional characteristics, usually with four differently sized cusps: two buccal shearing cusps, one lingual crushing cusp, and one distolingual cusp shortened at the marginal ridge. The central developmental groove with the main buccal groove forms the central pit. The mesial approximal marginal ridge is more pronounced and higher, almost straight, while the distal margin curves outward again.

The *maxillary third molar (dens serotinus)* is the most variable of all teeth: from a four-cusp form to a small peg tooth. The tooth can have three roots, but the peg forms often have only one root. Certain forms also have several root apices. The third molar appears to be in the process of regression, ie, the dentition is being reduced, with the third molar often not developing.

Details of the pulp cavity, roots, and occlusion of the maxillary posterior teeth are presented in Figs 4-57 to 4-59.

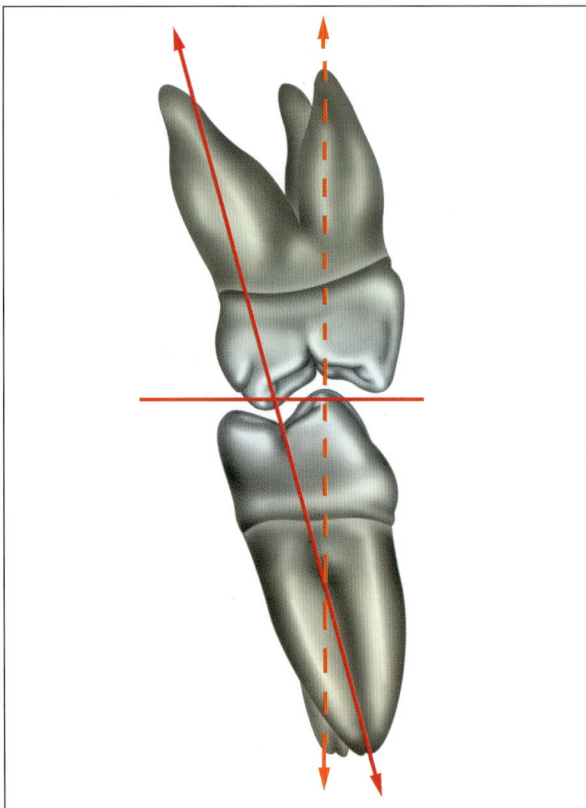

Fig 4-58 The roots of the maxillary posterior teeth have highly characteristic forms and a relatively large surface area in order to create a sturdy periodontium. The orientation of the roots follows the pattern of forces during mastication, as does the inclination of the teeth to the alveolar crests. This means that, in the maxillary molars, the palatal roots are splayed palatally and the buccal roots are spread mesially and distally; the roots of the mandibular molars are mesiodistally oriented.

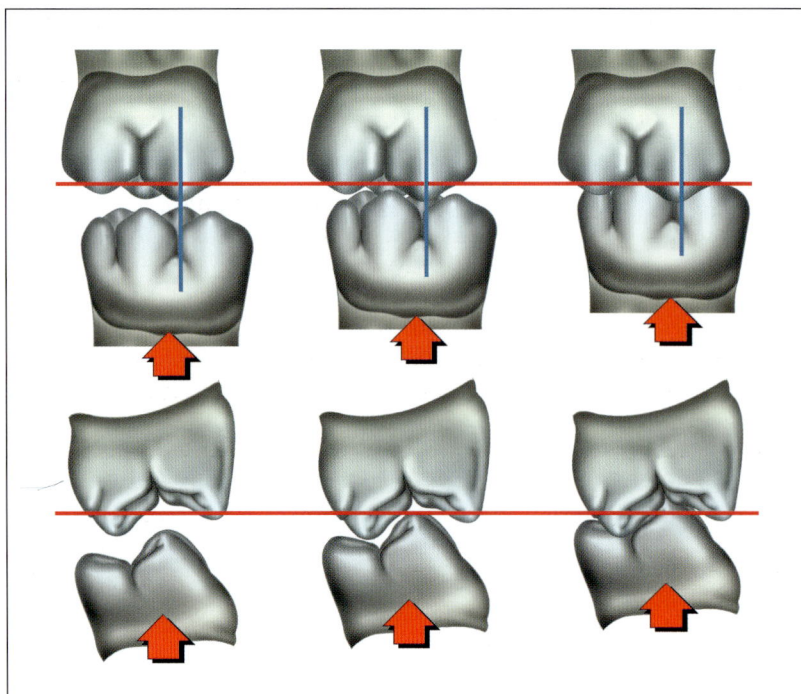

Fig 4-59 The occlusal patterns of the posterior antagonist teeth are matched to each other and engage in a sagittal and transverse direction in double intercuspation. In the position of terminal occlusion, the lingual and buccal tooth contours form a virtually closed area, against which the tongue lies vestibularly and the cheeks lingually.

Mandibular molars

The **mandibular first molar** (Fig 4-60) usually has a five-cusp crown with two lingual and three buccal prominences, which gives the tooth a long, rectangular outline. The roots are highly characteristic: there are only two roots, one anterior (mesial) and one posterior (distal). These roots are flattened and contain pronounced longitudinal depressions. The posterior root contains one canal; the anterior root contains two canals.

The average dimensions of the mandibular first molar are:

- Crown width (mesiodistal): 11.5 mm
- Crown depth (buccolingual): 10.2 mm
- Crown length: 8.3 mm
- Total apicocoronal length: 22.0 mm

The very large occlusal surface of the tooth enables it to withstand a large amount of masticatory pressure. The periodontium is correspondingly well developed: The roots mainly absorb sagittal forces but can also take transverse pressures because of the root flattening. The tooth is inclined slightly lingually, in accordance with the crown inclination. As the first accessional tooth, the mandibular first molar determines the height of the occlusion and the width of the dental arch at exfoliation.

The **vestibular (buccal) surface** has the three ridge-shaped, rounded cusps that are divided by slight longitudinal grooves. The tooth recedes distally, in keeping with the angle characteristic. A pronounced longitudinal and transverse convexity can be seen in the cervical area, where there are also slight cervical grooves. The line of the cervix appears to be wavy. The distal contact point lies far more apically than the mesial one, so that the mesial approximal edge has a greater longitudinal convexity than its distal counterpart.

The **lingual surface** is divided by a longitudinal groove; it shows both of the rounded, ridge-shaped cusps. The markedly smaller surface has only a slight transverse and longitudinal convexity. The cervical line is located more coronally on the lingual side than on the buccal aspect and is undulating. The lingual surface is slightly overhanging because of the tooth inclination.

The **approximal surfaces** are rhomboid in keeping with the tooth inclination. The vertical curvature of the buccal surface is greatest cervically, whereas the lingual surface contour appears to be overhanging occlusally and displays no appreciable curvature. The buccal cusps are shorter and more rounded than the lingual ones. The distal approximal surface is considerably smaller. The contact points are overhanging.

The **occlusal surface** is almost rectangular but rounded and becomes narrower distally. It is made up of five differently sized cusps, in order of decreasing size: mesiolingual, mesiobuccal, distolingual, centrobuccal, and distobuccal. The features of the cusps are typical, as is the pattern of the grooves. The central developmental groove is divided medially by a distinct main developmental groove, which produces a cross. This is where the central pit is located. Distally another distinct main groove branches off buccally, which separates the distobuccal cusp. The central groove divides into pronounced supplemental grooves before reaching the approximal marginal ridges.

The **mandibular second molar** (Fig 4-61) is very similar to the first molar, except that it is smaller overall and has only four cusps. It is very symmetrically structured, with roughly equally sized cusps that are divided by a cross-shaped groove. There are some mandibular second molars that have five cusps.

The average dimensions of the mandibular second molar are:

- Crown width (mesiodistal): 10.7 mm
- Crown depth (buccolingual): 9.8 mm
- Crown length: 8.0 mm
- Total apicocoronal length: 22.0 mm

The **mandibular third molar** shows great variability. It can be found with four or five cusps but also as a three- or six-cusp tooth. It normally resembles the mandibular second molar but is rather smaller. Its roots are often fused, with separate root canals. In many cases, this tooth is ectopic and often has to be extracted during the eruption phase because it presses against the mandibular second molar as it grows and causes severe pain.

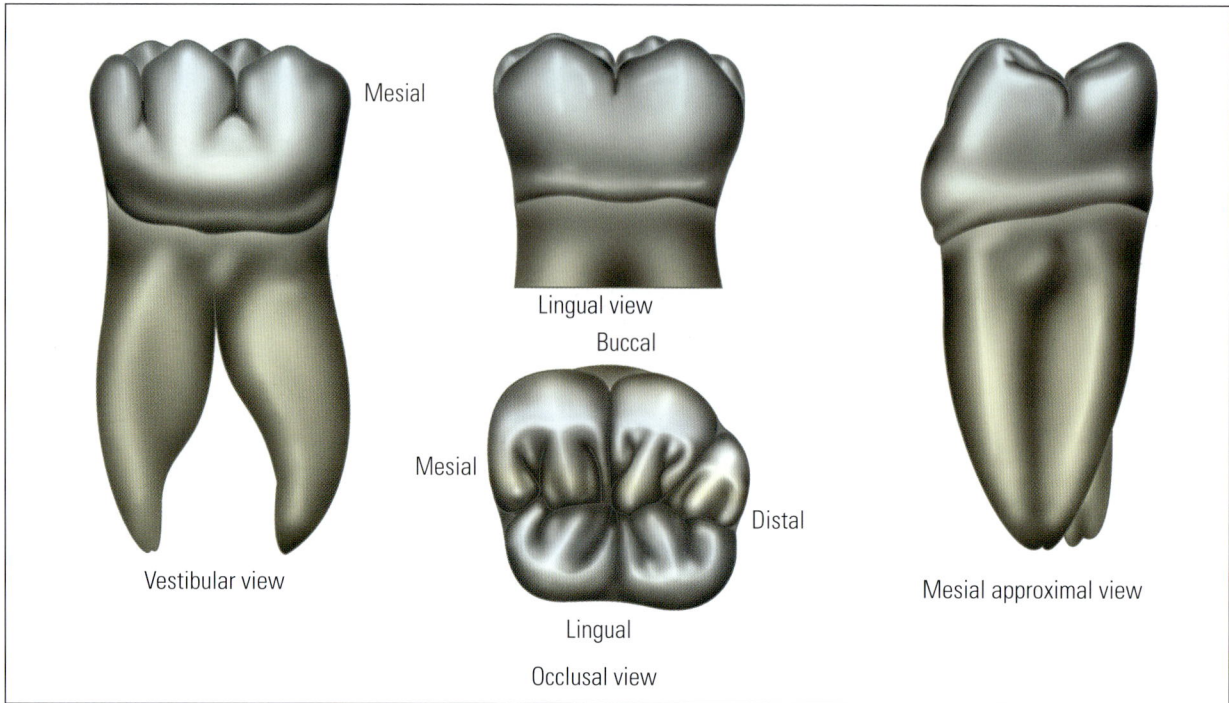

Fig 4-60 Morphology of the mandibular right first molar.

Mesial

Lingual view

Buccal

Mesial

Distal

Lingual

Occlusal view

Vestibular view

Mesial approximal view

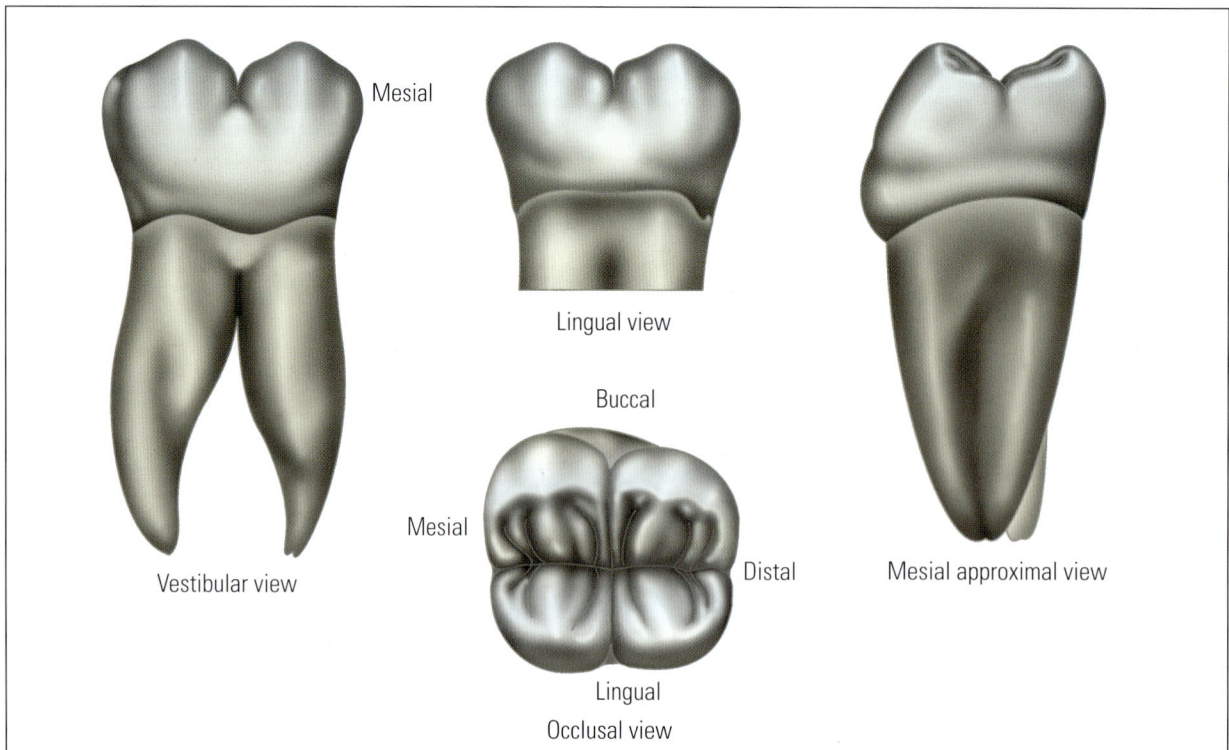

Fig 4-61 Morphology of the mandibular right second molar.

Mesial

Lingual view

Buccal

Mesial

Distal

Lingual

Occlusal view

Vestibular view

Mesial approximal view

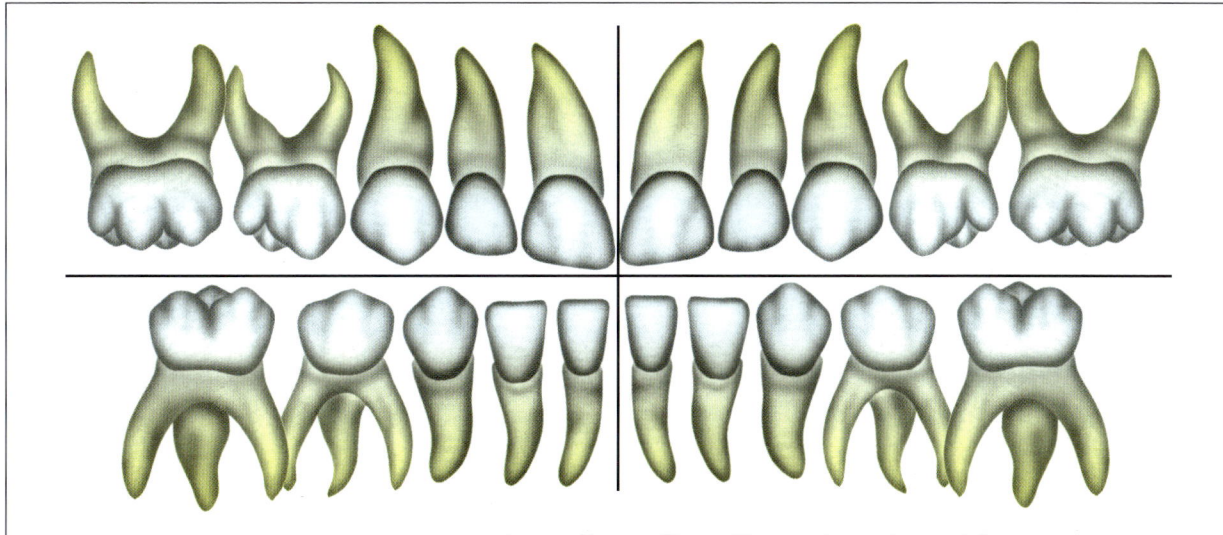

Fig 4-62 The vestibular view of the primary teeth shows their basic compact shape. The roots of the primary molars are flared; the tooth germs of the succeeding teeth lie between them.

Primary Teeth

The teeth of the **primary dentition** are known as *deciduous (dentes decidui)* or *primary teeth* as well as the *mixed* or *temporary dentition*, and they form the masticatory apparatus up to the sixth year of life. The primary dentition is made up of 20 teeth: eight incisors, four canines, and eight primary molars. The forms of these teeth match those of the permanent dentition, but there are no premolars (Fig 4-62).

The primary teeth that stand in place of the premolars bear a closer resemblance to the molars of the permanent dentition, which is why they are known as primary molars. The primary teeth are smaller and more delicate than the permanent teeth (2 to 4 mm smaller on average). They look bluish-white, in contrast to the yellowish color of the permanent teeth, because they contain less calcium.

One striking feature of the primary teeth is a thickening of the enamel margin cervically, so that they bulge outward over the gingival margin. The size ratio is an equally reliable characteristic: The primary teeth are far smaller but relatively broader than the permanent teeth in relation to their length; seen from the front, the primary dentition appears shorter than the permanent dentition. It should be noted that variations in the form of the primary teeth are very rare.

The **anterior teeth** of the primary dentition largely resemble the teeth with the same name in the permanent dentition. The incisors and canines are smoother than those in the permanent dentition, with less pronounced ridges. However, the central ridge is noticeably well developed labially, both in the maxilla and in the mandible. All the features, especially the angle characteristics, are strongly developed. The lingual surfaces in turn are less pronounced; ie, the dental tubercle is only slightly developed.

The **primary maxillary first molar** resembles a permanent premolar, but its pronounced rhomboid shape is noticeable. This tooth may also have a second cusp on the lingual half. The distinctive fissure separates the buccal and lingual cusps.

The **primary maxillary second molar** has some similarities with a permanent maxillary molar, but the rhomboid shape is predominant, while the mesiobuccal cusp overhangs a great deal buccally.

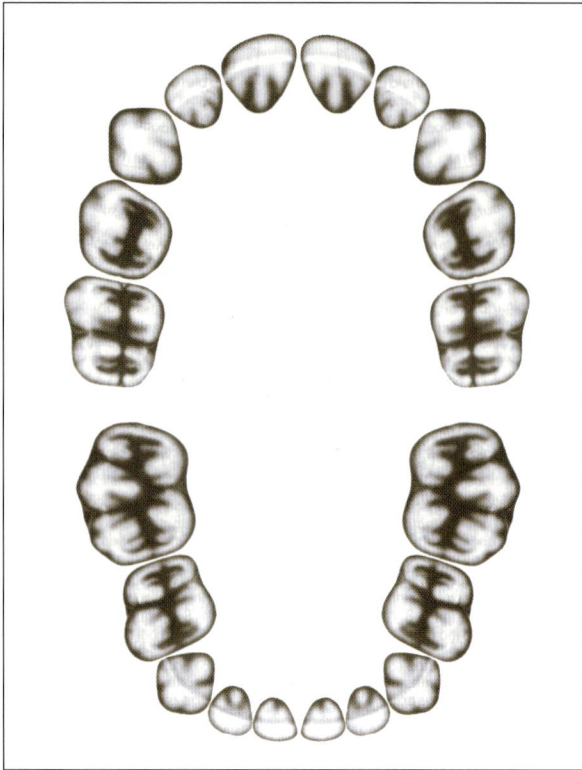

Fig 4-63 The primary dental arches of the maxilla and mandible are the same shape as in the permanent dentition: semicircular. The approximal contacts are lost immediately before exfoliation because the jaw grows.

The **roots** of the primary molars are widely flared because the tooth germs of the eventual premolars have to find space between them (see Fig 4-62). The pulp cavity and root canal of the primary teeth are spacious, and the walls of the teeth are correspondingly thinner. The roots of the primary incisors in the maxilla and in the mandible are quite flattened, whereas the roots of the primary canines are more evenly rounded. At exfoliation, the roots of the primary teeth are resorbed (*resorb* = to suck back) as a result of pressure from the growth of the permanent teeth.

The primary teeth are extremely susceptible to caries, which often leads to premature tooth loss or, in extreme cases, damage to the succeeding tooth. Because the primary teeth act as space maintainers for the permanent teeth, they should be retained for a long time. Any premature loss can influence the growth of the jaw, resulting in a lack of space for the permanent teeth and hence positional anomalies.

Eruption

Eruption refers to when the developing tooth breaks through the epithelial covering of the alveolar process in an occlusal direction. The development and the phase of eruption of the primary and permanent dentitions are linked to the growth in size of the skull and the jaws and hence to a person's general physical development. A distinction is made between the **primary dentition** and permanent dentition. The teeth of the **permanent dentition** comprise 20 successional and 12 accessional teeth; the latter originate from the same dental lamina as the 20 primary teeth and are the 12 molars of the permanent dentition.

The teeth of the permanent dentition are already developing during the primary dentition stage. The primary teeth require about 2 to 4 years for their development from tooth germs, from eruption through root formation; thereafter, they bear full masticatory function for approximately 4 years. Permanent teeth require approximately 12 years from tooth germ formation until the roots are completely formed: exfoliation is finished by age 10 to 13 years (Fig 4-64).

Movement phases in dental eruption occur as three changes in position:

The **primary mandibular first molar** bears no resemblance to the permanent premolar destined to replace it. It usually has four cusps on the occlusal surface, with the mesial cusps dominant. The cusp tips are sharp and pointed, as they are on all the primary molars. Ridge formation on the occlusal surfaces is prominent.

Among all the primary molars, the **primary mandibular second molar** bears the strongest resemblance to its succeeding molar, except that the middle buccal cusp protrudes slightly buccally and the cusps are more pointed and more prominent overall.

The **dental arch form** of the primary dentition is similar to that of the permanent dentition (Fig 4-63). The approximal tooth contacts are lost immediately before exfoliation of the teeth in approximately the sixth year of life because the jaws become larger.

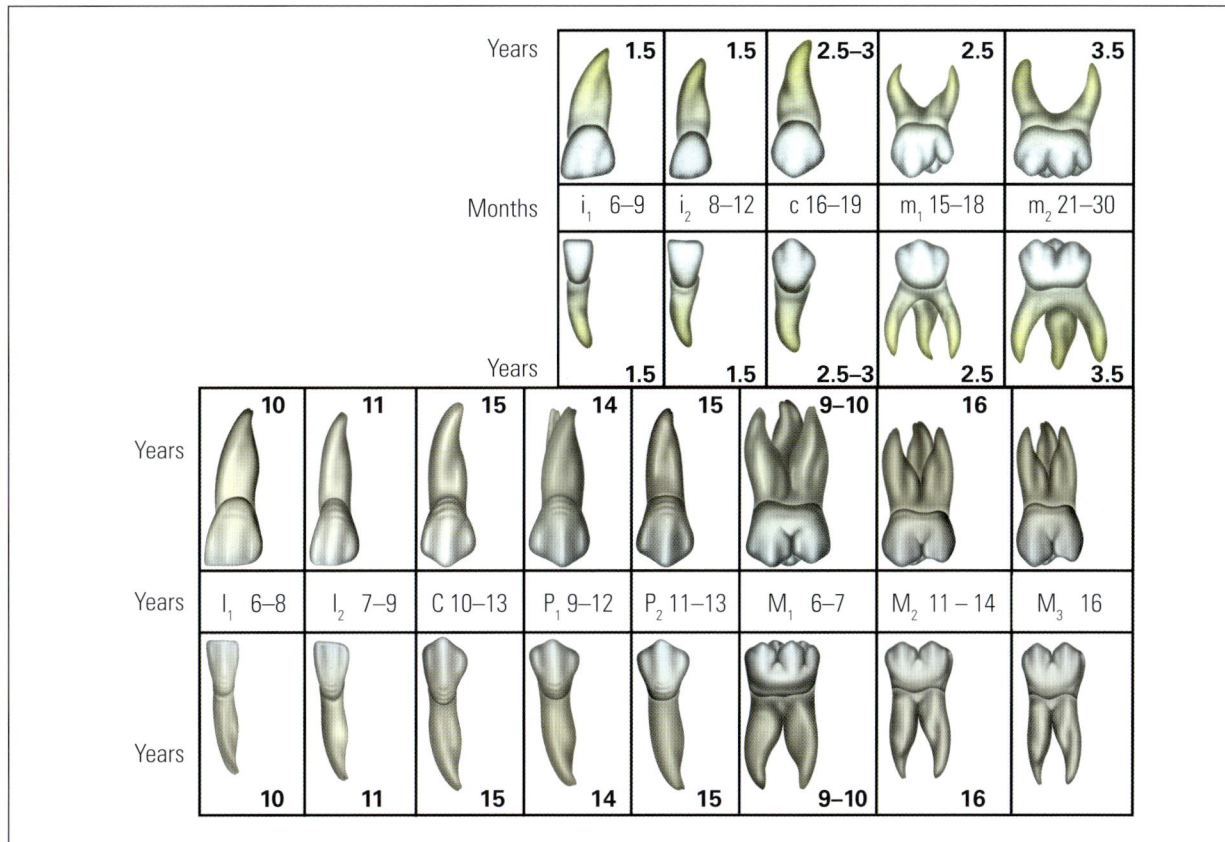

Fig 4-64 Eruption times for primary and permanent teeth. The average eruption times are given near the crown illustrations, while the average times required for root formation are given next to the root illustrations. i₁, primary central incisor; i₂, primary lateral incisor; c, primary canine; m₁, primary first molar; m₂, primary second molar; I₁, permanent central incisor; I₂, permanent lateral incisor; C, permanent canine; P₁, first premolar; P₂, second premolar; M₁, permanent first molar; M₂, permanent second molar; M₃, permanent third molar.

1. Changes in the position of the tooth germs during development (preeruptive movement)
2. Occlusal eruption of teeth as far as the occlusal plane (prefunctional eruptive movements)
3. Changes of position in the dentition (eg, mesial or occlusal migration)

The actual eruption of teeth in an occlusal direction starts as soon as the first edges of the roots are formed. Root growth and tooth eruption are synchronous, the length of eruption roughly corresponding to the length of root growth. The eruption length is only greater than root length in the case of the incisors and canines, because these tooth germs lie more deeply in the jaw. During occlusally directed growth, the alveolar crests grow in an occlusal direction as a result of bone formation.

In the primary teeth, there is dense connective tissue over the occlusal surfaces and incisal margins before eruption. The eruption of the primary teeth (ie, teething) can be associated with pain and fever because sharp edges cause injuries and inflammation in the maxillomandibular mucosa.

The germs and crowns of the accessional and successional teeth are covered with bone, which must be broken down during eruption. If the tooth is pushed through the connective tissue as far as the mucosal epithelium, slight inflammatory processes may occur.

During *root formation of the successional teeth*, the roots of the primary teeth are resorbed and

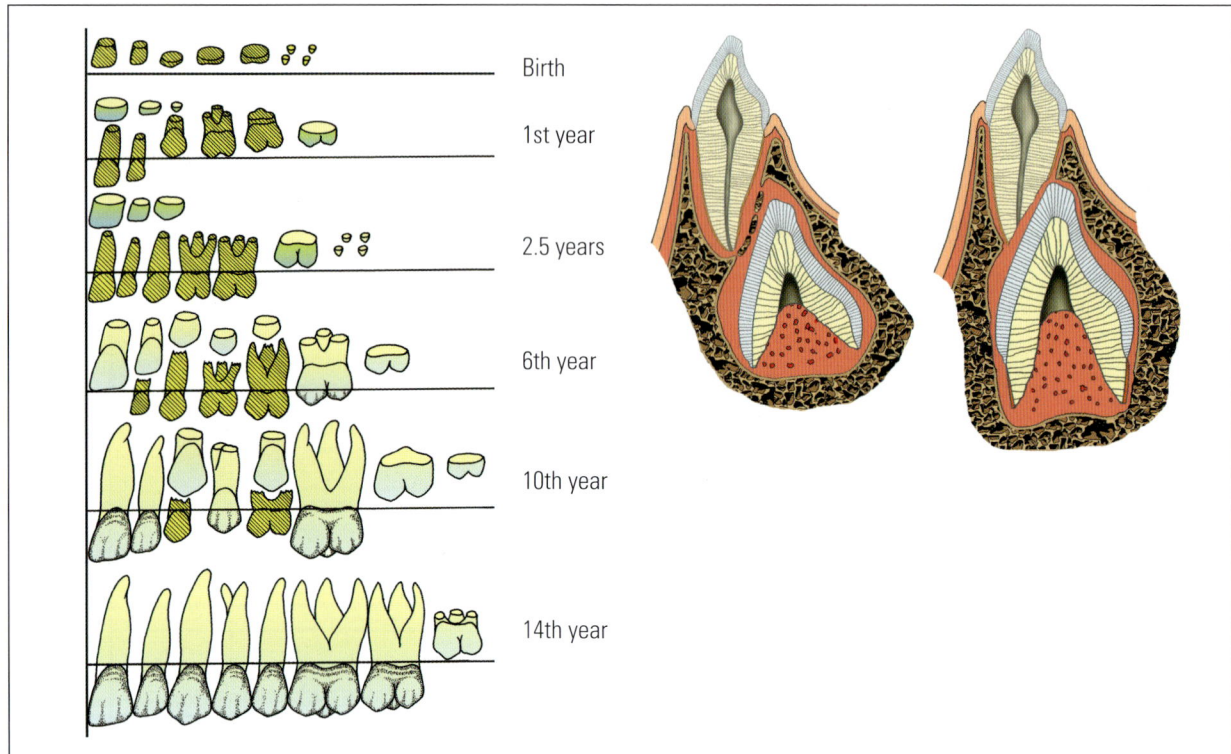

Fig 4-65 During root formation of the successional teeth, the crowns are pushed occlusally, and the primary roots are resorbed. At the same time, the alveoli of the primary teeth disappear as a result of bone resorption. When the succeeding tooth erupts and the primary tooth is shed, the alveolus for the permanent tooth develops through the formation of new bone material.

their crowns exfoliated (Fig 4-65). Eruption of the successional teeth also starts with early root growth, when root dentin and cementum are formed and the bone tissue is remodeled. Both processes are associated with the alveolar bone and the roots of the primary teeth being resorbed. The resorption starts a few years before a primary tooth is shed.

The **posterior successional teeth**, the premolars, are located between the flared roots of the primary teeth, whereas the **anterior successional teeth** are located anterior to the axis of the primary teeth. The primary tooth root is therefore resorbed at an angle from the lingual aspect. Later the successional teeth move directly inferior to the primary teeth, so that there is more space available for the successional teeth to grow. Growth and resorption processes are interrupted by resting phases.

The **pulp tissue** of the primary teeth is not dissolved but remains functional until the teeth are

shed. The coronal pulp retains its normal structure and remains fully functional until shortly before the crown is shed. In an inflammatory process, the pulp is transformed into granulation tissue at that time. As a result, the shedding of primary teeth happens without purulent inflammation or swelling. If coronal pulp has died, the resorption process may be slightly delayed.

The driving force for tooth eruption is mechanical growth pressure from root growth and the tensile force of the periodontal fibers already formed at the cervical root stump. The tooth is lifted out of the alveolar bone by the pull of bundles of fibers running in a coronal direction.

Eruption does not start until the periodontal ligament has developed at the coronal parts of the root. Later, physiologic tooth movements also take place as a result of the force of the periodontal fibers. Defective developments occur as a result of natural events, accidents, or dental interventions.

Morphology of the Dentition

Form and Function of the Dentition

Because teeth develop according to the law of form and function, the rows of teeth are defined in terms of their form and position in relation to each other as a functional dentition. Therefore, the forms should be interpreted as indications of their particular functions; ie, the form is the material expression of function.

A few geometric lines and figures can be used to describe the rows of teeth. They help to define the shape of the dental arches so that, in an edentulous jaw, the original tooth positions can be rediscovered. They are also useful in measuring the mandible and the maxilla. "Joint machines" (articulators) can be constructed with the data obtained to imitate the movement of the mandible.

The rows of teeth are described in the three anatomical planes of reference of the skull: the horizontal, sagittal, and frontal planes. The descriptive models can be taken from orthodontic model analysis and articulation theory.

Dental arch forms in the *horizontal plane* develop as a result of heredity, the number and form of the teeth, the influence of the muscles of the tongue and cheeks, and the structure of the facial part of the skull. In the primary dentition, the rows of teeth are semicircular. In the permanent dentition, the vestibular edges of the maxillary teeth form a semi-ellipse, whereas they follow the course of a parabola in the mandible. The maxillary and mandibular rows of teeth therefore do not have the same form; the maxillary arch is larger in the anterior area and extends over the mandibular arch, whereas this difference is evened out in the posterior region in favor of the mandibular arch. This difference in arch size arises because the mandibular anterior teeth are much narrower than the maxillary anterior teeth.

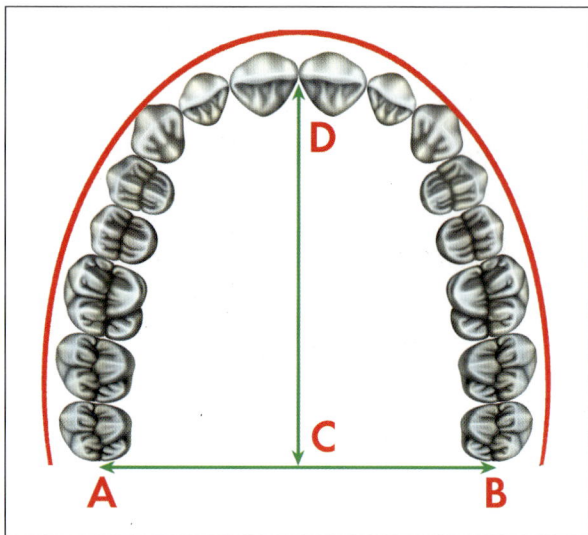

Fig 5-1 The maxillary dental arch is in the form of a semi-ellipse. The short axis of the ellipse measures 57 to 62 mm (A to B), while the half long axis measures 50 to 55 mm (C to D).

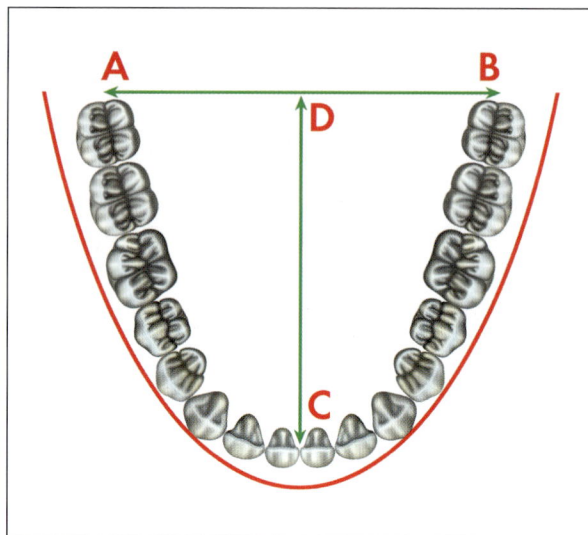

Fig 5-2 The mandibular arch is in the form of a parabola. The distance between the mesiobuccal cusps of the mandibular third molars is 55 to 60 mm (A to B), while the distance from the incisal point to this distance line is 48 to 52 mm (C to D).

The following are the average dimensions for the maxillary and mandibular dental arches: In the maxilla, the distance between the mesiobuccal cusps of the third molars is 57 to 62 mm; the distance from the contact point of the central incisors to the line marking the distance between the mesiobuccal cusps of the third molars is 50 to 55 mm (Fig 5-1). Transferred to an ellipse, the first distance line would be the short axis and the second line the half long axis. In the mandible, the distance between the mesiobuccal cusps of the third molars is 55 to 60 mm and hence is virtually the same as in the maxilla. However, the distance of the contact point of the central incisors to this distance line is only 48 to 52 mm (Fig 5-2).

As for the **dental arch width**, the ratio of tooth size to width of the dental arch is measured at two points in orthodontic model analysis. What is known as *Pont's index* (Figs 5-3 and 5-4) gives the average ratio between the width of all four incisors in the maxilla (sum of incisors = SI) and the width of the dental arch at two points, ie, the transverse distance between the first premolars (anterior arch width) and between the first molars (posterior arch width). To obtain actual figures, the numerator is multiplied by 100. Therefore, the dental arch width at the premolars (P) would be:

$$\frac{SI \times 100}{80} = P - P$$

while the dental arch width at the molars (M) would be:

$$\frac{SI \times 100}{64} = M - M$$

The **dental arch length** is derived from the ratio of tooth size to dental arch width. The length is measured as the vertical distance between the premolar arch width and the incisors. The dental arch lengths in the maxilla and in the mandible are the following:

- Maxillary dental arch length $= \dfrac{SI \times 100}{160}$

- Mandibular dental arch length $= \dfrac{SI \times 100}{160} - 2$

The symmetry of the dental arches can be determined through the midlines of the jaws. In the maxilla, the palatine raphe forms the axis of symmetry. The *raphe-papillary transversal* or *cross line* is another orientation line that runs at right angles to the median palatine raphe through the

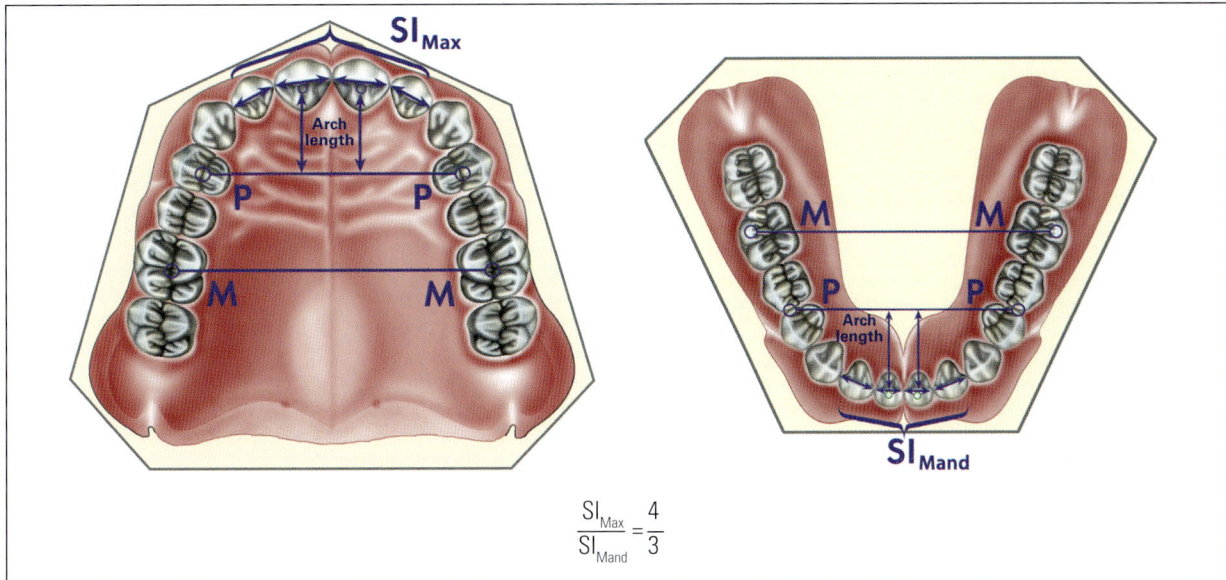

$$\frac{SI_{Max}}{SI_{Mand}} = \frac{4}{3}$$

Figs 5-3 and 5-4 The best-known method of model analysis in orthodontics is to determine Pont's index. A statistical average value establishes the ratio of the incisal widths in the maxilla to the dental arch width at two points. The sum of the incisors (SI) multiplied by 100 is divided by 80 to give the distance between the premolars (P) and is divided by 64 to give the distance between the molars (M). The dental arch length is the vertical distance from the incisors to the anterior arch width between the premolars and is calculated in the maxilla by multiplying SI by 100 and then dividing by 160. The mandibular posterior arch width between the premolars and molars as well as the mandibular arch length can also be calculated using an average ratio of the tooth widths of the mandibular anterior teeth to the maxillary anterior teeth.

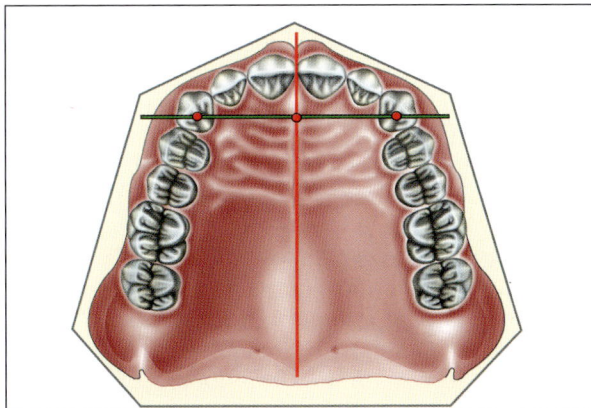

Fig 5-5 A measuring and orientation line that runs at right angles to the median palatine raphe is used in orthodontics. This line is the raphe-papillary transversal or cross line, which runs through the posterior area of the incisal papilla and through the canine points.

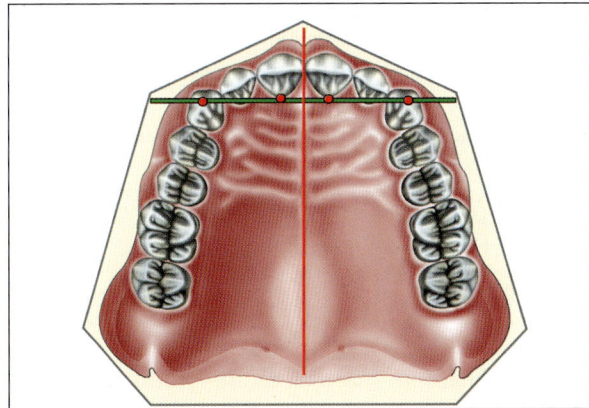

Fig 5-6 In complete denture prosthetics, this cross line is constructed through the middle of the incisal papilla and runs along the palatal surfaces of the central incisors to the tips of the canines; it is used for reconstructing the position of the anterior teeth.

posterior area of the incisal papilla and through the canines (Fig 5-5). In complete denture prosthetics, another cross line is constructed through the middle of the incisal papilla, also at right angles to the middle of the palate. It should run along the palatal surfaces of the central incisors to the tips of the canines; it is used for reconstructing the position of the anterior teeth (Fig 5-6).

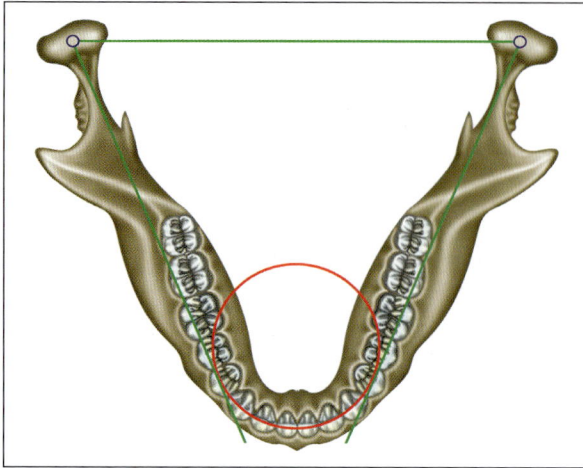

Fig 5-7 The Bonwill circle is a circular arch over the incisal edges of the mandibular anterior teeth and the buccal cusp tips of the mandibular first premolars. The tangents to this circle run over the buccal cusp tips of the posterior teeth to the midpoints of the condyle. The Bonwill circle and its tangents provide an initial approximation of the arch form of the mandibular teeth.

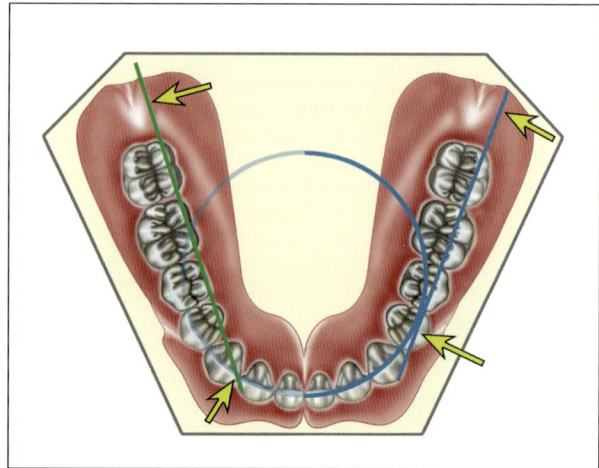

Fig 5-8 The tangents of the Bonwill circle *(blue)* start at the buccal cusp tips of the first premolars and run over the buccal cusps of the posterior teeth to the buccal contour of the mandibular alveolar tubercle. The Pound line *(green)* runs from the mesial contact point of the mandibular canine to the lingual contour of the tubercle; it runs through the tips of the lingual cusps of the mandibular posterior teeth.

The axis of symmetry of the dental arch has to be constructed in the mandible. It runs through the mandibular incisal point, which is the contact point between the two central incisors, and through the center-to-center distance of the two molar triangles.

Dentition in the Horizontal Plane

Geometric constructions can be used to describe the mandibular dental arch form. These include the Bonwill circle with its tangents, the Pound line, and the centers of the ridges.

The **Bonwill circle** (after William Gibson Bonwill) describes a circular arch that runs over the incisal edges of the mandibular anterior teeth and the buccal cusp tips of the mandibular first premolars (Fig 5-7). Tangents to this circle can be placed in the tips of the premolar cusps. These tangents run over the buccal cusp tips of the posterior teeth, over the buccal contour of the retromolar triangle (or mandibular alveolar tubercle), to the mid-

points of the condyles of the mandible (Fig 5-8). The Bonwill circle and its tangents provide an initial approximation of the arch form of the mandibular teeth.

The **Pound line** is a connecting line between the mesial contact point of the mandibular canine and the lingual contour of the retromolar triangle. The line runs through the tips of the lingual cusps of the mandibular posterior teeth (see Fig 5-8).

The **ridge or crest line** is the midline on the (edentulous) alveolar crests. In the mandible, it runs from the canine points to the middle of the mandibular alveolar tubercle; the central developmental grooves follow the course of this line. When setting up artificial posterior teeth, this line is essential for producing statically reliable tooth positions.

The position of the mandibular dental arch in the skull or facial area is determined by the occlusal plane, the Bonwill triangle, and the Balkwill angle. The Bonwill triangle defines the position of the occlusal plane in relation to the joints via the mandibular incisal point and the Balkwill angle. This establishes the average position of the mandibular teeth or the mandibular model at the joint points.

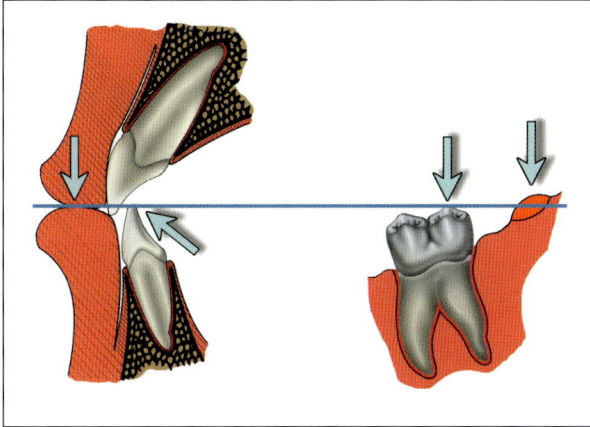

Fig 5-9 The *occlusal plane* is defined as a horizontal plane that runs through three points in the mandibular teeth: the mandibular incisal point and the distobuccal cusp tips of the mandibular second molars. This occlusal plane is level with the lip closure line and can bisect the retromolar triangle at half-height.

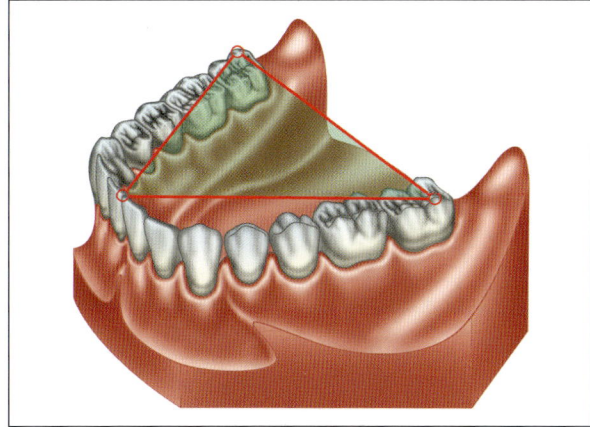

Fig 5-10 The occlusal plane forms a horizontal triangle through the three points in the mandibular dentition. Within this plane, the teeth meet in terminal occlusion. If the occlusal plane is extended forward and backward, it bisects the lip closure line at the front and the retromolar triangle at the rear.

The **mandibular incisal point** is the contact point between the mandibular central incisors. On the articulator, a mark is made that denotes the mandibular incisal point, either directly by means of an incisal pointer or indirectly with an adjustment tool for fixing the mandibular model.

The **occlusal plane** (or *bite plane*) is defined by three points in the mandibular dentition. It runs through the mandibular incisal point as far as the distobuccal cusps of the mandibular second molars (Fig 5-9). This forms a triangular shape. If the occlusal plane is extended forward and backward, the plane bisects the lip closure line at the front and the superior third of the retromolar triangle at the rear (Fig 5-10). The occlusal plane lies roughly parallel to the Camper plane (approximately 2 cm inferiorly) and parallel to the interpupillary line (Fig 5-11). Once the lip closure line on the occlusion rims and the half-height of the retromolar triangles on mandibular models are established, the course of the occlusal plane can be determined in edentulous jaws. The occlusal plane is a mean value for construction of articulators; it is permanently drawn onto average-value articulators and is hence an orientation guide when mounting the models in the articulator and when setting up the teeth.

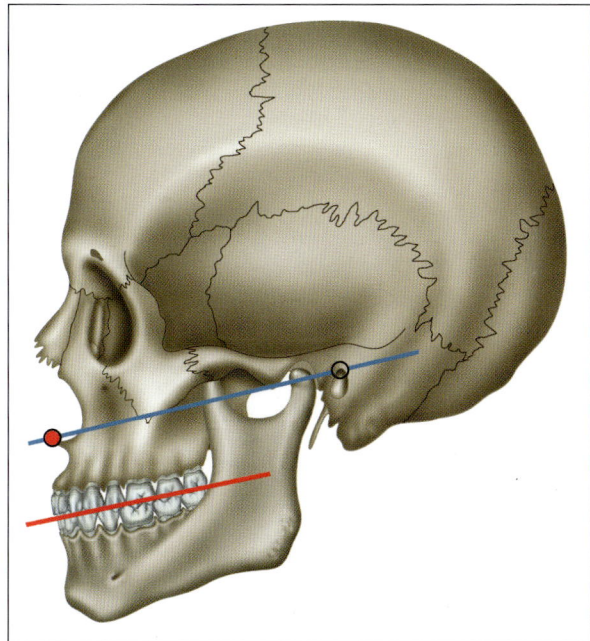

Fig 5-11 The occlusal plane lies roughly parallel to the Camper plane (approximately 2 cm inferiorly) and parallel to the interpupillary line. The occlusal plane is a mean value for construction of articulators; it is permanently drawn onto average-value articulators and is hence an orientation guide when mounting the models in the articulator and when setting up the teeth. The occlusal plane is sometimes called the *bite plane*.

119

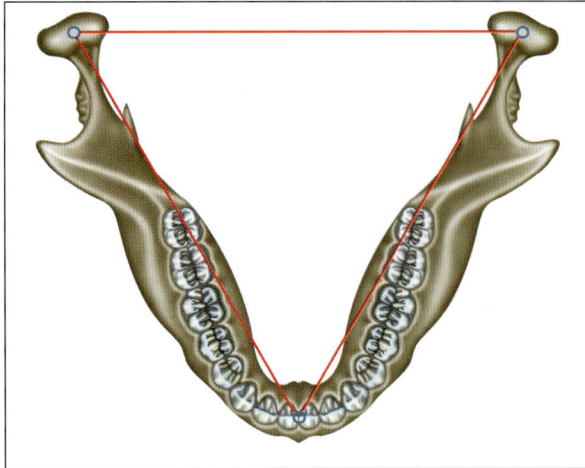

Fig 5-12 The Bonwill triangle is an equilateral triangle in which the 11.5-cm-long sides are statistically calculated and can stretch from the mandibular incisal point to the midpoints of the mandibular condyles. The Bonwill triangle defines the position of the occlusal plane in relation to the joints via the incisal point and the Balkwill angle. This enables the average position of the mandibular model at the joint points to be reconstructed.

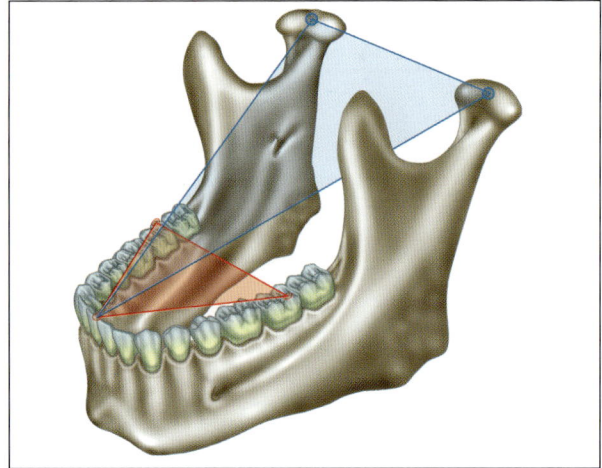

Fig 5-13 A perspective view of the Bonwill triangle with the occlusal plane shows the relationship between these geometric constructions.

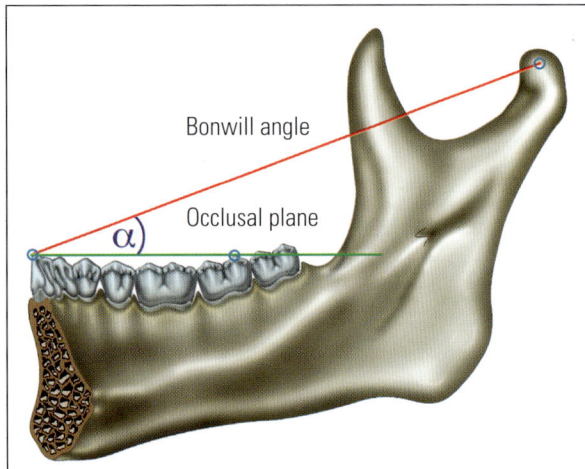

Fig 5-14 The Balkwill angle (α) denotes the incline of the Bonwill triangle to the occlusal plane or to the Camper plane; the angle of the Bonwill triangle to the occlusal plane at the incisal point is 22 degrees on average. This statistical mean is integrated into an average-value articulator and thus fixes the position of the mandibular incisal point and the occlusal plane at the joint points. In a joint-oriented interocclusal record using a facebow, the Balkwill angle is (indirectly) determined individually.

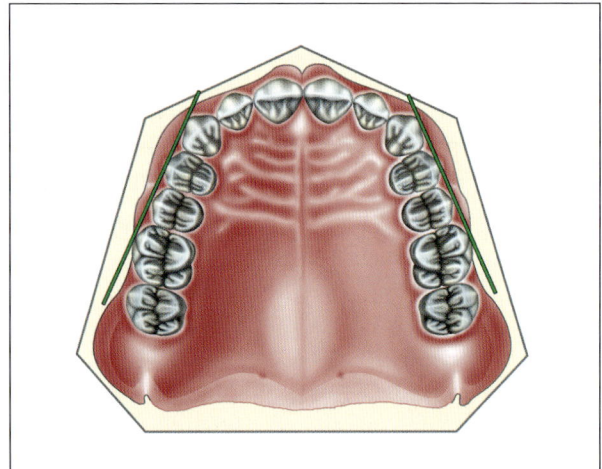

Fig 5-15 The premolar tangent in the maxilla runs from the labial medial ridge of the canine to the mesiobuccal cusp ridge of the first molar. Teeth must be set up in line with this tangent to meet an esthetic requirement: So that the mouth does not appear too full, the premolars must lie within this tangent.

The ***Bonwill triangle*** is an equilateral triangle in which the 11.5-cm-long sides (formerly 10 cm) are statistically calculated and can stretch from the mandibular incisal point to the midpoints of the mandibular condyles (Figs 5-12 and 5-13). The size of the Bonwill triangle is a statistical average

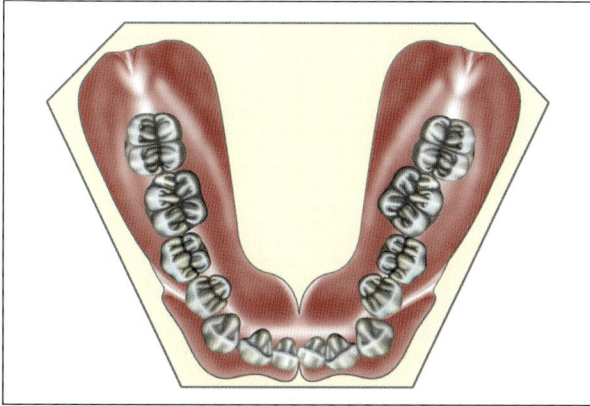

Fig 5-16 Malposition resulting from displacement of individual teeth or groups of teeth clearly reveals the deformation of the dental arch. The malposition is usually caused by crowding and only rarely by gaps in the dentition.

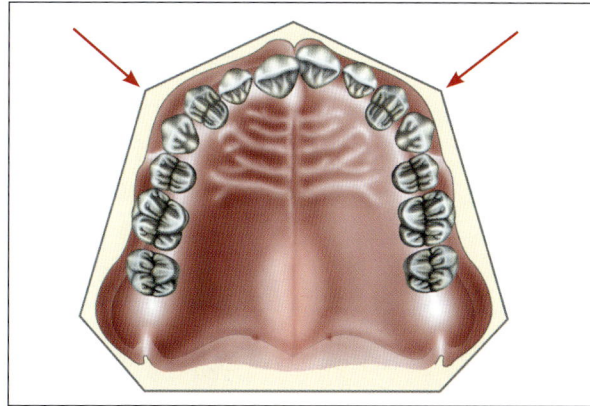

Fig 5-17 One striking malposition occurs when the canine has swapped places with the first premolar *(arrows)*.

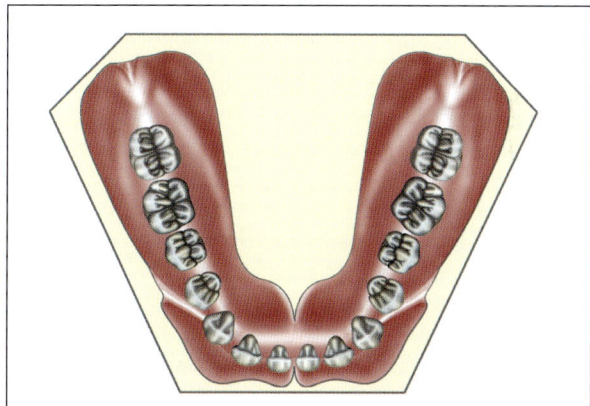

Fig 5-18 Severe crowding or large gaps between the teeth arise because of a mismatch between tooth size and jaw size.

that is constantly being reviewed and corrected. It enables the size of an articulator to be fixed in its key dimensions (distance between the joints and the incisal point).

The ***Balkwill angle*** denotes the angle between the Bonwill triangle and the occlusal plane (the Camper plane); the angle at the incisal point is 22 degrees on average (Fig 5-14). This statistical mean is integrated into an average-value articulator and thus establishes the position of the mandibular incisal point.

The lines and figures described above refer to the mandibular dental arch, but they also define the ellipsoid course of the maxillary teeth because the teeth have a definite positional relationship to each other as a result of their occlusal pattern. Once the mandibular tooth position has been clearly found with the aid of these lines, the dentition in the maxilla can be reconstructed on the basis of regular intercuspation.

The ***premolar tangent*** in the maxilla is a form characteristic of the maxillary arch that is seen as an esthetic requirement: So that the mouth does not appear too full, the premolars stand within a line that runs from the labial medial ridge of the canine to the mesiobuccal cusp ridge of the first molar (Fig 5-15).

Malposition of teeth in the horizontal plane

The development of the dentition may be disrupted, leading to variations from the normal positioning of teeth (Figs 5-16 to 5-18). A distinction is drawn between rotation, tipping, and displacement of teeth (Fig 5-19). An incorrect tooth position may be caused by displacement of a tooth germ, an incorrect tooth germ, or external influences during normal eruption, such as thumb sucking, lip biting, tongue thrusting, or persistence of primary teeth.

Rotation means a twisted tooth position relative to a vertical axis of rotation. A distinction is drawn between centric rotation (when the central

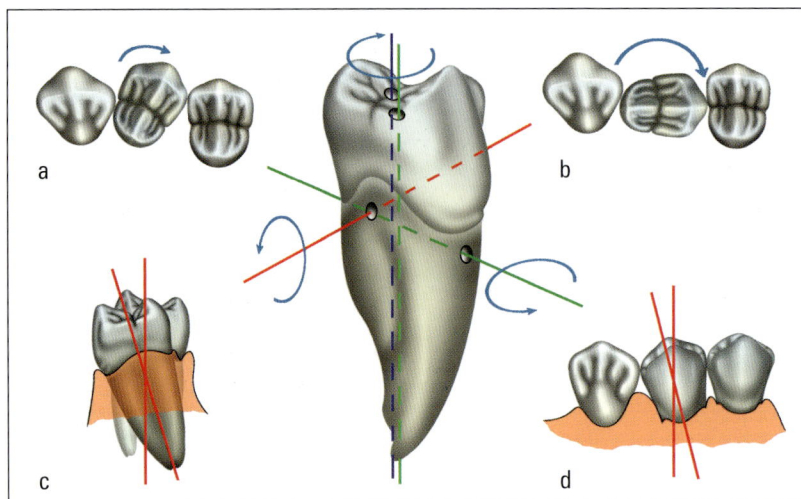

Fig 5-19 Deviations in the position of individual teeth can be defined as rotation or tipping. The following distinctions are made, depending on the position of the axis of rotation or tipping: *(a)* Rotation around an eccentric axis, when one edge of the tooth protrudes from the row of teeth. *(b)* Rotation around a central axis, usually the dental axis. *(c)* Tipping around a transverse axis, where the tooth is tipped in a vestibular or lingual direction. *(d)* Tipping around a sagittal axis, where the tooth is tipped in a mesial or distal direction.

tooth axis is the axis of rotation) and eccentric rotation (when the axis of rotation lies alongside the center of the tooth). A tooth rotated eccentrically out of the dental arch may be pushed back at the edge that is protruding; a centrically rotated tooth is twisted in the dental arch by diametrically opposed forces at its protruding edges. Rotation can be present with or without a lack of space. Severe rotation in a dentition with gaps often has a hereditary element, and the tooth will often rotate back into the incorrect position. This rotating back is stopped by surgical division of the marginal system of fibers. Rotation in a mouth with crowding, once the lack of space has been resolved, is usually rectified by the influence of the lips, cheeks, and tongue.

If a tooth is tipped beyond an axis that lies within the dental arch, or beyond an axis that is perpendicular to the arch, this gives rise to vestibular, oral, mesial, or distal tipping.

Vestibular tipping of the maxillary anterior teeth may be inherited or caused by thumb sucking. In the posterior region, a persistent primary tooth or displacement of a tooth germ may produce vestibular tipping.

Oral tipping of the maxillary anterior teeth is an inherited characteristic of the complete vertical overlap. Oral tipping of the mandibular anterior teeth occurs after premature loss of primary canines in association with considerable lower lip tension. Oral tipping of the posterior teeth arises from incorrect germ positioning and disrupted exfoliation.

Mesial tipping of the incisors often results from a lack of space. If the lack of space is resolved, the incisors usually right themselves again. Mesial and distal tipping in the posterior region can arise because of teeth displaced into a gap.

Tooth displacement means the shifting of individual teeth or groups of teeth. If a tooth exceeded the occlusal level at eruption or if the occlusal line is not reached, this is deemed to be tooth displacement (high or low). Displacements usually accompany tipping or rotation.

Tooth retention is present when a tooth lies correctly in the jaw but remains buried beyond the normal eruption time. Semiretention arises if a tooth has only managed half of its eruption path because it is squeezed by crowding or because root and alveolar bone are fused.

Crowding can have various causes and take various forms. In the case of primary crowding, there is often a mismatch between tooth size and jaw size, for example, in the form of restricted development in the growth of jaw width and length. Secondary crowding results from pronounced mesial migration of the posterior teeth, so that the anterior teeth twist to form a flat front. A lack of space will produce local tipping and rotation when the crowding affects parts of the dentition or the entire arch. A temporary lack of space will result from primary tooth persistence.

Spaces or gaps can have a hereditary cause, where the teeth are too small in jaws that are too large (see Fig 5-18). A localized space between the central incisors or in other parts of the dental arch

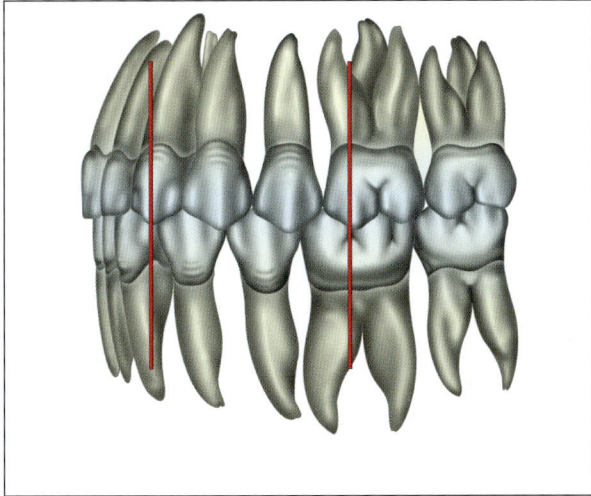

Fig 5-20 The antagonists rule describes the regular intercuspation within the rows of teeth, whereby each tooth has two antagonists (occlusion of cusps, fossae, and marginal ridges). The mandibular central incisors and the last maxillary molars are the exception to the rule, with only one antagonist each. Antagonists fit into the approximal depressions of the opposing teeth.

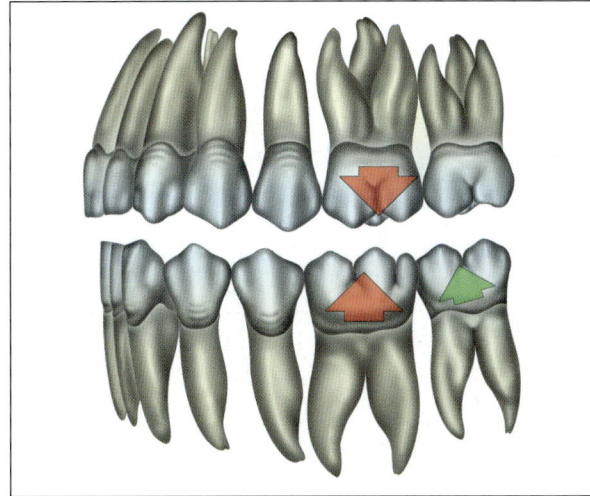

Fig 5-21 A distinction is made between the primary and secondary antagonists. The primary antagonist is the tooth of the same name in the opposing jaw *(red arrows)*. Secondary antagonists lie mesial to the primary antagonist in the mandible and distal to it in the maxilla *(green arrow)*.

is called a *diastema*. Gaps can arise because of external influences such as supernumerary teeth or cysts intervening, but also when the tongue or foreign bodies are incorporated as a result of habit. Spaces between all the teeth can be resolved if all the teeth are pushed forward toward the midline. Gaps in the maxillary anterior teeth as a result of thumb sucking are reversible if the child gives up the habit. Spaces in the mandibular anterior teeth can be caused by overdevelopment or faulty functioning of the tongue. Tongue function can usually be relearned with the aid of appliances. In the case of overdevelopment, surgical reduction of the tongue may become necessary. Dysgnathia caused by lack of space is more common than faulty development caused by dentitions with gaps.

Dentition in the Sagittal Plane

In the sagittal plane, the rows of teeth can be described in their state of intercuspation. Different views of the teeth become visible, depending on which sagittal plane is chosen: The medial plane shows the rows of teeth from the lingual; if the sagittal plane lies outside the dental arches, the rows of teeth are seen from the vestibular view. The intercuspation of the teeth can be seen in each view and follows a regular pattern.

The *antagonists rule* (occlusion of cusps, fossae, and marginal ridges) denotes the regular intercuspation of the rows of teeth, whereby each tooth has two antagonists (Fig 5-20). The mandibular central incisors and the maxillary third molars (or second molars in the absence of third molars) are the exception to the rule, with only one antagonist each.

The *antagonist* (opposing tooth) denotes the tooth that occludes with the corresponding teeth in the opposing jaw when biting down. A distinction is made between the primary and secondary antagonists. The primary antagonist is the tooth of the same name in the opposing jaw. Secondary antagonists lie mesial to the primary antagonist in the mandible and distal to it in the maxilla (Fig 5-21).

Neutro-occlusion denotes the state of intercuspation in the normal occlusion, when the tip of

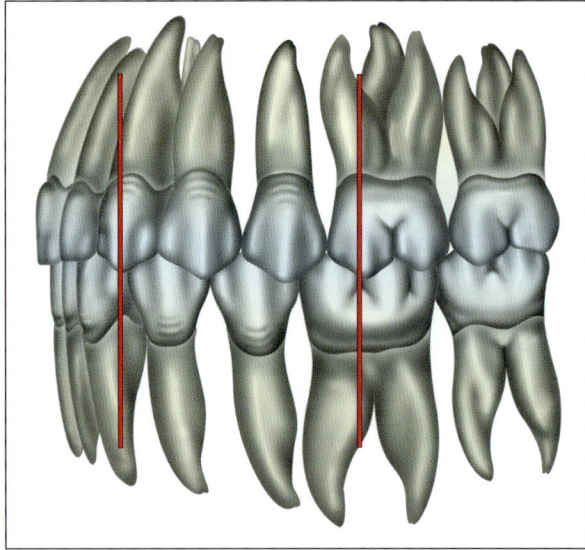

Fig 5-22 Neutro-occlusion denotes intercuspation in the normal sequence of antagonists in relation to the fixed points: The maxillary canine lies between the mandibular canine and first premolar, while the mesiobuccal cusp of the first molar occludes with the middle of the mandibular first molar. Angle's classification provides a descriptive model of the malpositions of teeth and dental arch deformation, which makes treatment planning simpler. This classification refers to malocclusions in the sagittal direction.

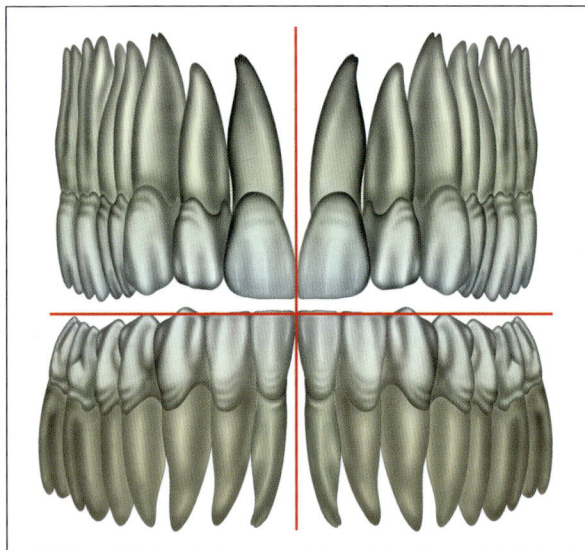

Fig 5-23 The frontal view of the dentition in neutro-occlusion shows the symmetric arrangement of the teeth in relation to the middle of the face; all the teeth are slightly inclined mesially. The maxillary anterior teeth are level with the horizontal occlusal plane; the posterior teeth follow the path of the sagittal curve of occlusion.

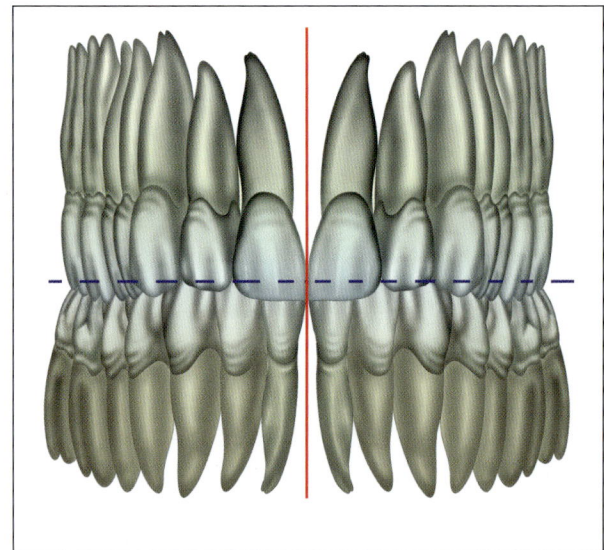

Fig 5-24 Intercuspation according to the antagonists rule can be seen in the frontal view of neutro-occlusion; the mandibular central incisors only have one antagonist. The maxillary anterior teeth fit over the mandibular antagonists; the buccal cusps of the maxillary posterior teeth also fit over their mandibular antagonists.

the maxillary canine lies between the mandibular canine and the first premolar, while the mesiobuccal cusp of the maxillary first molar fits into the buccal fissure of the mandibular first molar (Figs 5-22 to 5-24). In the medial plane, neutro-occlusion displays the regular intercuspation of the anterior teeth in the form of the normal (or scissors) occlusion. The horizontal overlap and protrusion of the maxillary teeth in relation to the mandibular anterior teeth can be seen here; this

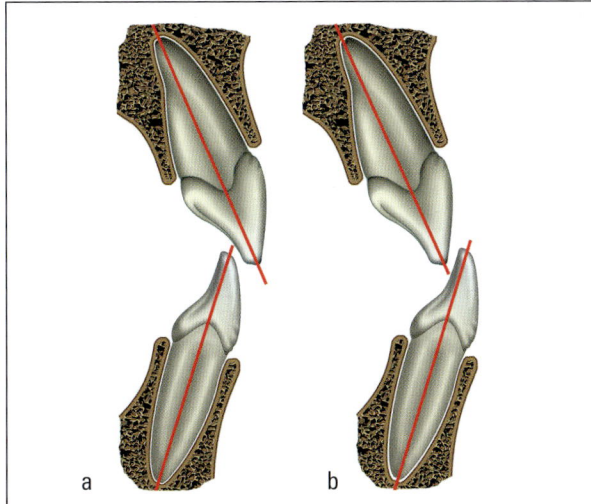

Fig 5-25 *(a)* The vertical overlap of the maxillary anterior teeth over the mandibular anterior teeth gives rise to a scissors effect of the anterior teeth, which is why the normal occlusion is also sometimes called a *scissors bite*. The mandible is pushed forward to achieve the scissors effect or to bite food more efficiently. *(b)* A vertical overlap of the mandibular anterior teeth in front of the maxillary anterior teeth is less favorable because the mandible can only be forcibly retracted a small amount for a better scissors effect.

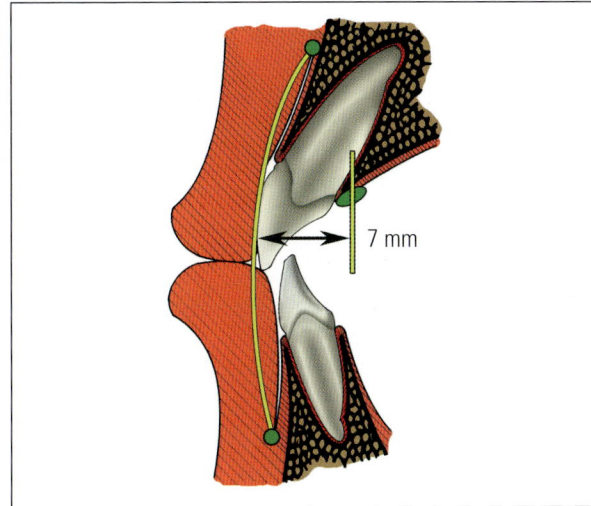

Fig 5-26 The vertical anterior dental arch is a flat section of a circular arc from the maxillary to the mandibular vestibular fornix. The arc runs an average distance of 7 mm from the middle of the incisive papilla and defines the natural shape of the mouth externally. The labial contours of the maxillary incisors lie on this section of the arc and support the upper lip. With their incisal edges, they turn the lower lip outward slightly.

is also known as the *overjet*. The scissor effect of the incisors is achieved by the mandible being pushed forward when biting food (Fig 5-25).

The **vertical anterior dental arch** describes the vestibular angulation of the anterior teeth. Viewing tooth position and inclinations of the alveolar ridge in the medial plane, a circular arc can be drawn from the maxillary to the mandibular vestibular fornix, the contour of which runs 7 mm from the middle of the incisive papilla. The labial contour of the maxillary anterior teeth lies on this arc, so that these teeth support the upper lip with their labial surfaces and the bottom lip with their incisal edges (Fig 5-26). For prosthetic work, the position of the anterior teeth should be reconstructed in keeping with the vertical anterior dental arch.

The **vestibular inclination of the anterior teeth** can be interpreted as a rudimentary snout formation of the dentition. The protruded part of the mouth allows the teeth to bite food more efficiently without requiring so much force because of the advantageous effect of the scissor action of the relatively sharp incisors. The canines and premolars are used for biting very tough food.

The sagittal plane reveals yet another characteristic form of the dentition: The mandibular teeth are inclined mesially on the jaw, as are the maxillary anterior teeth and premolars; only the maxillary first molar stands almost vertically, while the subsequent maxillary molars appear to be tipped distally (Fig 5-27). This means that the teeth form a curve in the line in which they occlude (Fig 5-28).

The **sagittal curve of occlusion** (occlusal line) is the continuous connecting line along the occlusal surfaces of the posterior teeth in the maxilla and the mandible in the sagittal direction. It starts at the tip of the mandible, falls away caudally, reaches its lowest point at the first molar, and rises again with the last molars; the distobuccal cusp of the second molar lies at the same level as the tip of the canine. If the sagittal curve of occlusion is drawn along both the mandibular and maxillary buccal cusp tips and is projected onto the sagittal plane, the two lines run parallel, but the maxillary curve is displaced caudally in comparison with the mandibular curve, according to the depth of intercuspation or cusp height. The sagittal curve of occlusion divides the occlusal plane

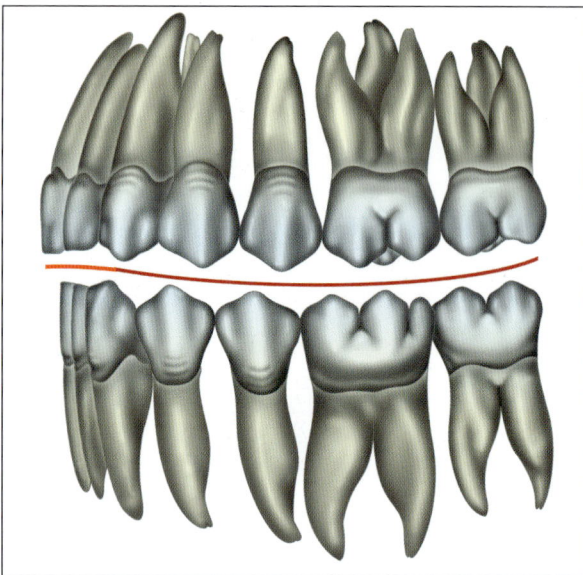

Fig 5-27 The typical mesial inclination of the teeth can be seen in the vestibular view. The first molar, which stands vertically, and the maxillary second and third molars, which are inclined distally, are the exceptions.

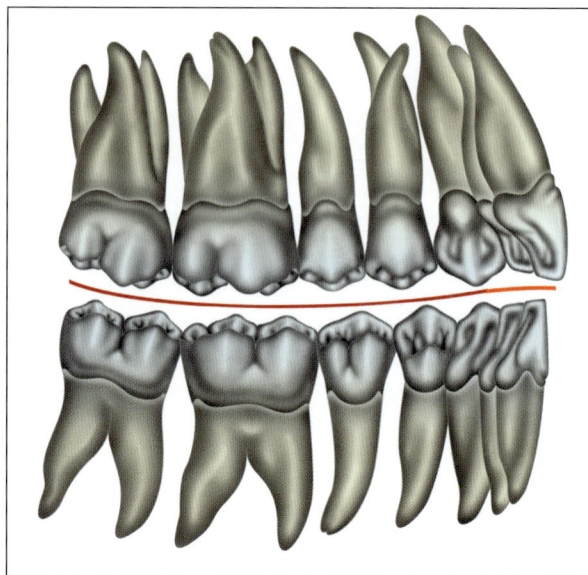

Fig 5-28 The mesial inclination and the root characteristic—the distal curvature of the roots—form vertical curves that produce a harmonious match with the pattern of masticatory forces.

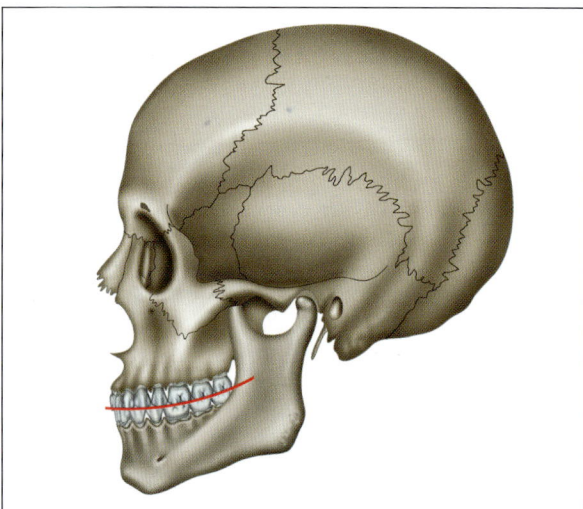

Fig 5-29 The sagittal curve of occlusion is a line curving slightly caudally.

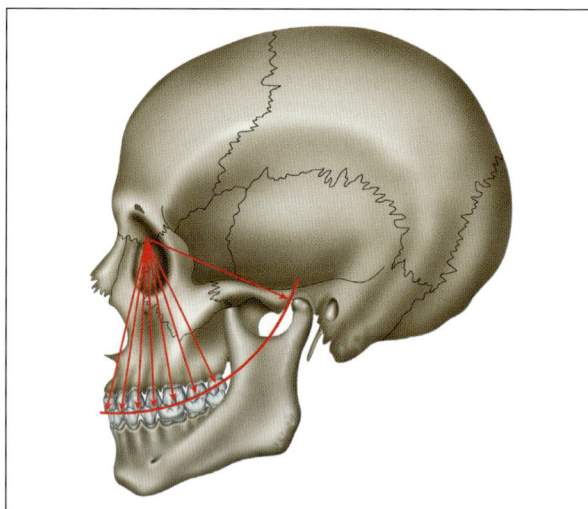

Fig 5-30 The curve of Spee must be seen as a special form of the sagittal curve of occlusion. According to Spee, the dental axes are inclined so that their projections meet in the orbital cavity as radii of the curve of Spee. The dorsal projection of the curve of Spee is supposed to be at a tangent to the anterior surface of the condyle of the mandible. Spee assumed that this curve, which was named after him, corresponded to the path of movement of the mandible in protrusive excursions. He believed that the teeth would always maintain sliding contact in any movement along this curve. However, more detailed analysis has shown that these contacts do not exist in the normal bite.

Fig 5-31 An Angle Class II malocclusion is described as disto-occlusion of the mandibular dentition. The antagonists are displaced by at least one-fourth of a premolar's width in relation to the fixed points.

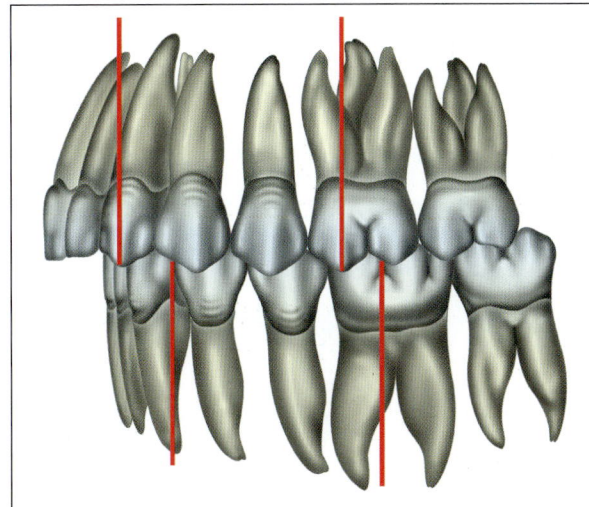

at four common points: on the right and left at the distobuccal cusp of the second molar and at the tips of the right and left canines. If the path of the occlusal plane is known, the sagittal curve of occlusion can be reconstructed.

The **curve of Spee** (named after Count Ferdinand Spee) is a sagittal curve of occlusion that bends sharply downward, its dorsal projection touching the anterior surface of the condyle (Figs 5-29 and 5-30). The tooth axes are inclined so that their projections meet in the orbital cavity as radii of the curve of Spee. According to Spee, the forward movement (protrusive excursion) of the mandible runs along this curve, with all the teeth maintaining sliding contact. This is not true of the normal occlusion. The sagittal curve of occlusion follows a flatter course and enables separation of the posterior teeth during protrusive excursions.

Malposition of teeth in the sagittal plane

Occlusal anomalies in the sagittal direction can be described as malocclusions according to Angle's classification. Starting with neutro-occlusion (Class I), a distinction is made between unilateral or bilateral disto-occlusion (Class II) and unilateral or bilateral mesio-occlusion (Class III).

Disto-occlusion or *posterior occlusion* means retrusion of the mandibular teeth in relation to the fixed points: The maxillary canine and the

maxillary first molar are pushed anteriorly by one-fourth of a premolar's width from the position of neutroocclusion (Fig 5-31). All possible malpositions of individual teeth can be seen here. One noticeable defect of this occlusal displacement is the position of the anterior teeth in relation to each other. This gives two more groups of divergent anterior relationships.

The **anterior open bite** with protrusion of the maxilla (Angle Class II, division 1) takes the following forms:

- Labial tipping of the maxillary incisors
- Lingual tipping of the mandibular incisors
- Lengthening of the maxillary dental arch (tapered front)
- Shortening of the mandibular dental arch to produce a flattened front
- Sagittal overdevelopment of the maxilla (prognathism)
- Sagittal underdevelopment of the mandible (micrognathism)

In combined forms, the vertical overlap of the incisors can be very large so that the lips are not closed when in their relaxed position, and the incisal margins of the maxillary anterior teeth lie in front of the bottom lip. The resultant open-mouth breathing affects the bacterial flora in the oral cavity and increases the susceptibility to caries. If the bottom lip presses behind the maxillary anterior teeth when swallowing to ensure an air-tight

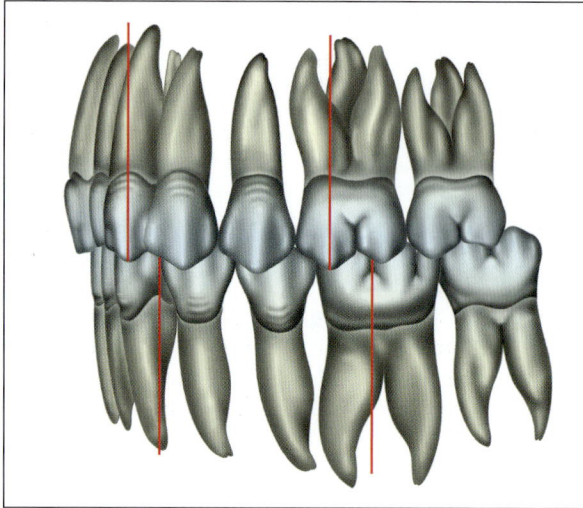

Fig 5-32 A key sign of an Angle Class II, division 2 malocclusion is the vertical overlap, which is caused by steep inversion of the incisors with anterior crowding.

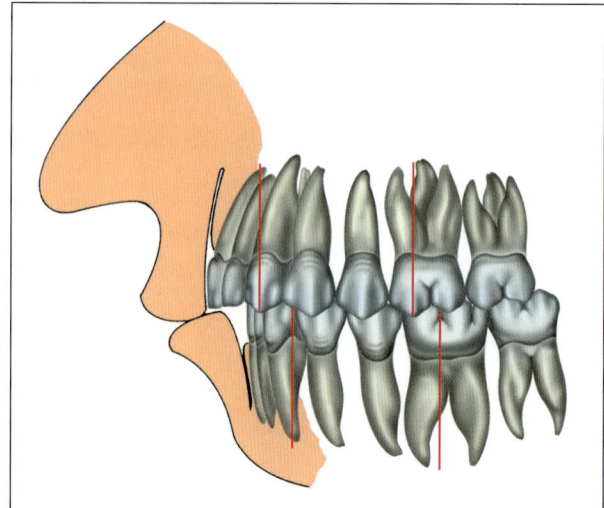

Fig 5-33 The sagittal overdevelopment of the maxilla (prognathism) or sagittal underdevelopment of the mandible (micrognathism) brings with it extraoral changes, such as the impression of a receding chin with a large midface (prominent nose profile), seen here.

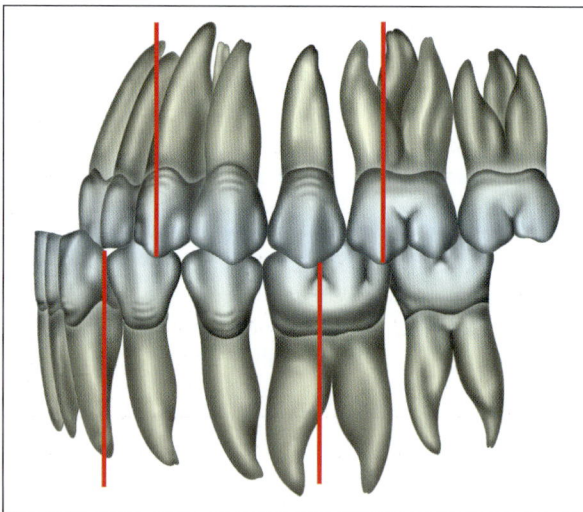

Fig 5-34 An Angle Class III malocclusion is described as mesio-occlusion or prognathism, in which the mandibular dentition is displaced mesially by one-fourth of a premolar's width in relation to the fixed points; this gives the chin a jutting appearance.

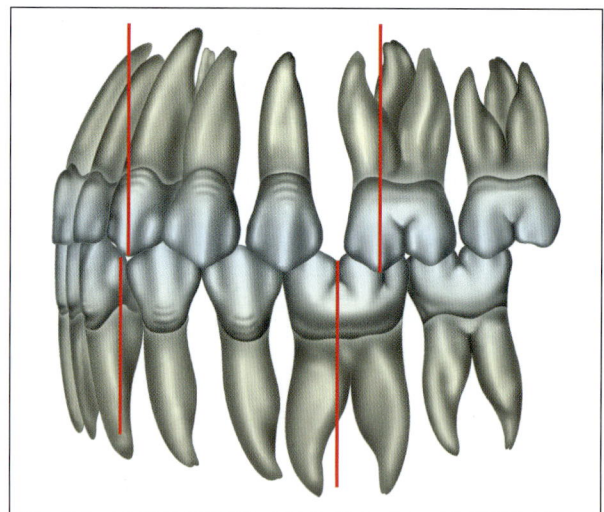

Fig 5-35 An occlusal variant of mesio-occlusion with normal vertical overlap of the anterior teeth develops because of gaps between the anterior teeth as well as between the posterior teeth.

seal, the protrusion is increased. This dentition anomaly is usually hereditary and less often due to exogenous factors such as thumb sucking, nasal breathing, or incorrect sleeping position.

A *deep bite* or *steep bite* (Angle Class II, division 2) exists if the maxillary incisors are positioned extremely steeply in the jaw and cover the

mandibular anterior teeth to a variable width without sagittal protrusion (Fig 5-32). The more inverted the teeth (tipped inward), the more pronounced is any anterior crowding. The lateral incisors sometimes overlap the central incisors or the canines in a flattened anterior dentition. If the alveolar ridges are lengthened, the maxillary incisors reach the mandibular gingival margin or vestibular fornix. Here both the maxillary and mandibular anterior teeth go beyond the normal occlusal plane. A vertical overlap may also exist in combination with neutro-occlusion. The profile appearance of a vertical overlap is a deepened mentolabial sulcus over a prominent chin and a shortened lower face. It gives the impression of overdevelopment of the midface with a large nose (prominent nose profile) (Fig 5-33). In the case of deep bites, the sideways movement of the mandible under tooth contact is impeded or impossible. The masticatory movements then tend to follow a chopping masticatory pattern. Forward movements lead to excessively wide distances between posterior teeth.

Mesio-occlusion denotes the mesial displacement of the mandibular dentition by at least one-fourth of the premolar's width, in relation to the fixed points (Fig 5-34). The anterior teeth may have a normal vertical overlap, and gaps between the maxillary anterior teeth are common (Fig 5-35); edge-to-edge occlusion, in which the incisal margins of the maxillary and mandibular anterior teeth meet, is possible. If the inclination of the axes of the teeth is correct, this results in protrusion of the mandibular anterior teeth in front of the maxillary teeth. This malposition of the teeth is known as an *anterior reverse articulation*, *reverse vertical overlap*, or *mandibular protrusion*. If brought into the neutro-occlusion position, a mesio-occlusion can have entirely normal intercuspation of the posterior teeth and incisors with a normal vertical overlap.

Prognathism denotes the sagittal protrusion of the mandibular anterior teeth without the presence of mesio-occlusion. The extraoral symptom of prognathism is a pronounced, protruding, prominent chin, hence the alternative name *progenia* (*geneion* = chin). Prognathism can take the following forms:

- Tipping of the maxillary anterior teeth in a palatal direction
- Tipping of the mandibular anterior teeth in a labial direction
- Lengthening of the mandibular alveolar arch
- Shortening of the maxillary dental arch to produce a flattened front
- Overdevelopment of the mandible in a sagittal direction

- Underdevelopment of the maxilla (micrognathism)

The degree of prognathism ranges from an edge-to-edge position of the anterior teeth through to the mandibular anterior teeth completely covering the maxillary anterior teeth, which is always associated with a reverse articulation situation. The rows of teeth can cross at the canines or the lateral incisors. In prognathism, the incisal position cannot be adopted or only with force. Sideways movements are possible without slip interferences, provided a reverse vertical overlap is not present. Prognathism is hereditary and can be accentuated by exogenous factors.

Dentition in the Frontal Plane

The symmetric arrangement of the teeth in relation to the middle of the skull or face can be seen in the frontal view of the dental arches. All the teeth in the maxillary and mandibular dentitions have a characteristic inclination (Figs 5-36 and 5-37). The maxillary teeth are inclined in a vestibular direction, while the mandibular teeth and their masticatory surfaces are inclined lingually (except the mandibular incisors). The alveolar ridges also have this inclination. The inclination of the teeth and alveolar ridges is a definite requirement because it means the masticatory forces are mainly transmitted axially to the periodontium: When food is being ground by the posterior teeth, the mandible glides from outward (out of a lateral position) into the terminal occlusal position. Therefore, food tends to be crushed by the mandible gliding from buccal to lingual, the direction of forces corresponding to the inclination of the alveolar ridges.

The **transverse curve of occlusion** is the continuous connecting line along the occlusal surfaces of the posterior teeth of the jaws in the frontal plane, which arises from the lingual inclination of the mandibular posterior teeth (see Fig 5-36). A transverse curve of occlusion can be produced by drawing a line that would connect the idealized occlusal surfaces; this gives a curve that bends caudally and runs vertically to the sagittal curve.

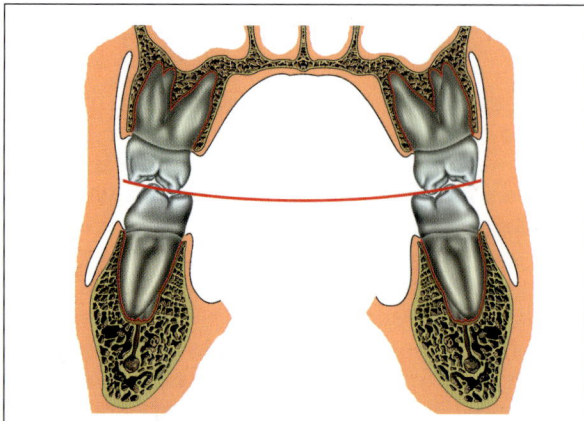

Fig 5-36 A characteristic inclination of the maxillary teeth in a vestibular direction and the mandibular teeth in a lingual direction can be seen from the approximal view. The alveolar ridges are also inclined in the same directions. As a result, the masticatory surfaces in the mandible are inclined toward the floor of the mouth, which gives rise to the so-called transverse curve of occlusion.

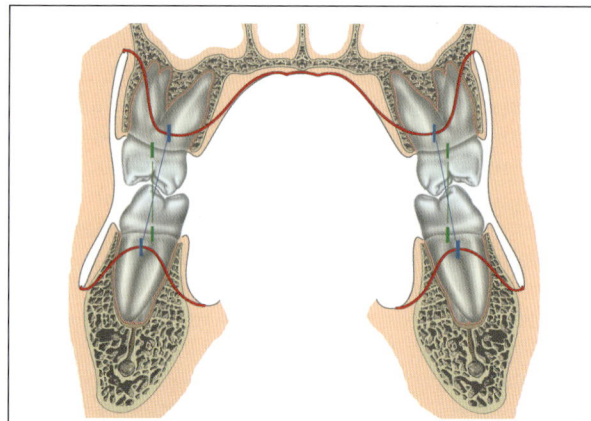

Fig 5-37 Following tooth loss, the jaws shrink in the direction of inclination. As a result, the centers of the alveolar ridges are displaced so that the outline of the maxillary alveolar ridge becomes smaller and that of the mandibular alveolar ridge becomes larger. This fact has implications for the stability of a complete denture.

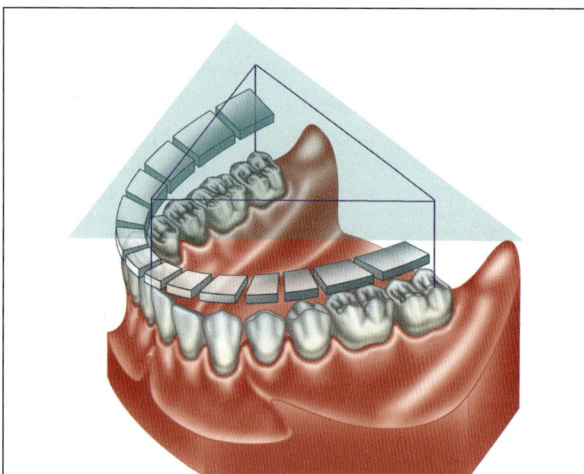

Fig 5-38 The masticatory surfaces of the posterior teeth are arranged together at the occlusal plane in the sagittal and transverse curve of occlusion, which creates a section of a sphere (calotte). This fact should be exploited when setting up complete dentures so that teeth are set up according to a calotte shape.

The bending of the two *curves of occlusion* is almost identical. Both curves therefore span an area that forms a section of the surface of a sphere, a *calotte* (Fig 5-38). The calotte is interrupted in the area where the maxillary anterior teeth occlude over the mandibular anterior teeth.

The *function of the curves of occlusion* is to separate the rows of teeth selectively in respect of masticatory function: The mandible is pushed forward to bite food, and the incisors come into shearing contact. If the food is broken up in the posterior region, this always takes place on one side, while no load is placed on the other side. When chewing with the posterior teeth, the mandible glides out of a lateral position into the terminal occlusal position, and the food is crushed. If the opposite side also had cusp contact during this chewing impact, the teeth would be under transverse and hence nonphysiologic stress at those points.

Fig 5-39 In neutro-occlusion, there is normal intercuspation of the posterior teeth in the transverse direction. Positional anomalies in the transverse direction are referred to as *reverse articulations*.

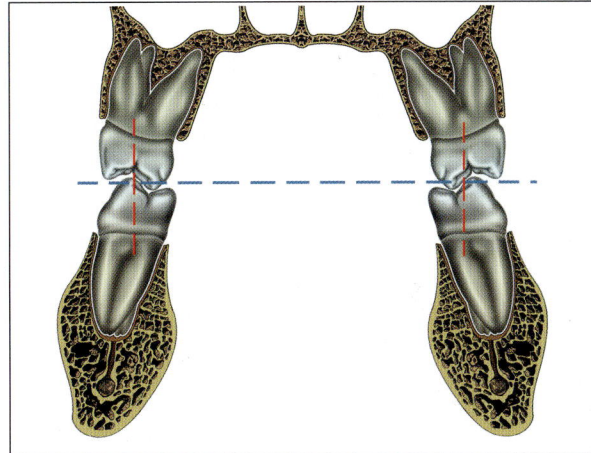

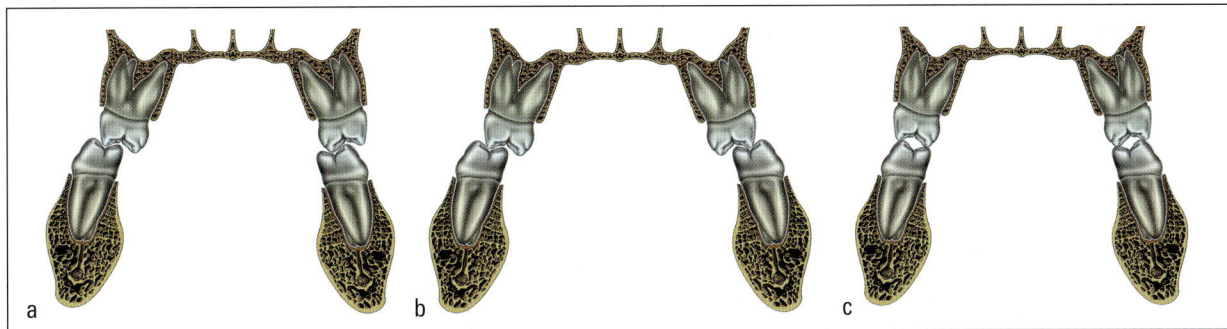

Fig 5-40 Displacements of occlusion in the transverse direction usually occur as symptoms accompanying other dysgnathias. These malocclusions mainly arise in the posterior segment. The cusps of the posterior teeth are no longer in their normal cusp-fossa intercuspation, but the mandibular dentition is *(a)* unilaterally migrated in the vestibular direction or *(b)* bilaterally displaced in the vestibular direction. *(c)* The edge-to-edge situation of the cusps can be seen as a microsymptom of the reverse articulation.

Malposition of teeth in the frontal plane

The malpositions in the frontal plane are the various forms of reverse articulation or transverse malocclusions, when the dental arches are deformed in the transverse direction and cross over in occlusion. These occur both as localized occlusal variations and as symmetric anomalies. Reverse articulations are usually symptoms that accompany other forms of dysgnathia and rarely occur in isolation. The term *reverse articulation* is generally used to denote a malocclusion in the area of the posterior teeth, when the mandibular posterior teeth have migrated in a vestibular direction and do not lie in their normal cusp-fossa relationships. This reverse articulation of the occlusion of the posterior teeth may be bilateral or merely unilateral (Figs 5-39 and 5-40).

Bilateral reverse articulations are symmetric anomalies that arise when there is overdevelopment of the mandible in the transverse direction; in this case, the mandibular posterior teeth occlude over the maxillary posterior teeth vestibularly.

Unilateral reverse articulations are asymmetric deformations of the jaws. They can be caused by deformation of the temporomandibular joint (TMJ) or by forced guidance of individual groups of teeth. The malposition of groups of teeth can give rise to reverse articulation situations, such as the reverse vertical overlap of prognathism or crowding in the anterior and posterior segments.

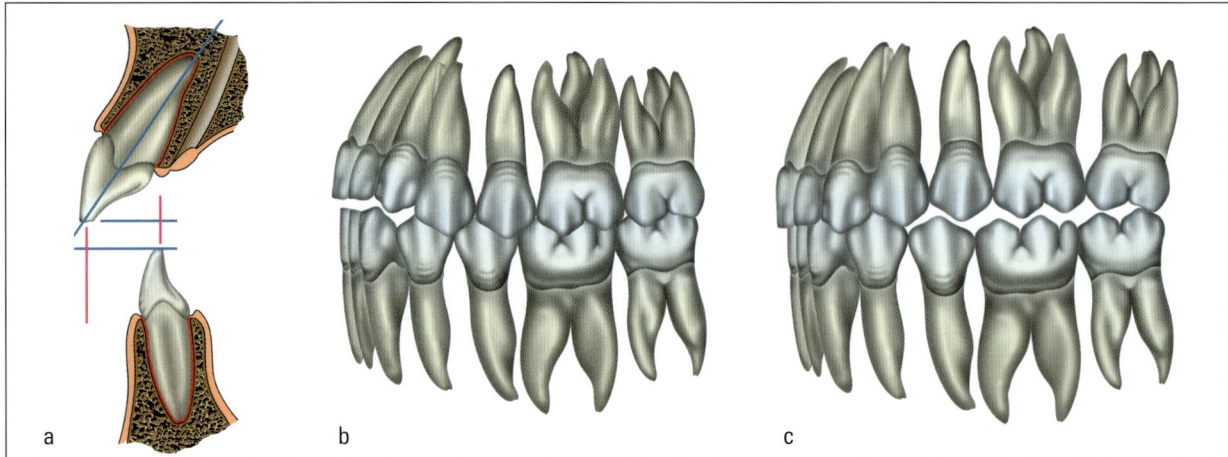

Fig 5-41 An open bite occurs as a localized malocclusion when certain segments of the dentition have no antagonist contact in terminal occlusion, such as the anterior open bite shown here *(a and b)*, in which the lips may not come together in a relaxed position. An open bite may also occur in the area of the posterior teeth *(c)*.

If the dental arches have been displaced as a whole in relation to each other because of exogenous factors, there may simply be a reverse articulation situation in the anterior region, but the malposition is found in both halves of the jaw.

Lateral forced guidance usually causes displacements in the lower face, such as the middle of the chin deviating to the side. Otherwise there are no striking extraoral symptoms of the reverse articulation. The causes of reverse articulations are mainly linked to causes of the accompanying forms of dysgnathia. Congenitally narrow jaws can create natural reverse articulation situations as much as hereditary malpositioning of groups of teeth; while the former produces a bilateral reverse articulation, a unilateral anomaly can occur with the latter. A unilateral reverse articulation can develop because of thumb sucking if this causes one-sided compression in the mandible. Asymmetry of the head and the TMJs due to disease should also be considered as possible causes of a reverse articulation.

In the frontal plane, malpositioning of the teeth can occur in the vertical direction as localized malocclusions, where certain parts of the dentition have no antagonist contact in terminal occlusion or where segments of the dentition are lengthened beyond the occlusal line. A distinction is made between the open bite and the deep bite.

An *open bite* exists if a few teeth do not come into occlusal contact in terminal occlusion because they do not reach the normal occlusal plane (Fig 5-41). The open bite can affect both anterior and posterior teeth. If the teeth are still erupting, the open bite is only temporary. The open bite in the anterior segment can be seen directly by gaping of the incisal margins. An open anterior bite is often accompanied by sagittal tipping of the anterior teeth in a labial or lingual direction if thumb sucking is the cause of the anomaly. In severe defects, the mouth is often held in an open position, which leads to increased mouth breathing and thereby a change in the bacterial flora in the mouth and a susceptibility to caries. Deformation of the periodontium may also be expected where teeth have no antagonists.

Severe forms of open bite will impair biting function and general masticatory function. They impede swallowing because the labial closure of the oral cavity is absent (lip incompetence); speech defects may also arise.

The *causes* of anterior open bite include the following:

• *Sucking* fingers and other objects, tongue thrusting, and lip biting. These bad habits can lead to an open bite. The nature and duration as well as the intensity of the habits determine the

Fig 5-42 The deep bite is mainly found as a symptom accompanying sagittal malocclusions. *(a)* There is severe overlapping (X) of the maxillary anterior teeth over the mandibular anterior teeth and the lip closure line or occlusal plane; in this case, the mandibular teeth may have a relatively normal approximal inclination. *(b)* A very steep deep bite extending to the cervical margin of the mandibular anterior teeth can be caused by increased steepness of the axial inclination of the maxillary anterior dentition.

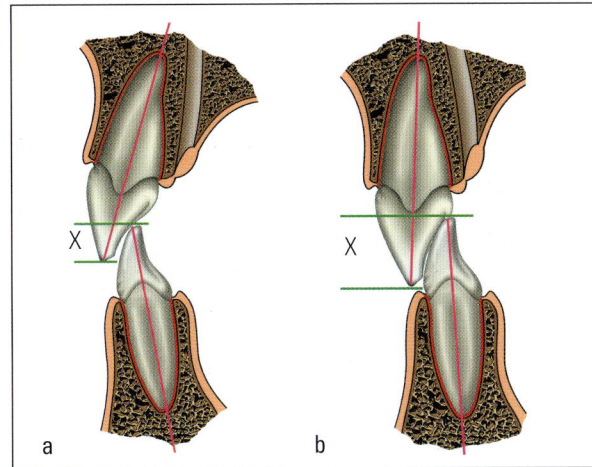

severity of the occlusal deformation. Not everyone with a long-standing sucking habit will develop an open bite. The open bite is made worse if biting on the sucked object predominates during sucking.

- *Rickets* caused by vitamin D deficiency. This affects the mineralization of bones and hard dental tissue and can lead to softening of the bone. The reduced resistance of the bone to muscular impact produces growth disturbances. In the dentition, the mandibular anterior dental arch is flattened and the maxillary anterior sections bend, even in response to moderate sucking.
- *Mouth breathing*. This often leads to narrowing of the maxillary dental arch, anterior crowding, and growth impairment in the anterior alveolar region.
- *Inheritance* of a particular cranial structure and skull development. This can lead to an open bite with a receding profile and open mouth breathing.

An *open bite in the posterior segment* exists if individual or several pairs of antagonists do not make contact in the anterior region when vertical overlap conditions are normal. This deformation of the dentition is not noticeable extraorally, even if it occurs symmetrically on both sides.

This defect can arise as a result of a skeletal growth anomaly where the posterior segment of the mandible is more developed than the anterior. The habit of interposing the edges of the tongue can produce a lateral open bite.

A *deep bite* means that the incisors overlap the opposing teeth by more than 3 mm (Fig 5-42). The functional disadvantages of this defect are that mandibular movement is impaired (chopping masticatory pattern) and strain is placed on the periodontium if the mandibular incisors bite into the gingiva. A deep bite is rarely found in the posterior region because extreme reverse articulation situations would need to be enforced for the broad masticatory surfaces of the molars to be able to glide past each.

The deep bite, as a vertical malocclusion, occurs if both anterior pairs of opposing teeth have erupted beyond a theoretical occlusal plane. Whereas in a vertical overlap the overlap arises from increased steepness of the dental axial inclination, in a deep bite there is lengthening of the maxillary incisors, and the mandibular anterior teeth touch the palatal mucosa. Otherwise, the deep bite may exist as a secondary symptom of a vertical overlap.

A deep bite situation also exists if the patient has to bite down deeply out of the physiologic rest position to achieve the terminal occlusal position, ie, when the interocclusal distance is very large. A deep bite arises because of a lack of contact between the incisors at eruption, which is accompanied by lengthening of the alveolar areas in this region.

Box 5-1 summarizes the various malocclusions and malpositions of teeth.

Box 5-1   Summary of the various malocclusions and malpositions of the teeth

Normal intercuspation

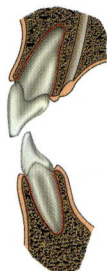

The *normal occlusion* involves a small vertical overlap and protrusion of the maxillary teeth over the mandibular anterior teeth, usually without contact and with an incisal vertical overlap. Labial surfaces of the maxillary anterior teeth support the upper lip, while incisal margins support the bottom lip; this gives rise to a vertical anterior dental arch.

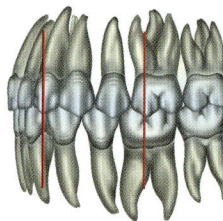

In *neutro-occlusion*, intercuspation follows the rule of antagonists: The fixed points are the maxillary canine and the first molar with their corresponding antagonists.

Disto-occlusion

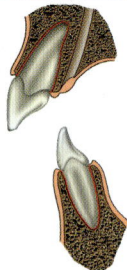

Disto-occlusion means the mandibular teeth lie in a posterior (distal) position by at least one-fourth of a premolar's width; it is described as prognathism if the maxillary anterior teeth protrude considerably, with an adverse esthetic effect and receding chin. There is scarcely any detrimental effect on masticatory function.

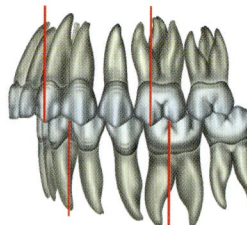

Disto-occlusion with the maxillary incisors forming a *tapered front* and open mouth position is hereditary or is caused by habitual thumb sucking or tongue biting.

Mesio-occlusion

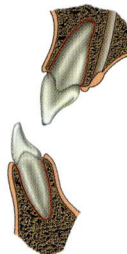

Mesio-occlusion means protrusion of the mandibular dentition in a mesial direction by at least one-fourth of a premolar's width; the relationship of the anterior teeth varies, usually with protrusion of the mandibular anterior teeth and jutting chin (progenia or prognathism), normal vertical overlap with gaps in the maxillary teeth, or an edge-to-edge occlusion.

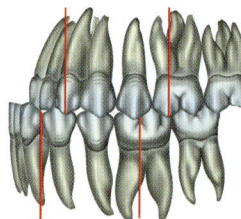

Prognathism takes the form of a reverse vertical overlap of the mandibular anterior teeth, identified by a prominent chin. This type of occlusion has adverse effects on masticatory function.

Malposition vertically

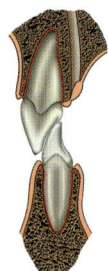

Deep bite means a pronounced vertical overlap of the maxillary anterior teeth over the mandibular anterior teeth, often extending as far as the cervical margin of the mandibular anterior teeth. It gives rise to pronounced sagittal development of the upper face with a pronounced mentolabial sulcus.

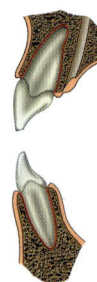

Open bite is a localized malocclusion in which individual teeth in terminal occlusion have no contact in the anterior or posterior segment. If severe, it leads to open mouth breathing together with a susceptibility to caries. It is usually temporary as a result of tooth retention.

Malposition horizontally

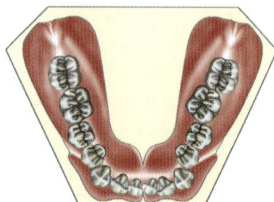

Crowding arises because of a mismatch between tooth size and jaw size. The lack of space produces localized tipping and rotation.

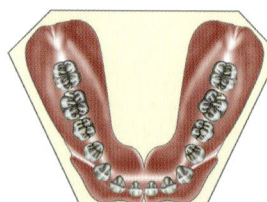

Spaces arise when teeth are too small in jaws that are too large. Gaps will also form if the tongue or foreign bodies are habitually interposed between the teeth.

Box 5-1 *(cont)* Summary of the various malocclusions and malpositions of the teeth

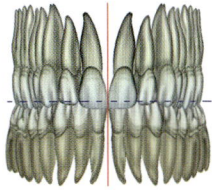

The *anterior teeth* should be arranged regularly to the right and left of the midline. The midlines of the jaws coincide. The sequence of antagonists is regular.

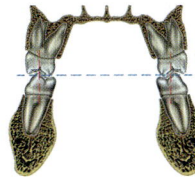

The *buccal shearing cusps* of the maxillary posterior teeth overlap the buccal occluding cusps of their mandibular antagonists. The lingual cusps of the maxillary posterior teeth fit into the central developmental grooves of the mandibular posterior teeth; this produces the transverse curve of occlusion.

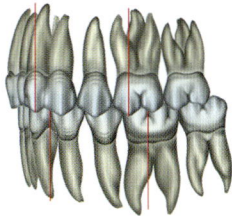

Vertical overlap, with steep anterior teeth and overlapping of the mandibular anterior teeth as far as the vestibular fornix, means a poorly functioning deep bite, in which only a chopping masticatory pattern is possible and protrusive excursion is impeded.

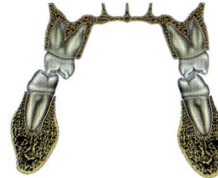

The *reverse articulation*, as a localized occlusal deviation in the posterior segment, can be bilateral or unilateral. A unilateral reverse articulation occurs if there is deformation of the jaws/dental arches with joint damage.

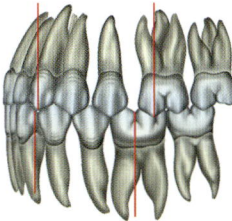

Mesio-occlusion with normal vertical overlap of the anterior teeth arises because of gaps between the anterior teeth as well as between the posterior teeth.

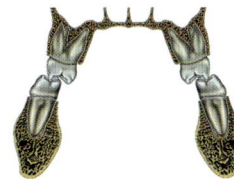

In *bilateral reverse articulation*, the buccal cusps of the maxillary posterior teeth occlude with the central developmental grooves of the mandibular posterior teeth on both sides. The mandibular dental arch is wider than the maxillary dental arch with overdevelopment of the mandible in the transverse direction.

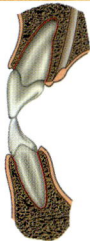

In the *edge-to-edge* or *end-to-end occlusion*, the incisal margins of the anterior teeth meet each other in the occlusal position. The consequence is severe abrasion of the cutting edges. The incisors have no cutting effect. The occlusal height will be reduced if abrasion becomes advanced.

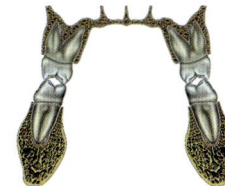

Edge-to-edge occlusion in the posterior segment is a type of reverse articulation. Here the cusps of the posterior antagonists touch each other.

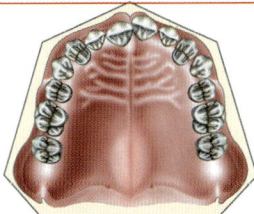

Displacement is the incorrect positioning of individual teeth and groups of teeth. Displacement usually accompanies tipping or rotation.

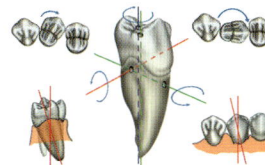

Rotation and tipping are distinguished by the position of the axis of rotation or tipping, with rotation around eccentric or central axes and tipping around sagittal or transverse axes.

135

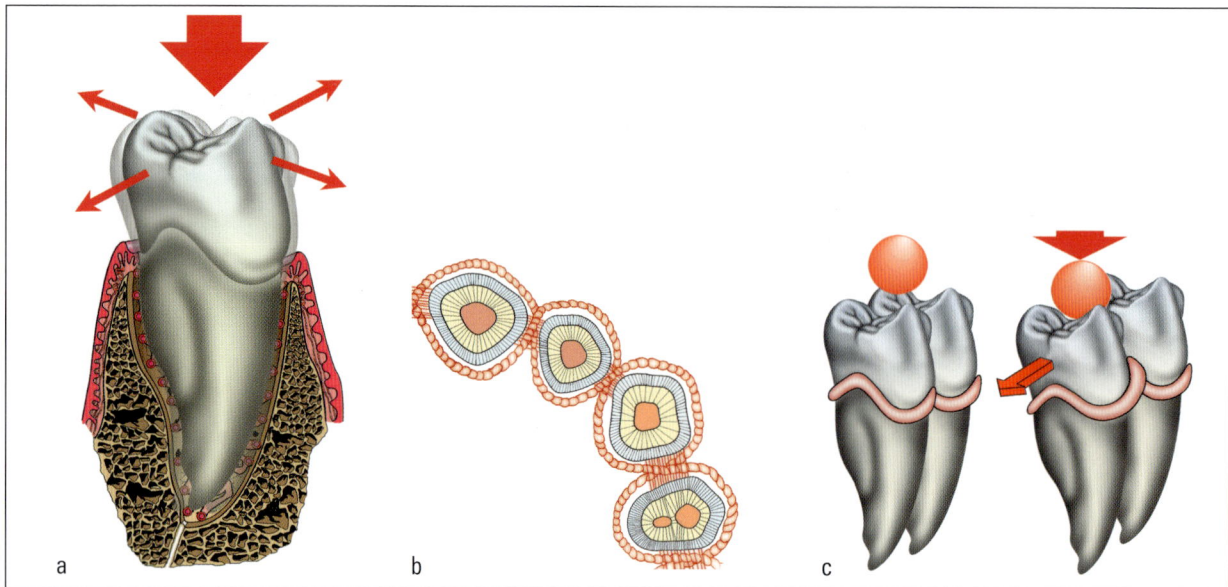

Fig 5-43 *(a to c)* The tooth can be tipped in all directions in space by forces acting axially. Via the contact points, the tooth within the dentition is supported against forces acting sagittally. The so-called tissue linkage, which means the tooth is connected to its neighboring teeth by a ligamentous apparatus, protects against forces that tip the tooth outward.

Function of the Closed Dentition

Why the dentition is made up of individual teeth needs to be explored. A permanently fused ridge of bone, for example, would be a feasible alternative. However, the individual teeth are anchored in the bone with ligaments, and the teeth are able to tip. Why the teeth are arranged in a curved arch also needs to be explained; an angular dental arch could indeed be conceivable.

The first consideration is the teeth under stress. The predominant force component acting on each tooth is directed apically, but each tooth can be tipped in sagittal and transverse directions by the sloping surfaces of the cusps (Fig 5-43). To a certain extent, this is a good thing because this redirection of forces transfers a large proportion of the energy to the neighboring teeth.

Tipping in a sagittal direction within the dental arch pushes the tooth against the adjacent teeth. As a result, the vertical component of masticatory forces is redirected horizontally and, similar to an elastic impact, is passed on from crown to crown until the energy is absorbed by all the periodontal tissues of the teeth. This is only possible if there are no gaps between teeth and all the teeth are connected by approximal contact points. In an angular dental arch, a sagittally directed elastic impact could not be smoothly transferred without interruption. Within a round dental arch, this transfer of forces is far easier. This is why restoration of the gap-free pattern of the dental arch ought to be clearly identified as a primary aim of prosthetic measures.

Lingual tipping of the tooth is only possible if the neighboring teeth are pressed mesiodistally, because a tooth is basically broader in its vestibular aspect than lingually. The tooth is wedged in the dental arch, or the transverse impact can be passed on to the neighboring teeth via the contact points as a sagittal force component (Fig 5-44). Once again, the rounded arch form of the dentition is therefore advantageous. Transverse thrusts in a lingual direction can be well compensated for by a multirooted tooth when the roots are flared. The roots of the maxillary molars are flared in just such a functionally advantageous manner (Fig 5-45).

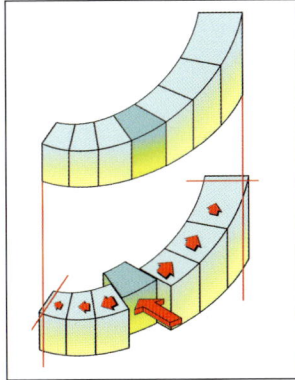

Fig 5-44 When a force acting transversally tips the tooth lingually, the tooth becomes wedged within the row of teeth because each tooth, as part of an arc of a circle, is narrower lingually than buccally. The neighboring teeth move apart, and the force is transferred via the contact points in the row of teeth.

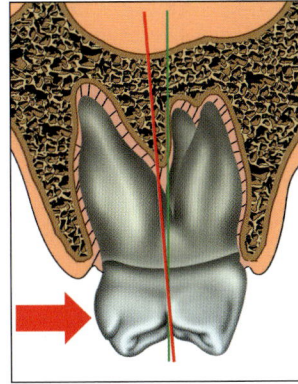

Fig 5-45 Transverse thrusts in a lingual direction can be well compensated for by a multi-rooted tooth when the roots are flared. The roots of the maxillary molars are flared in just such a functionally advantageous manner.

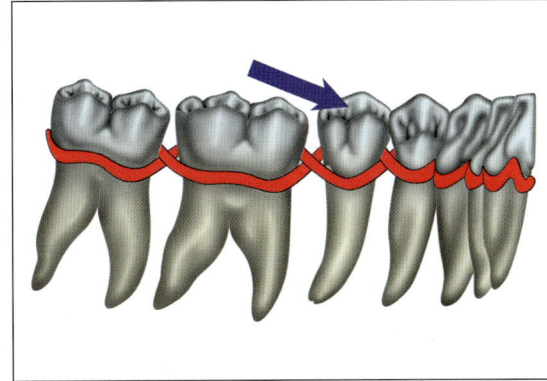

Fig 5-46 The tissue linkage of the teeth with each other also functions when forces are acting sagittally. A tooth that is tipped within the row of teeth transfers the force that causes tipping to its neighboring teeth, partly in the form of an elastic impact via the contact points and partly via the ligamentous apparatus.

Vestibular tipping of the tooth is absorbed by the marginal fibers. The teeth are linked to each other by the fibers of the marginal periodontium encircling the teeth, so that any movement of a tooth pulls the subsequent teeth in the same direction and the teeth support one another. This can be referred to as *tissue linkage*, and it also operates in the sagittal direction (Fig 5-46). A tooth that is tipped inside the row of teeth passes that tipping on to its neighboring teeth, partly in the form of an elastic impact via the contact points and partly via the ligamentous apparatus. The ligamentous apparatus is most effective when the teeth are tipped outward: In this situation, tissue linkage is usually the only form of support. The complex structure of the ligamentous apparatus can be interpreted as the ligaments running around the teeth in loops. If a tooth is tipped, the ligaments tense up and the tooth is supported.

However, this *linkage* alone is not enough. During the chewing process, the mandible slides out of a lateral position into terminal occlusion, in which the buccal cusps of the maxillary teeth enclose the mandibular teeth like a reinforcing ring, so that support here is provided by the antagonists. At the same time, the mandibular teeth offer the maxillary teeth support in the same way because the lingual cusps of the maxillary teeth fit into the central developmental grooves of the mandibular teeth and are thus "wedged."

These observations primarily apply to the terminal occlusion or a position directly before it. The masticatory force is generally greatest in terminal occlusion because beforehand the most masticatory force is used for reshaping the food. Furthermore, as the mandible slides into terminal occlusion, the direction of the force acting on the maxillary dental arch is directed lingually in its transversally acting portion.

Another effective protection against excessive transverse stresses is provided by the nerve supply to the periodontium in the form of a pain warning system. The nerves of the periodontium with the conduction nerves of the masticatory muscles form a reflex path that works as follows: When the critical stress limit for the periodontium is reached as a result of masticatory pressure, the masticatory muscles are "short-circuited" and the masticatory force immediately diminishes. This is a familiar feeling to anyone who has ever had the misfortune to bite onto a cherry stone. Before any awareness of pain, the mouth has already reopened as a reflex action.

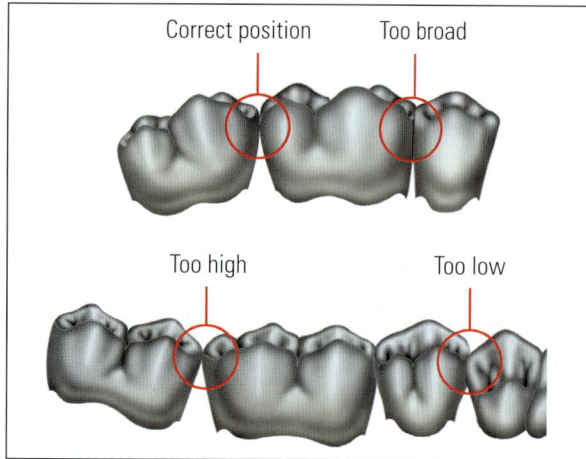

Correct position   Too broad

Too high   Too low

Fig 5-47 The overhanging approximal ridges form the interdental embrasure between two teeth, a functional part of the masticatory area. The contact points lie deep in the embrasure. The contact points are meant to protect the interdental papilla and therefore must be accurately reproduced; ie, they should lie directly below the occlusal level but not too high in order to form an adequate interdental embrasure. They should also not lie too low because, if they do, food can slip into the resulting recess or the interdental papilla can be squeezed. The same can happen if the contact point is too broad and flat.

Contacts of the Teeth

An essential distinction is made between two fundamentally different contact situations in relation to the teeth. First, there are the approximal contacts of the teeth within the dentition, which happen in the contact points. The second type lies occlusally between the maxillary and mandibular dentitions when occluding.

The **approximal contact points** lie deep in the interdental embrasure between the teeth. The overhanging approximal ridges of adjacent teeth form the *interdental embrasure*, a functional part of the masticatory area (Fig 5-47). As all the teeth taper down toward the root, the approximal contact points lie directly below the occlusal level. These contacts render the masticatory area closed, which has the function outlined above.

The **contact points** are meant to protect the interdental papilla and therefore must be accurately reproduced. They should lie below the occlusal level but not too high in order to form an adequate interdental embrasure. They should not lie too low because, if they do, food can slip into the resulting recess or the interdental papilla can be squeezed. The same can happen if the contact point is too broad and flat.

As a result of the natural movement of the teeth over time, the **contact points** are worn away, starting as punctiform, then eventually becoming linear and flat contacts. This gives rise to various contact situations and the teeth crowding to-

gether in a mesial direction. This process is also known as *physiologic mesial migration* of the teeth. Seen occlusally, the contact points on the anterior teeth are located vestibularly, whereas the points on the posterior teeth are increasingly displaced toward the middle of the tooth until, in the case of the molars, they lie on the line of the central developmental grooves (Fig 5-48). This produces recesses between the teeth that can be kept clean by self-cleaning. Seen from the vestibular view, the position of the contact points, as they line up next to each other, follows the course of the sagittal curve of occlusion; ie, in the anterior region, the points lie along a straight line (Fig 5-49). In the mandible, they fall downward as far as the first molar, then rise up again; in the maxilla, the mesial contact point of the first molar is already higher again.

Occlusal contacts are the tooth contacts of the opposing rows of teeth brought together in terminal occlusion. When masticatory surfaces are anatomically shaped and nonabraded, the occlusal contacts are punctiform. Flat occlusal contacts only develop as a result of abrasion.

Centric stops denote the occlusal contacts on the occluding cusps in the case of occluding masticatory surfaces. Where there is anatomical "double interlocking," in which the supporting occluding cusps always lie between two cusps of the antagonists in the intercuspation position, just this cusp touches the opposing teeth centrically. *Centric* means the occlusal contacts meet the antagonists in the middle, so that the acting

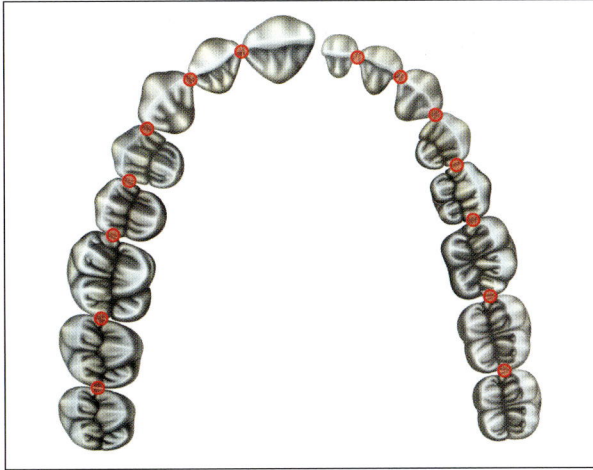

Fig 5-48 In the anterior region, the contact points are vestibularly located; more distally, the points are increasingly displaced toward the line of the central developmental grooves. The contact points lie so that the recesses between the teeth are kept as small as possible, which means that no gaps can form where debris might accumulate.

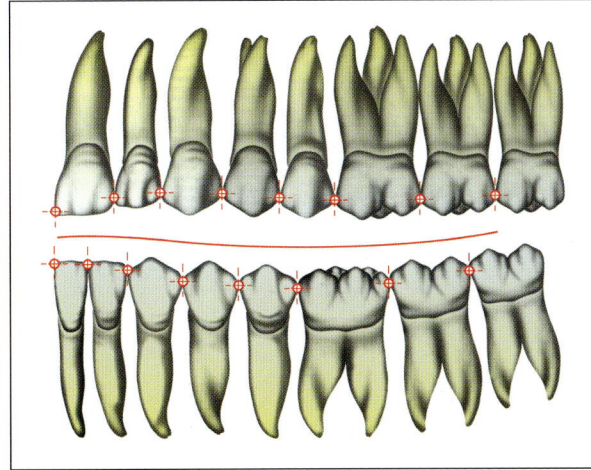

Fig 5-49 Seen from the vestibular view, the contact points follow the course of the sagittal curve of occlusion; ie, on the anterior teeth, the points lie along a straight line. In the mandible, they fall downward as far as the first molar, then rise up again.

masticatory forces are passed on in the direction of the tooth axes and the periodontium is stressed in the center.

Contact areas are the middle occlusal contacts into which the centric stops fit on the antagonist. This means that for each tooth there are both centric stops on the supporting occluding cusps as well as contact areas in the fossa area and on the approximal marginal ridges.

Regular interlocking in the transverse direction is seen on the posterior teeth as a cusp-fossa relationship. Based on the principle of technical "single interlocking," anatomical "double interlocking" of the teeth arises from the arrangement of the cusps in a double row (Fig 5-50). This means that the masticatory surfaces interlock according to the two-cusp principle; ie, the lingual cusps of the maxillary teeth interlock into the central fossa of the mandibular antagonists, while the buccal cusps of the maxillary teeth slide over the antagonists in a vestibular direction. For the buccal cusps of the mandibular teeth, this results in positioning in the central fossa of the maxillary antagonists; for the lingual cusps of the mandibular teeth, it results in overlapping over the lingual cusps of the maxillary teeth.

The **antagonist situation** in the sagittal direction shows that the cusps of the posterior teeth always

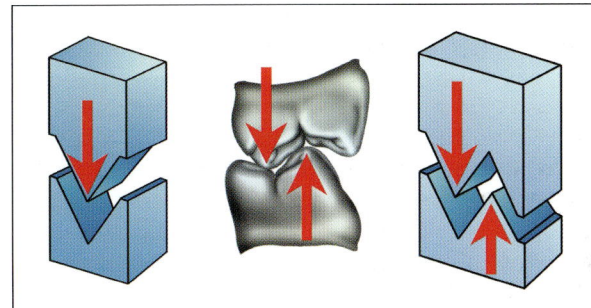

Fig 5-50 The anatomy of the occlusal contacts can be interpreted as follows: The principle of technical "single interlocking" becomes anatomical "double interlocking" due to the arrangement of the cusps in a double row. The masticatory surfaces interlock following the two-cusp principle; ie, out of four antagonizing cusps involved, two are active and two are passive.

interlock into the interdental embrasures of the opposing teeth. As a result of the sloping surfaces of the cusps, the antagonists are driven apart as if by a wedge. In an interlocking relationship where the teeth are tipped in a sagittal direction, the masticatory pressure is not only absorbed axially by the teeth involved in the chewing act at the time but also passed on to the neighboring teeth via the approximal contact points.

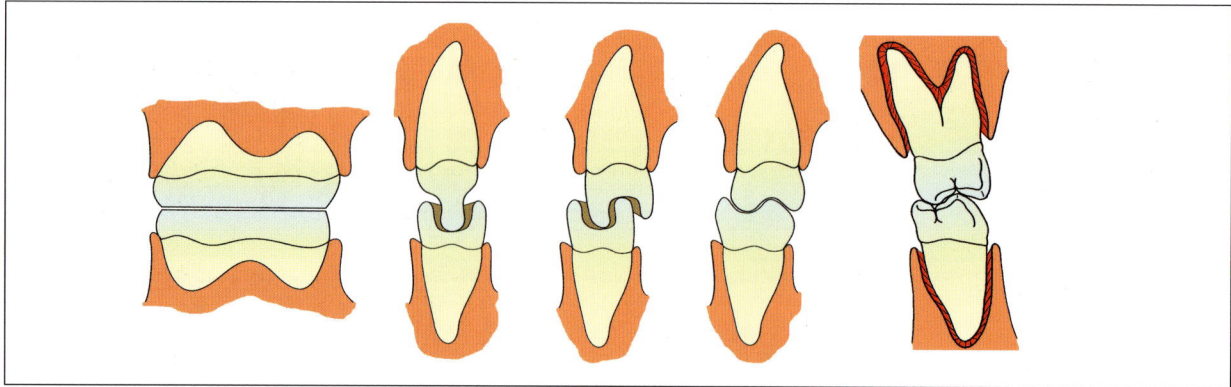

Fig 5-51 Very large, flat masticatory surfaces would be only slightly loaded eccentrically out of the centric position during friction movements, but they are unsuitable for crushing grainy food. A cusp-bearing surface is better suited to crushing fibrous and tough food as well as grainy foods. According to the pestle-and-mortar principle, full refinement of the occlusal relief leads to the anatomical form of opposing masticatory surfaces.

Form and position of occlusal contacts

One conceptual model would be to represent opposing cusps as spheres laid out in the pattern of occlusion. The spheres would lie in the deepest areas of the masticatory surfaces, the contact areas. Given a pronounced occlusal relief, a sphere rests in a stable position and thereby displays three-point (tripod) contact. If the tooth had no cusps, the sphere would roll to and fro. Thus, *centric stops* in their contact areas do not contact the antagonists at a single point, but each tooth has at least two contact areas on which centric stops of the opposing teeth lie.

These contact areas basically lie on the line of the central developmental grooves, with a lingual tendency in the mandible and a rather buccal tendency in the maxilla. The centric stops lie on the buccal cusps in the mandibular dentition and on the lingual cusps in the maxillary dentition. This produces a *double row* made up of the contact areas and the centric stops on the occlusal surfaces of the rows of teeth. The sum of forces that occur will load each individual tooth centrically.

Cusp-fossa-marginal ridges occlusion means an occlusal relation in which the centric stops do not contact the opposing tooth centrically in a tooth-to–two tooth relationship, but the opposing cusps occlude in the contact areas in both the interdental embrasures and the central fossae. Cen-

tric occlusion only comes about when the row of teeth is closed within itself and forces can be transferred via the approximal contacts. Although the majority of centric stops do not contact the opposing teeth centrically, the sum of the acting forces nevertheless puts centric load on the teeth within the closed row of teeth.

Cusp-fossa occlusion denotes a contact relationship in a constructed tooth-to-tooth relation in which one tooth only contacts its antagonist. This can result in axially directed, stable loading.

To clarify this, further observations are first made based on an individual tooth. Teeth with totally flat masticatory surfaces would be conceivable. To achieve centric loading, these teeth would have to be guided exactly in full surface contact, or the masticatory surfaces would have to be so large that grinding movements out of this central position would have only minimal influence on any centric loading. These tooth forms can be found in ruminants: short teeth with a large, flat surface. However, this makes it very difficult to process tough food. A surface with cusps is better suited to crushing fibrous and tough as well as grainy foods. With a cusp-bearing chewing surface, the food a person eats can be chewed up more efficiently. After all, humans are omnivores, which means we do not favor a single, specific type of food.

The simplest intercuspation would thus be an opposing pair of teeth, comprising one tooth

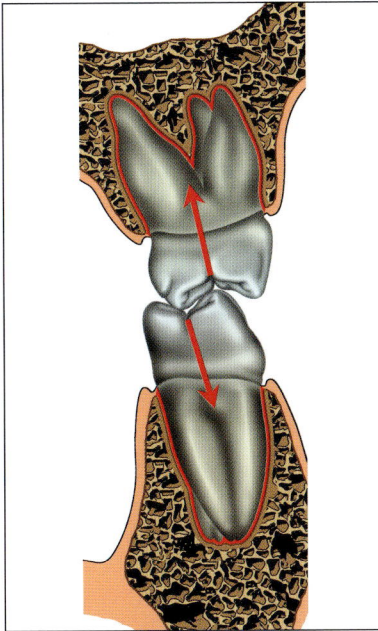

Fig 5-52 The well-developed pattern of occlusion forms a punctiform contact with the opposing teeth. The occlusal contacts are positioned so that centric loading of the teeth can be achieved. Centric loading means that force is directed toward the center of the periodontal tissues.

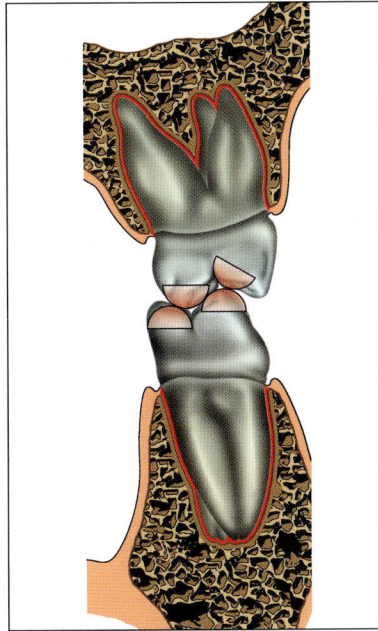

Fig 5-53 The occluding cusps can be represented as hemispheres that have punctiform contact. In the case of anatomical double intercuspation, the supporting cusps (lingual in the maxilla, buccal in the mandible) lie between two antagonizing cusps according to the cusp-fossa contact relationship.

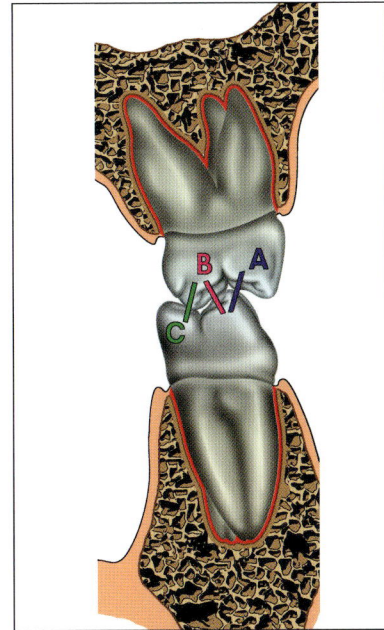

Fig 5-54 Occlusal contacts between the cusps are referred to as A, B, and C contacts in the buccolingual direction. A-contacts are found between the buccal cusps of the opposing teeth, B-contacts between the supporting cusps, and C-contacts between the lingual cusps.

with one cusp, that occluded in a trough-shaped antagonist—similar to a pestle and mortar arrangement. If the single-cusp tooth were then far smaller than the trough-shaped tooth, food could be crushed and ground up by large lateral movements to and fro. However, this food could still escape to the sides and would have to be propelled back by the tongue and cheek. The greater the difference in shape, the more the periodontium is stressed during lateral movements.

Therefore, a structural shape in which the opposing teeth represent both pestle and mortar is more favorable. This results in the anatomical form of masticatory surfaces as the occlusal relief becomes fully refined (Fig 5-51). The grinding or frictional area is doubled, and the two tooth surfaces can be shaped to fit together more closely. A lateral movement from the outside inward simply needs to be performed, in which the outer pestle grinds the food and pushes it into the inner mortar, where the food can also be crushed. The tongue then pushes the food back between the pestle and mortar surfaces. To compensate for the transverse forces during lateral movement, the teeth merely need to be appropriately tipped against the direction of movement.

The efficiency of such a pestle and mortar system can be further enhanced if the contact areas do not interdigitate as flat planes but only touch at a few points. The well-developed natural pattern of occlusion displays punctiform contact with the opposing teeth (Fig 5-52). The occlusal contacts are positioned so that centric loading of the teeth can be achieved.

Figs 5-53 to 5-59 further illustrate the form and position of occlusal contacts.

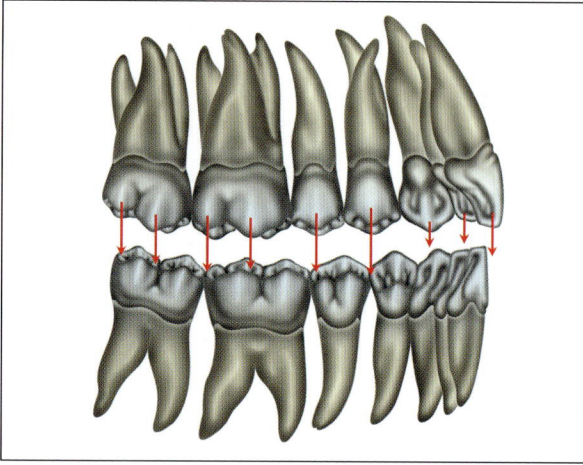

Fig 5-55 All the lingual cusps of the maxillary dentition fit into the areas of the central developmental grooves of the mandibular dentition. The maxillary anterior teeth fit labially over the mandibular anterior teeth. In this kind of regular intercuspation, there are simultaneous and uniform occlusal contacts.

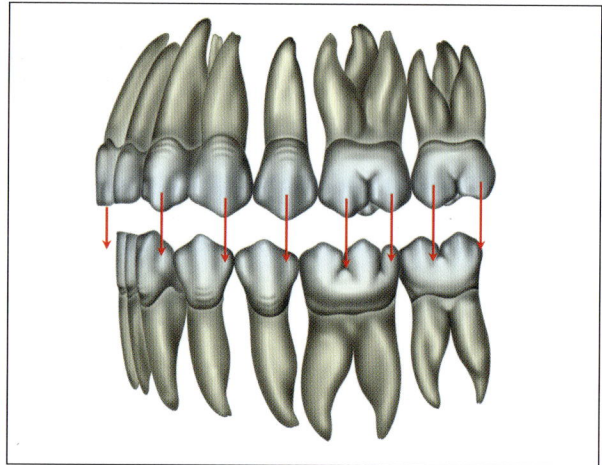

Fig 5-56 The tips of the buccal cusps of the premolars and the distobuccal cusps of the maxillary molars fit into the approximal areas of the mandibular posterior teeth. The mesiobuccal cusps of the maxillary molars fit into the buccal longitudinal groove between the cusps of the mandibular molars.

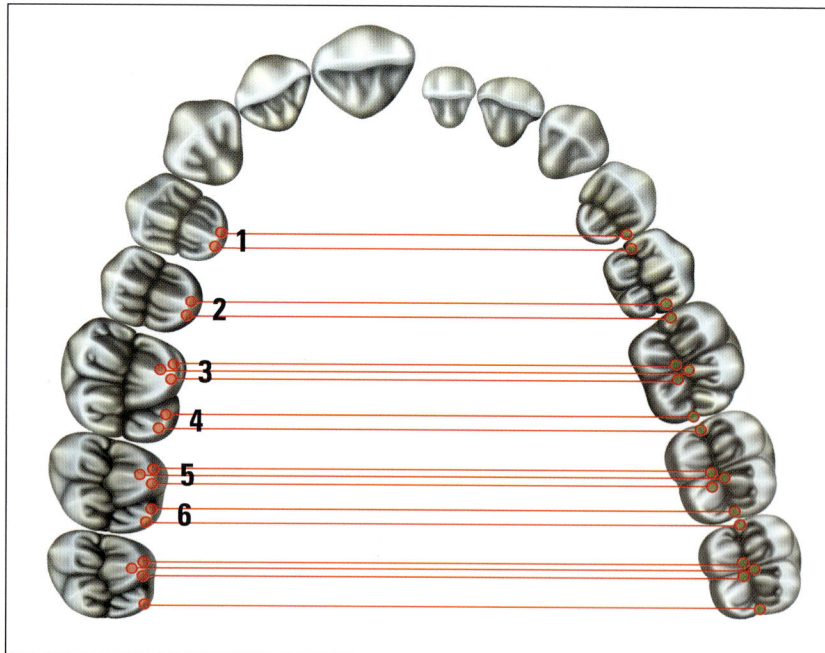

Fig 5-57 The centric stops in the maxilla and the contact areas in the mandible are arranged as follows:
1. The lingual cusp of the maxillary first premolar fits onto the approximal marginal ridges of the mandibular premolars.
2. The lingual cusp of the maxillary second premolar fits onto the approximal marginal ridges of the mandibular second premolar and first molar.
3. The mesiolingual cusp of the maxillary first molar fits into the central fossa of the mandibular first molar.
4. The distolingual cusp of the maxillary first molar fits onto the approximal marginal ridges of the mandibular molars.
5. The mesiolingual cusp of the maxillary second molar fits into the central fossa of the mandibular second molar.
6. The distolingual cusp of the maxillary second molar fits onto the distal marginal ridge of the mandibular second molar.

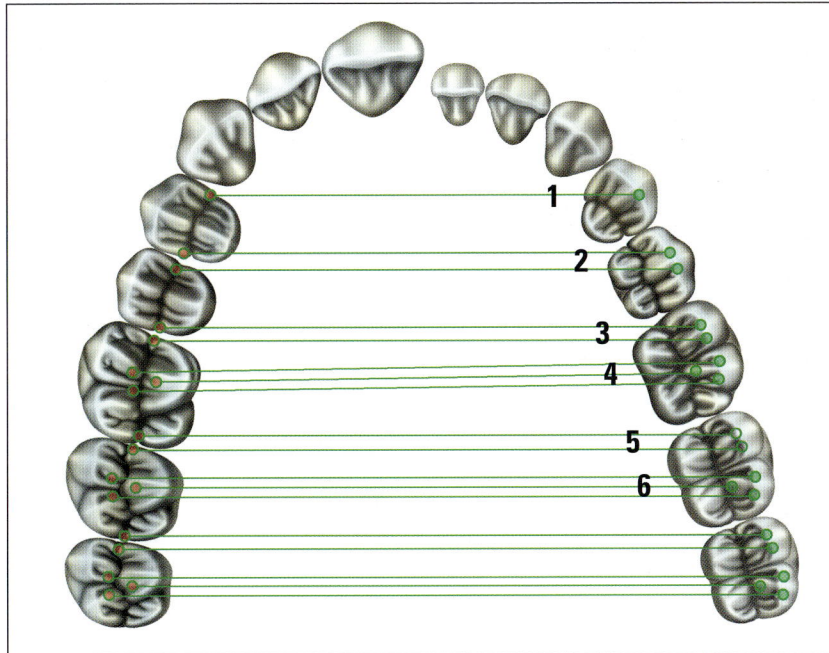

Fig 5-58 The centric stops in the mandible and the contact areas in the maxilla are arranged as follows:
1. The buccal cusp of the mandibular first premolar fits into the mesial marginal ridge of the maxillary first premolar.
2. The buccal cusp of the mandibular second premolar fits into the approximal marginal ridges of the maxillary premolars.
3. The mesiobuccal cusp of the mandibular first molar fits into the approximal marginal ridges of the maxillary second premolar and first molar.
4. The distobuccal cusp of the mandibular first molar fits into the central fossa of the maxillary first molar.
5. The mesiobuccal cusp of the mandibular second molar fits into the approximal area between the maxillary first molar and second molar.
6. The distobuccal cusp of the mandibular second molar fits into the central fossa of the maxillary second molar.

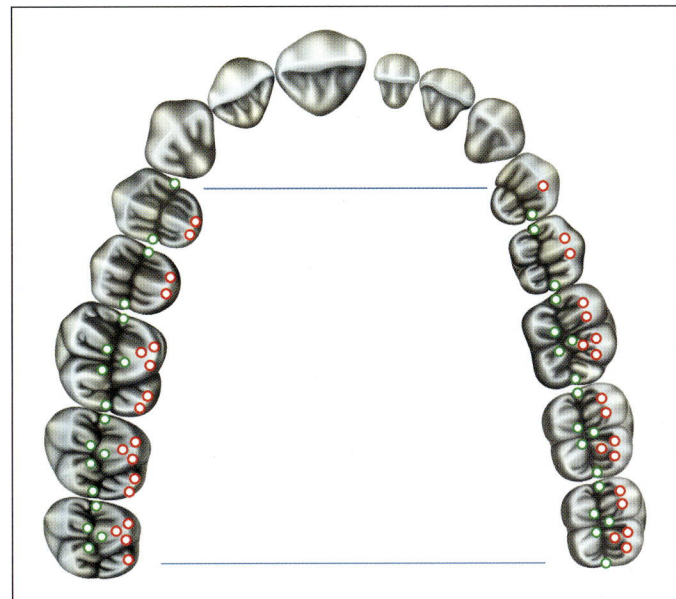

Fig 5-59 The occlusal contacts and occlusal areas on the premolars and molars are arranged as follows: The centric stops are marked in *red* and the contact areas in *green*. The contact areas are located on the triangular ridges and on the approximal marginal ridges, while the centric stops are found on the cusp ridges close to the cusp tips and on the cusp crests. The occlusal contacts are on the masticatory surfaces arranged in the form of a double row. One row of contacts lies in the region of the central developmental grooves of the teeth, while the other row is on the buccal cusps in the mandible and on the lingual cusps in the maxilla.

Advantages of punctiform occlusal contacts

Punctiform contacts are the best form of occlusion. This explanatory model is primarily intended to show why the occlusal contacts must be created as punctiform during systematic reconstruction of masticatory surfaces. The main advantages of punctiform occlusal contacts include the following:

- During sideways (lateral) movements, the contact points are constantly changing from one moment to the next, as if the round cusp surfaces were rolling against each other (Figs 5-60 and 5-61); in this case, the anatomical shape of the cusps is assumed.
- Consequently, the momentary surface pressure for identical masticatory pressure is far greater with punctiform contacts, and hence the actual masticatory activity is more efficient (see Fig 5-60). In other words, when a contact covers a large area, more masticatory pressure has to be expended to obtain the same surface pressure per portion of that area.
- This in turn means that lateral movement leads to relatively low transverse stresses on the teeth when the contacts are punctiform. This is because the same crushing work can be done with less masticatory pressure (similar to a sharp knife, which requires very little force to cut efficiently).
- The small, alternating grinding area reduces excessive wear on the teeth.
- When there are several punctiform contacts, the contact area is "rougher," so the food can be broken up and crushed more effectively (Figs 5-62 and 5-63).
- With punctiform contacts, the progression of force is clearly defined; ie, force is transferred to a definite point and not to a large area where it might result in uncontrolled tilting.
- The three-point (tripod) contact of a cusp in its contact area is mechanically stable and well defined. This stable position is a prerequisite for centric occlusion (Fig 5-64).

In this *illustration of punctiform contacts*, abrasion areas on teeth would seem to be signs of wear that diminish the value of the system, following the analogy of the sharp knife as a technical tool. However, comparison between a technical and a physiologic system ends here. In a physiologic system, the sharp-cusped chewing surfaces help to ensure that all the parts of the system can differentiate.

As the teeth grow, their position is guided by the occlusal patterns of their antagonists; then the roots and the periodontal tissues differentiate in response to the arising masticatory forces until they reach their optimal form. In the process, the TMJ, muscles, and habits of movement all develop into a harmonious system. In a normal masticatory system, areas of abrasion will grind equally harmoniously, and this should not be seen as diminishing the efficiency of the system. When reconstructing masticatory surfaces, it is easier, more accurate, and hence more physiologic to create punctiform contacts, irrespective of whether the above-mentioned advantages can be achieved. This cannot be achieved with the same certainty if the contacts are flat.

The above outline of the advantages of punctiform contacts requires further clarification. The momentary contact point on a model can be used to do this, because the cusps are idealized as spherical surfaces. On contact, the spherical surfaces are directed past each other. The spheres do not turn but rub against each other. However, no contact point on the spherical surfaces can constantly be in contact throughout the whole movement. By contrast, if two flat surfaces glide over each other, some areas of the surfaces will have frictional contact throughout the whole movement.

Where masticatory pressure is identical, frictional resistance and hence transverse stress will be the same for punctiform as for flat-surface contact. However, punctiform contact has the advantage of requiring less masticatory force for chewing activity than is needed with a flat contact. This means that transverse stress will always be less with punctiform contacts. For this to be true, the contacts must lie exactly inside the physiologic system. Incorrect positioning of contact points leads to faulty contacts during lateral movements, which interfere, are more prone to grinding, and place more stress on the periodontal tissue. Areas of abrasion on replacement crowns are an indication of such faulty contacts.

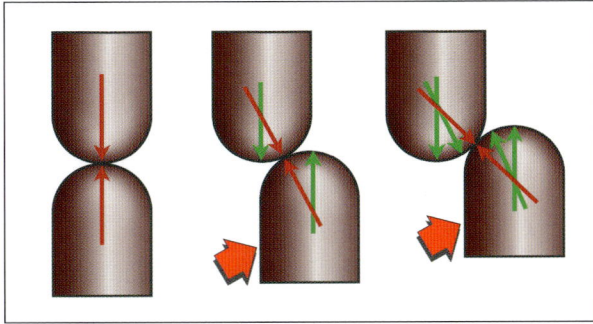

Fig 5-60 If cusps are round, the contact points are constantly changing from one moment to the next during lateral movements. With punctiform contacts on round cusps, the progression of force is clearly defined. The surface pressure for identical masticatory pressure is far higher with punctiform contacts on round cusps than with flat-plane contact. This means that actual food-crushing activity is more efficient or that, with punctiform contact, less masticatory pressure needs to be expended to achieve the same crushing activity. This results in lower transverse stresses on the teeth with punctiform contacts.

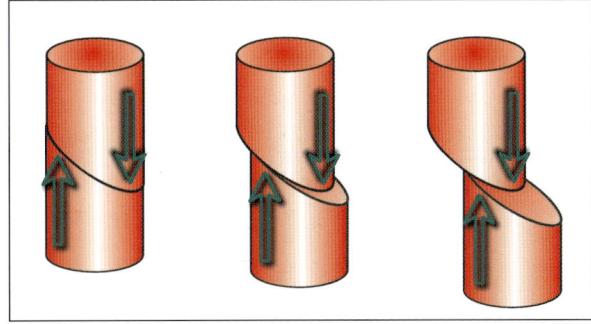

Fig 5-61 In the case of flat-plane contact, certain portions of the surface are constantly under frictional contact during lateral movement, which means greater abrasion.

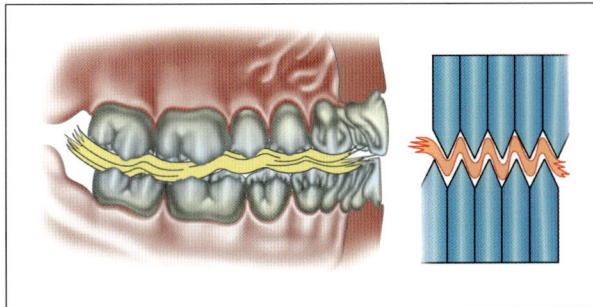

Fig 5-62 A cusped masticatory surface with several punctiform contacts is "rougher," so food can be torn up more effectively.

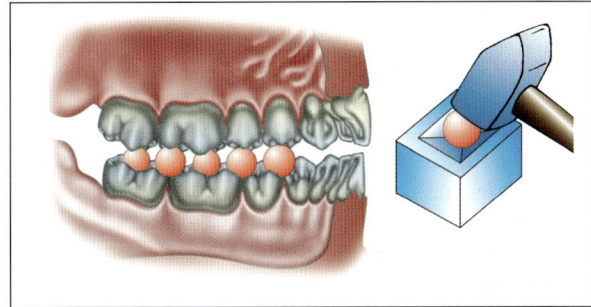

Fig 5-63 During crushing, grainy food is held and ground up in the cusped masticatory surface.

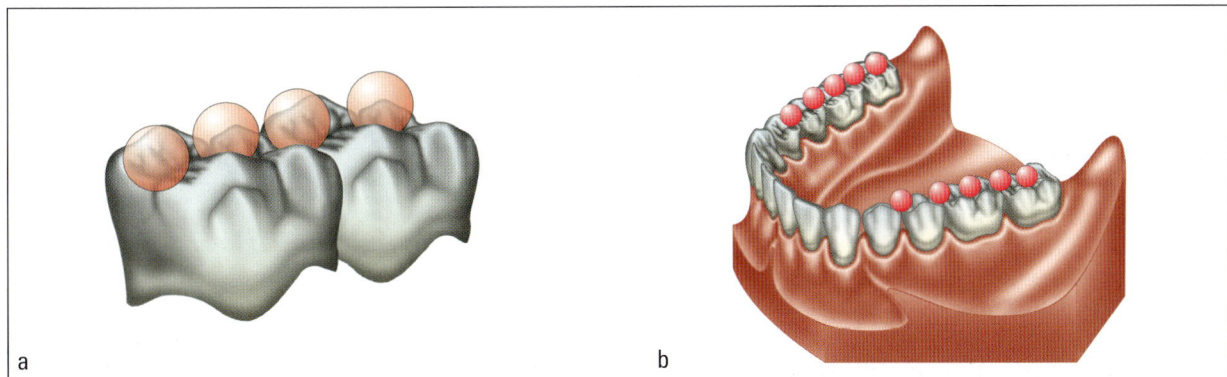

Fig 5-64 *(a and b)* The round cusps usually lie in three-point contact in their contact area. A three-point contact is mechanically stable, similar to a sphere that rests in a stable position in an occlusal relief with pronounced cusps, whereas it would roll to and fro in a relief without any cusps.

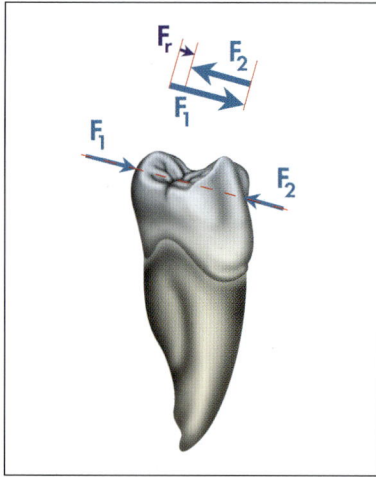

Fig 5-65 Forces (F_1, F_2) can be interpreted as vectors and geometrically added together. Forces acting on a rigid body and lying on a line of action are added together or subtracted from each other. The sum or the difference is then the resultant force (F_r).

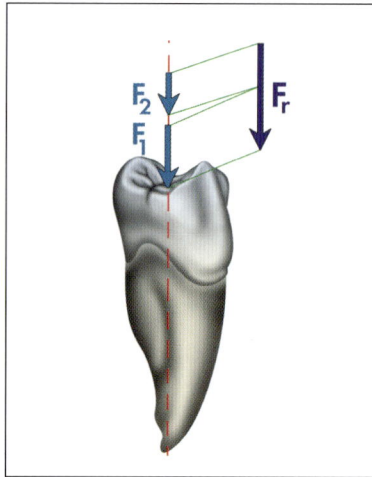

Fig 5-66 The geometric addition of forces (F_1, F_2) is done with the aid of a parallelogram of forces. The forces are displaced along their lines of action until the vectors lie behind each other. The connecting line between the ends of the vectors gives the resultant force (F_r).

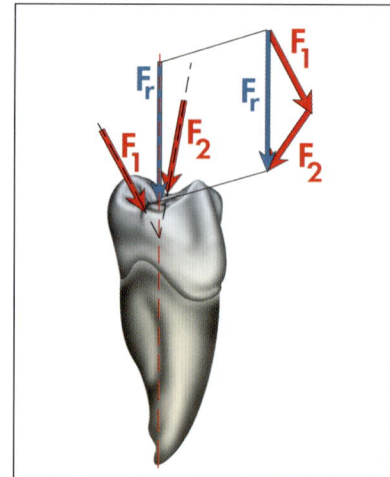

Fig 5-67 The geometric addition applied to one tooth, which is loaded on its approximal marginal ridges. To simplify matters, it is assumed that the intersecting point of the lines of action of the two forces lies at a point on the line of action of the resultant force.

Defined force progression

Punctiform contacts clearly define the progression of force or how the incorrect position of a contact can put transverse load on a tooth. Before a description of how forces act on a tooth is given, here follows a brief explanation of the physical principles governing forces and how they are combined: Forces can be represented as vectorial values; ie, they can be illustrated as arrows. The length of the arrow is a measure of the size of the force, and the direction of the arrow is the direction of the force. The forces on a rigid body (in this case, the tooth) can only be displaced along their line of action, ie, on a line that is an extension of the (force) vector; parallel displacement is not possible.

When several forces act on a tooth (or a rigid body), they can be combined to produce a resultant force (equivalent force). The individual forces are known as *components*. These individual components can be combined by geometric addition to produce a resultant (Fig 5-65). If several forces are located on a collective line of action, the sum or difference of these forces is the resultant. If two (or more) forces have a collective working point,

a parallelogram of forces can be constructed and they can again be combined by geometric addition to produce a resultant force (Figs 5-66 and 5-67). The resultant can be calculated according to the trigonometric law of cosines.

If more than two forces act on one point, a parallelogram of forces or a polygon of forces has to be created several times in order to add the forces together geometrically (Fig 5-68). Forces with different working points are displaced along their line of action up to an intersecting point, which produces a normal parallelogram of forces. A resultant force with the correct total and the correct direction, but not the exact position, is obtained. However, because the resultant can also be displaced in its line of action, the midpoint of a rigid body can be assumed to be the working point. In the case of a tooth, the point where the line of action of a resultant force intersects the tooth surface can be taken as a first approximation of the working point.

During static loading of the teeth in terminal occlusion, a tooth is physiologically (ie, centrically to its periodontium) loaded by the sum of forces, despite forces acting eccentrically. As masticatory pressure is absorbed during a movement when

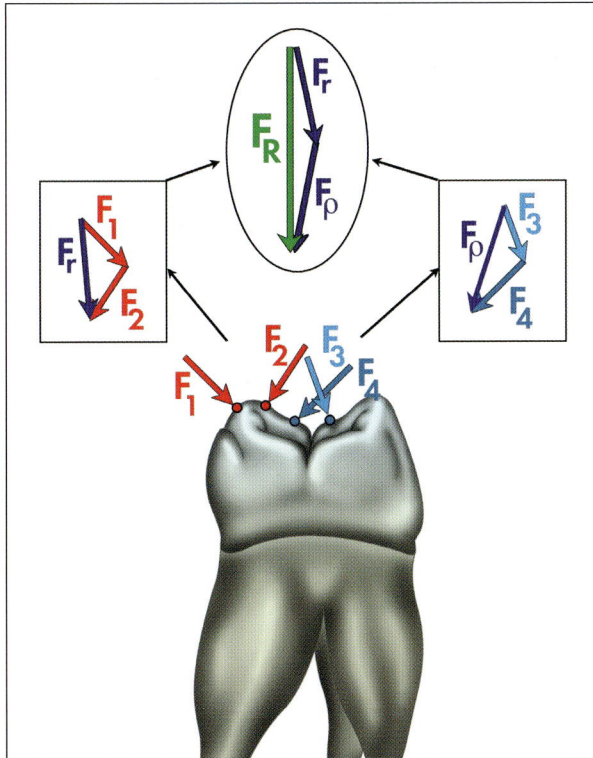

Fig 5-68 When several forces act upon a tooth, the geometric addition has to be performed several times by means of a parallelogram of forces. The aim here is to reduce the real loading situation to a single area. This does not affect the principle of addition of forces because forces can also be combined in three-dimensional space. A parallelogram of forces is created with the forces F_1 and F_2 and with the forces F_3 and F_4. The intersections of the lines of action denote the position of the resultant forces (F_r and F_p). Another parallelogram is then drawn with the resultant forces. The resultant force of all the acting forces (F_R) then loads the tooth centrically if it follows the direction of the tooth axis.

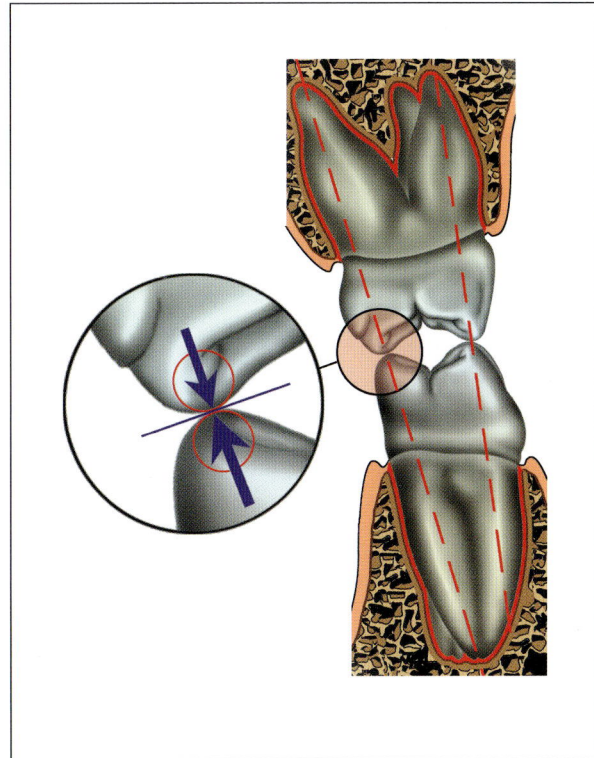

Fig 5-69 The progression of forces in the extreme lateral position lies within the periodontal tissue of the teeth involved. If the occluding surfaces are roughly spherical, the forces act in a defined direction: They are actually perpendicular to the tangents of the spherical surfaces. As a result, when in a lateral position where the buccal and lingual cusps of the antagonists make contact, the loading on the teeth is still centric.

teeth are in contact, the forces alternate in their direction if not in total. An extreme lateral position shows how the progression of force takes place there. All the positions between these extremes and terminal occlusion will show resultant forces whose lines of action lie somewhere between the lines of action of those two positions. If the forces of the two positions are absorbed by the periodontium, the intervening forces would also have to be compensated.

The progression of force in the extreme lateral position lies within the periodontium of the teeth involved, if the occluding surfaces are roughly spherical. The forces act in a defined direction

because they are perpendicular to the tangents of the spherical surfaces (Fig 5-69). This means that in a lateral position, in which the buccal and lingual cusps of the opposing teeth contact, the loading on the teeth will still be centric.

Flared or splayed roots of multirooted teeth are ideally suited to absorbing forces that arise during lateral movement with tooth contact. Such transverse forces are more likely to occur with posterior teeth (molars), which are multirooted.

The real progression of forces during movements is not entirely covered by this illustration of extreme positions, but this does provide a good approximation. In particular, it clearly shows the need for punctiform contacts to be retained even during lateral movements. If just one contact is lost during the movement, the relationships alter, or uncontrolled faulty stresses will result. Therefore, when contouring occlusal surfaces, it is always important to check contacts by means of lateral movements in an articulator.

Principles of mechanics are applied here to explain the characteristic features of form of a physiologic system. The explanatory model should merely be seen as a guide to illustrate the advantages of punctiform contacts or as an aid in understanding why it is so necessary to reconstruct the masticatory area based on certain formal considerations. This model does not take into account other influential factors that may play a role in the development of these characteristic features.

Abrasion of occlusal contacts

As the teeth erupt, they have prominent cusps and ridges, by which they align themselves with each other in occlusal contact until optimal contact is achieved. The prominent functional surfaces are abraded as a result of masticatory function. The degree of wear depends on:

• The strain caused by the nature of the food
• The age of the dentition
• The resistance of the enamel
• The nature of the occlusal contact

The last of these conditions makes it clear that the correct positioning of a tooth within the dentition is not merely an esthetic requirement but a functional necessity. Only when the teeth are accurately positioned and have the correct inclination within the dentition can exact, optimal occlusal contact be achieved with minimal wear. This situation can be referred to as *physiologic abrasion*, whereby the functional surfaces are "ground in," depending on the path of movements during chewing.

This is a **process of adaptation** whereby the relief of the masticatory surfaces adapts to the particular mandibular movements, which are determined by the inclination of the path followed during movement of the TMJs. The abrasion surfaces of the teeth are the "worn-in" tracks of mandibular movements. Conclusions can be drawn from these abrasion surfaces (also known as *ar-*

ticulation surfaces) about the paths followed by the TMJs. Depending on the degree of wear, different occlusal contacts can be found in a natural dentition (Fig 5-70):

• Full-surface contact in an abraded normal occlusion with considerable friction resistance during movement contacts
• Partial-surface contact, which offers precise support and minimal friction resistance during horizontal forward movement
• Supporting cusp contact with imprecise guidance and virtually free sliding movements, which can result in nonphysiologic loading of the periodontal tissue caused by tipping and can damage the TMJ
• Punctiform occlusal contact with centric periodontal loading and the slightest of horizontal friction resistance. This occlusal contact is regarded as the physiologic contact and needs to be reconstructed when artificially restoring the masticatory surface. The contacts should, of course, be checked while lateral movements are carried out.

Once again there is a connection with the law of form and function: The course of movements of the mandible during chewing are determined by the musculature and guided by the TMJs, like a railroad car being guided by the tracks. This guidance by the joints is matched by the way in which the abrasion surfaces on the teeth are ground in, which in turn alters the joint guidance. Pathologic forms of movement, such as tooth grinding and a nervous chewing motion with the mouth empty, lead to abrasion surfaces that may produce eccentric loading of teeth during normal chewing processes. This will lead to pathologic changes to the periodontal tissue and the TMJ.

The aim of systematically reproducing the masticatory area with punctiform contacts, in which the functional surfaces of the teeth meet evenly at several points, is to rebuild pathologic abrasion surfaces in order to achieve centric transmission of forces and to reduce friction resistance during horizontal movements. This balanced sliding situation cannot be technically created because, for instance, the reconstruction of masticatory surfaces cannot be done accurately under loading exerted by masticatory pressure. Therefore, contacts of the lingual cusps should be avoided

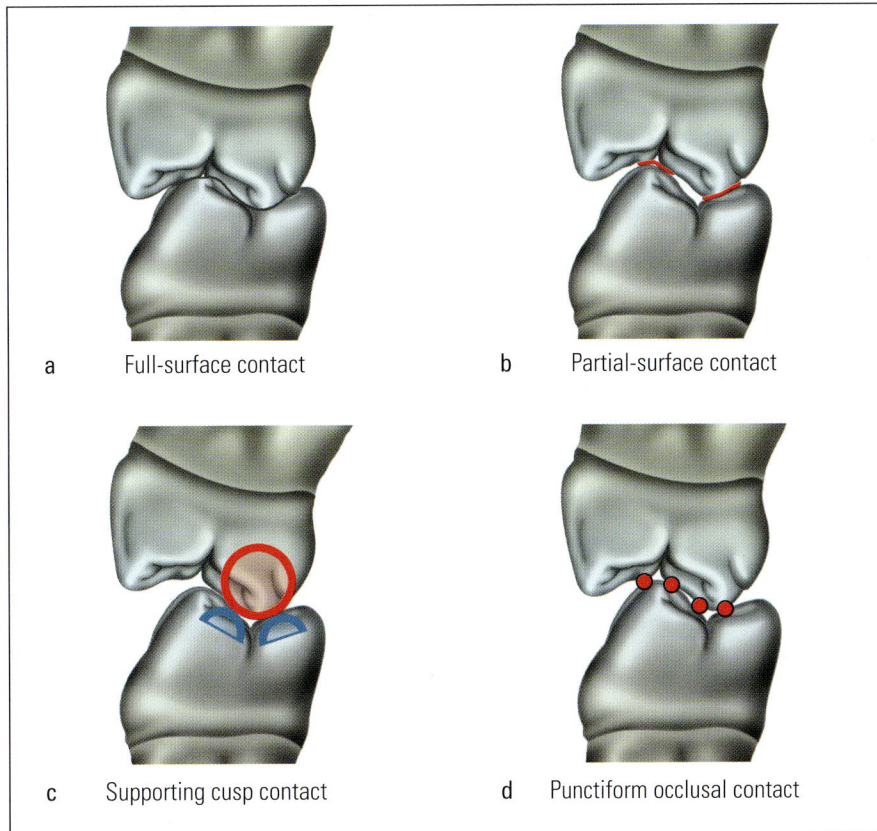

a   Full-surface contact   b   Partial-surface contact

c   Supporting cusp contact   d   Punctiform occlusal contact

Fig 5-70 *(a to d)* Different forms of occlusal contact are identified, depending on the degree of abrasion of the masticatory surfaces. Punctiform occlusal contact *(d)* is the best because it means that roughly axial loading of the tooth by masticatory force can take place. This occlusal contact is regarded as the physiologic contact and should be reconstructed during artificial restoration of the masticatory surface. These contacts must, of course, be checked while lateral movements are being performed.

and removed when checking movements in the articulator. The buccal cusps are able to absorb enough loading from masticatory pressure.

In terms of differentiating the normal tooth position in the normal occlusion, the teeth will incline until this sliding contact is achieved during lateral movement. This is because an excessive lingual contact would force the mandibular teeth into lingual tipping. It is interesting to note in this respect that there is a pronounced lingual inclination of the masticatory surfaces on all the mandibular posterior teeth.

Another advantage of reconstructing punctiform occlusal contacts is that further abrasion can be reduced, preventing permanent damage to the periodontium and the TMJ. Frequently, dysfunctional changes may even be reversed, especially damage to the TMJ.

6

Cranial Anatomy

The **bony skull** *(cranium)* forms the basic bony structure (skeleton) of the head. It is balanced on the first cervical vertebra or the spinal column. It is the point of origin and attachment of many muscles, which in turn partly defines its shape. The shape of the skull is mainly determined by its contents. For instance, there is a connection between the brain and the structure that houses the brain; if the brain grows excessively, the cranium surrounding it becomes enlarged. Equally, premature ossification of the cranium leads to malformations of the brain. A similar relationship exists in the facial part of the skull, where special functions such as that of the masticatory system enforce a specific shape on the jaws, the temporomandibular joints (TMJs), and the teeth.

The **cranium** is made up of 29 cranial bones, which are fitted together like a mosaic to make a roughly spherical shape (Fig 6-1). The individual bones are fused together by sutures, cartilage, and bony connections. The exceptions are the mandible, which is fixed to the skull by two joints, and the hyoid bone, which does not articulate with and is not firmly fixed to any bone in the body but is suspended freely between muscular tracts.

If the skull is divided by a circular, horizontal cut at its widest circumference, the result is the high-vaulted roof of the skull *(calvaria)* and the base of the skull. On the inside of the calvaria as well as the cranial sutures, there are impressions, fossae, and depressions that are produced by blood vessels and by the surface of the brain.

The **skull cap** *(calvaria)* forms the superior, closed, spherical shell of the skull, which is formed by the parietal bones, the frontal bone, and the occipital bone. The calvaria is made up of lamellar bony plates and extends from the orbital margins to the midpart of the occipital bone and at the sides to the temporal bones.

From the cut surface of the skull cap, the structure of a typical bony plate is visible, with an outer layer *(lamina externa)* and an inner layer *(lamina interna)*; between the two compact laminae lies spongy or cancellous material of varying thickness, which contains the bone marrow and numerous blood vessels. Very thin-walled veins run from the bone

Cranial vault
(neurocranium)

1 occipital bone (*os occipitale*)
1 sphenoid bone (*os sphenoidale*)
1 frontal bone (*os frontale*)
2 parietal bones (*ossa parietalia*)
2 temporal bones (*ossa temporalia*)

Skull
(*cranium*)

Facial bones
(*cranium faciale*)

1 ethmoid bone (*os ethmoidale*)
2 nasal bones (*ossa nasalia*)
2 lacrimal bones (*ossa lacrimalia*)
2 inferior nasal conchae
   (*conchae nasales inferiores*)
1 vomer
2 zygomatic bones (*ossa zygomatica*)
2 palatine bones (*ossa palatina*)
2 maxillary bones (*ossa maxillae*)
1 mandibular bone (*os mandibula*)

Visceral cranium
(*splanchnocranium*)

Auditory ossicles
(*ossicula auditus*)

2 hammers (*mallei*)
2 anvils (*incudes*)
2 stirrup bones (*stapedes*)
1 hyoid bone (*os hyoideum*)

Cranial vault (*neurocranium*)

Frontal bone
(os frontale)

Parietal bone
(os parietale)

Sphenoid bone
(os sphenoidale)

Temporal bone
(os temporale)

Ethmoid bone
(os ethmoidale)

Occipital bone
(os occipitale)

Lacrimal bone
(os lacrimale)

Nasal bone
(os nasale)

Zygomatic bone
(os zygomaticum)

Vomer

Palatine bone
(os palatinum)

Inferior nasal
concha
(concha nasalis
inferior)

Maxilla

Mandible
(mandibula)

Visceral cranium (*splanchnocranium*)

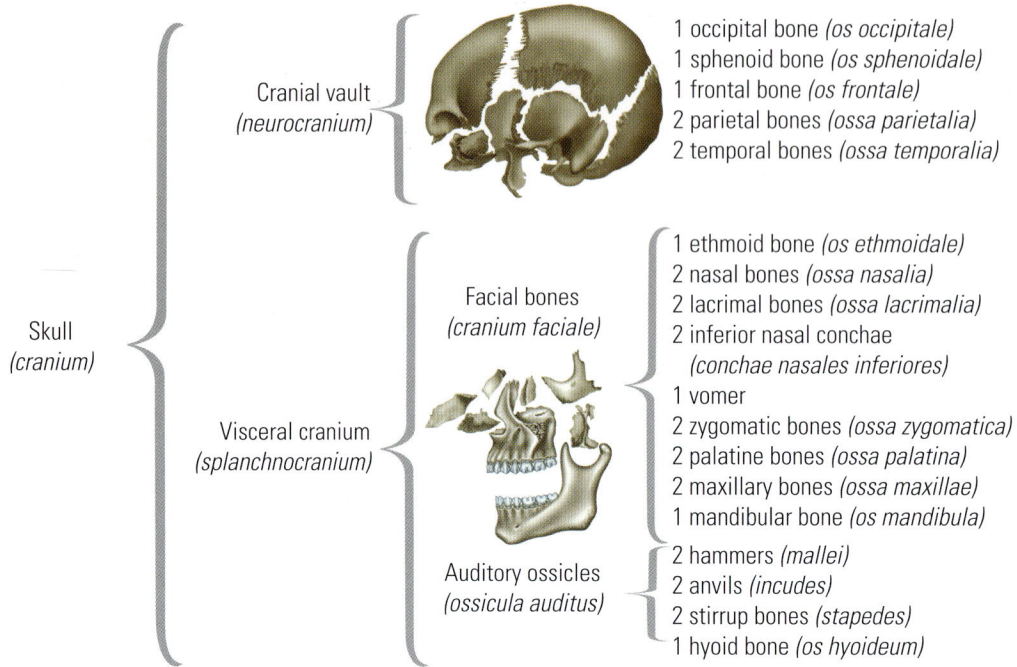

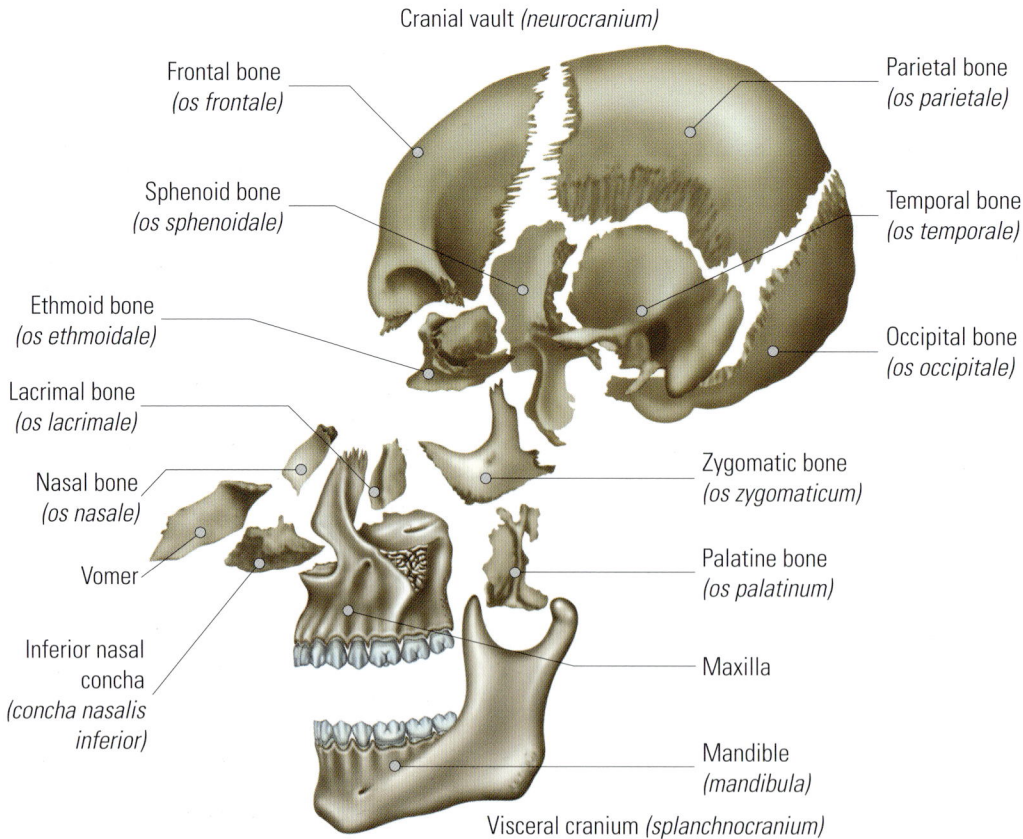

Fig 6-1 Bones of the bony skull.

Fig 6-2 In the bones of the cranium and the facial area, the static loading caused by masticatory pressure produces increased pull on cancellous substance, which is identified as trajectories. These can be seen in the basal arch of the mandible, in the processes of the maxilla, and in the bones of the cranial vault. The trajectories are shown here in the lateral view of the skull.

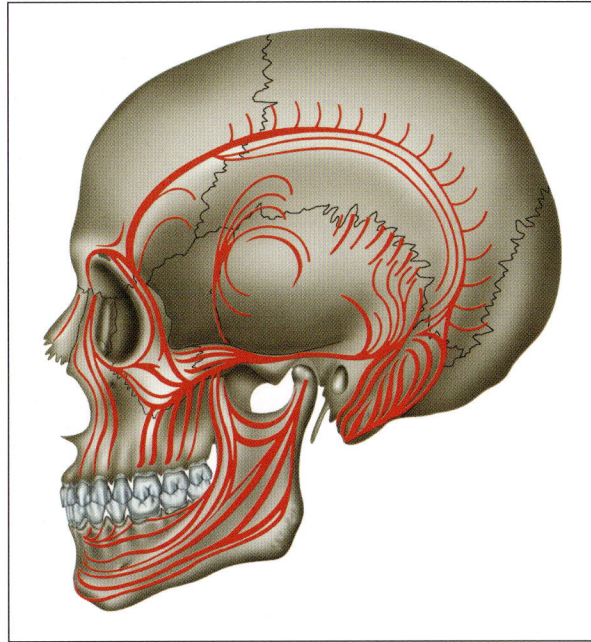

marrow in and out through special bone canals. The outer surface of the skull cap is covered by a relatively thick layer of periosteum, the *pericranium*. On the interior surface, the periosteum is represented by the dura mater of the brain, which adheres to the bone.

The skull, as the top of the body, encases the brain and the sensory organs and contains openings for the digestive tract and the airways. The different functions of the skull determine the differentiated form of its two different areas: the cranial vault and the facial bones.

This division into the cranial vault and the visceral cranium is most marked when viewed from the side. The border between the two parts runs roughly around the root of the nose, over the supraorbital margin, and out to the outer auditory orifices.

The **cranial vault** *(neurocranium)*, formed by the temporal bones, the sphenoid bone, the frontal bone, the parietal bones, and the occipital bone, is virtually round and relatively smooth. The external auditory canal plus the zygomatic bone (also running from the temporal bone), as well as

a prominent muscle attachment to the temporal bone (the mastoid process), are the most striking features on the lateral surface of the skull.

The **facial bones**, or the visceral cranium *(splanchnocranium;* Greek, *splanchnos;* Latin, *viscus* = viscera), are mainly formed by the dominant maxilla and mandible. They also include the zygomatic bones, nasal bones, lacrimal bones, ethmoid bones, inferior nasal conchae, vomer, palatine bones, hyoid bone, and the auditory ossicles (hammer, anvil, and stirrup). The zygomatic bone forms the lateral orbital margin as well as the attachment to the zygomatic arch. The maxilla forms the inferior edge of the orbit and the lateral borders of the nasal cavity. The frontal bone forms the bulging superior orbital margin.

Pronounced cancellous tracts, known as *trajectories*, can be seen in the facial bones and the bones of the cranial vault. These develop from the static loading caused by masticatory pressure (Fig 6-2). They can be seen in the basal arch of the mandible, in the processes of the maxilla, and in the bones of the cranial vault.

Base of the Skull

The separation of the skull into the facial part and the cranial vault can be seen from the **outer surface of the base of the skull** (Fig 6-3). Removing the mandible to view the base of the skull *(basis cranii)* reveals the very highly differentiated anterior facial part and the clearly defined neurocranial part. The anterior area is formed by the two maxillary bones, to which the palatine bones are attached at the rear. To either side of that are the zygomatic bones *(zygomata)*, which join the temporal bones to form the zygomatic arch *(arcus zygomaticus)*. The middle connection between the roof of the palate *(palatine vault)* and the body of the sphenoid is formed by the vomer; the lateral connections between the sphenoid and the maxilla are formed by the pterygoid processes of the sphenoid bone.

The **area of the cranial vault**, formed by the sphenoid bone, the temporal bones, and the occipital bone, contains several holes and fissures as openings through which blood vessels and nerves pass. The large occipital foramen *(foramen occipitale magnum)*, where the articular eminences of the occipital condyles *(condyli occipitales)* are located anterolaterally, is noticeable. The joint surfaces of the TMJs are found on the temporal bones, right at the roots of the zygomatic arch near the external auditory orifices.

The **inner surface of the base of the skull** (Fig 6-4) is smooth with delicate depressions formed by the cerebral gyri *(impressiones digitatae)*. Fine sulci and holes can also be seen as well as canals that can be traced as the course of blood vessels and nerves.

Three fossae can be seen on the inside of the base of the skull: an anterior fossa, middle fossa, and posterior fossa. The **anterior cranial fossa** *(fossa cranii anterior)* is mainly formed by the frontal bone, which lets through a sharp lamella of the ethmoid bone in the middle. The floor of the anterior cranial fossa is made up of extremely thin bony plates that form the roof of the orbits and, anteriorly and vertically, the walls to the frontal sinuses.

The **middle cranial fossa** *(fossa cranii media)* is halved in the middle of the skull by the sella turcica of the sphenoid bone. The sphenoid and temporal bones form the base of the middle cranial fossa. This middle area of the base of the skull is where the most openings for nerves and blood vessels are found.

The **posterior cranial fossa** *(fossa cranii posterior)* contains the striking occipital foramen in the occipital bone, which, with parts of the temporal bones, forms the bony base of the posterior cranial fossa.

Figures 6-5 and 6-6 show the topographic details of the skull from anterior and lateral views.

The **cranial sutures** join together the bones of the cranium. In the cranial sutures, the bones are indented and contain narrow strips of connective tissue, which give the bony vault of the skull a certain elasticity. As growth areas, the sutures allow cranial growth up to the age of 40 or 50 years. This is because the brain continues growing until this stage of life, which forces the cranium to grow with it. Age-induced ossification of the cranial sutures only happens once the brain has stopped growing. The individual sutures are the following:

- The **coronal suture** *(sutura coronalis)* runs crosswise over the skull cap and joins the frontal bone to the parietal bones.
- The **sagittal suture** *(sutura sagittalis)* is the suture between the parietal bones and runs from the coronal suture to the lambdoid suture.
- The **lambdoid suture** *(sutura lambdoidea)* runs between the occipital bone and the parietal bones; the continuation between temporal bone and occipital bone is known as the *occipitomastoid suture (sutura occipitomastoidea)*.
- The **sphenofrontal suture** *(sutura sphenofrontalis)* joins the frontal bone to the wings of the sphenoid.
- The **squamous suture** *(sutura squamosa)* joins the parietal and temporal bones to the skull at the sides.

The suture between the two squamae of the frontal bone *(sutura frontalis)* closes by the end of the sixth year of life; sometimes a fine residual suture is left above the root of the nose. In the skull of the newborn, the cranial sutures, such as the coronal, sagittal, and lambdoid, are permeated by sections of connective tissue and are elastic. The sutures are open in the form of fontanels so that the brain can be seen pulsating beneath *(fonticulus;* Latin, *fons* = fountain) (Fig 6-7).

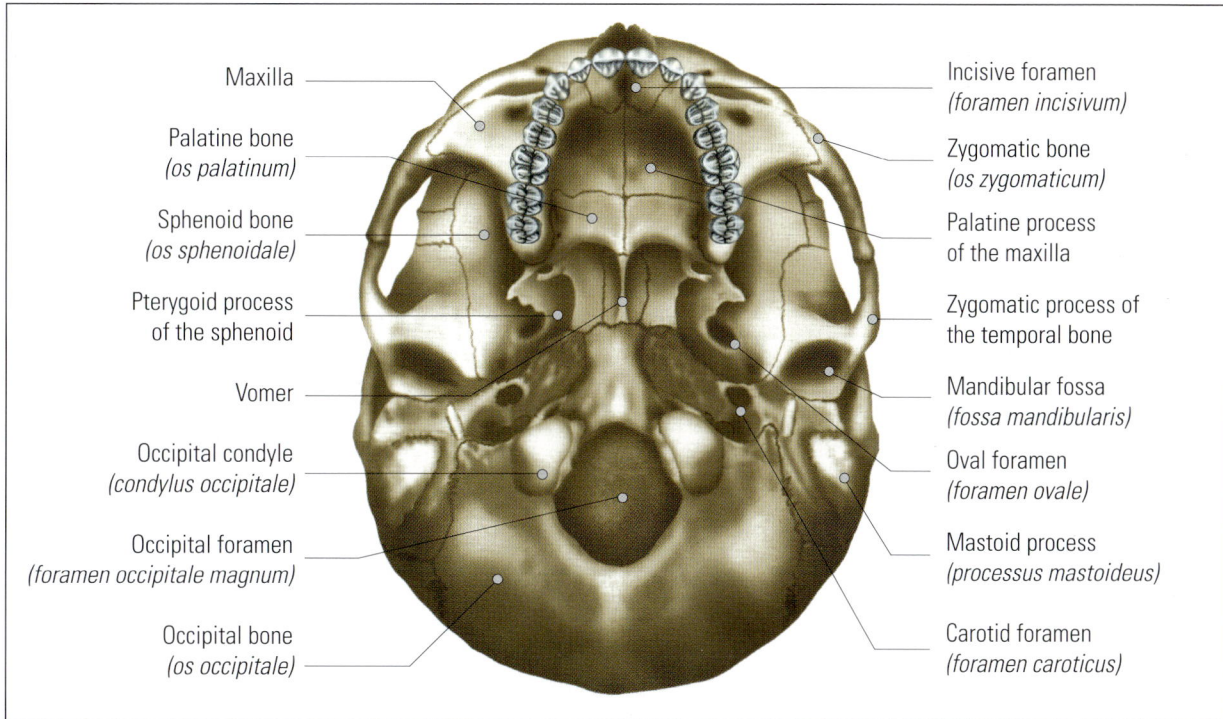

Fig 6-3 Topographic details of the outer surface of the base of the skull.

Maxilla
Palatine bone (os palatinum)
Sphenoid bone (os sphenoidale)
Pterygoid process of the sphenoid
Vomer
Occipital condyle (condylus occipitale)
Occipital foramen (foramen occipitale magnum)
Occipital bone (os occipitale)
Incisive foramen (foramen incisivum)
Zygomatic bone (os zygomaticum)
Palatine process of the maxilla
Zygomatic process of the temporal bone
Mandibular fossa (fossa mandibularis)
Oval foramen (foramen ovale)
Mastoid process (processus mastoideus)
Carotid foramen (foramen caroticus)

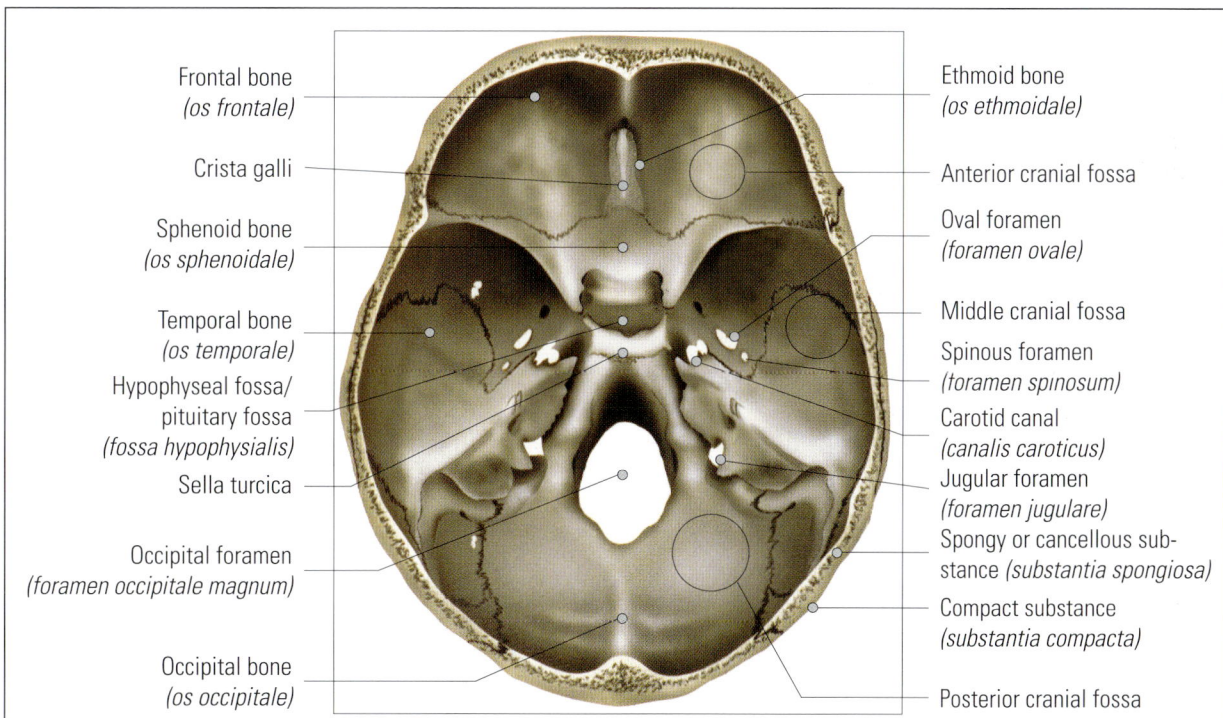

Fig 6-4 Topographic details of the inner surface of the base of the skull.

Frontal bone (os frontale)
Crista galli
Sphenoid bone (os sphenoidale)
Temporal bone (os temporale)
Hypophyseal fossa/ pituitary fossa (fossa hypophysialis)
Sella turcica
Occipital foramen (foramen occipitale magnum)
Occipital bone (os occipitale)
Ethmoid bone (os ethmoidale)
Anterior cranial fossa
Oval foramen (foramen ovale)
Middle cranial fossa
Spinous foramen (foramen spinosum)
Carotid canal (canalis caroticus)
Jugular foramen (foramen jugulare)
Spongy or cancellous substance (substantia spongiosa)
Compact substance (substantia compacta)
Posterior cranial fossa

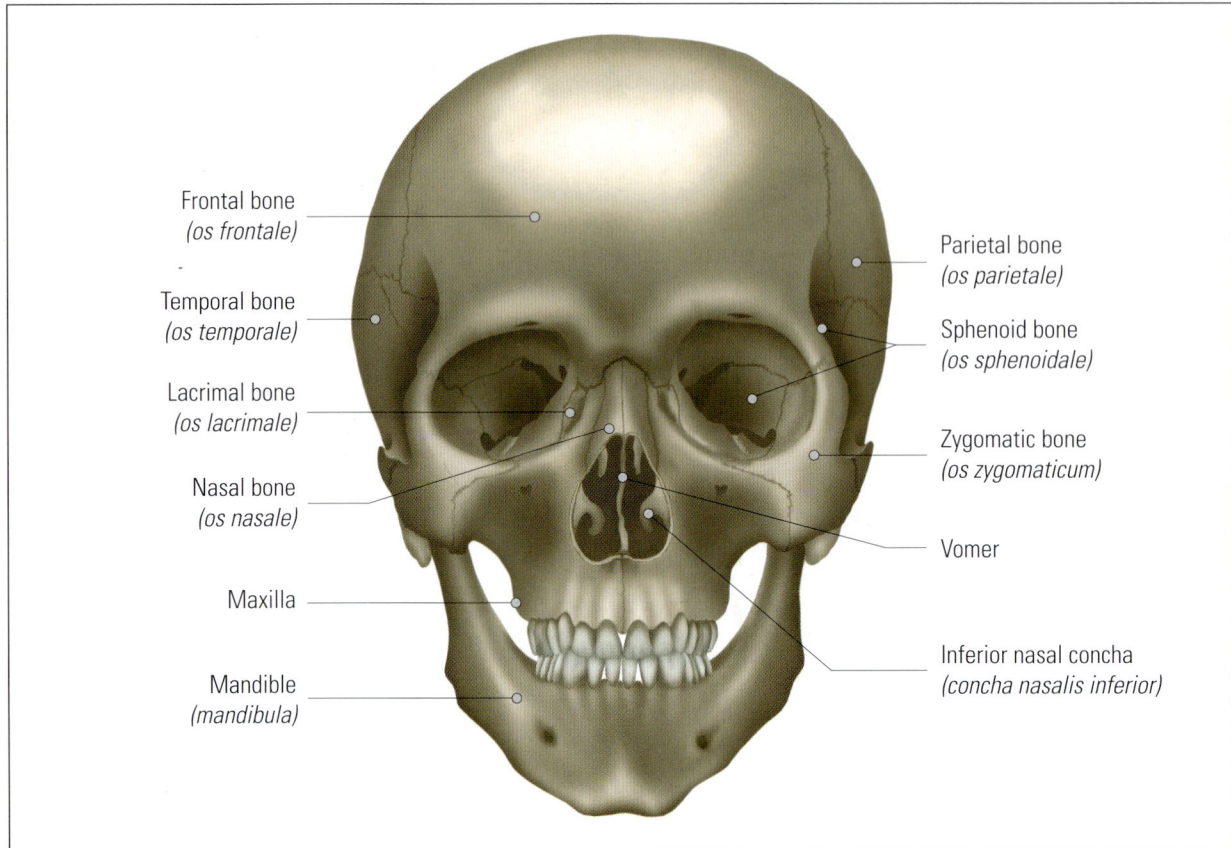

Fig 6-5 Topographic details of the anterior view of the skull.

There are two central and two lateral fontanels, with the lateral ones being less important (Fig 6-8). The large, anterior fontanel is formed by the frontal bone and the parietal bones; the posterior fontanel lies at the crossover point with the lambdoid suture. The fontanels only close fully during the second year of life. In the fontanels, the individual cranial bones can move against each other so that the relatively large skull is able to change shape safely as it passes through the narrow birth canal.

Coronal suture
(sutura coronalis)

Frontal bone
(os frontale)

Sphenoid bone
(os sphenoidale)

Lacrimal bone
(os lacrimale)

Nasal bone
(os nasale)

Zygomatic bone
(os zygomaticum)

Maxilla

Mandible
(mandibula)

Parietal bone
(os parietale)

Squamous suture
(sutura squamosa)

Occipital bone
(os occipitale)

Occipitomastoid suture
(sutura occipitomastoidea)

Temporal bone
(os temporale)

Sphenoid bone
(os sphenoidale)

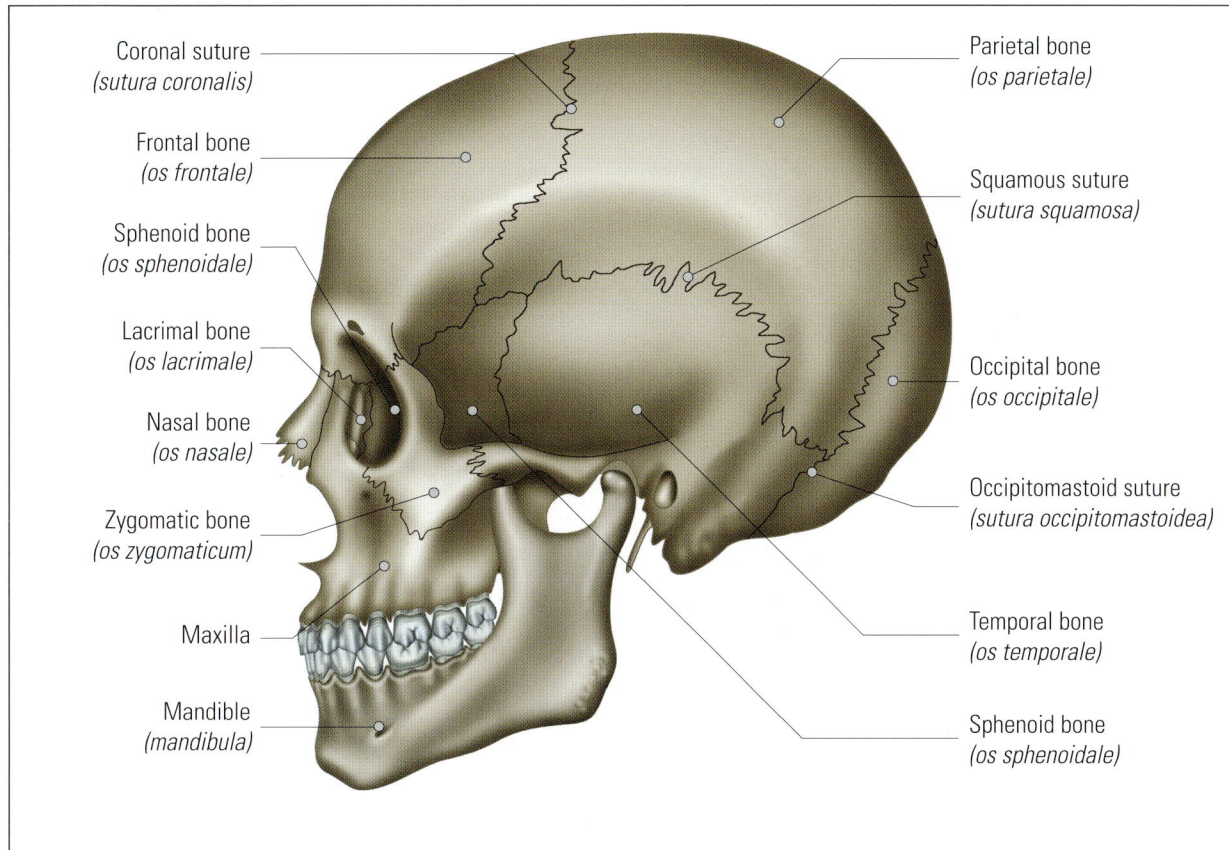

Fig 6-6 Topographic details of the lateral view of the skull.

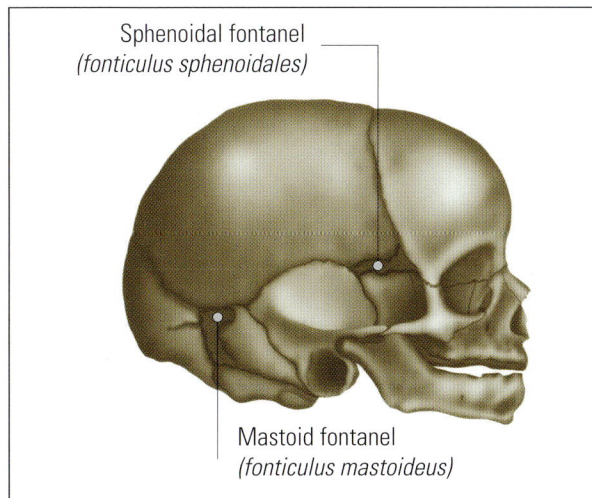

Sphenoidal fontanel
(fonticulus sphenoidales)

Mastoid fontanel
(fonticulus mastoideus)

Fig 6-7 The sutures in the skull of a newborn infant take the form of fontanels (*fons* = fountain; *fonticulus* = small fountain), under which the pulsating of the brain can be seen, which resembles the welling up of a torrent of water in a fountain.

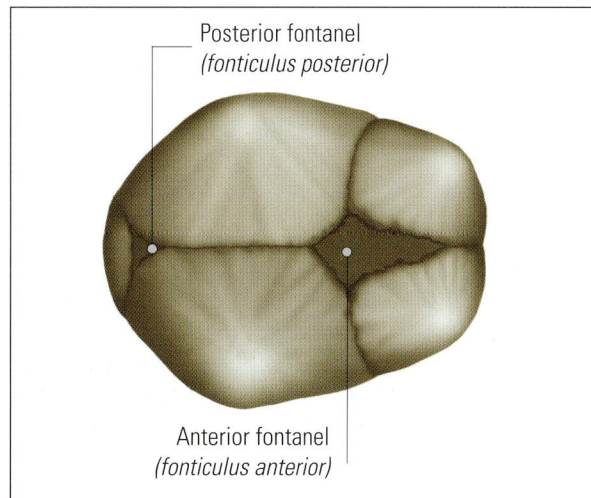

Posterior fontanel
(fonticulus posterior)

Anterior fontanel
(fonticulus anterior)

Fig 6-8 Two important fontanels in the skull cap are the central suture openings. The growth tracts of the bony squamae of the frontal and parietal bones can be clearly seen in a superior view of the neonatal skull.

Bones of the Cranial Vault

The **frontal bone** *(os frontale)* arises from a paired arrangement where two parts are fused into one bone in the adult (Fig 6-9). The frontal bone forms the anterior area of the cranium and the roof of the orbits. Behind the prominent orbital swellings are the frontal sinuses, which are air-filled and lined with mucous membrane. These sinuses are connected to the actual nasal cavity as paranasal sinuses. The nasal part *(pars nasalis)* of the frontal bone, on which the nasal skeleton grows, lies between the two roofs of the orbits.

The **occipital bone** *(os occipitale)* forms the back of the head (the occiput) and the bony casing for the cerebellum and parts of the cerebral hemispheres (Fig 6-10). The occiput is where the muscles of the neck attach. The large occipital foramen *(foramen occipitale)* at the base of the skull is the opening through which the spinal cord, located in the spinal canal, passes. The articular eminences at the front next to the occipital foramen are the joint surfaces of the atlanto-occipital and atlanto-axial joints. The occipital bone comprises four elements that are grouped around the occipital foramen and form one unified bone: at the front, the unpaired piece of bone called the *basilar part (pars basilaris)*; at the sides, the lateral parts *(partes laterales)*; and, at the back, the occipital squama *(squama occipitalis)*.

The **parietal bone** *(os parietale)* forms the roof of the skull in its middle section and is hence the superiormost aspect of the cranium. The sutures to the adjacent bones, the frontal bone, the occipital bones, and between the parietal bones themselves ossify very late and thus enable the skull to enlarge.

The **sphenoid bone** *(os sphenoidale)* is a symmetric bone at the base of the skull (Fig 6-11), from whose transverse bodies run two horizontal pairs of wings *(alae majores* and *alae minores)* and a vertical pair of wings, the pterygoid processes *(processus pterygoidei;* Greek, *pteryx* = wing).

Pterygoid processes can be divided into one lateral and one middle lamella, which serve as the points of origin for the pterygoid muscles for mandibular movement. These pterygoid processes are joined to the infratemporal surfaces of the body of the maxilla and contact the vertical plates of the palatine bones. The greater palatine canal *(canalis palatinus major)* is formed by these three bony parts and opens into the palatine foramina. Blood vessels and nerve pathways run through the canal into the posterior palatine region.

The two horizontal pairs of wings contain important openings through which nerves from the oral cavity and the orbits pass. The optic canal *(canalis opticus)* is located in the small wing *(ala minor)* and allows the optic nerve to pass through from the cranial cavity to the orbit. The large wing *(ala major)* is the site of the round foramen *(foramen rotundum)*, a roundish canal that carries the second branch of the trigeminal nerve (maxillary branch). The oval foramen *(foramen ovale)*, the oval hole for the third branch of the trigeminal nerve (mandibular branch), is also located in the ala major.

The **temporal bone** *(os temporale)* is the part of the skull on which the head mainly rests during sleep (Fig 6-12). It takes its name (literally "time bone") from the fact that the hairs at the temples are the first to go gray, hence indicating the passage of time in life. The structure of the temporal bone is very complex. The temporal bone houses a bony capsule for the organ of hearing and balance (the ear), which is why this bone has numerous cavities and canals. The temporal bone is divided into three parts: the petrous, tympanic, and squamous parts.

The **petrous part** *(pars petrosa)* is the posterior region of the temporal bone and is made up of very hard bone. The mastoid process is a bony bulge projecting downward from the petrous part that arises because of the pulling effect of turning the head.

The **tympanic part** *(pars tympanica)* forms the external auditory canal (or external auditory meatus) as a tube, at the inner end of which the eardrum is stretched.

The **squamous part** *(pars squamosa)* is the actual body of the temporal bone and forms the lateral wall of the skull. The zygomatic process extends forward from this squamous part and, together with the temporal process of the zygomatic bone, forms the zygomatic arch *(arcus zygomaticus)*. On the underside of the temporal squama lies the socket *(fossa mandibularis)* for the TMJ, which is bounded anteriorly below the root of the zygomatic process by the articular tubercle *(tuberculum articulare)*. The styloid process *(processus styloideus)*, which can vary in length, is the bony attachment for the stylomandibular ligament.

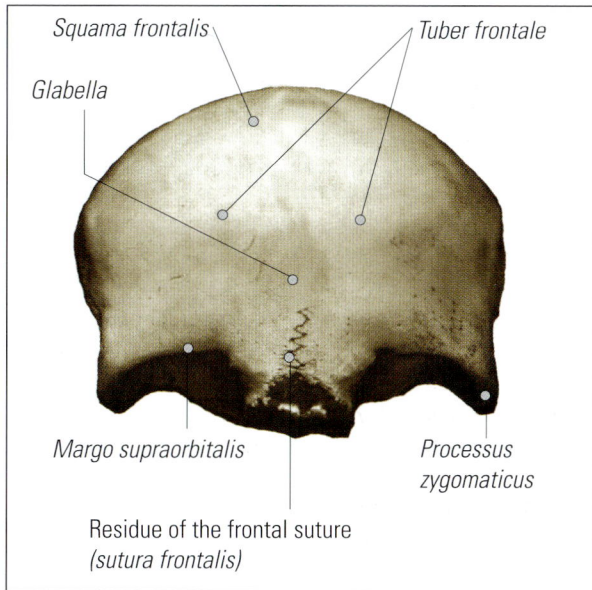

Fig 6-9 Frontal bone, anterior view *(facies externa)*.

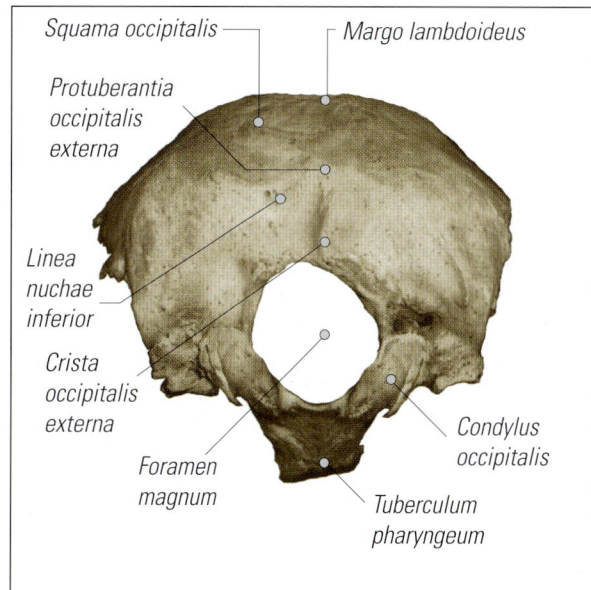

Fig 6-10 Occipital bone, basal view.

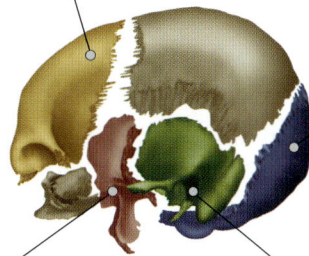

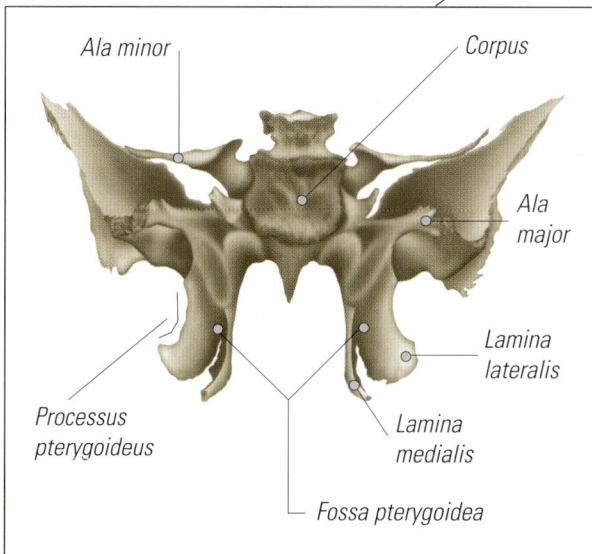

Fig 6-11 Sphenoid bone, posterior view.

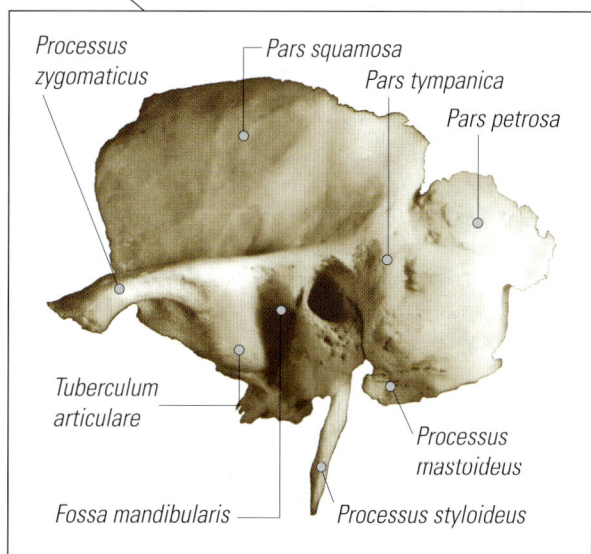

Fig 6-12 Temporal bone, external lateral view.

159

Facial Bones

The **ethmoid bone** is a sievelike, perforated, air-filled bone with a number of cavities known as *ethmoidal cells (cellulae ethmoidales)*, which feed into the nasal cavity and are part of the paranasal sinuses. A plate of the ethmoid bone projecting downward, known as the *perpendicular* or *vertical plate (lamina perpendicularis)*, forms the superior part of the nasal septum. The superior edge of the perpendicular plate forms a cockscomb-like crest *(crista galli)* extending into the cranial cavity. A narrow bony plate forms the roof of the ethmoid bone (cribriform plate; *lamina cribrosa*), which is perforated with numerous holes like a sieve. The lateral walls of the ethmoid bone are smooth, paper-thin bony plates (orbital lamina; *lamina orbitalis*) that form one part of the medial orbital wall. The ethmoidal labyrinth is located on either side of the nasal septum and, with its curved, twisted lamellae of bone (superior and middle nasal conchae), forms the branched passages of the nasal cavities and the paranasal sinuses.

The **superior nasal concha** *(concha nasalis superior)*, like the middle nasal concha *(concha nasalis media)*, lies at the medial surface of the ethmoidal labyrinth; from this surface a narrow, hook-shaped uncinate process *(processus uncinatus)* is projected backward and lies in front of the maxillary hiatus *(hiatus maxillaris)*.

The **inferior nasal concha** *(concha nasalis inferior)* is a shell-shaped or turbinate bone that lies along the lateral wall of the nasal cavity and covers part of the opening to the maxillary sinus. At its superior aspect, the inferior nasal concha meets the ethmoidal labyrinth. A process *(processus lacrimalis)* is directed upward to the lacrimal bone and, together with that bone, forms the medial wall of the nasolacrimal canal.

The **nasal bone** *(os nasale)* is a small, rectangular bone that forms the bridge or dorsum of the nose. It attaches to the frontal process of the maxilla and at its superior aspect borders the frontal bone.

The **lacrimal bone** *(os lacrimale)* is located at the anterior medial wall of the orbit and contains a vertical depression (the lacrimal sulcus), which with the lacrimal sulcus of the frontal process on the maxilla forms a connecting passage to the nasal cavity. This is where the lacrimal sac is located.

The **vomer** resembles the blade of a plow and forms the inferior aspect of the nasal septum. The vomer borders on the perpendicular process of the ethmoid bone superiorly and the sphenoid bone posteriorly. The posterior, free edge of the vomer separates the two posterior nares *(choanae)* from each other.

The **zygomatic bone** or cheekbone *(os zygomaticum)* is a rectangular bone that presents two processes: the temporal and the frontal processes. It forms the bony foundation of the cheek. The bone forms a bridge between the facial part of the skull and the lateral walls of the cranium via the zygomatic arch, which is shaped by the temporal process and the zygomatic process of the temporal bone. Via these two processes, the zygomatic bone transfers masticatory forces from the maxilla to the cranial vault. The **palatine bone** *(os palatinum)* is paired and forms the posterior part of the bony or hard palate as well as the lateral wall of the nasal cavity. The palatine bone is made up of a horizontal plate and a perpendicular plate of bone. The horizontal plate *(lamina horizontalis)* forms the posterior part of the hard palate and is joined to the palatine processes of the maxilla via a transverse palatine suture.

The mobile soft palate *(velum palatinum)*, which separates the oral cavity and the nasal cavity in the pharyngeal area, attaches to the dorsal part of the horizontal plate. The surfaces of the two palatine bones turned toward the oral cavity form the palatine crest *(crista palatina)* at their juncture, which posteriorly forms the short, blunt posterior nasal spine *(spina nasalis)*. The perpendicular plate *(lamina maxillaris)* attaches to the nasal surface of the maxilla and to the medial surface of the pterygoid process of the sphenoid bone. The perpendicular plate of the palatine bone covers the posterior part of the maxillary hiatus and runs vertically up to the orbit.

Figure 6-13 illustrates the facial bones of the skull individually.

The **hyoid bone** *(os hyoideum)* is a small, bracelet-shaped bone that is suspended freely between various muscles (Fig 6-14). In other words, it does not articulate with and is not permanently joined to any other bone. Muscles and ligaments of the floor of the mouth and the throat are fixed to the hyoid. Two processes projecting upward sit on either side of the body of the hyoid: the large, dorsally placed greater horns *(cor-*

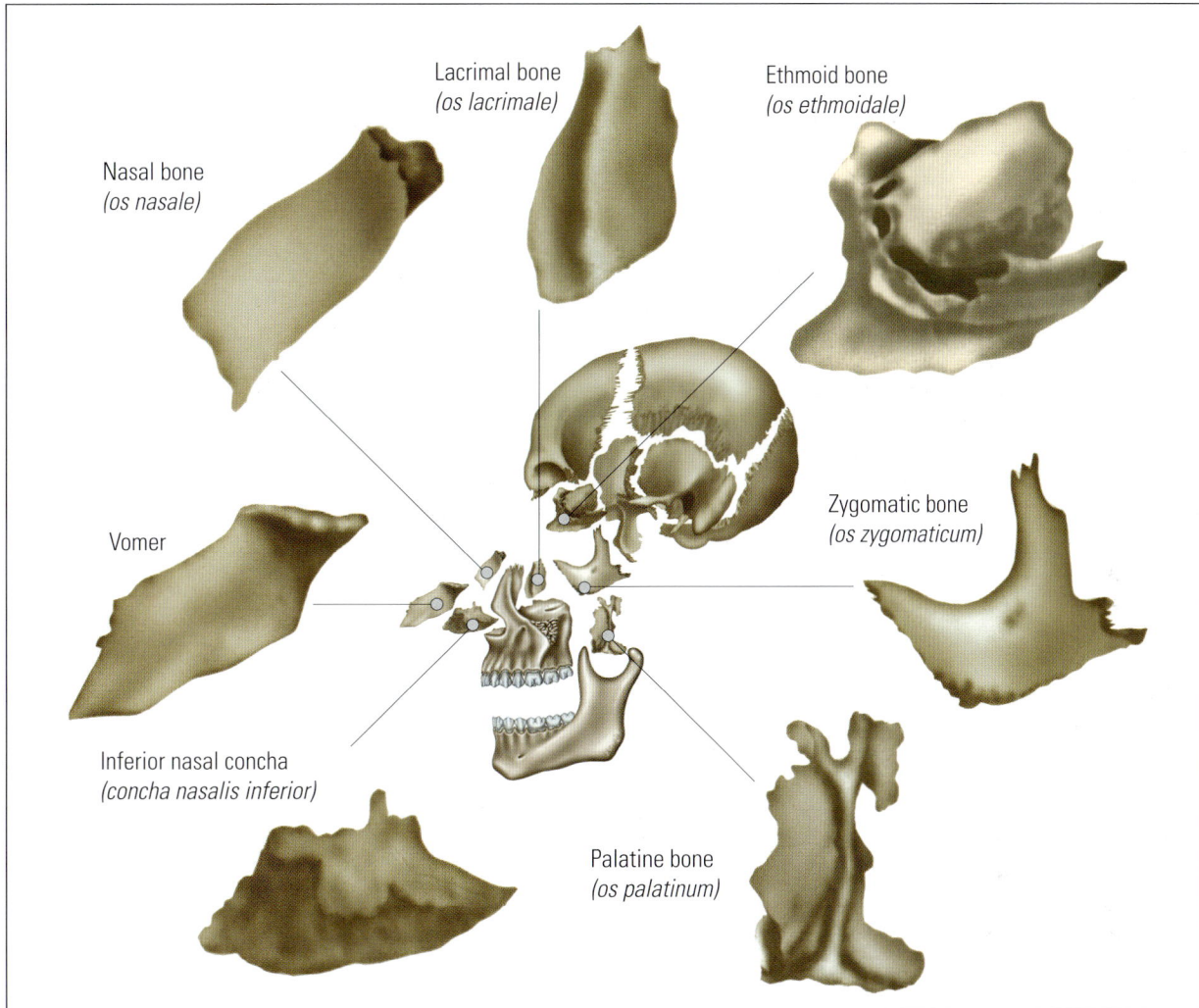

Fig 6-13 Facial bones with the skull separated out.

Nasal bone
(os nasale)

Lacrimal bone
(os lacrimale)

Ethmoid bone
(os ethmoidale)

Vomer

Zygomatic bone
(os zygomaticum)

Inferior nasal concha
(concha nasalis inferior)

Palatine bone
(os palatinum)

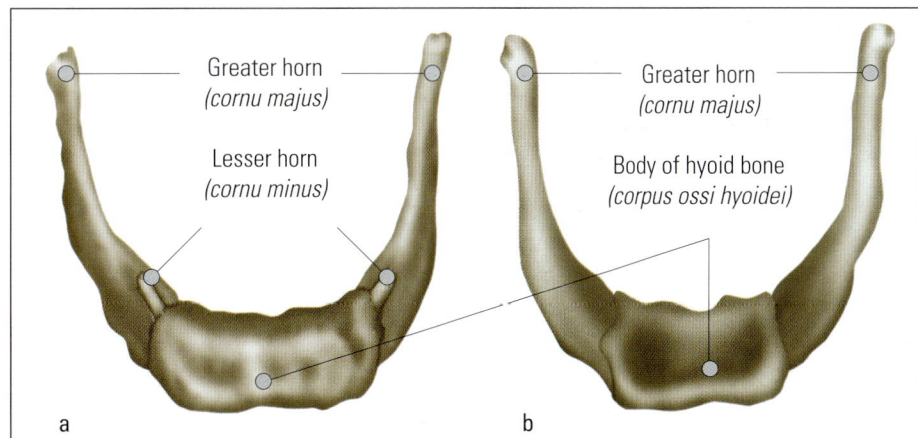

Greater horn
(cornu majus)

Greater horn
(cornu majus)

Lesser horn
(cornu minus)

Body of hyoid bone
(corpus ossi hyoidei)

Fig 6-14 Hyoid bone. *(a)* Anterior view. *(b)* Posterior view.

a

b

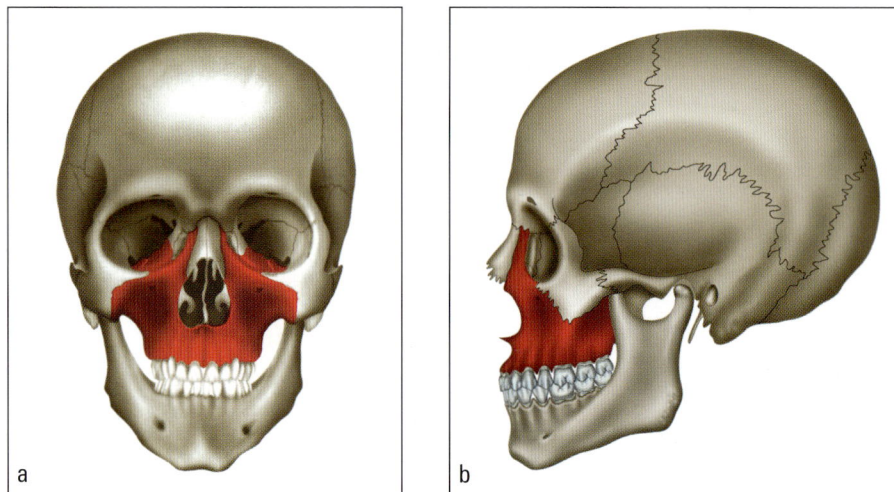

Fig 6-15 *(a and b)* Arrangement of the maxilla in the facial part of the skull.

nu majus) and the small, cartilaginous, centrally placed lesser horns *(cornu minus)*. This is where the stylohyoid ligament attaches, which extends to the styloid process of the temporal bone.

Maxilla

The maxilla is a paired bone; ie, there are two maxillary bones that are joined by a bone suture. However, the individual maxillary bones also have a paired arrangement. Thus, it is still possible to detect the development from one maxillary process and the frontal process, giving rise to the unified maxillary bone for each half of the face.

The maxilla, like the mandible, is described as one bone because functionally it represents a single structure. It lies centrally in the facial or visceral cranium and thus forms the bony foundation of the face (Fig 6-15); the shape and size of the face are determined by the dimensions of the maxilla. A compact body of the maxilla, from which the four maxillary processes project, can be identified in each maxillary bone. The walls of the orbit, the nasal cavity, and the palatine vault are formed by the maxilla. It holds the maxillary dentition and transfers masticatory pressure via the processes to the cranial vault.

The **body of the maxilla** *(corpus maxillae)* is made up of thin bony plates and contains the maxillary sinus *(sinus maxillaris)*. Four surfaces can be identified on the three-sided body resembling a truncated pyramid: the facial surface, the nasal surface, the orbital surface, and the infratemporal surface.

The **facial surface** *(facies anterior)* is the anterior surface of the body of the maxilla, which is bordered superiorly by the infraorbital margin *(margo infraorbitalis)* and posterolaterally is divided from the infratemporal surface by the infrazygomatic crest *(crista infrazygomatic)*. A few millimeters below the infraorbital margin lies the infraorbital foramen *(foramen infraorbitale)*, which is the exit for the infraorbital canal *(canalis infraorbitale)* that emerges from the orbit. The canine fossa *(fossa canina)* is a flat depression located roughly at the root apex of the canine, below the infraorbital foramen and the root of the zygomatic process. It is named after the canine tooth and is the origin of a mimic muscle (muscle of facial expression).

The **infratemporal surface** *(facies infratemporalis)* is demarcated from the facial surface by the infrazygomatic crest. The protuberance-like bulging of the maxillary tuberosity *(tuber maxillae)* at the inferior edge of the surface is striking; its rough areas border the palatine bone and the pterygoid processes. Toward the cheek are located the alveolar foramina *(foramina alveolaria)*, tiny holes that are openings for parts of the maxillary branch of the trigeminal nerve for the dental nerves of the molars. A groove running from a posterior-superior to an inferior-anterior position

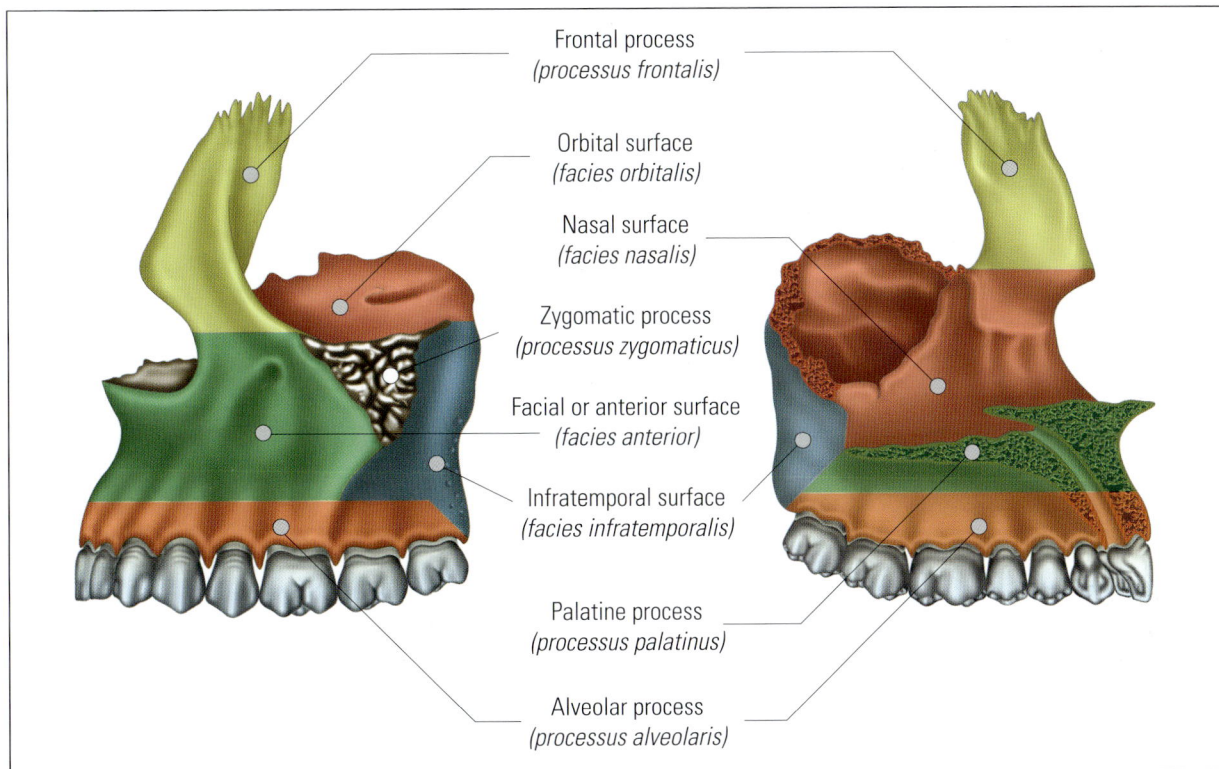

Fig 6-16 The surfaces and processes of the maxilla, highlighted by color.

over the tuberosity toward the palate, together with the sulcus of the palatine bone *(sulcus ptery-gopalatinus)*, form the pterygopalatine canal *(canalis pterygopalatinus canalis*; in the palatine area, also known as the *greater palatine sulcus*, ie, *canalis palatinus major)*.

The **orbital surface** *(facies orbitalis)* forms the largest part of the orbital floor. A groove runs from the posterior orbital margin and anteriorly becomes the infraorbital canal. It is the infraorbital sulcus *(sulcus infraorbitalis)*, the course of which is followed by the infraorbital nerve, part of the maxillary branch of the trigeminal nerve. In the bottom of the sulcus and the canal there are tiny holes through which nerves from the maxillary anterior teeth pass.

The **nasal surface** *(facies nasalis)* forms the inner surface of the corpus and the lateral wall of the nasal cavity. This surface contains a long, narrow, five-sided window known as the *maxillary hiatus (hiatus maxillaris)*, which marks the

entrance to the maxillary sinus. This maxillary hiatus is covered posteriorly by the perpendicular plate of the palatine bone, inferiorly by the inferior nasal concha, and superiorly by the ethmoidal labyrinth. There is a prominent ridge to which the inferior nasal concha attaches *(crista conchalis)*. The lacrimal sulcus *(sulcus lacrimalis)* becomes the lacrimal canal or duct where it is covered by the lacrimal bone.

The **maxillary sinus** *(sinus maxillaris)* is a cavity in the corpus of the maxilla that is lined with mucous membrane and filled with air. It is the largest paranasal sinus and is connected to the frontal sinus via the other paranasal sinuses. The apices of the roots of the molars and possibly the premolars project into the sinus and are generally covered with thin bony plates. Sometimes the bony covering over a root apex may be missing so that the root protrudes freely into the sinus.

Figure 6-16 illustrates the surfaces and processes of the maxilla.

Maxillary Processes

The **frontal process** *(processus frontalis)* rises vertically between the lacrimal bone and the nasal bone up to the frontal bone. It forms a closed bony connection with the cranial area so that masticatory forces can be transferred to the cranium while bypassing the nasal and orbital cavities.

The **zygomatic process** *(processus zygomaticus)* is a short process with a triangular cross section that runs along the side of the orbital surface to the zygomatic bone. A convexity of the maxillary sinus may be found inside the process. This process also transfers masticatory pressure vertically to the cranium, while bypassing the eye socket, but also laterally via the zygomatic bone to the temporal bone. The infrazygomatic crest *(crista infrazygomatica)* runs caudally from the zygomatic process to the alveolar jugum *(jugum alveolare)* of the distobuccal root of the maxillary first molar.

The **alveolar process** *(processus alveolaris)* is directed vertically and downward and, with the process on the opposite side, forms the alveolar ridge. It bears the teeth, and its shape is dictated by the dental arch, which is why it is also known as the *dental process*. This maxillary process is strongly functionally designed and is resorbed following tooth loss. This involves irreversible, resorptive disuse atrophy, in which the tissue is broken down by osteoclasts. As a result, the alveolar ridge shrinks in the direction of inclination. All of the other processes are also subject to this process of disuse atrophy, but their shape does not alter as markedly as that of the alveolar process.

At the wide inferior edge of the alveolar process lie the dental alveoli or **tooth sockets** *(alveoli dentales)*. There are eight tooth sockets, which are separated by interdental or interalveolar septa *(septa interdentale, septum interalveolare)*. These thin sheets of bone can also emerge between individual root tips in the case of multirooted teeth and then form **interradicular** or **alveolar septa** *(septa interradicularia* or *septum alveolare)*. In keeping with the shape of the roots, the alveoli are roughly funnel-shaped and, following the path of the roots, are curved distally. The outer and inner edges, which mark the boundary of the alveoli and also form the free marginal arch of the alveolar process, are together known as the *limbus alveolaris*.

On the external surface of the alveolar process, long prominences can be seen as far as the surfaces of the maxillary body; these correspond to the roots of the teeth and are called **alveolar juga** *(juga alveolaria, jugum alveolare)*. These are particularly well developed in the anterior area and only slightly noticeable in the area of the posterior teeth. When a denture body is being shaped, the alveolar juga are reproduced in the anterior area.

The **palatine process** *(processus palatinus)* starts as a horizontal plate at the inferior edge of the nasal surface and extends to the middle of the skull to unite with the process on the other side to form the anterior palatine vault. This vault is the floor of the nasal cavity in its anterior part. At the point where the two palatine processes run into each other to form a palatine suture, the processes thicken into a ridge projecting into the nasal cavity; this is the nasal crest *(crista nasalis)*, which tapers in front into a point known as the **anterior nasal spine** *(spina nasalis anterior)*. The vomer attaches to the nasal crest, forming the nasal septum and extending as far as the frontal bone or the sphenoid bone. This is how the palatine vault is statically supported against the cranial area.

The oral surface of the palatine process is rough, whereas the nasal surface is smooth. At the suture site, directly at the attachment to the alveolar process, there is a depression that runs vertically and, with the process on the opposite side, forms a canal known as the **incisive canal** *(canalis incisivum)*. Toward the palate, this canal has one exit hole, the **incisive foramen** *(foramen incisivum)*. Toward the nasal cavity, this canal divides into two exit holes; it holds nerves and blood vessels to supply the anterior part of the palate.

A fine suture often runs at the side from the **incisive foramen** to the interdental area between the canine and the lateral incisor. This suture demarcates the **incisive bone** *(os incisivum;* also known as the *premaxilla* or *intermaxillary bone)* from the maxilla proper. The incisive bone holds the incisors and may be present as a separate bone in some animals.

Figures 6-17 and 6-18 illustrate the topographic details of the maxilla.

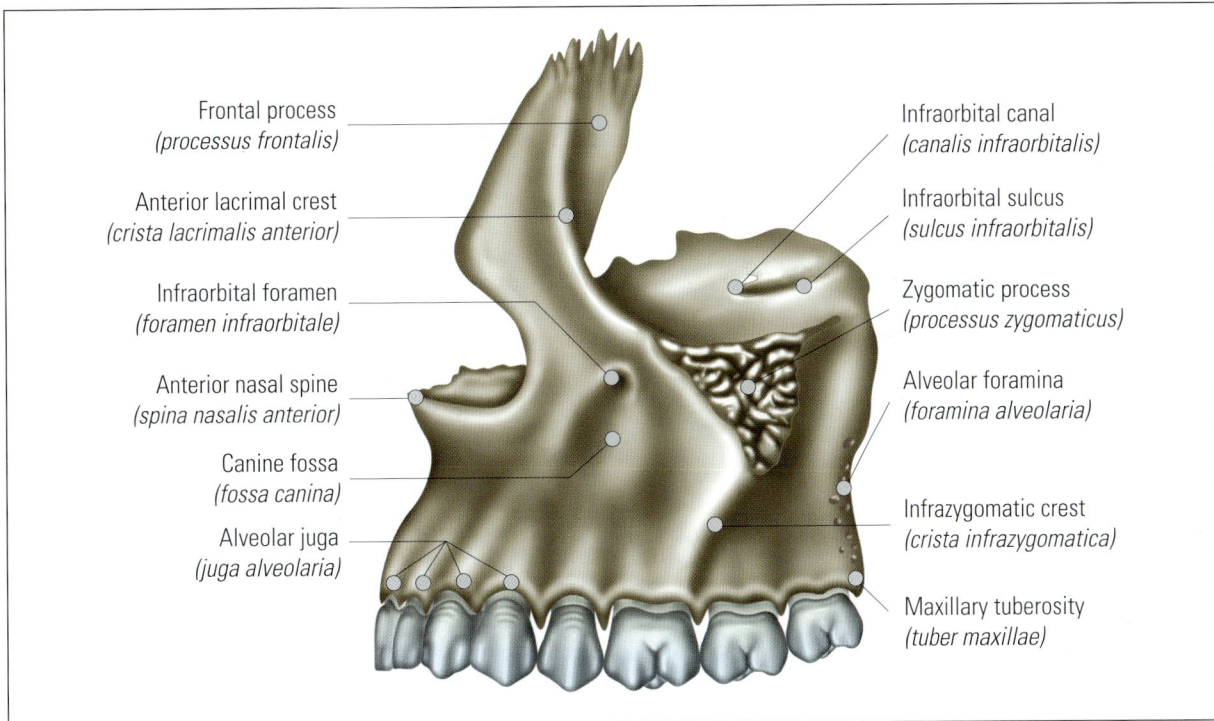

Fig 6-17 Topographic details of the maxilla, exterior sagittal view.

Frontal process (processus frontalis)

Anterior lacrimal crest (crista lacrimalis anterior)

Infraorbital foramen (foramen infraorbitale)

Anterior nasal spine (spina nasalis anterior)

Canine fossa (fossa canina)

Alveolar juga (juga alveolaria)

Infraorbital canal (canalis infraorbitalis)

Infraorbital sulcus (sulcus infraorbitalis)

Zygomatic process (processus zygomaticus)

Alveolar foramina (foramina alveolaria)

Infrazygomatic crest (crista infrazygomatica)

Maxillary tuberosity (tuber maxillae)

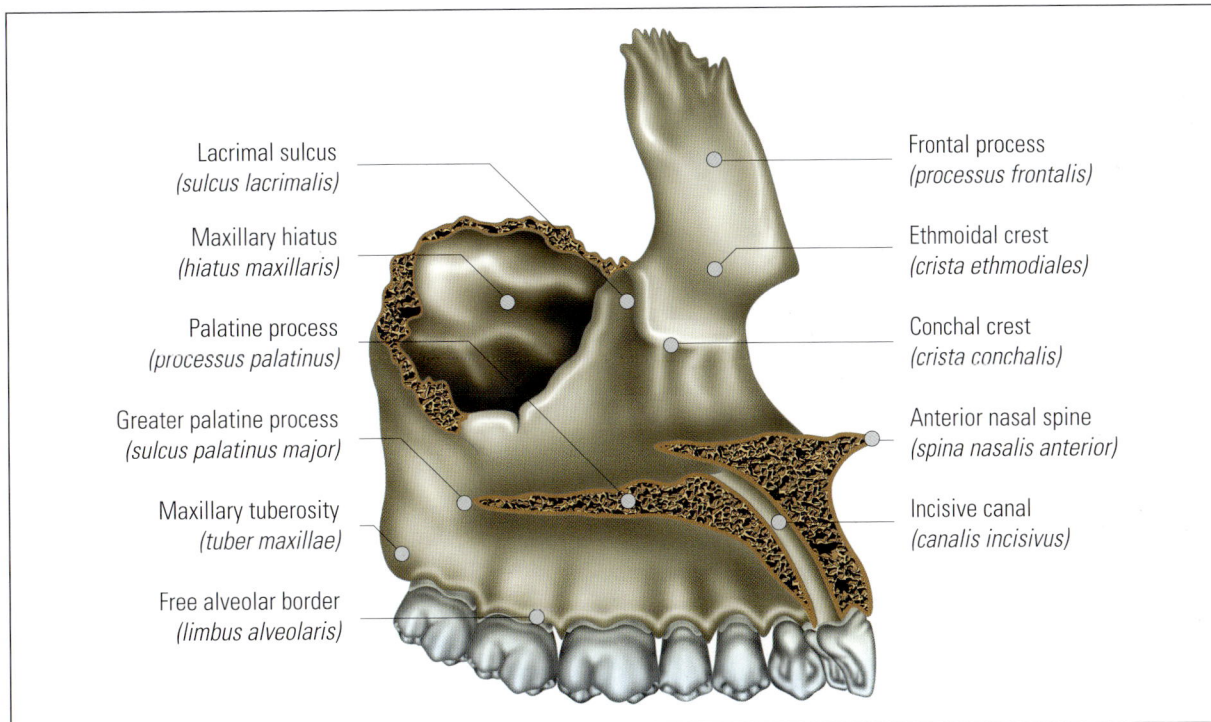

Fig 6-18 Topographic details of the maxilla, interior sagittal view.

Lacrimal sulcus (sulcus lacrimalis)

Maxillary hiatus (hiatus maxillaris)

Palatine process (processus palatinus)

Greater palatine process (sulcus palatinus major)

Maxillary tuberosity (tuber maxillae)

Free alveolar border (limbus alveolaris)

Frontal process (processus frontalis)

Ethmoidal crest (crista ethmodiales)

Conchal crest (crista conchalis)

Anterior nasal spine (spina nasalis anterior)

Incisive canal (canalis incisivus)

Bony Palate

The bony palate *(palatum osseum)* forms the roof of the oral cavity and the floor of the nasal cavity (Fig 6-19). It is made up of the palatine processes of the maxillary body; the incisive bone, which forms a bony fusion with the maxilla in adults; and the horizontal plates of the palatine bones, the backward projection of the palatine processes (Fig 6-20). The bony palate is held together by the following **sutures**:

- Median palatine suture *(sutura palatina mediana)*
- Transverse palatine suture *(sutura palatina transversa)*
- Incisive suture *(sutura incisiva)*

The **median palatine suture** runs exactly in the midline of the skull from the anterior to the posterior nasal spine. In the region of the alveolar processes, the median palatine suture is referred to as the *intermaxillary suture*—the suture between the maxillae. The median palatine suture joins the palatine processes and the alveolar processes of the maxilla or the incisive bone and the horizontal plates of the palatine bones to each other. In the dorsal area, the palatine suture may be swollen into a ridge-shaped prominence; if so, it is known as the *torus palatinus*. The mucosal covering over this torus is very thin and not very soft; a denture may rock back and forth over this torus if the other parts of the palate are more yielding.

The **transverse palatine suture** crosses the median palatine suture vertically at the level of the interdental spaces between the second and third molars, deviates dorsally before the alveolar process, and then runs around the tuberosity of the maxilla. This suture can continue to be traced as the division between the maxilla and the pterygoid processes of the sphenoid bone.

The **incisive suture** runs on both sides from the incisive foramen between the lateral incisors and canines through to the nasal cavity. This suture links together the incisive bone and the maxillae.

The **openings in the bony palate** allow nerves and blood vessels to pass through to supply the palatal mucosa. The incisive foramen is the exit point for the incisive canal. In the mucosal covering, this incisive foramen can be identified as the incisive papilla *(papilla incisiva)*, which often has to be hollowed out on the base of a denture. Third molars are found here as well as one greater palatine foramen *(foramen palatinum majus)* and, behind that, two or three lesser palatine foramina *(foramina palatina minora)*. The greater palatine foramen is the exit point from the pterygopalatine canal for vessels and the greater palatine nerve *(nervus palatinus major*; part of the maxillary branch of the trigeminal nerve), which supply the glandular area and the anterior part of the palate. The lesser palatine foramina are secondary openings of the pterygopalatine canal and contain vessels and nerves to supply the posterior part of the palate.

Developmental abnormalities in the formation of the bony palate mainly arise at the sutures between the different parts of the palate. One common abnormality is cleft lip, jaw, and palate (cheilognathouranoschisis; cheilognathopalatoschisis), which occurs when the incisive suture and the median palatine suture have failed to fuse. As a result, the oral and nasal cavity are not separated so that, when a baby is breastfeeding, the milk is forced back out through the nose or the infant cannot suckle at all because he or she is unable to create negative pressure in the oral cavity by suction. This cleft deformity is often bilateral. A *cleft palate* is the common name for the condition in which the incisive sutures and the median palatine suture are not fused. A *harelip* is the term used when only the incisive suture has not fused to the nasal cavity. In both cases, the lip of the maxilla has not grown together so that a cleft up to the nose is visible.

These developmental abnormalities, which are dominant inherited disorders, can be corrected by surgical repair while the child is still an infant. Prosthetic treatment to close the opening to the nasal cavity can be provided with what are known as *obturators*.

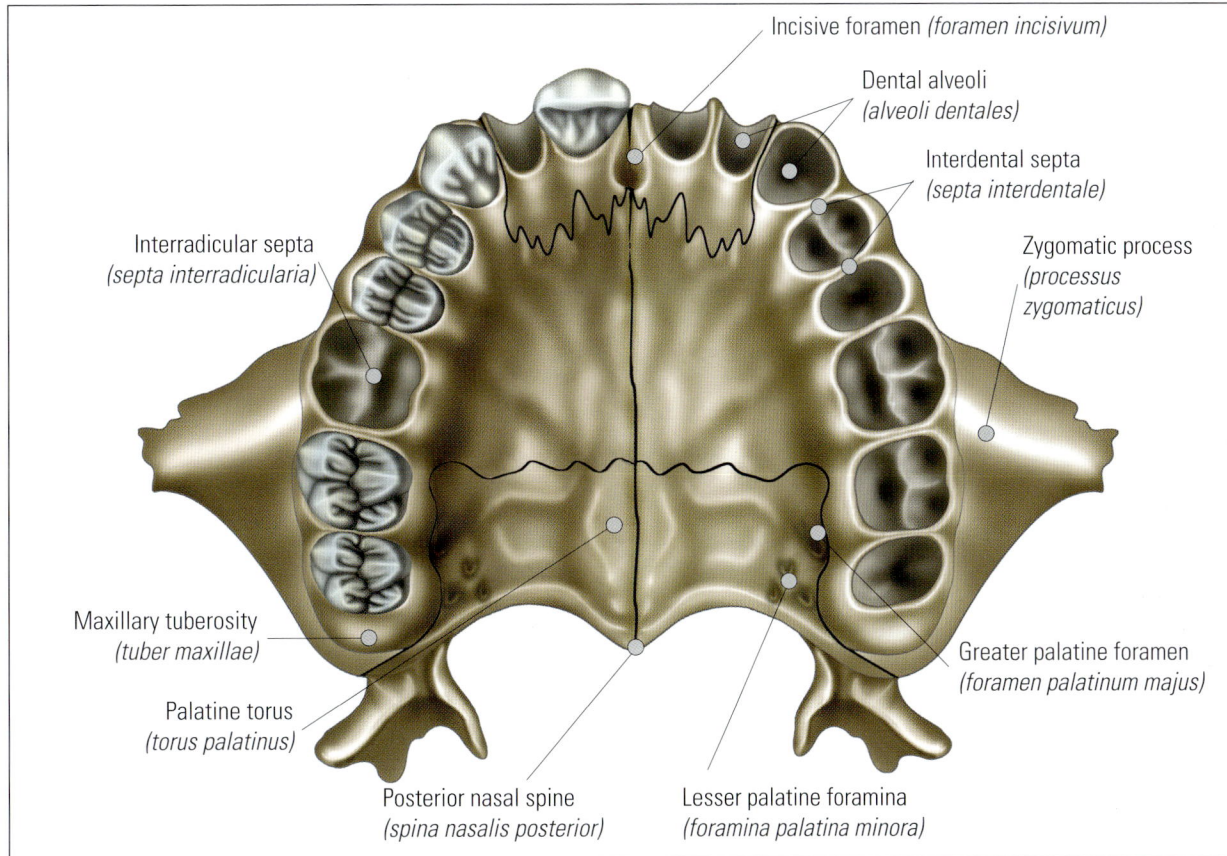

Fig 6-19 Topography of the bony palate with its openings and sutures.

Incisive foramen (foramen incisivum)

Dental alveoli (alveoli dentales)

Interdental septa (septa interdentale)

Zygomatic process (processus zygomaticus)

Greater palatine foramen (foramen palatinum majus)

Interradicular septa (septa interradicularia)

Maxillary tuberosity (tuber maxillae)

Palatine torus (torus palatinus)

Posterior nasal spine (spina nasalis posterior)

Lesser palatine foramina (foramina palatina minora)

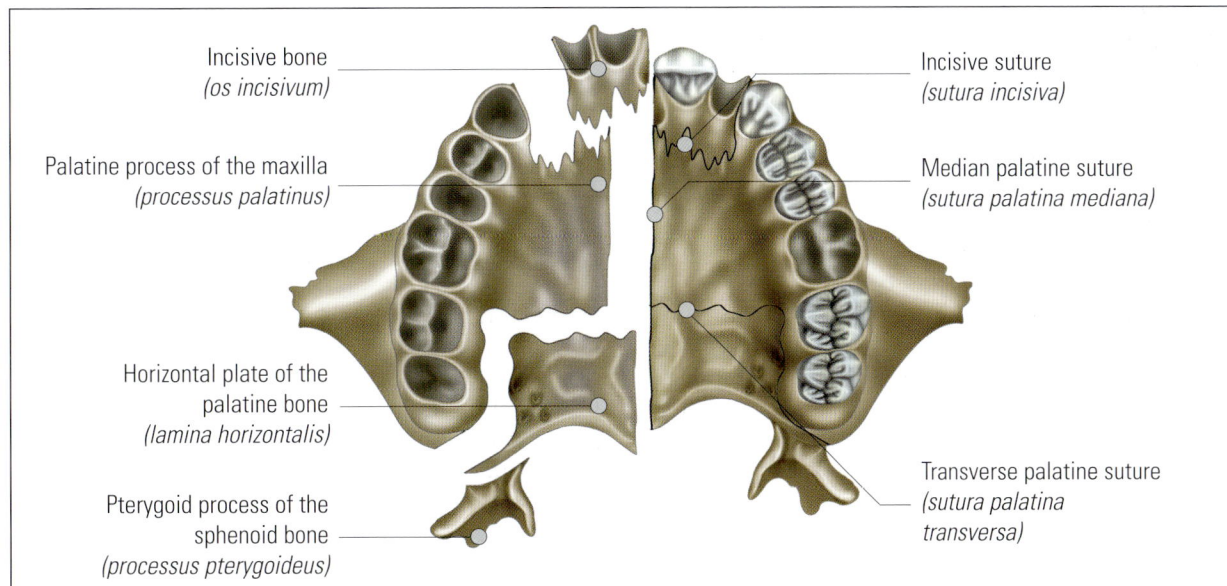

Fig 6-20 The separated bones of the bony palate.

Incisive bone (os incisivum)

Palatine process of the maxilla (processus palatinus)

Horizontal plate of the palatine bone (lamina horizontalis)

Pterygoid process of the sphenoid bone (processus pterygoideus)

Incisive suture (sutura incisiva)

Median palatine suture (sutura palatina mediana)

Transverse palatine suture (sutura palatina transversa)

Mandible

The mandible (*mandibula*; Latin, *mandere* = to chew) is a paired bone that is fused at the symphysis before birth. *Symphysis* means the bony site where the two halves of the mandible are fused, which lies on the midline of the symmetric bony plate. The parabolically shaped bony plate, as the largest of the facial bones, determines the shape and size of the lower part of the face. The main parts of the mandible are the body and the rami of the mandible.

As a single bone, the mandible is attached to the skull by two true joints (TMJs) in a mobile fashion, and it bears the mandibular dentition. Movement of the mandible takes place in these two joints. The TMJs connect the mandible to the temporal bone and guide it in its movements against the maxilla.

The **functional construction** of the mandible comprises the basal arch, formed by the condylar process *(processus condylaris)*, the middle part of the ramus of the mandible, and the body of the mandible, which is enlarged in front by the chin (Fig 6-21). The formation of the alveolar part *(pars alveolaris)* on the mandible results from direct functional stress caused by the teeth; the coronoid process *(processus coronoideus)* results from the pull of the temporal muscle, and the angle of the mandible results from the pull of the medial pterygoid muscle internally and the masseter muscle externally.

The **body of the mandible** *(corpus mandibulae)* is made up of the base of the mandible *(basis mandibulae)* and the alveolar part; it starts at the angle of the mandible (*angulus mandibulae*; submaxillary angle) or at the last molar and runs via the symphysis with the opposite side right up to the other angle of the mandible.

The **mandibular canal** *(canalis mandibulae)* runs through the body of the mandible, starting at the mandibular foramen on the inner surface of the ramus and extending as far as the symphysis. Blood vessels and nerves supplying the mandibular teeth run through the canal. Some of the vessels and nerves exit at the mental foramen, while the remainder run as far as the symphysis. These nerves are part of the mandibular branch of the trigeminal nerve.

The **alveolar part** *(pars alveolaris)* is the bony foundation of the tooth-bearing alveolar ridge and displays the typical bony structure: a dense outer bony plate covered with periosteum, an inner bony layer lining the alveoli, and the cancellous bone lying between the compact layers (Fig 6-22). The bony alveolar ridge is where the compact layers of the outer surface and those of the alveoli merge. The outer layer of the alveolar bone is the typical substantia corticalis and is relatively thick here. The cancellous tissue is missing at the roots of the incisors so that external and internal compact tissue layers combine with the alveolar compact tissue to form a uniform bony mass.

The **cancellous tissue** is made up of narrow trabeculae with mainly red, blood-forming (hematopoietic) bone marrow. The cancellous trabeculae display noticeable functional alignment based on lines of traction and pressure initiated by tooth and muscle stresses. This means that the arrangement of the cancellous trabeculae adapts to changing stresses.

The **internal alveolar wall** to the tooth sockets is a rigid but greatly perforated cortical layer. This bony layer is known as the *cribriform plate (lamina cribriformis)*. It is particularly highly perforated in the cervical and apical areas. The openings correspond to the Volkmann canals and connect the periosteum to the bone marrow spaces through which blood and lymph vessels pass. Bundles of Sharpey fibers are embedded in the cortical layer of the alveolus, similar to the situation in the cementum.

The **composition** of the alveolar bone is the same as that of other bones: 45 parts by weight inorganic hydroxyapatite (calcium phosphate), 30 parts by weight organic matrix comprising collagen fibers, and 25 parts by weight water.

The shape and position of the alveolar bone is determined by the teeth and their function: The mandibular incisors are inclined in a vestibular direction, the mandibular canine stands rather perpendicular, and the mandibular molars and premolars have a tendency to a lingual positioning. Following tooth loss, the osseous lamellae of the alveoli are resorbed as the thin bony parts shrink considerably (Fig 6-23). It appears as if the alveolar ridges are shrinking in the direction of inclination, which changes the path of the mandibular alveolar ridge into a trapezoidal, tapering shape.

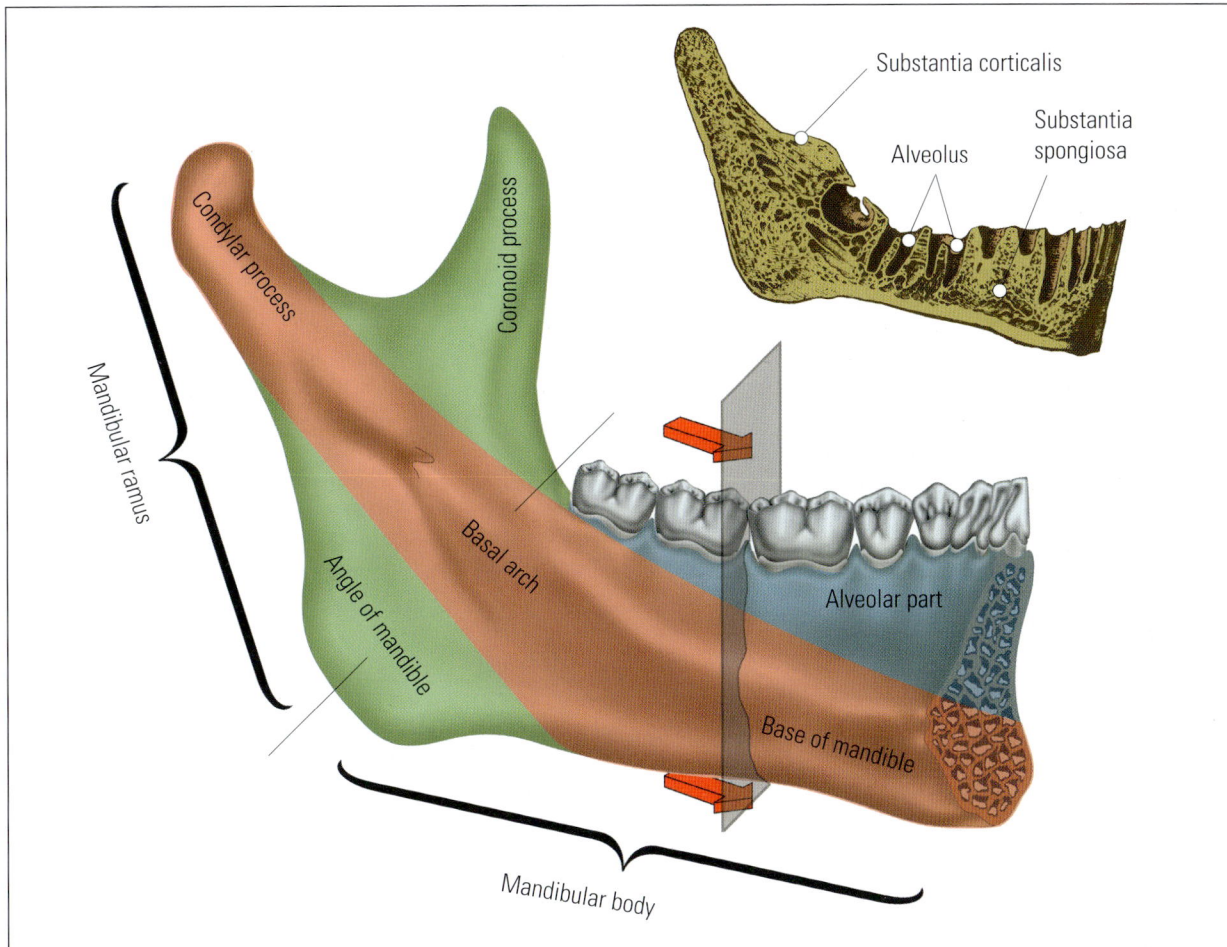

Fig 6-21 Functional construction of the mandible.

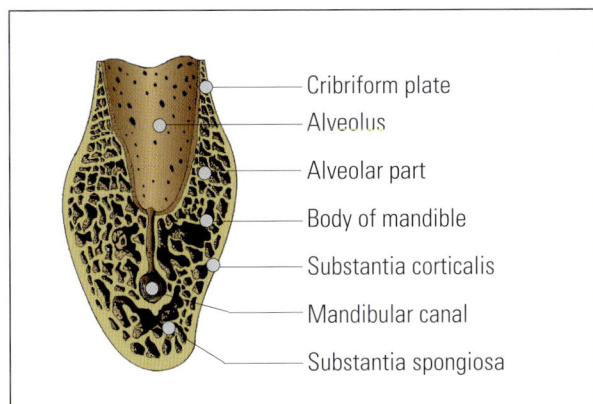

Fig 6-22 Structure of the mandibular bone.

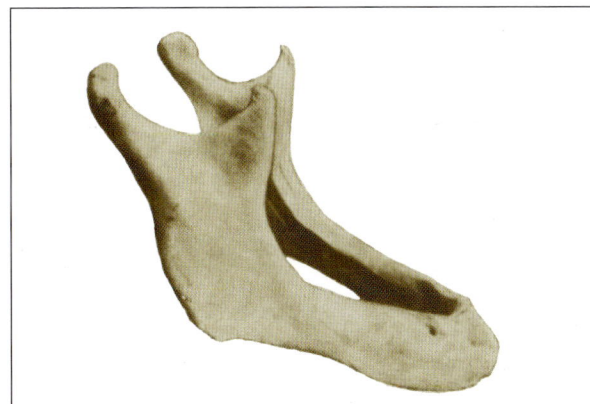

Fig 6-23 After tooth loss, the functionally oriented parts of the mandible as well as the alveolar part, the angle of the mandible, and the coronoid process shrink. This can result in a thin strip of bone that does not provide adequate denture support.

The *root apices of the molars* lie inferior to the border of the floor of the mouth. The root apices of the anterior teeth are the most distant from the mandibular canal, while the distance is smaller with the posterior teeth. Consequently, the roots of the third molars are very close to the mandibular canal and may even encompass it.

Body of the Mandible

External surface topography

The *mental trigone (trigonum mentale)* is located in the region of the symphysis as a triangular bony support that strengthens the symphysis and safeguards against transverse stresses. The inferior corners of the mental trigone lying on one side are formed by the *mental tubercles (tuberculum mentale)*.

The *mental foramen (foramen mentale)*, despite its name, is not directly in the chin but rather at the apices of the premolar roots. It is an exit point for blood vessels and nerves from the mandibular canal, some of which supply the chin area. The mental foramen generally lies at the level of the vestibular fornix and, when the alveolar part is resorbed following tooth loss, may lie on the alveolar ridge; as this can be associated with a risk of pressure points, it should be covered during prosthetic treatment.

The *oblique line (linea obliqua)* forms the anterior projection of the mandibular ramus into the body of the mandible *(corpus mandibulae)*. This thickened ridge of bone is the attachment site for the buccinator muscle *(musculus buccinator)*. The border of a mandibular denture must be shortened in keeping with the oblique line because, if not, pressure points may arise during muscle movements or the denture may be levered off. In this case, denture reduction is a necessity.

The *alveolar juga (juga alveolaria)* are the prominences in the alveolar part caused by the roots. They are particularly pronounced in the region of the anterior teeth and ought to be reproduced on an anterior denture body for esthetic reasons. However, they should be omitted in the posterior region because, if this is not done, deposits may form on the denture. This usually means calcu-

lus deposits in the region of the posterior teeth because this is where exit points for the salivary glands are located.

The *free alveolar border (limbus alveolaris)*, as an arcuate free border of the alveolar part, marks the superior boundary of the mandibular body.

The external surface topography of the mandible is shown in Fig 6-24.

Internal surface topography

The *digastric fossa (fossa digastrica)* is a flat depression on the inferior border of the mandibular body at the symphysis. It is the attachment point for the digastric muscle.

The *mental spines (spinae mentales)* lie very close to the symphysis, directly above the digastric fossa. These four bony projections are divided into the lower spines *(spinae musculi geniohyoidei)* for the geniohyoid muscle and the upper spines *(spina musculi genioglossi)* for the genioglossus muscle.

The *mylohyoid line (linea mylohyoidea)* is a ridge of bone that, starting very close to the mental spines, extends diagonally in a posterosuperior direction. It is the attachment for the geniohyoid muscle and forms the border of the floor of the mouth. When the floor of the mouth rises during swallowing, a mandibular denture whose border is too deep can cause pressure points; the denture border should therefore be shortened in keeping with the mylohyoid line. Once again, denture reduction is a necessity.

The *sublingual fovea (fovea sublingualis)* is the flat impression of the sublingual gland in the region of the premolar roots above the mylohyoid line. The *submandibular fovea (fovea sublingualis)* is the slight impression of the submandibular gland in the region of the molars below the mylohyoid line.

The *alveolar part (pars alveolaris)* of the mandibular body bears the mandibular set of teeth and has the same topographic features as the alveolar process of the maxilla: alveoli, interalveolar septa, interradicular septa, and the aforementioned alveolar juga. The alveolar part is inclined lingually in line with the inclination of the posterior teeth.

The *retromolar trigone (trigonum retromolare)* demarcates the alveolar part from the mandibular

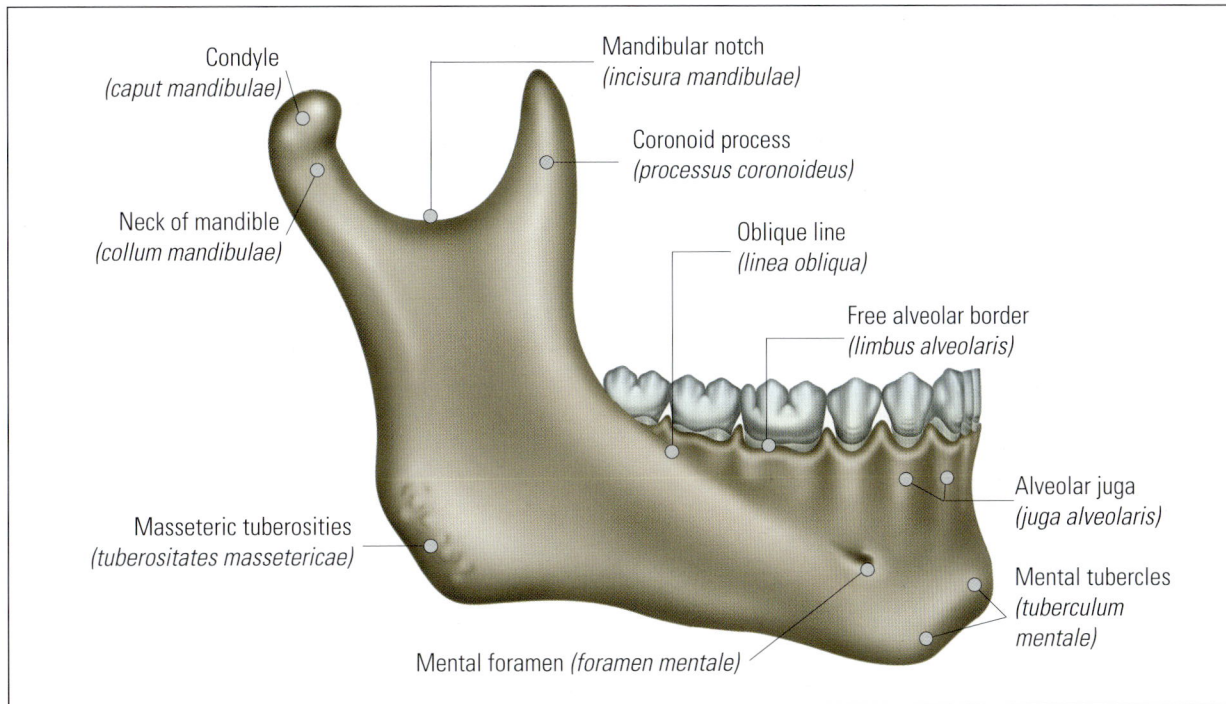

Fig 6-24 External surface topography of the mandible.

ramus. The trigone is a small, porous bony support posterior to the last molar on the alveolar ridge. After tooth loss, this portion of bone is not resorbed, much like the tuberosity of the maxilla. This area of bone can also be used to support a denture base. The topographic border of the retromolar trigone is marked by the temporal ridge, which starts on the internal surface of the mandibular ramus and is divided into two limbs or crura: the lateral crus *(crus laterale)* and the medial crus

(crus mediale), which runs beside the oblique line. The elevation of mucous membrane over the retromolar trigone is often given the same name, which can be confusing when this variable mucosal elevation is used as a reference point for the occlusal plane. The retromolar trigone lies about 2 to 3 mm below the occlusal plane.

The internal surface topography of the mandible is shown in Fig 6-25.

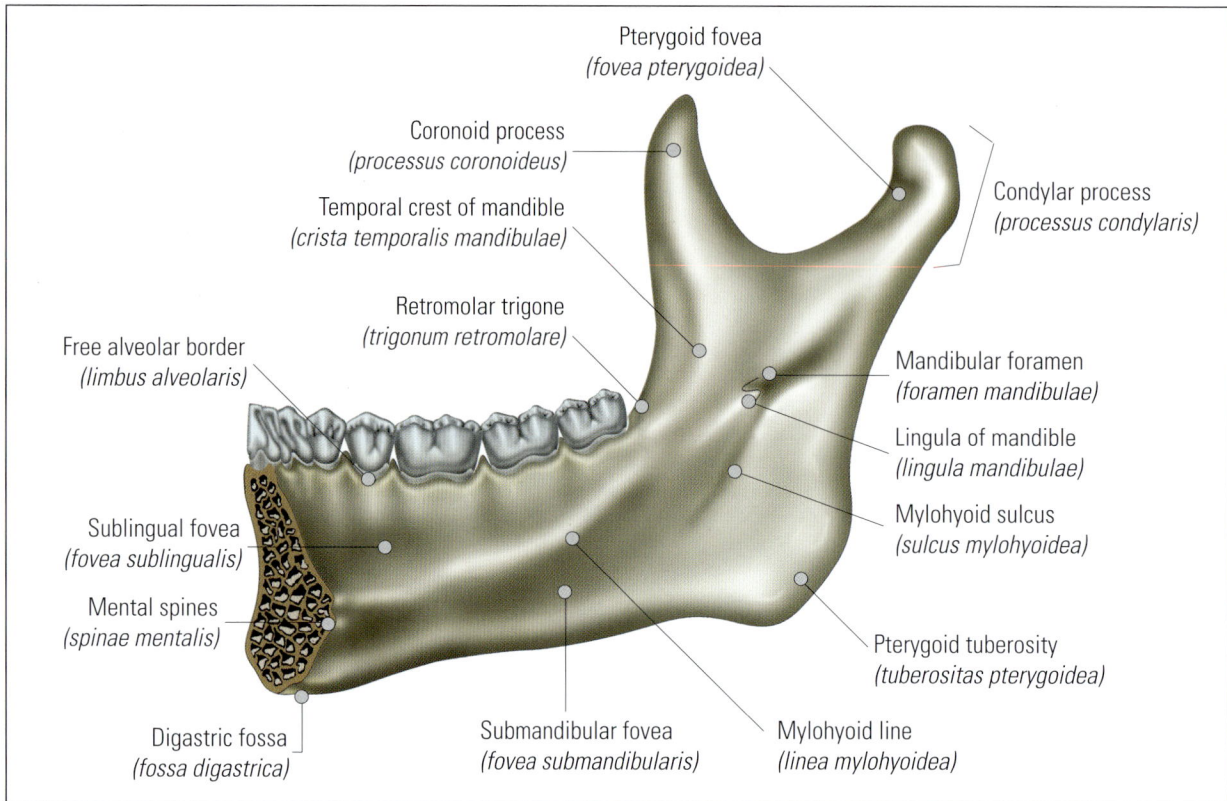

Fig 6-25 Internal surface topography of the mandible.

Rami of the Mandible

The rami of the mandible (*rami mandibulae*; singular: *ramus mandibulae*) are the extensions of the mandibular body rising vertically in a dorsal direction. The constructive foundation is the basal arch, from which the functionally oriented parts such as the angle of the mandible and the condylar and coronoid processes arise (Figs 6-26 and 6-27).

The **angle of the mandible** (*angulus mandibulae*; submaxillary angle) joins the posterior border of the ramus to the inferior margin of the mandibular body. The large masticatory muscle (*musculus masseter*) attaches to the external surface of the angle of the mandible. Here it produces the **masseteric tuberosities** (*tuberositates massetericae*), whereas on the internal surface the middle pterygoid muscle (*musculus pterygoi-*

deus) produces the **pterygoid tuberosities** (*tuberositas pterygoidea*).

The shape of the angle of the mandible is characterized by the function of these two strong muscles of mastication. In newborn babies, these muscles are not yet fully active so that the angle of the mandible is still not very pronounced. The angle is around 120 degrees in adults and between 140 and 160 degrees in neonates and the elderly (Fig 6-28). In elderly or edentulous patients, the muscles are only under slight stress, which means that the bony tissue of the attachment is resorbed and the angle of the mandible loses its pronounced shape. It looks as if the angle between the body and the ramus has changed, but in reality it is the bone mass that is altered.

The rami divide into two processes, the condylar process posteriorly and the coronoid process anteriorly. The **condylar process** (*processus articularis* = articular process; also *processus con-*

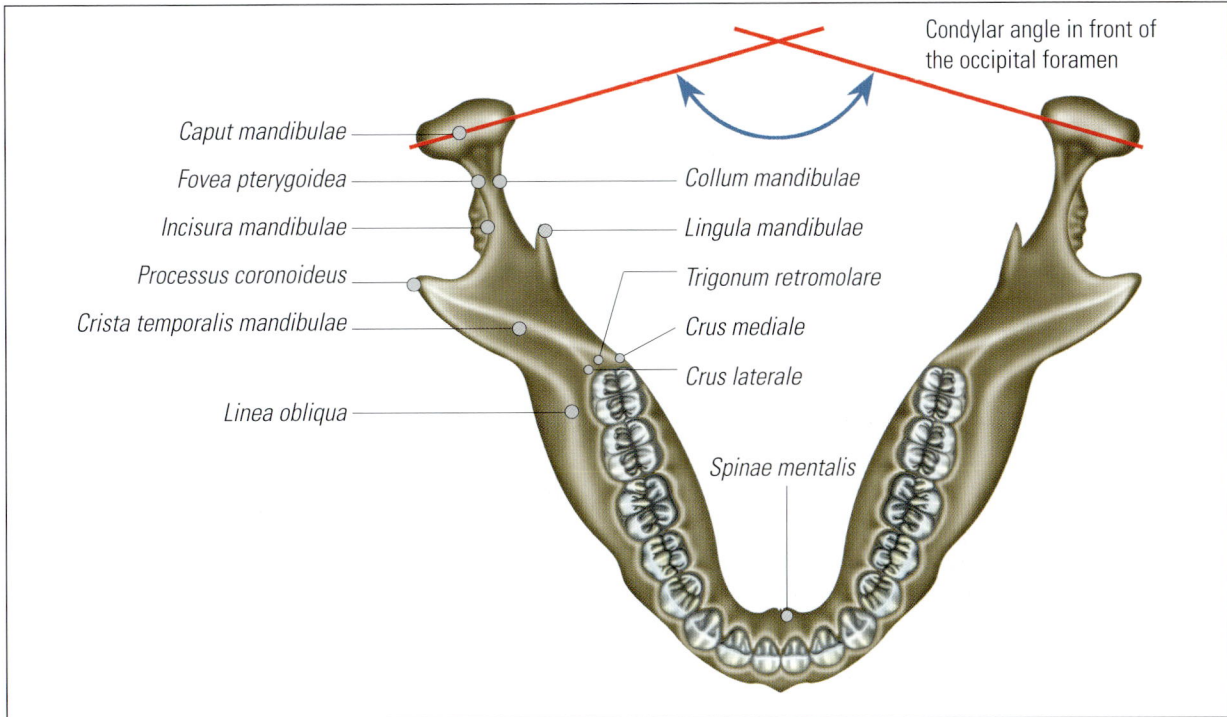

Fig 6-26 Topography of the mandible, occlusal view.

Caput mandibulae
Fovea pterygoidea
Incisura mandibulae
Processus coronoideus
Crista temporalis mandibulae
Linea obliqua

Condylar angle in front of the occipital foramen
Collum mandibulae
Lingula mandibulae
Trigonum retromolare
Crus mediale
Crus laterale
Spinae mentalis

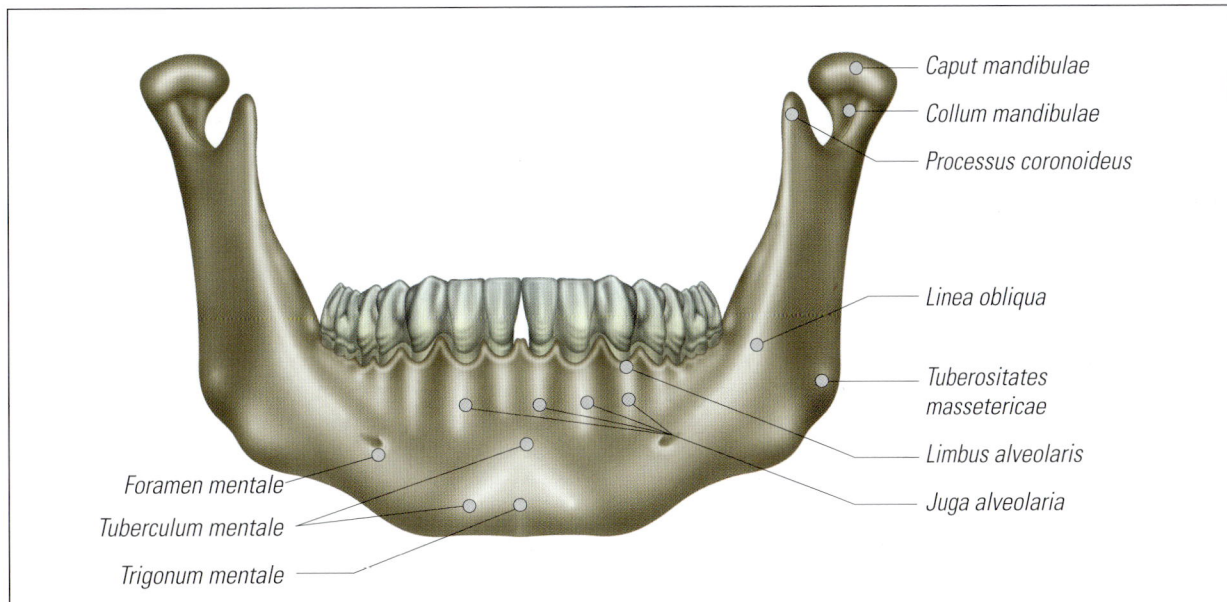

Fig 6-27 Topography of the mandible, anterior view.

Caput mandibulae
Collum mandibulae
Processus coronoideus
Linea obliqua
Tuberositates massetericae
Limbus alveolaris
Juga alveolaria
Foramen mentale
Tuberculum mentale
Trigonum mentale

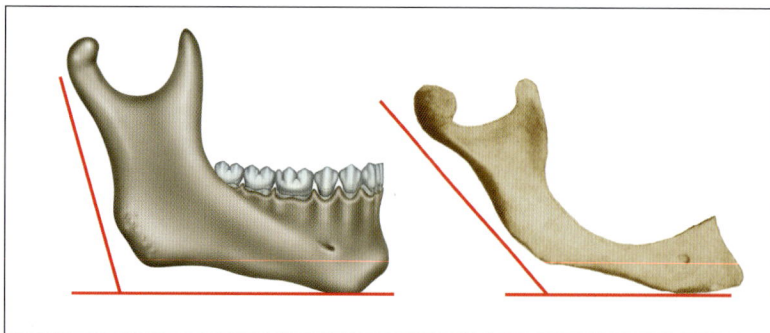

dylaris) comprises the neck of the mandible *(collum mandibulae)*, on which the condyle of the TMJ sits. The articular condyle is also known as the head of the mandible *(caput mandibulae)*. It is made up of a kidney-shaped roll of tissue whose longitudinal axis meets up with the axis of the condyle on the opposite side in front of the occipital foramen.

The **coronoid process** *(processus coronoideus)* is actually the ossified insertion tendon of the large temporal muscle *(musculus temporalis)*.

The **mandibular notch** *(incisura mandibulae)* is a roundish notch between the two processes of the mandibular rami. This relatively narrow rim of bone broadens on the condylar process to a small depression directly below the condyle. The lateral pterygoid muscle attaches in this small depression, which is why it is called the **pterygoid fovea** *(fovea pterygoidea)*.

The **mandibular foramen** *(foramen mandibulae)* is located in the middle on the internal surface of the mandibular ramus roughly level with the occlusal surfaces of the molars. The mandibular foramen serves as an entry point into the mandibular canal for the third branch of the trigeminal nerve. The position of the mandibular foramen changes during growing and aging processes. A complete half of the jaw can be anaesthetized by injecting anesthetic into the immediate vicinity of the mandibular foramen.

During mandibular movements, this mandibular foramen is in a relative resting state, which is why it is often interpreted as the pivotal point of the mandible. This interpretation is also justified by the fact that an opening at a nonresting point would endanger the vessels entering at that point

and would therefore have been selected against during evolution.

The **lingula mandibulae** is found at the mandibular foramen as a small bony projection to which a tendon attaches, namely the sphenomandibular ligament. This tendon holds the mandible at the same distance from the base of the skull during movement because it cannot stretch. This means, of course, that the mandibular foramen is only able to perform slight relative movements.

The **mylohyoid sulcus** *(sulcus mylohyoidea)* is a shallow groove running forward and downward from the mandibular foramen into the floor of the mouth and carrying nerves and blood vessels for the floor of the mouth *(nervus* and *arteria mylohyoidea)*.

The **mandibular torus** *(torus mandibulae)* is a pronounced bony bulge on the internal surface of the body of the mandible in the region of the premolars, which is seen in roughly 3% of patients examined. In extreme cases, the torus may interfere with the seating of a mandibular denture, in which case it must be surgically removed.

Types of Joints

A distinction is made between joints (junctions or *juncturae)* and true joints (synovial joints or articulations) in terms of the way bones are joined together. *Juncturae* are the solid bony connections such as sutures (Fig 6-29), synchondroses (cartilaginous joints), and ossified connections. These are defined according to the nature of the connecting material:

Fig 6-29 Example of a bone suture: lambdoid suture between the parietal bones and the occipital bone. In sutures, the jagged edges of the bones are fused by connective tissue fibers.

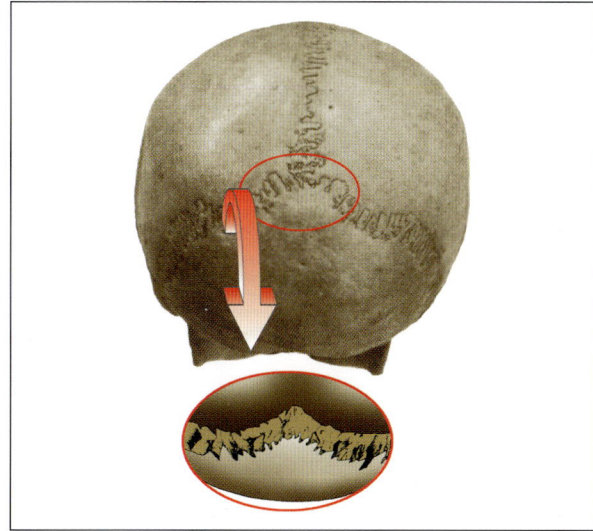

- The **fibrous joint** *(junctura fibrosa)* denotes two bones united by connective tissue fibers in the bone sutures; the two bones are "sewn together" by fibers (eg, the cranial sutures).
- The **cartilaginous joint** *(junctura cartilaginea)* denotes two bones united by fibrocartilage, such as the symphysis of the pelvic bones.
- The **osseous joint** *(junctura ossea)* can develop from the ossification of a fibrous joint. Examples of this type are cranial sutures, the symphysis in the mandible, and the sacral vertebrae.
- **True joints or articulations** *(juncturae synovialis, articulationes)* permit the movement of two bones against each other; they can be divided into freely movable (diarthroses) joints and rigid joints (amphiarthroses). The rigid joints with a fixed joint capsule and short, strong ligaments permit only slight mobility or simply have a cushioning effect (eg, the tarsals and carpals of the feet and hands).

Structure

Joint bodies at the ends of the bones that are to be connected bear the articular surfaces with a 3- to 4-mm-thick layer of hyaline or fibrocartilage as the articular cartilage (Fig 6-30). Articular surfaces can be divided into the convex condyle and the concave socket. The purpose of the articular cartilage is to achieve considerable closeness of fit, to

act as a shock absorber due to its elasticity, and to save the bone from splintering in response to mechanical strain. It is noticeable in some joints that the surfaces do not fit together exactly; in other words, they display incongruence that is compensated for by articular discs (eg, *meniscus articularis* in the knee or *discus articularis* in the TMJ).

The **joint capsule** *(capsula articularis)* is made up of a strong coating of connective tissue that provides an airtight seal to the joint cavity. The joint capsule is fixed to both articulating bones and is made up of two layers. The outer fibrous layer (*membrana fibrosa*; fibrous membrane) consists of crosswise collagen fibers that are reinforced by ligaments. The inner layer (*membrana synovialis*; synovial membrane) is a thin layer through which blood vessels and nerves pass and whose processes, known as *synovial folds* or *villi*, secrete the synovial fluid.

Synovial fluid *(synovia)* is a tough, stringy substance made up of tissue fluid, dead epithelial cells, and other cell fragments that reduces friction between the joint surfaces like a lubricant.

A **joint cavity** (joint space; *cavum articulare*) is a capillary space in a living joint that is squeezed together by external tissue pressure. This joint space is the characteristic feature of a true (synovial) joint.

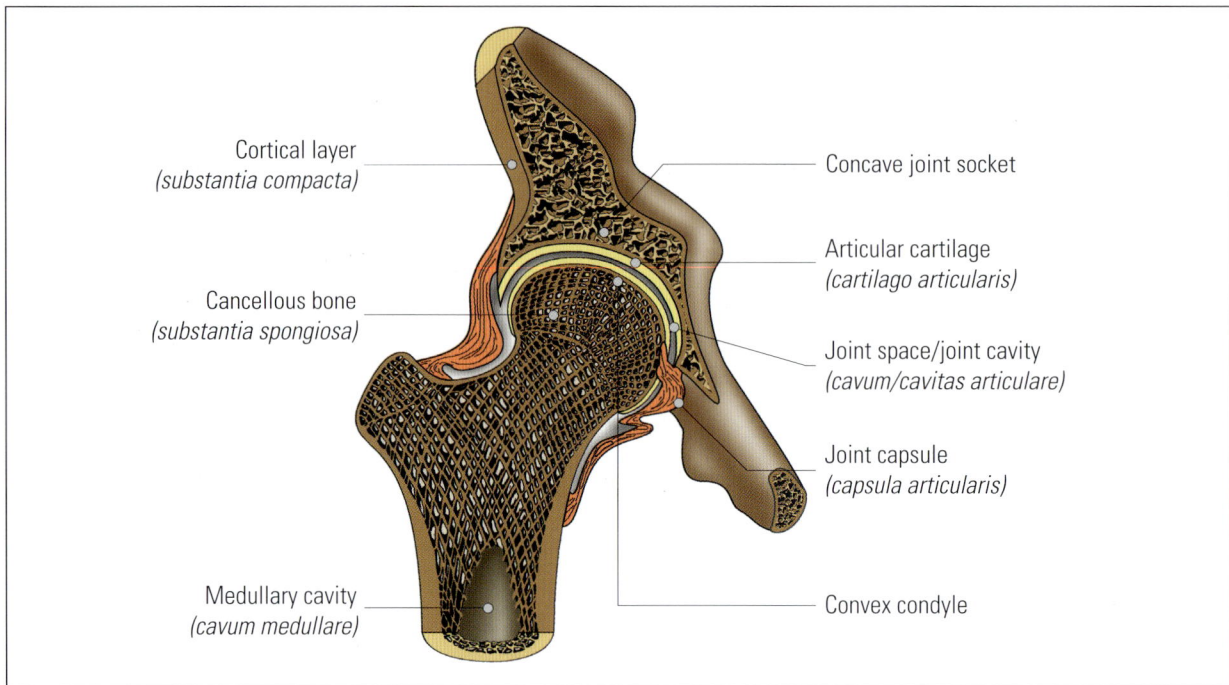

Fig 6-30 Schematic diagram of a joint with joint bodies and joint capsule.

The **synovial bursae** protect the tendons against particular stress when they slide over the bones as a result of the movement of the joints. The usual location of these bursae is the tissues of the joint capsule, ie, where tendons attach to the bone in a wide angle and where strong shearing movements against the skin and bone take place.

Tendon or synovial sheaths are bundles of collagen fibers that extend between the tendons running in different directions to ensure that the tendons are guided alongside each other. Connective tissue membranes are also found enclosing long tendons, guiding the tendons and carrying vessels that feed the tendons.

The **mobility of the joints** depends on the shape and closeness of fit of the articular surfaces (bone guidance), the arrangement and strength of the articular ligaments (ligament guidance), and the arrangement and functional direction of the muscles acting on the movable bones.

The particular geometric shape of the articular surfaces determines the direction of motion of a joint, ie, the number of degrees of freedom. There are six basic types—hinge, ellipsoidal, spheroidal

(or ball-and-socket), saddle (or sellar), pivot, and plane—depending on the geometric shape and the principal directions of motion (Fig 6-31).

The **hinge joint** (or *ginglymus*) permits rotation around one axis, which lies perpendicular to the movable parts. A hinge joint has only one degree of freedom. The knee and the interphalangeal joints in the hands are examples of hinge joints.

The **ellipsoidal joint** permits movement around two axes of rotation (biaxial). The condyle is egg-shaped (ellipsoid) and fits into the matching joint socket. Examples of this type are the joints between the wrist and the forearm bones and the joints between the occiput and the first vertebrae.

The **spheroidal** or **ball-and-socket joint** has three degrees of freedom; ie, movements are possible in all spatial axes. Examples are the hip and shoulder joints.

The **saddle** or **sellar joint** permits movements around two spatial axes, which means it has two degrees of freedom as a result of two arched articular surfaces with matching curves. One of the joints in the thumb is an example of this type.

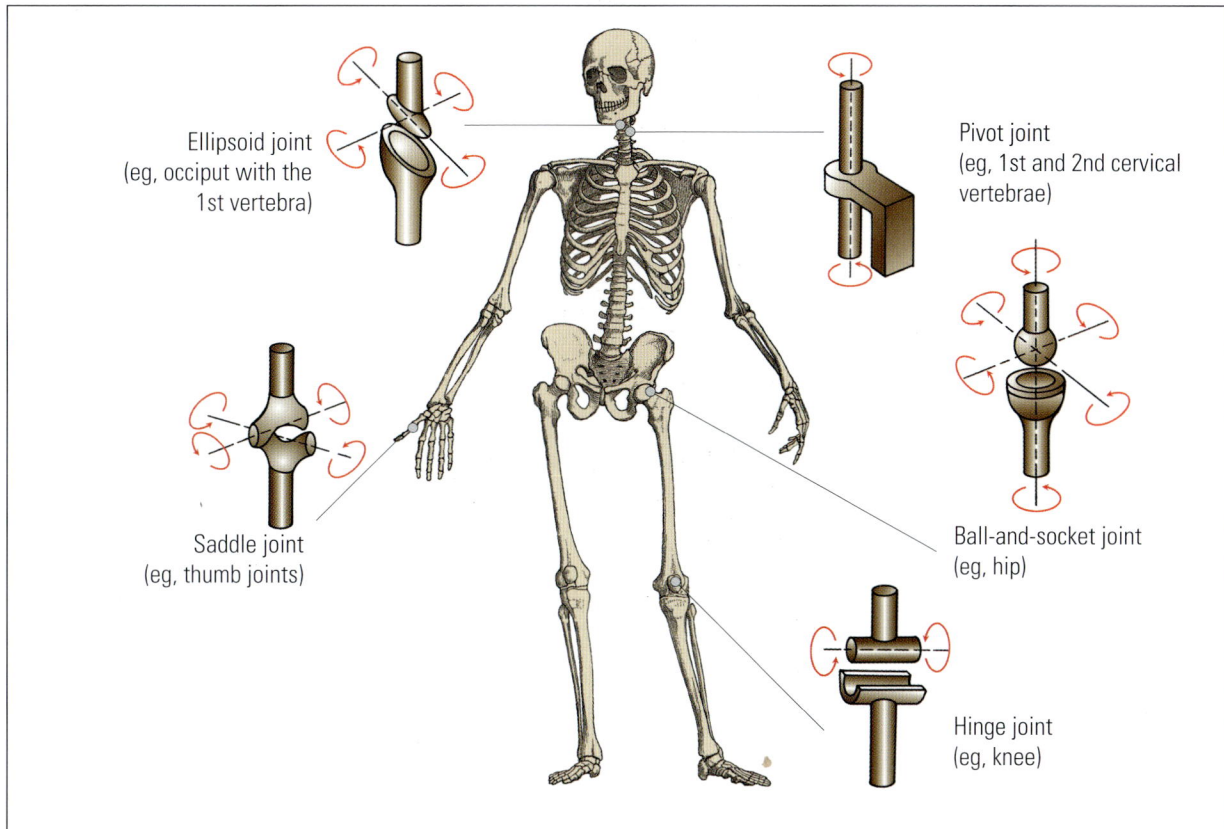

Fig 6-31 The six types of joints can be differentiated according to their degrees of freedom (plane joint not shown here).

The **pivot joint** occurs when a ring-shaped bone surrounds a peg or pivot of bone, making rotation around the axis of the pivot possible. Both the bony ring and the peg of bone are able to rotate in this case. The joint between the first and second cervical vertebrae (atlanto-axial joint) is an example of a pivot joint.

The **plane joint** permits a sliding movement by the flat articular surfaces against each other.

Temporomandibular Joint

The mandible as a single bone is fixed to the skull by two true (synovial) joints. The two joints are entirely separate from each other, but because they are identical in structure and because movement of the mandible always takes place simul-taneously in both joints, they are often merely referred to as a single joint (*articulatio temporo-mandibularis*; Latin, *articulatio* = joint). Therefore, the topographic description can be applied to a single TMJ.

The TMJ is located directly anterior to the opening of the outer auditory canal (*porus acusticus externus*). A distinction is made between the bony and the connective tissue parts of the joint.

The **bony parts** of the TMJ (Fig 6-32) include the:

- Mandibular fossa *(fossa mandibularis)*
- Articular tubercle *(tuberculum articulare; eminentia articularis)*
- Retroarticular process (*processus retroarticulare*; or tympanic tubercle: *tuberculum tympanicum*); these parts belong to the squamous part of the temporal bone and are the fixed parts of the joint

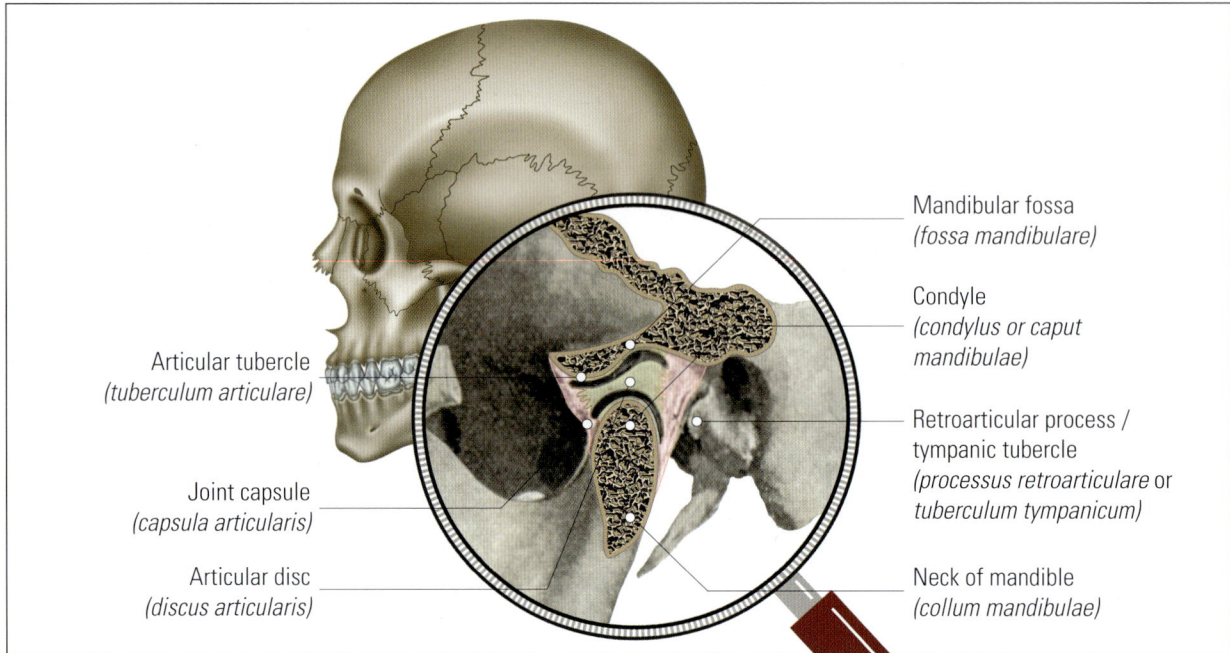

Fig 6-32 Bony parts of the TMJ, lateral view.

Articular tubercle
(tuberculum articulare)

Joint capsule
(capsula articularis)

Articular disc
(discus articularis)

Mandibular fossa
(fossa mandibulare)

Condyle
(condylus or caput
mandibulae)

Retroarticular process /
tympanic tubercle
(processus retroarticulare or
tuberculum tympanicum)

Neck of mandible
(collum mandibulae)

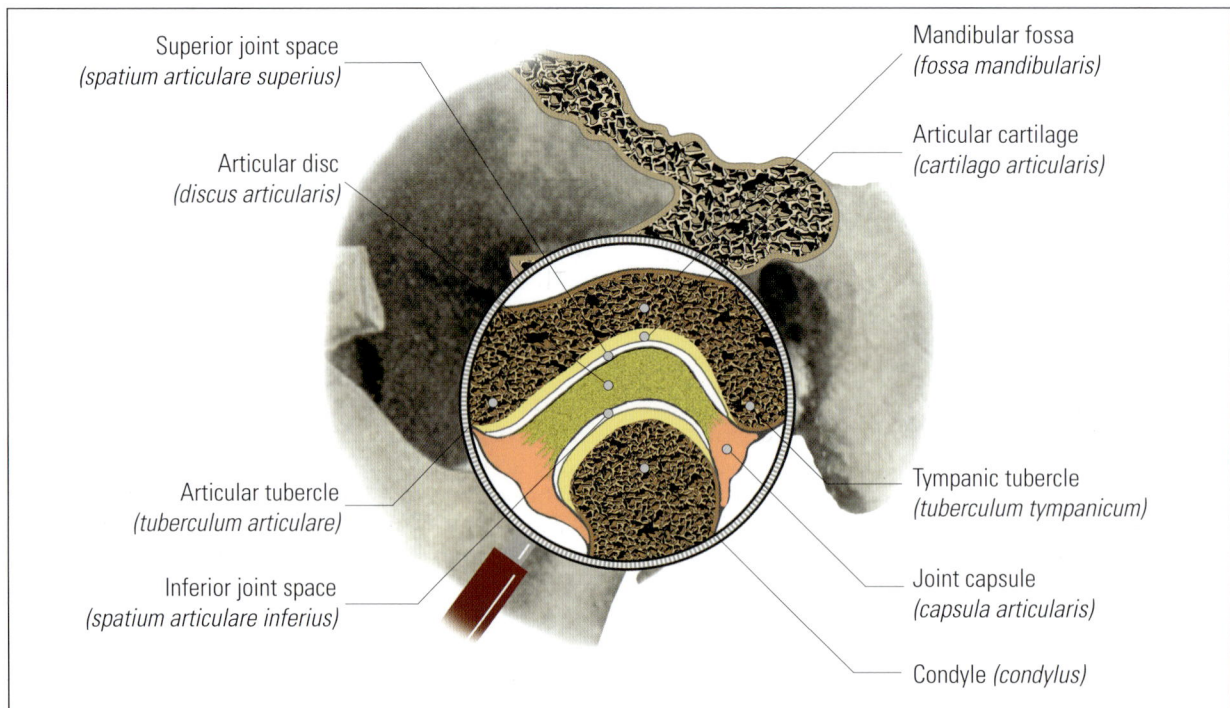

Fig 6-33 Connective tissue parts of the TMJ in relation to joint structure.

Superior joint space
(spatium articulare superius)

Articular disc
(discus articularis)

Articular tubercle
(tuberculum articulare)

Inferior joint space
(spatium articulare inferius)

Mandibular fossa
(fossa mandibularis)

Articular cartilage
(cartilago articularis)

Tympanic tubercle
(tuberculum tympanicum)

Joint capsule
(capsula articularis)

Condyle (condylus)

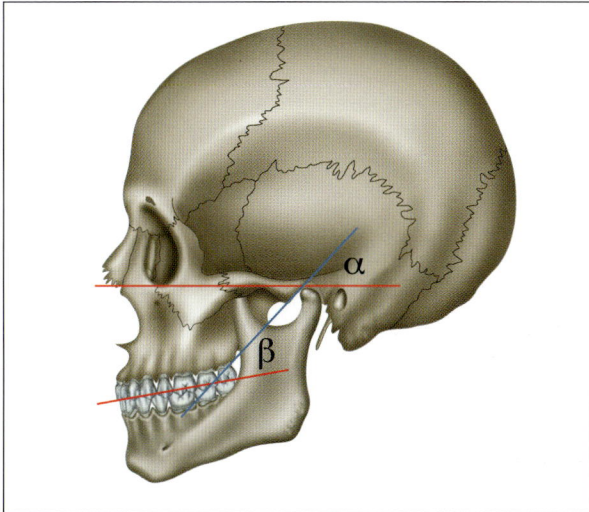

Fig 6-34 The slope of the condylar path in the sagittal direction: This inclination can be related to various reference planes; the angles of inclination α to the auriculo-infraorbital plane and β to the masticatory plane are shown here.

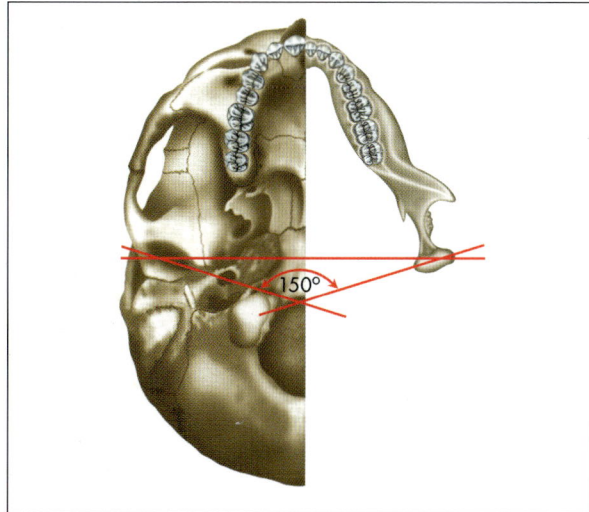

Fig 6-35 In the horizontal plane, the transverse condylar axes and the articular fossa axes meet in front of the occipital foramen. The angle between the hinge axes and the real horizontal axis is approximately 150 degrees.

• Condyle *(condylus* or *caput mandibulae)*, a part of the mandible and the movable part of the joint

The **connective tissue parts** of the TMJ (Fig 6-33) include the:

• Joint capsule *(capsula articularis)*
• Articular disc *(discus articularis)*
• Articular cartilage *(cartilago articularis)*
• Articular ligaments *(ligamenta)*

Form and position of the individual parts of the joint

The **articular surface** belongs to the squamous part of the temporal bone so that the joint actually permits movement between the temporal bone and the mandible, hence the name *temporomandibular joint*. The actual mandibular fossa is bounded posteriorly by the root of the zygomatic process of the temporal bone. This part is known as the *retroarticular process* or *tympanic tubercle*. The anterior border of the mandibular fossa forms the articular tubercle *(tuberculum articulare)*.

The articular surface is a long depression whose transverse axis meets the transverse axis of the opposing joint at an obtuse angle in front of the occipital foramen. In addition, the articular surface viewed laterally forms an S-shaped curve, where the concave surface from the depth of the mandibular fossa is inclined anteriorly, sloping downward, and becomes a convex section. This surface is known as the *condylar path*. The inclination of the condylar path in the sagittal plane (Fig 6-34) can be determined as the horizontal condylar inclination in relation to various reference planes (auriculo-infraorbital plane, Frankfort plane, Camper plane).

The **articular surface** is covered with smooth, elastic fibrocartilage that reduces pressure and friction. In the bottom of the mandibular fossa, the articular surface is made up of only a thin bony plate, which can scarcely be loaded by pressure; this indicates that masticatory pressure is not transferred in the mandibular fossa but to other bony parts of the joint. The articular tubercle and the inner and outer marginal ridges are the most suitable for functional loading.

The **condyle** *(caput mandibulae; condylus)* is located on the articular process of the mandible. It resembles a kidney-shaped roll of bone whose transverse axis is adapted to the articular surface (Fig 6-35); ie, the transverse axes of the two condyles do not form a line but intersect at an obtuse angle (approximately 150 to 165 degrees).

The anterior part of the condyles is covered with cartilage and is much smaller than the mandibular fossa. The resulting lack of closeness of fit is known as *incongruence*.

The *articular disc (discus articularis)* lies between the mandibular fossa and the condyle and compensates for the incongruence between these parts of the joint. This disc divides the joint into two parts because it is connected to the joint capsule all the way around.

The *articular capsule (capsula articularis)* is a loose casing of connective tissue that forms an airtight seal around all parts of the joint so that slight negative pressure is created inside the joint and the joint components are pressed together. The external layer of the capsule *(membrana fibrosa)* is made up of bundles of collagen fibers, while the internal layer *(membrana synovialis)* carries blood vessels and nerves and secretes the synovial fluid. The joint capsule is fixed around the articular surface on the temporal bone and on the condyle.

Articular Disc

The *articular disc (discus articularis)*, also known as the *joint disc*, is made up of tight connective tissue fibers in which fibrocartilage is embedded. It is a curved disc that is thickened at the edges; it is 1 to 1.5 mm thick in the middle and 3 to 4 mm thick at the edges. The articular disc is fused throughout to the joint capsule, so that it divides the joint into two compartments and makes it into a double joint.

There is a capillary gap between the articular disc and the condyle, which is known as the *inferior joint space (spatium articulare inferius)*. As the articular disc rests on the condyle like a cap, rotary movement can take place in the inferior joint space. Sliding movement is permitted by the *superior joint space (spatium articulare superius)* between the disc and the mandibular fossa. Viewed as a double joint, the superior joint space can be seen as a sliding joint in which the disc is able to slide forward and backward with the condyle on the articular surface sloping forward and downward. In the inferior joint space, which can be seen as a hinge joint, the condyle rotates in the concave surface of the disc. This means that if one

part of the joint is unable to function, the functioning of the other part is still guaranteed.

The *lateral pterygoid muscle* with a few tendinous fibers radiates into the joint capsule and into the disc, which is then pulled forward during forward and lateral movements.

The *functions of the articular disc* are as follows:

- It divides the joint cavity into two functional compartments, which makes the special functional movement of the mandible possible.
- Compressive forces are cushioned by the disc or distributed to a larger area to protect the mandibular fossa and condyle.
- The separation into a pivot (rotary) joint and a sliding joint means that friction is distributed over twice the area.
- The incongruence is balanced out by the articular disc.

The TMJ permits all movements that enable humans as omnivores to process both plant and animal food. Furthermore, the TMJ enforces a separation of the dentition into a working side and a nonworking side. Lateral jaw movements are necessary to prepare the food, and the bites of food are always processed on one side of the dentition only. This makes it necessary to separate the nonworking side so that there is no interference with gliding movement on this no-load side. This separation is achieved by:

- The slope of the condylar path in two directions in space, namely in the horizontal and vertical planes
- The inclination of the teeth within the occlusal curves
- The particular direction of pull of the muscles, especially of the lateral pterygoid muscle, which enforces Bennett movement
- The articular tubercle, on which the condyle glides during lateral and forward movement

The structure of the human TMJ permits complex movements of the mandible, in contrast to the limited movement possibilities in animal jaws. The *jaw joints* in pure carnivores will only allow its cylindric joints, which are firmly held by the close-fitting joint fossa, to perform simple hinge movements; these allow very simple vertical opening and closing movements. The pointed, sharp-edged teeth of these animals slide past each other when the mandible is closed, and they interlock closely with each other. Carnivores only need to tear their food or crush bones; they do not require any lateral or forward movement.

In *herbivores*, the jaw joints have very flat, convex joint cavities, in which flat condyles sloping in a transverse direction come to rest. This joint structure permits flat, lateral grinding movements. The noncanine chewing surfaces are designed for crushing raw, solid plants.

Jaw joints of rodents have narrow, groove-shaped joint cavities in which narrow cylindric joints are set in a sagittal direction; these permit forward and backward movement. The rodents' teeth are very flat and inclined in accordance with the type of movement performed: the maxillary teeth inclined outward and the mandibular teeth inward.

Joint Capsule and Articular Ligaments

The articular capsule *(capsula articularis)* forms an airtight seal around the joint so that slight negative pressure can be created inside the joint cavity. The negative pressure in the joint cavity means that the bony joint components are firmly pressed together. The joint capsule is attached around the mandibular fossa and is loose and wide enough to ensure that the movements of the joint cannot be impeded.

This tendinous coating of connective tissue is made up of a dense outer tissue layer and an inner epithelial layer, known as the *synovial layer*. The synovial fluid is produced here, which consists of protein, salts, tissue fragments, and water. In the event of a ruptured capsule, the synovial fluid would be an ideal nutrient for bacteria. The thick posterior wall of the capsule arises at the petrotympanic fissure *(fissura petrotympanica)*, while the anterior wall is attached to the horizontal surface of the articular tubercle.

The fibers of the joint capsule converge at the neck of the mandible and thus surround the condyle at the rear, roughly 5 mm below the edge of the articular surface; anteriorly the fibers surround the condyle directly at the edge of the joint surface because this is where the lateral pterygoid muscle attaches. The joint capsule of the TMJ is so loose that, if the joint is dislocated, rupture of the capsule will only rarely occur, if at all.

The functions of the capsule are to:

• Hold the parts of the joint together
• Create an airtight seal on the joint cavity
• Produce synovial fluid

To support the loose joint capsule, there are three articular ligaments that have to reinforce the capsule while limiting the movements of the jaw (Figs 6-36 and 6-37). These ligaments are the temporomandibular, sphenomandibular, and stylomandibular ligaments.

The *temporomandibular ligament (ligamentum laterale* or *temporomandibulare)* arises from the external surface of the zygomatic process on the temporal bone, close to the articular tubercle, and runs obliquely down and backward to the back of the neck of the mandible; a few vertical fibers are firmly attached to the capsule.

The *sphenomandibular ligament (ligamentum sphenomandibulare)* has its origin at the spine of the sphenoid bone and the middle edge of the mandibular fossa, from where it projects downward and forward to the inner surface of the neck of the mandible and to the lingula at the mandibular foramen.

The *stylomandibular ligament (ligamentum stylomandibulare)* comes from the styloid process of the temporal bone *(processus styloideus)* and runs around to the posterior edge of the ramus of the mandible and as far as the angle of the mandible. It has little importance in terms of joint stability, but in the event of dislocation it prevents the mouth from being closed in order to avoid greater damage.

Joint diseases

As a result of overload or strain, the joints can sustain diseased changes of varying severity. These can be divided into sprains, dislocations, arthritis, and osteoarthritis.

A *sprain* (distortion) denotes overextension of the joint capsule and articular ligaments, which can result in effusion of blood in the joint and can cause the joint capsule to swell up because of increased secretion of fluid.

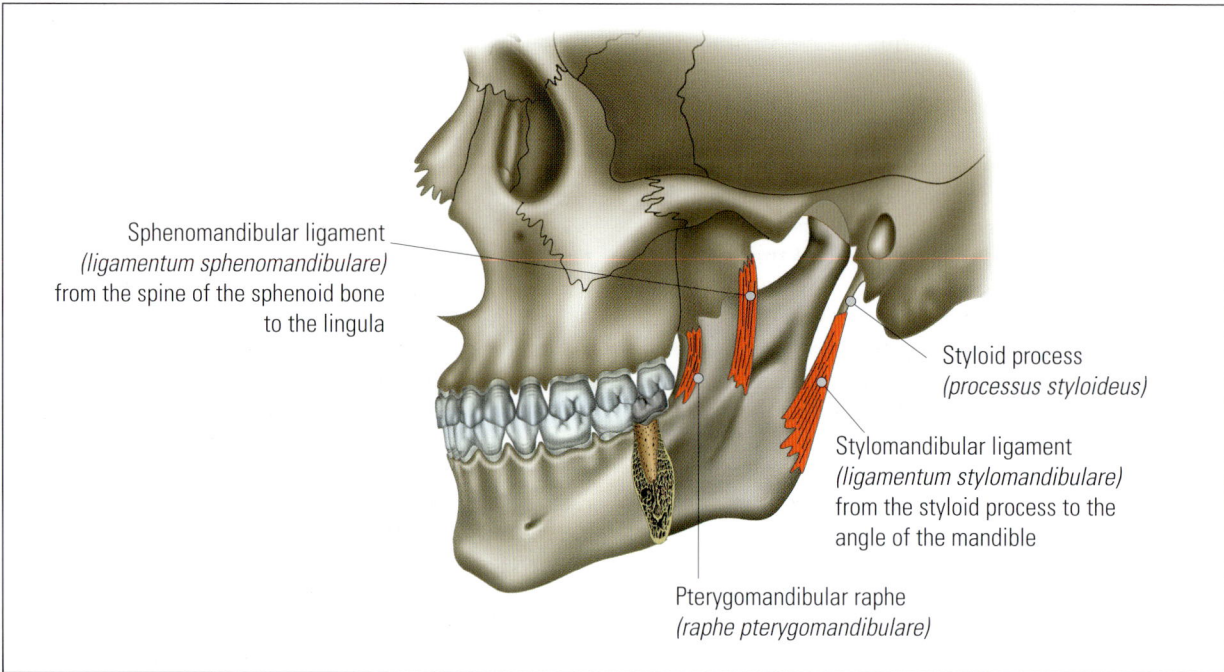

Sphenomandibular ligament
(ligamentum sphenomandibulare)
from the spine of the sphenoid bone
to the lingula

Styloid process
(processus styloideus)

Stylomandibular ligament
(ligamentum stylomandibulare)
from the styloid process to the
angle of the mandible

Pterygomandibular raphe
(raphe pterygomandibulare)

Fig 6-36 The articular ligaments, interior view. The articular ligaments of the TMJ support and reinforce the relatively slack joint capsule while limiting the movements of the jaw.

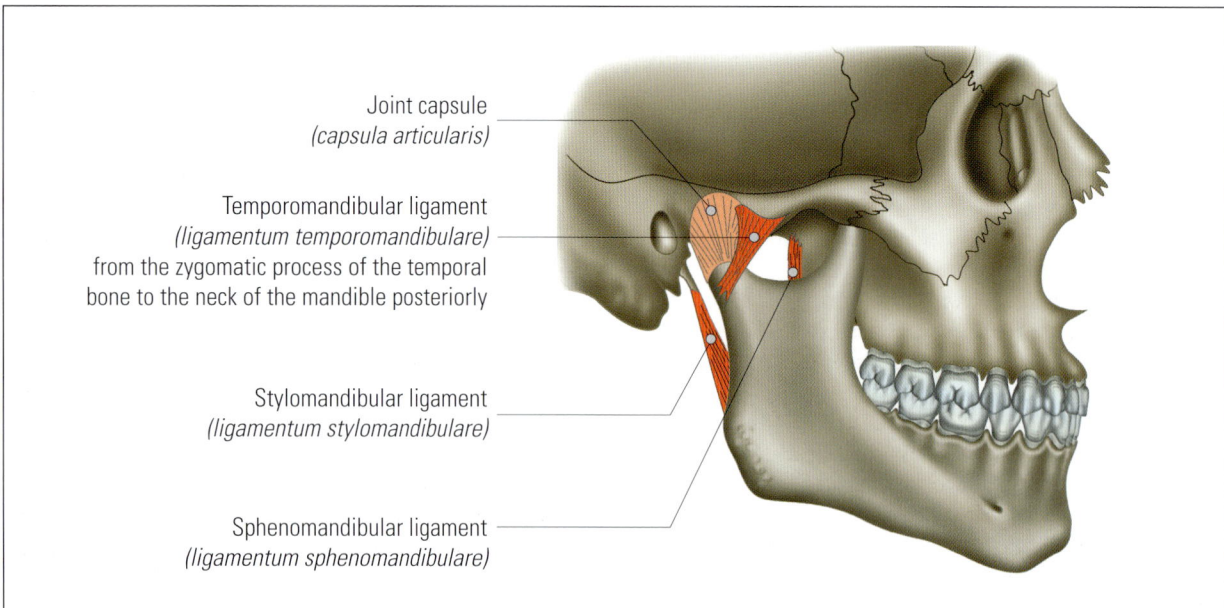

Joint capsule
(capsula articularis)

Temporomandibular ligament
(ligamentum temporomandibulare)
from the zygomatic process of the temporal
bone to the neck of the mandible posteriorly

Stylomandibular ligament
(ligamentum stylomandibulare)

Sphenomandibular ligament
(ligamentum sphenomandibulare)

Fig 6-37 The articular ligaments, exterior view.

A *dislocation* (luxation) refers to the situation where the condyle comes out of the joint socket or fossa and articular ligaments are often torn. The less the condyle is held by the socket, the easier it is for dislocations to happen. In the case of the TMJ, the condyle may slide out of the mandibular fossa when the mouth is opened very wide, without the ligaments being stretched or torn. In the TMJ, if the condyle slides in front of the articular tubercles, for instance, this can cause a painful occlusal lock. The joint can be put back into place (reduced) by firmly applying backward and downward pressure on the mandibular dentition.

Arthritis is an inflammatory change to the joints in which purulent fluid is often secreted into the joint cavity, leading to painful swelling of the joint capsule. It can result in permanent damage to bone and cartilage tissue.

Osteoarthritis is a degenerative joint disease that usually involves wear of the cartilage and fibrillation of the bone, mainly as a sign of aging but also as a result of inappropriate stress on particular joints.

Skin

The skin *(cutis)* covers the outer surface of the body and, in an adult, is an organ measuring roughly 1.6 m^2, with an average thickness of 1 to 4 mm. The veins can show as a bluish color through very thin areas of the skin. The skin is a contact organ, meaning that physical events and the environment can come into contact with it. The functions of the skin are outlined in the following paragraphs.

Passive protective function: Owing to its strength and elasticity, the skin protects the bodily tissues against harmful influences from outside, such as mechanical effects (eg, knocks, tearing, pressure, and blows), chemical hazards, and heat. However, it also protects against loss of moisture caused by severe evaporation of water from inside the body.

Active protective function: The skin prevents disease-causing organisms from penetrating inside the body; invading infectious pathogens are destroyed by specially stored defensive sub-

stances that are partly produced by the skin (acid mantle), or the constant exfoliation of the skin actually makes it difficult for pathogens to penetrate.

Sensory function: There are about half a million touch receptors on the surface of the skin, around a quarter of a million cold receptors, and roughly 30,000 heat receptors. With these sensory nerves, the skin develops excellent surface sensibility in order to enhance the general quality of the body's senses and improve the body's orientation in its surroundings. Sensations can be perceived as pleasant or unpleasant, depending on the strength of stimulus on the different receptors, which cannot objectively reproduce the strength of a stimulus but merely the differences in stimulus. The sensation of pain may also be viewed as a protective function.

Function of heat regulation: The skin radiates heat. The heat given off can be reduced or increased as a result of variations in the blood flow, whereby the skin expands or contracts. The release of heat can be increased as the energy of evaporation is withdrawn due to increased sweat secretion and evaporation of the skin's liquid content. Heat release can also be curtailed when the hairs on the body become erect (gooseflesh) and form an insulating cushion of air.

Secretory function: A considerable proportion of bodily excretions pass through the skin, harmful substances being excreted in the sweat (around 1 liter a day). These harmful substances are mainly sodium chloride, potassium, calcium, and magnesium salts but also include urea and uric acid, lactic acid, and amino acid. As well as these substances, the skin also secretes sebum by means of special glands. Sebum keeps the skin supple. In conjunction with sweat, it forms an emulsion film on the skin, which acts as an acid mantle thanks to the elimination of harmful acidic substances (uric acid and lactic acid). The acid mantle also provides active protection for the skin because it inhibits the growth of bacteria.

Respiratory function: As well as secreting sweat, harmful substances, and sebum, the skin can also give off carbon dioxide. A gas exchange with oxygen also happens because around 1% to 2% of oxygen exchange is regulated by the skin.

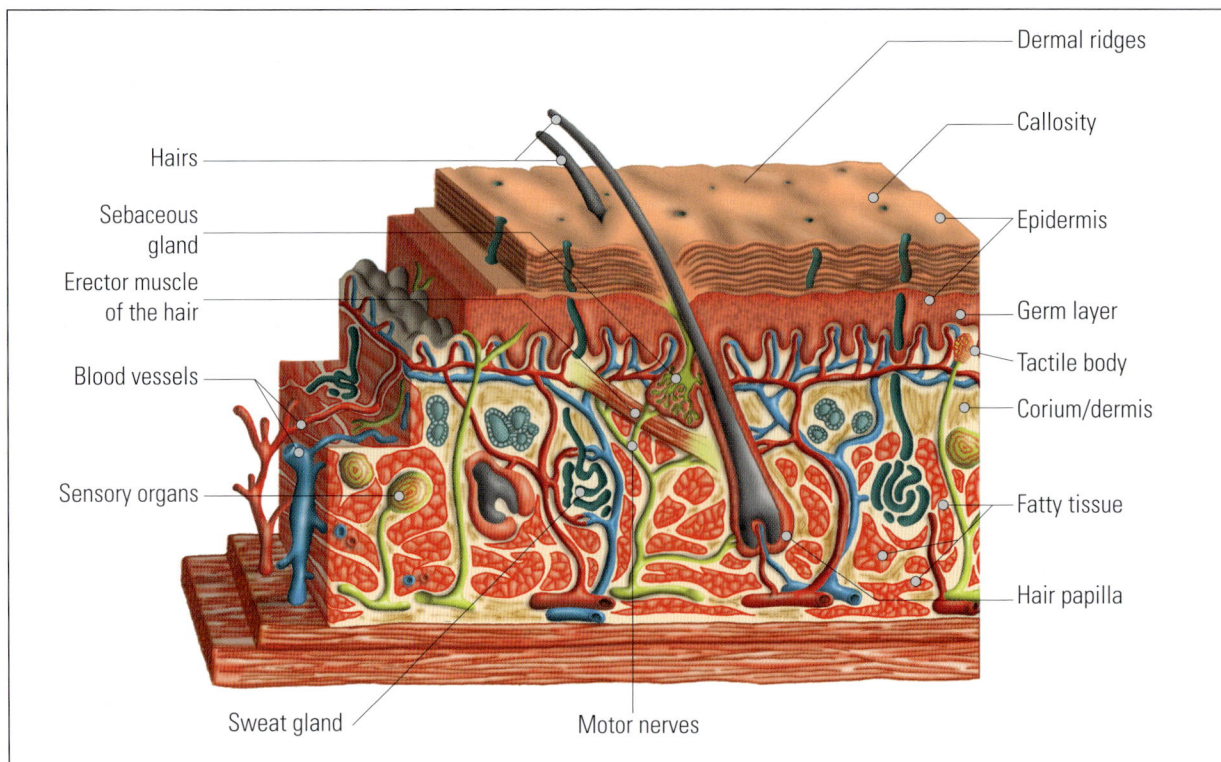

Fig 6-38 Structure of human skin.

Structure

The skin can be divided into three layers, which can be firmly attached to the lower tissue layers by tight bands of connective tissue (Fig 6-38).

The **epidermis** is the cuticle or outer layer, with its outermost horny layer made up of dead, multilayered squamous epithelial cells. It regenerates constantly and has a good healing tendency. The outer horny layers are constantly being worn away and are replaced by squamous epithelial cells in the underlying basal layer as they divide and work their way to the surface within 28 days.

The **dermis** (corium) is made up of dense connective tissue of collagen and elastic fibers, in which vascular bundles and nerve endings are located. It is the connecting layer between the epidermis and the subcutis. The interwoven, feltlike connective tissue fibers give this layer of the skin its flexibility, tensile strength, and elasticity.

The **subcutis** (subcutaneous or subdermal layer) is not strictly classified as belonging to the skin, even though functionally it is part of the skin because it forms the connection with the deeper-lying tissues, such as the tendons or bones. The subcutis is made up of loose connective tissue in which fat cells are lodged. The thickness of the subcutaneous fatty tissue differs depending on where it is located, while the laying down of depot fat is hormonally regulated. The stored fat forms the mantle of fat and the skin's padding of fat.

Skin Appendages

The skin is flexible and elastic to permit tension-free movements, especially at the joints. Its secretions make it particularly resistant. Pigments contained in the germ layer determine the color of the skin. The skin adapts to the mechanical strain on the different areas of the body. The dermal ridges (a special marking on the surface of the skin) develop individually as a hereditary pattern in each person so that impressions of the pads of the fingers and toes as well as the balls of the feet and hands enable a person to be identified (dactyloscopy, ie, finger print analysis).

The skin appendages are the hair and nails as well as the glands in the skin, namely sweat, sebaceous, olfactory, and mammary glands.

Hair and nails are formed by the epidermis and take on protective and tactile functions. *Hairs* are long keratin filaments that grow from the hair bulb out of the subcutaneous tissue through the epidermis. The hair bulb is supplied with tactile nerves, muscle fibers, and sebaceous glands. The hairs can be involved in the sense of touch because of the nerve supply; as a result of the muscle supply, the hairs may become erect (gooseflesh) and thus be used for heat regulation.

Nails are horny extensions of the epidermis and correspond to the claws or hooves of animals. They provide protection for the finger pads but also act as an opposing surface to enhance the sense of touch in the fingertips. The sense of touch is reduced when a nail is lost. The nails are formed as horny plates in the matrix of the nail bed. Destruction of the nail bed leads to growth abnormalities or loss of the nail.

Skin glands (dermal glands) comprise the sebaceous glands as well as small sweat glands and olfactory glands. The olfactory glands are particularly large sweat glands, which include the ceruminous glands (which secrete ear wax). The skin contains around 20 million small, knot-like sweat glands. The dermal glands are single-cell or multicellular acinous (berrylike) or tubular glands in the skin that secrete their products directly outward (exocrine glands). These mucous, sweat, and sebaceous glands form a protective film for the skin. The mammary glands are transformed sweat glands. The ceruminous and lacrimal glands are special kinds of dermal glands.

Skin atrophy (wasting or thinning of the skin) develops as a normal sign of aging because of the breakdown of the skin's constituents, their individual layers, and elastic fibers, which causes a decrease in skin tone. The skin becomes pale, gray, dry, thin, and wrinkled; the blood vessels in the skin stand out more distinctly because of thinning of the overlying layers.

Skin bacteria are the bacteria living on healthy skin as a main constituent of the skin flora, which are found on more moist areas of skin such as the scalp, the face, the palms of the hands, the armpits, between the toes, and in the glandular ducts and hair follicles. They cannot be completely removed by washing or strong disinfectants and they repeatedly spread out quickly from the channels in the skin. The most important skin bacteria are aerobic and anaerobic bacteria such as staphylococci, corynebacteria, sarcinae, streptococci, mycobacteria, as well as fungi.

Working in the laboratory with *dental technology materials* (active and auxiliary materials) can result in skin hazards that particularly affect the hands, forearms, neck, and facial areas. This can cause irritation and dryness of the skin or sensitization (development of an allergy) originating from plastic monomers, dust from metal grinding (chromium, nickel), and acrylic mixing fluids (eg, for artificial stone).

Frequent hand-washing and working with wet hands as well as metal, plaster, and acrylic dust are *particularly stressful to the skin*. People who suffer from hay fever, neurodermatitis, or generally dry skin are especially at risk. Regularly using skin protection and skin care products and avoiding contact with occupational materials that irritate the skin are important protective measures. Chemical or mechanical irritation of the skin through constant exposure will break down the skin barrier. When working with such occupational materials, dental technologists should take the following precautions:

- Protect the skin with skin care products including moisturizing cream
- Avoid contact with irritants
- Wear protective gloves, clothing, and glasses/mask
- Use suction cleaning tools

Glands

The glands are organs made up of specialized cells of the epithelium that produce a specific substance: a secretory product. Glands that release their secretion through a separate secretory duct or directly to an external or internal surface are known as *exocrine glands* (*exo* = outside; *krinein* = secrete). These are distinguished from endocrine glands, which release their internal secretion (hormone) directly to the bloodstream. Glands can be classified according to the nature of their *secretion*:

• Serous glands produce a thin secretion containing protein, such as the lacrimal glands.
• Mucous glands produce a viscous, slimy secretion as a transporting mucus.
• Mixed glands produce both a serous and a mucous secretion (eg, saliva) that also contains digestive enzymes.

The *structure* of a gland can be traced back to invaginations (turning inward) of the surface epithelium. These invaginations can be shaped like tubes (tubular form) or small hollows (alveolar form). Branched glandular ducts with a main excretory duct, secondary excretory duct, connecting pieces, and endpieces develop from these basic forms (Fig 6-39).

The *glandular cells* release their secretory product in a wide variety of ways, which means a further classification of glands can be made:

• Apocrine glands discharge their secretion— once it has formed and accumulated in the apex of the cell—together with a piece of cytoplasm (eg, mammary glands).
• Holocrine glands discharge whole cells as their secretory product (eg, sebaceous glands in the skin).
• Merocrine glands release a fine-grained, droplike secretion through the surface of the cell.

Saliva

Saliva is a secretion of either a watery (serous) or slimy (mucous) consistency that is formed by salivary glands and is released into the oral cavity. The following distinctions are made:

• Serous saliva is the watery diluting or rinsing saliva; it is rich in salt and protein and contains digestive enzymes.
• Mucous saliva is the slimy lubricating saliva; it is viscous, stringy, and poor in salt and protein.
• Seromucous saliva is a mixed saliva made up of varying proportions of serous and mucous saliva.

The saliva from the parotid gland, mandibular gland, sublingual gland, and the glands of the oral mucosa is a mixed saliva. Its chemical composition and quantity (normally 1.0 to 1.5 liters a day in humans) depend on the diet and on psychologic and nervous factors: Dry foods lead to the release of a mucous lubricating saliva; acids and alkalis cause a watery diluting or rinsing saliva to be produced.

Functions of saliva: The food is moistened, made slippery, and diluted by the saliva to make it easier to swallow; the constant production of saliva helps with self-cleaning of the mouth and leads to constant empty swallowing. Salivary amylase (ptyalin) brings about predigestion in which starch and glycogen are split. The saliva provides a good nutrient medium for microorganisms in the mouth.

The *composition of saliva* differs considerably from that of blood plasma. Saliva contains the following:

• *99% water* to thoroughly wet and dissolve foods
• *0.6% solids*, which shed epithelial cells and bacteria
• *Mucins* as lubricants in the oral area; they make food particles slippery and ease tongue and cheek movements
• *Enzymes* (ptyalin) for predigestion of carbohydrates
• *Salts* in the form of sodium, potassium, chloride, and bicarbonate ions

Saliva has a pH of 7 to 8 and has a bactericidal action due to leukocytes. It is usually weakly acidic, clear, odorless, colorless, and viscous.

Mineral components of saliva have the effect of healing (remineralizing) the hydroxyapatites attacked by lactic acid on the tooth surface. They also form deposits of tartar, particularly on the lingual surfaces of the mandibular incisors and the buccal walls of the maxillary molars, while salivary stones (known as *sialoliths*) may block the excretory ducts of the salivary glands. The electrolytes contained in saliva have corrosive effects on metals in the mouth.

Fig 6-39 Structure of an exocrine gland, with several endpieces and an excretory duct.

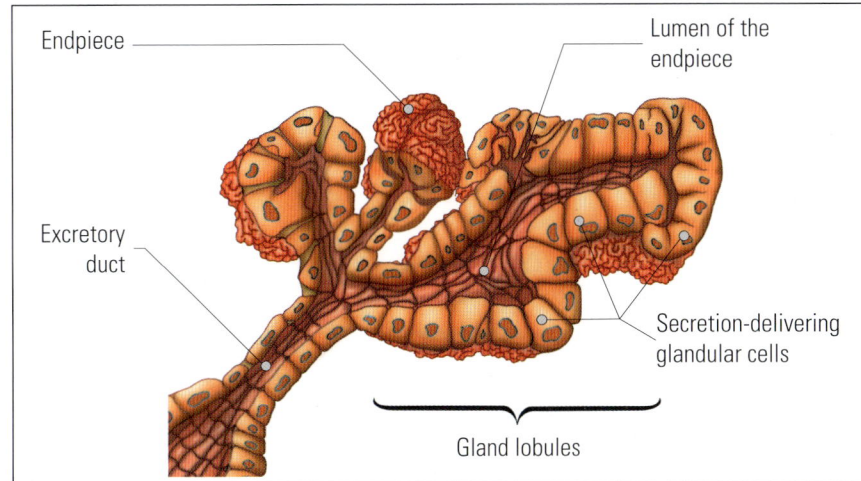

Endpiece

Lumen of the endpiece

Excretory duct

Secretion-delivering glandular cells

Gland lobules

Mucous Membrane

The mucous membrane (mucosa, *tunica mucosae*) forms the epithelial lining of the inner surface of the digestive tract (intestinal mucosa), oral and nasal cavity, airways, respiratory organs, and urinary and sexual organs.

Layers of the mucous membrane

The ***mucosal epithelium*** (epithelium mucosa) is mostly nonhorny squamous epithelium or ciliated epithelium, which is constantly kept moist and slippery by a mucous secretion made up of mucus cells (goblet cells) or by mucous glands. The mucus also acts as a chemical buffer. The oral cavity is lined with multilayered squamous epithelium, the intestine with single-layered prismatic epithelium, the respiratory tract with multiple rows of ciliated epithelium, and the urinary tract with transitional epithelium.

Mucosal connective tissue (*lamina propria*) lies directly below the mucosal epithelium and ensures that substances are transported between the surface and the vessels. Blood and lymphatic vessels as well as autonomic nerve fibers run through this layer.

The ***mucosal muscle layer*** (*lamina muscularis mucosae*) is only found in the digestive tract, starting in the esophagus and extending to the rectum.

Submucous connective tissue (*tela submucosa*) is the innermost layer, in which blood and lymph vessels and autonomic nerve fibers are brought closer to the mucous membrane. The other layers are supported on the submucous connective tissue in a free-moving way.

Functions of the mucous membrane

The functions of the mucous membrane include the following:

- *Protective function:* In this case, effective protection against bacteria, viruses, and parasites; however, the mucous membrane also ensures mechanical and chemical protection as well as biologic protection. These functions are mainly performed by the multilayered squamous epithelium and ciliated epithelium.
- *Sensory function:* In this case, perceiving pain in response to temperature differences and mechanical effects.

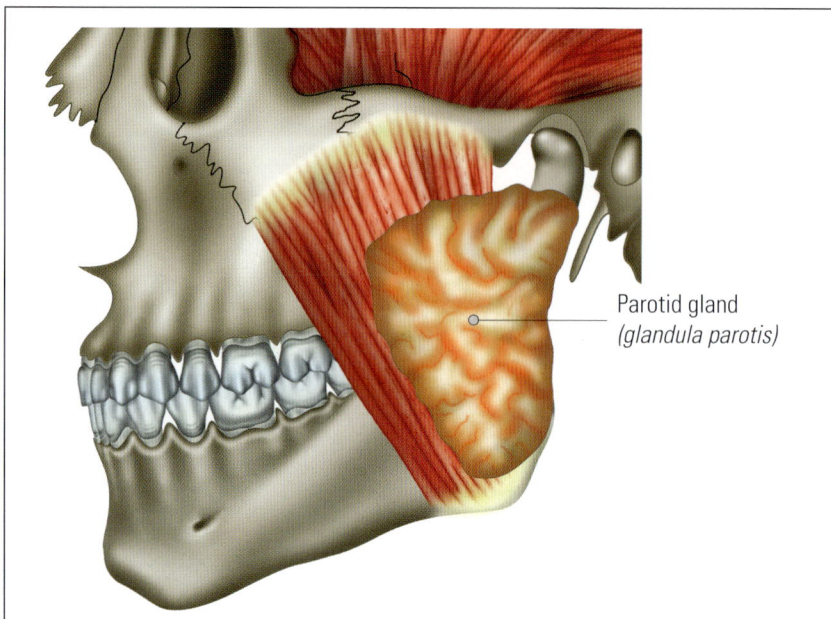

Fig 6-40 The parotid gland *(glandula parotis)* lies in front of the ear on the large masticatory muscle (masseter), which it encloses from the dorsal.

Parotid gland
(glandula parotis)

- *Production of mucus:* As a transporting mucus or as glandular products containing digestive enzymes.
- *Absorptive function:* Absorbing nutrients in the digestive tract. These functions are undertaken by highly prismatic epithelial cells.

  Mucous membranes do not have any hairs or sweat glands, while sebaceous glands are only found in the transitional epithelium of the lip mucosa. Generally the mucosa is free-moving on its connective tissue support. The exception is the oral mucosa, which is fixed in a (relatively) immobile way onto the bony jaws, the mucosal epithelium being interwoven with the mucosal connective tissue. Here the connective tissue lamina propria functions as an adhesive layer for the mucosal epithelium. The mucosa is normally nonhorny, but a horny layer (callosity) may develop at mechanically stressed sites.

  The **mucosa of the oral cavity** is made up of multilayered, nonhorny squamous epithelium, which is translucent. Except in the gingiva (the mucosal area of the alveolar ridges as far as the teeth) and the area of the anterior hard palate, a large amount of mixed mucus and salivary glands are located in the oral mucosa.

Salivary glands lie in the oral cavity and produce saliva. They can be classified according to their size.

Small salivary glands in the mouth are mucous and serous glands and include the following:

- Labial glands *(glandulae labialis)*
- Buccal glands *(glandulae buccalis)*
- Molar glands *(glandulae molares)*, which open into the vestibular area of the mouth
- Palatine glands *(glandulae palatinae)*
- Lingual glands *(glandulae linguales)*, which open into the oral cavity

Large salivary glands include the following:

- **Parotid gland** *(glandula parotis)*, a serous gland that lies in front of the outer ear and exits in the cheek, level with the second molar (Fig 6-40)
- **Sublingual gland** *(glandula sublingualis)*, a mixed gland that lies in the sublingual fossa of the mandible and exits in the sublingual caruncle, a papilla of mucous membrane next to the frenulum of the tongue (Fig 6-41)
- **Submandibular gland** *(glandula submandibularis)*, a mixed gland that lies in the mandibular

Fig 6-41 The sublingual gland *(glandula sublingualis)* lies in the sublingual fossa of the mandible on the floor of the mouth. The submandibular gland *(glandula submandibularis)* lies in the mandibular fossa under the mylohyoid muscle (here cut away), which it encloses from the dorsal.

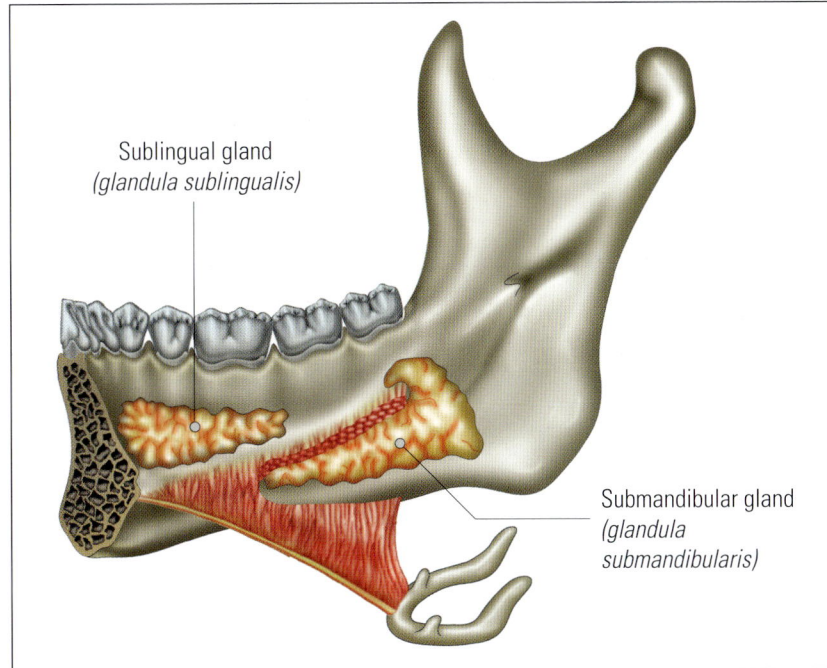

Sublingual gland
(glandula sublingualis)

Submandibular gland
(glandula submandibularis)

fossa of the mandible and also exits in the sublingual caruncle (see Fig 6-41).

All of these glands perform an important metabolic function and produce a specific secretion that altogether make up saliva.

Mucosal Covering in the Maxilla

The whole of the palatal area can be occupied by a denture base wherever there is a bony support underneath. In the area of the palatal folds, the palatal mucosa is firm and, without submucosa, is fused to the bone over a wide area; it is permeated by a latticework of collagen fibers and elastic fibers, which gives the palatal mucosa a high degree of strength and deformability.

In the posterior part of the palate, the mucosa is softer and has a submucosa with fatty and glandular tissue in addition to elastic fibers. The palatine glands *(glandulae palatinae)* guarantee the slidability of the mucosa. With age, these mucosal glands become increasingly replaced by fat.

The mucosa can be compressed to varying degrees on its bony base; it is elastic and resistant to stress. It forms pads that are elastic under pressure and act like water cushions. These areas of varying compressibility can be referred to as *resilience zones*. These variably resilient zones of mucosa (Fig 6-42) include the following:

- The **fibrous marginal zone** is the area of the alveolar ridge. Here the outer layer of mucosa is firmly fused to the periosteum. The zone is broad at the front, becomes narrower dorsally, and has very low resilience.
- The **fibrous median zone** is the median palatine suture with the torus from the incisive foramen to the posterior nasal spine. The mucosal layer here is also fused to the periosteum with connective tissue fibers. This zone has very low resilience.

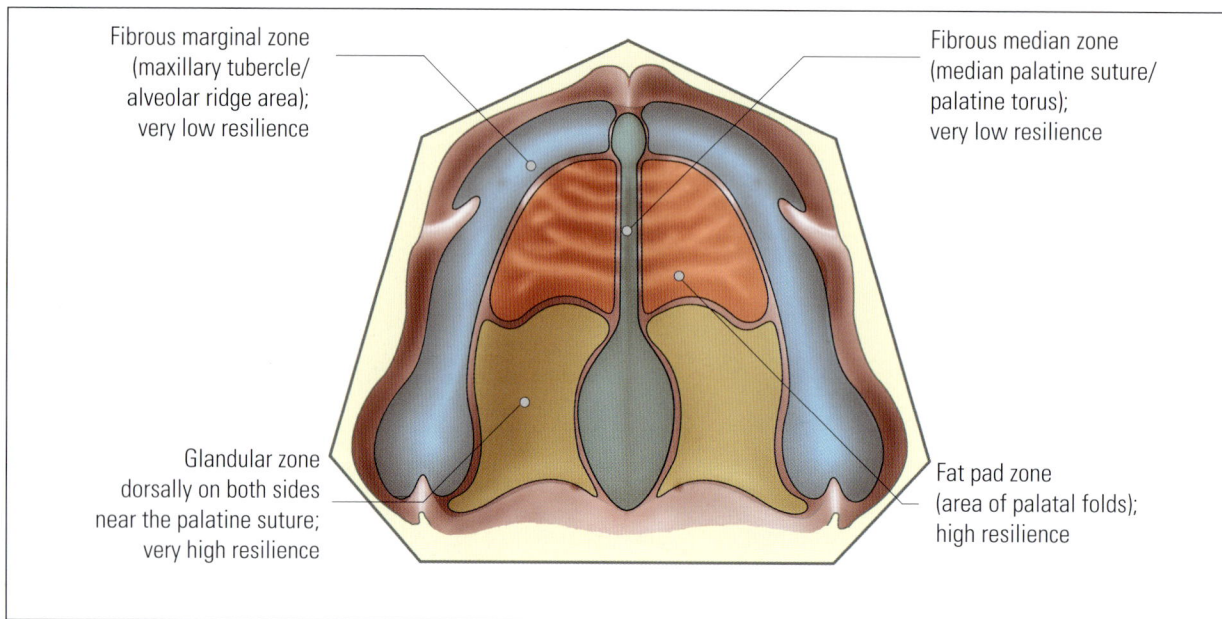

Fibrous marginal zone
(maxillary tubercle/
alveolar ridge area);
very low resilience

Fibrous median zone
(median palatine suture/
palatine torus);
very low resilience

Glandular zone
dorsally on both sides
near the palatine suture;
very high resilience

Fat pad zone
(area of palatal folds);
high resilience

Fig 6-42 Resilience zones in the maxilla.

- The *glandular zone* lies in the dorsal part of the palate near the median palatine suture and has very high resilience.
- The *fat pad zone* is the pressure and fricative field of the palate, generally the area of palatal folds with relatively high resilience. The fatty tissue is distributed over the whole of the palatine vault, except in the fibrous zones.
- The *maxillary tuberosity*, as part of the fibrous marginal zone, has very low resilience.
- The *incisive papilla* is compressible but sensitive.
- The *vestibular fornix* cannot be described in terms of its resilience because it only has bony support at the infrazygomatic crest.

The very yielding glandular and fat pad zones allow a denture to sink in more markedly when loaded by masticatory pressure. These areas do take on prosthetic significance if so-called etchings are to be made on the denture base.

The transition from hard to soft palate, namely the *vibrating line*, is particularly important. This borderline is difficult to locate clearly. However, if the soft palate joining the bony palate at this point is made to vibrate by the nose-blowing effect or by pronouncing a vowel during the impression-taking process, the precise course of the border can be traced.

The *course of the border* runs in an arch from one tuberosity to another. In 90% of cases, this arch is curved dorsally because of the pronounced posterior nasal spine. The vibrating line then runs in a double arch from one tuberosity to another, passing through the two pronounced palatine foveolae *(foveola palatina)* and enclosing the posterior nasal spine.

The muscle attachments and paths of the cheek and lip muscles also have to be taken into account. Thus, the orbicular muscle of the mouth, the levator and depressor muscles of the angle of the mouth, the greater zygomatic muscle, and the buccinator form a knot of muscles lying in the region of the angle of the mouth. If a canine is incorrectly positioned or the occlusal height is too small, the angle of the mouth will fall inward, which produces a crease in the mouth through which saliva escapes. The corners of the mouth become moist and can become inflamed.

The *muscle attachments* and course of the muscles in the area of the anterior teeth above the vestibular fornix are strained if the edges of

Fig 6-43 The anatomical and topographic features of the mucosal covering of the jaws demand that the outline of the denture border makes allowance for the muscle attachments and ligaments and uses undercut areas of the alveolar ridge as mechanical retentions. The dentures projected in this elderly skull show the differentiated shaping of the denture flange, which serves to retain a denture.

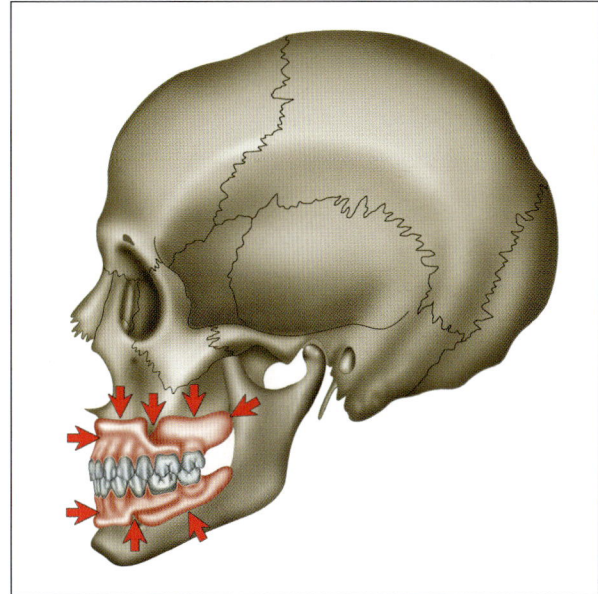

the denture are too overhanging, so that the mucosa in the lip area is pulled inward, the redness of the lips disappears, and a narrow oral fissure results. In addition, a thick denture flange will raise the outer mouth above the upper lip; it looks as if the patient has a roll of cotton wool in the fornix. As well as the feeling of tightness and the altered appearance, pressure points can also develop. To ensure that correct edge shaping is achieved, the impression of the functional edge must allow for the attachment of the buccinator in the tubal/buccal cavity and in the area of the subjugal crest (Fig 6-43).

Denture-Bearing Area in the Maxilla

As a result of resorption of the alveolar processes due to tooth loss, the maxillary alveolar ridge line is narrowed because the ridges are resorbed in the direction of inclination. The setup of teeth for complete dentures can interfere with the statics. The gap from the vestibular fornix to the ridge line will vary in size, depending on the degree of

bone reduction. Where the ridges are highly developed, there may be vestibular undercut areas that are suitable as mechanical retentions for the denture base. There is usually a firm, immobile, poorly compressible mucosa on the rounded alveolar ridge. The mobile mucosa of the cheek and lip area extends in the arch as far as the alveolar process and forms the vestibular fornix.

Vestibular fornices (fornix vestibuli superioris and *inferioris)* are the superior and inferior limits of the vestibule, which can be interrupted by ligaments, can be moved only tangentially to the alveolar ridge by cheek and lip muscles, and may be slightly widened. In the vestibular fornix, the denture border should form what is known as a *valve-type seal*, which prevents air from getting underneath the denture. The exact path of the fornix, given the variable arrangement of the different forms of mucosa, can only be recorded by means of a functional impression so that the denture border will not cause interference even during movement. The denture base should not impinge on ligaments and muscle attachments in the vestibular sulcus as areas for reduction (Fig 6-44). The features to be avoided are described in the following paragraphs.

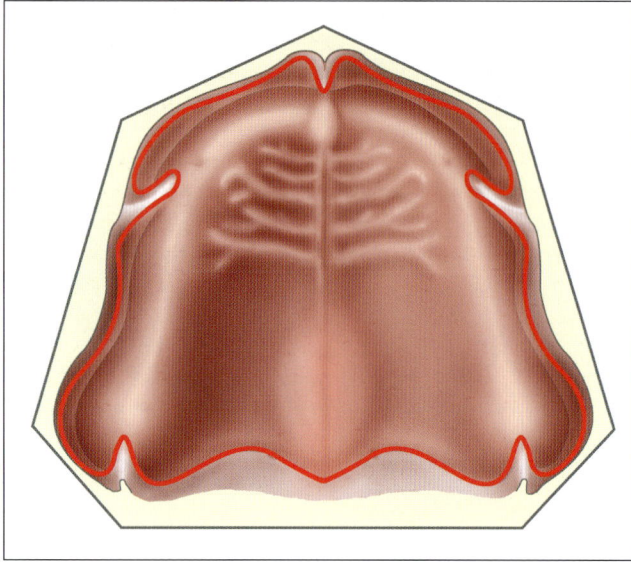

Fig 6-44 The anatomical and topographic features of the denture-bearing area in the maxilla demand that the outline of the denture border is shaped to avoid impinging on the ligaments and muscle attachments. In the maxilla, the denture border can be repositioned over the whole vestibule in the depth of the fornix and extended as far as the path of the vibrating line. The border of the denture shown here must be taken into consideration even when fabricating individual impression trays.

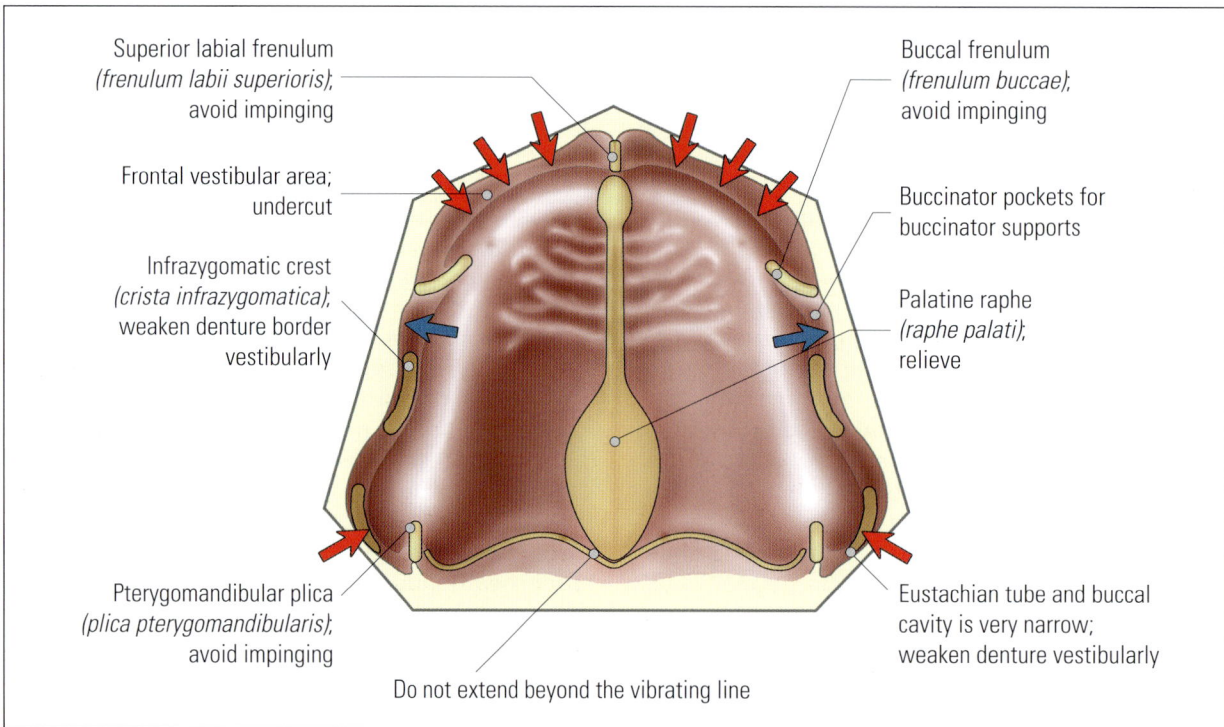

Superior labial frenulum
(frenulum labii superioris);
avoid impinging

Frontal vestibular area;
undercut

Infrazygomatic crest
(crista infrazygomatica);
weaken denture border
vestibularly

Pterygomandibular plica
(plica pterygomandibularis);
avoid impinging

Buccal frenulum
(frenulum buccae);
avoid impinging

Buccinator pockets for
buccinator supports

Palatine raphe
(raphe palati);
relieve

Eustachian tube and buccal
cavity is very narrow;
weaken denture vestibularly

Do not extend beyond the vibrating line

Fig 6-45 Denture-bearing area in the maxilla.

The **superior labial frenulum** *(frenulum labii superioris)* must be avoided throughout its height. If it attaches at the middle of the alveolar ridge, it can be surgically shortened.

The **buccal frenula** *(frenulum buccalia)*, left and right and sometimes two frenula on each side, which can be located level with the premolars or the canine, must not be restricted in their movement; if they are, serious pressure points can develop.

The **infrazygomatic crest** *(crista infrazygomatica)*, as a bony base in the fornix, can give rise to pressure points if the edge of the plate is too long or too thick.

The **eustachian tube/buccal cavity** is the area of the fornix at the maxillary tuberosity that is often very narrow and undercut. The denture flange here must not be worked too prominently and thickly because the cheek muscles will narrow the space even further when the mouth is opened and during lateral movements.

The **maxillary tuberosity** *(tuber maxillae)* is not resorbed during tooth loss. The denture base should fully cover this part of the palate because it can provide support to the denture. Furthermore, pronounced tubes offer excellent mechanical retention. In extreme cases, a maxillary tuberosity can be surgically smoothed if it protrudes too much.

The **pterygomandibular plica** *(plica pterygomandibularis)* is a distinct fold of mucosa that attaches in the middle behind the maxillary tubercle and must be avoided by the denture base because it is tightened during mouth opening and will lift up the denture.

The **vibrating line** is the borderline in the transition from hard to soft palate, beyond which the denture border should not extend; if it does, sensitive patients may experience a retching sensation.

The **median raphe of the palate** *(raphe palati)* is the counterpart to the bony palatine suture, which is only covered by a thin, poorly compressible mucosal layer. It may be thickened in the dorsal area into a palatine torus *(torus palatinus)*. A raphe with a torus should be covered or relieved if it is prominent; the palatine torus must always be relieved or, in the case of skeletal plates, completely avoided because otherwise the denture will rock, cause pressure points, and may even break.

The **incisive papilla** *(papilla incisiva)*, as the anterior tip of the palatine raphe, must be relieved on the denture base, and skeletal plates must be completely avoided. If not, pressure points can arise. If the nerves are constricted at the papilla, this can impair the patient's subjective sense of taste. This clouding of the sense of taste can occur because pressure on the papilla interferes with the sense of smell, which, combined with the tongue's sense of taste, makes up the whole sensation of taste.

The **alveolar jugae** *(juga alveolaris)* should be reproduced in the area of the anterior teeth for esthetic reasons but, in the posterior area, should not be impinged on for reasons of oral hygiene.

Figure 6-45 illustrates the denture-bearing area in the maxilla.

Denture-Bearing Area in the Mandible

The mandibular denture does not rest on a large bony foundation, unlike the support provided by the palate in the maxilla. Owing to the small area available (only the alveolar ridge with the dorsally positioned trigones), the retaining effect is also considerably reduced. The bony foundation in the mandible is highly variable in its atrophied forms. From a relatively well-developed, high, sharp alveolar ridge to a totally flat alveolar ridge that may even lie inferior to the floor of the mouth, all forms are possible.

After **tooth loss**, the alveolar ridge of the mandible is also resorbed in the direction of inclination, which gives rise to the particular form of the alveolar line: The straight alveolar lines bend sharply at precisely the canine point; the alveolar line of the posterior teeth widens out, while it sinks down in a lingual direction in the anterior area. A trapezoid open at one side is formed by the parabolic alveolar line.

As well as the relatively small denture-bearing area of the alveolar ridge, the complicated marginal course of the movable buccal mucosa and especially the highly mobile floor of the mouth impede retention of a complete denture. In addition, the shape, size, and mobility of the tongue have an influence on shaping of the denture. A

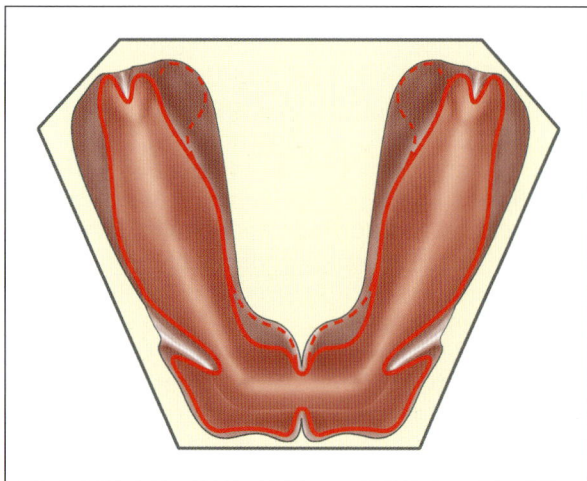

Fig 6-46 The denture-bearing area in the mandible is far smaller than that in the maxilla, and the outline of the denture border is more differentiated. In the mandible, only the frontal vestibule is usable for the outline of the denture border; the lateral areas are moved too much by muscle attachments. The sublingual and paralingual areas can be included in the denture-bearing area in a few cases. The illustrated border demarcation is taken into consideration even when fabricating individual impression trays.

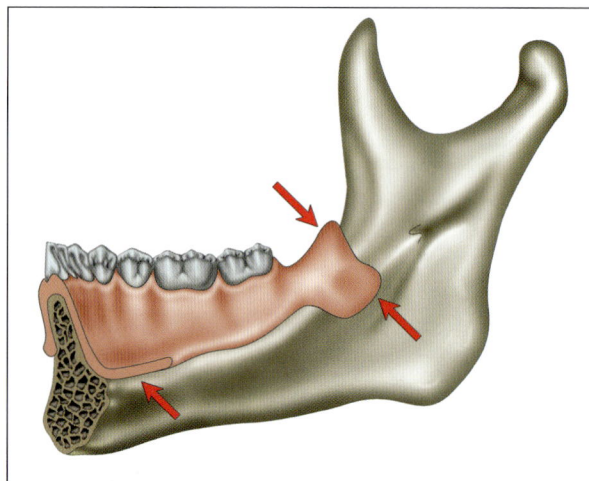

Fig 6-47 The retromolar trigone *(trigonum retromolare)* is recorded on both sides as a denture support. The anterior sublingual area can be used to extend the denture base horizontally (sublingual roll) under the tongue. The lateral sublingual spaces (paralingual pockets), located lingually under the trigones, offer mechanical retention as undercut areas together with the undercut anterior alveolar ridge area.

mandibular denture is much more exposed to the muscle activities of the cheeks, lips, tongue, and floor of the mouth than a maxillary denture.

The outward course of the bony wall of the mandibular body means that the vestibular fornix is usually underlaid with bone in the vestibular area. In the lingual region, the sturdy mylohyoid ridge marks the limit of the denture border. As a result, the border of the mandibular denture has very definite areas requiring reduction (Fig 6-46).

The *inferior labial frenulum (frenulum labii inferioris)* and *buccal frenulum (frenulum buccae)* should not be impinged, as in the maxilla, so as not to impede movement of the ligaments.

The *mental foramen (foramen mentale)* may lie on the alveolar ridge if there has been severe atrophy, and it must then be avoided or covered. If there are pressure points in this area, the patient may experience pain from teeth that are no longer there.

The *oblique line (linea obliqua)*, as the insertion of the buccinator muscle, forms the buccal boundary of the base, from which premolars run

dorsally. The denture border must be shortened in keeping with this line.

The *pterygomandibular plica* (*plica pterygomandibularis* or *raphe pterygomandibularis*; *plica* = fold; *raphe* = seam) runs from the posterior border of the retromolar trigone dorsally and upward to the maxillary tuberosity and must not be impinged, as in the maxilla.

The *mylohyoid line (linea mylohyoidea)*, as the insertion of the mylohyoid muscle and the boundary of the floor of the mouth, also demarcates the border of the denture plate. This is because during swallowing the floor of the mouth is raised along this line, and a plate border that extends beyond this line in the floor of the mouth will cause severe pressure points. The patient will often be unable to swallow without difficulty. The edge of the plate, from the premolars onward, should therefore be shortened dorsally as far as the retromolar trigones in keeping with this line.

The *frenulum of the tongue (frenulum linguae)* must not be impinged because, if impinged, the mobility of the tongue will be impeded. If the denture base is to be reground, only the insertion of

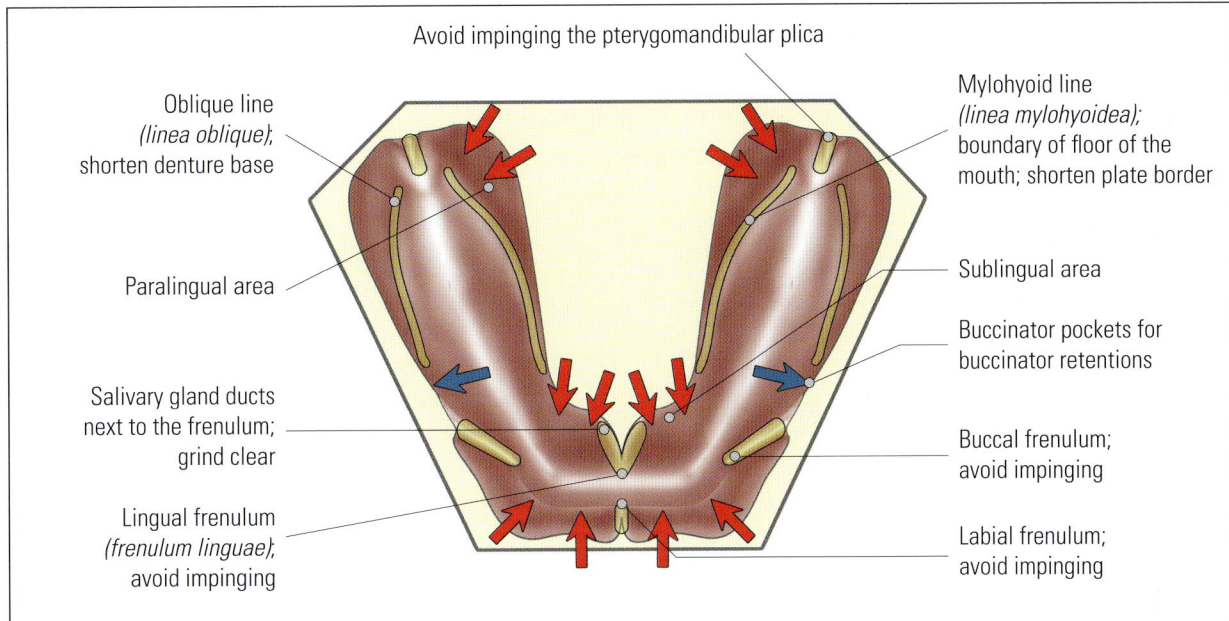

Avoid impinging the pterygomandibular plica

Oblique line
(linea oblique);
shorten denture base

Mylohyoid line
(linea mylohyoidea);
boundary of floor of the
mouth; shorten plate border

Paralingual area

Sublingual area

Buccinator pockets for
buccinator retentions

Salivary gland ducts
next to the frenulum;
grind clear

Buccal frenulum;
avoid impinging

Lingual frenulum
(frenulum linguae);
avoid impinging

Labial frenulum;
avoid impinging

Fig 6-48 Denture-bearing area in the mandible.

the frenulum needs to be avoided. The denture border should not be widened along the course of the frenulum because that will impede the suction capacity of the denture base.

The **sublingual caruncles** *(carunculae sublingualis)* are small papillae on the left and right next to the frenulum of the tongue and are openings of the salivary glands. An impression must not be taken of these openings because they can become blocked, preventing the flow of saliva. The result for the patient is a dry mouth, with the salivary gland swelling up and causing an unpleasant feeling of tightness. The impressions of the papillae can be created in the denture border by grinding out slightly.

The **alveolar tubercle of the mandible** *(tuberculum alveolare mandibulae)* is a bulge of mucous membrane over the retromolar trigone *(trigonum retromolare)* that can arise because of particular muscle attachments. The denture base can be extended as far as this (Fig 6-47), but the pterygomandibular plica must not be impinged.

The **alveolar jugae** *(juga alveolaria)* are prominences over the roots of the teeth, which should only be reproduced in the mandible in the area of the anterior teeth, whereas the dorsal area of the

outer edge of the denture should be kept smooth for hygiene reasons. Any manipulation of the denture border should be done by the dentist and not by the dental technician.

Figure 6-48 illustrates the denture-bearing area in the mandible.

Tongue

The tongue *(lingua;* Greek, *glotta* or *glossa)* is an oval muscular organ covered with mucosa that is mainly made up of highly developed striated musculature with extremely variable mobility. The tongue is highly perfused with blood and carries nerves for the senses of taste and touch. It helps in eating and during chewing, sucking, and swallowing, and it is used for the purposes of speech because it is highly mobile. The tongue almost completely fills the oral cavity and extends at the rear as far as the epiglottis. The body of the tongue can be divided into the root, dorsum, and apex (or tip), while the surfaces and edges are described as the superior surface *(facies superior)*, the lateral margins *(margines laterales)*,

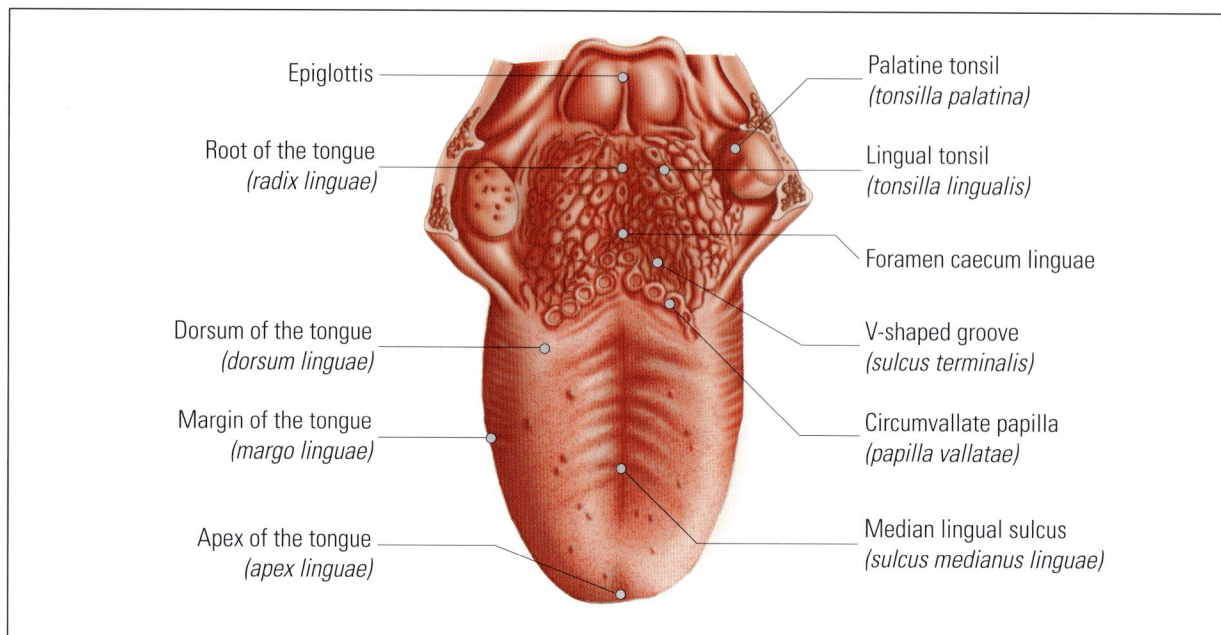

Fig 6-49 The dorsum of the tongue displays a differentiated structure.

and the inferior surface *(facies inferior)*. Lifting up the tongue reveals the anterior apex and lateral margins on the underside, while the central part at the root is seen to be fused to the floor of the mouth over a wide area.

The ***frenulum of the tongue*** *(frenulum linguae)* is a thick fold under the tongue that extends forward to the mandible and is moved powerfully during tongue movements. Because the frenulum of the tongue is moved a great deal during speaking, chewing, and swallowing, a denture border must not restrict the frenulum.

The ***root of the tongue*** *(radix linguae)* is the posterior part of the body of the tongue, which is divided from the dorsum by a V-shaped groove, the terminal sulcus *(sulcus terminalis)*. At the posteriorly directed apex of the sulcus, there is a depression *(foramen caecum linguae)*, a rudimentary remnant of the thyroglossal duct.

The ***dorsum of the tongue*** carries not only the free nerve endings for the sense of touch but also numerous differently shaped papillae mainly for the sense of taste (Fig 6-49). The mucosa on the

dorsum is firmly (hence immovably) joined to the inner musculature of the tongue by bundles of fibers. Based on form and function, there are four different types of papilla on the mucosa of the body and root of the tongue (Fig 6-50):

1. ***Filiform papillae*** *(papillae filiformes)* are distributed over the whole of the dorsum and give it a velvety, rough, or coarse surface. The posteriorly directed papillae are horny at their tip and contain tactile nerves for mechanical functions, temperature sensation, and pain sensitivity.

2. ***Reddish, fungiform papillae*** *(papillae fungiformes)* are mainly located at the margins and apex of the tongue and contain taste buds, while special mucous glands known as *gustatory glands* are absent. Instead, these papillae contain a lot of lymph cells.

3. ***Circumvallate papillae*** *(papillae vallatae)* are wart-shaped taste papillae that lie mainly in a V-shaped formation in front of the terminal sulcus. Each papilla is surrounded by a circular groove in whose epithelium the taste buds

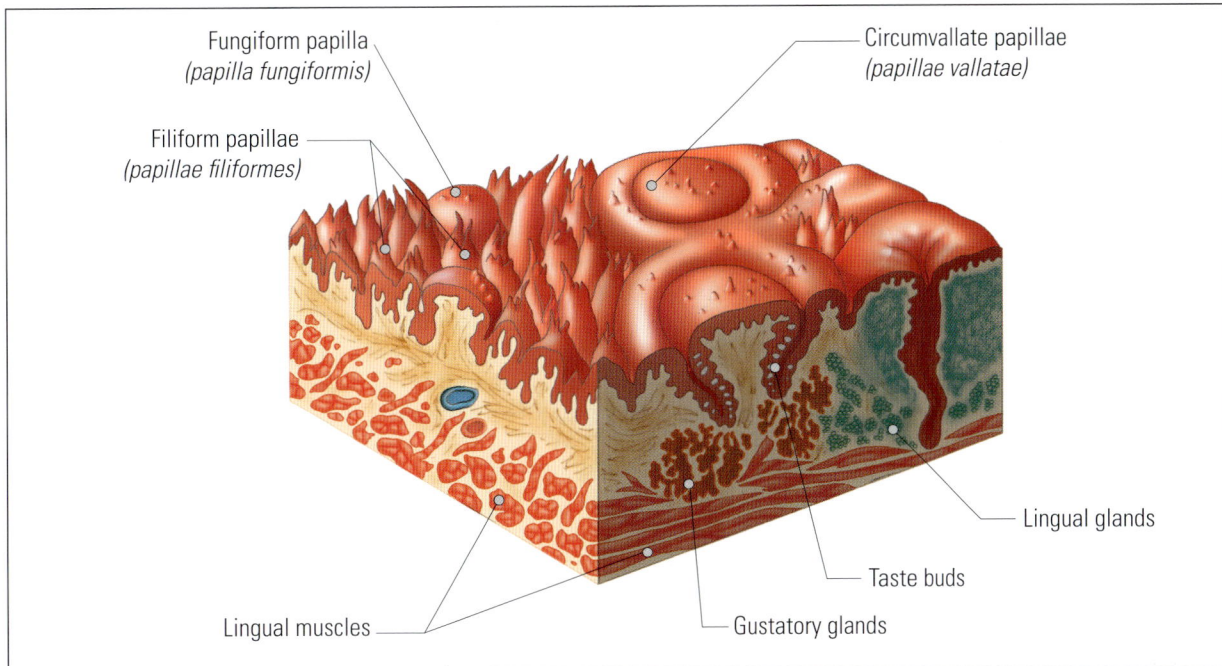

Fig 6-50 Diagram of a section through the tongue surface, showing the various papillae.

lie and where ducts from mucous glands end. There are branches of the taste nerve *(nervus glossopharyngeus)* located in the taste buds, and a few fibers of the nerve also run between the taste buds.

4. **Foliate papillae** *(papillae foliatae)* are mucosal folds running roughly crosswise along the posterolateral border of the tongue. Taste buds are densely distributed in these foliate papillae, with openings from serous gustatory glands.

The **four taste qualities** are sweet, sour, salty, and bitter, and each is assigned to a specific region of the tongue surface. As well as enabling the sensation of foodstuffs, the sense of taste also helps in the detection of harmful and inedible substances. Sweet is perceived as a pleasant stimulus from edible substances and functionally is checked preferably with the tip of the tongue, while salty is checked at the anterior margin, both by fungiform papillae; sour is checked at the middle margin by foliate papillae, while bitter is checked by circumvallate papillae at the base of the tongue. Poisons (eg, alkaloids such as strychnine) taste bitter, and the stimulus threshold for this taste nuance is therefore low, triggering protective reflex reactions. Because most of the taste buds sensitive to bitter tastes are located at the base of the tongue, the protective reflex is often retching.

The **sense of taste** is a chemically active sense, which means that the taste receptors react to substances dissolved in saliva. The finely graduated taste sensations are based on the interaction of the sense of smell and taste, which is why a head cold will dull the sense of taste. The tactile and temperature sensations as well as the sense of pain in the lips, tongue, and palate can also influence the sensation of taste, for instance with crunchy foods, alcohol, or excessively strong spices.

Musculature of the Tongue

The musculature of the tongue is divided into two halves by the septum of the tongue *(septum linguae)*, a sheet of connective tissue at the midline. The position of this septum can be seen from the superior surface of the tongue as the median sulcus *(sulcus medianus linguae)*. Two groups of tongue muscles can be identified by their course, namely those that originate from parts of the skeleton and end in the tongue and those that have their origin and ending in the tongue itself. The first group are known as *extrinsic* (originating outside the tongue), while the muscles entirely within the tongue are referred to as *intrinsic*.

Extrinsic muscles (which may also be known as *skeletal muscles of the tongue*) originate from the mandible, the hyoid bone, and the styloid process (Fig 6-51). The fiber bundles of these muscles run into the tongue, are arranged in the three planes in the body of the tongue, and merge into the intrinsic musculature. The internal muscles are mainly responsible for changing the shape of the tongue (deformability) as they interact antagonistically and force the antagonists to relax.

Extrinsic muscles of the tongue

- The *genioglossus muscle (musculus genioglossus)* originates as a paired muscle at the mental spine and fans out to both the apex and the base of the tongue. This muscle draws the base of the tongue forward with its lower fibers, while the other fibers draw the tongue to the floor of the mouth.
- The *hyoglossus muscle (musculus hyoglossus)* originates as a thin plate of muscle from the greater horn of the hyoid bone and from parts of the adjacent body of the hyoid. Its parallel fibers lie along the outer side of the genioglossus muscle, and it is able to draw the tongue downward and backward with the hyoid bone fixed.
- The *styloglossus muscle (musculus styloglossus)* radiates from the styloid process of the temporal bone over the lateral margin of the tongue to the apex. The muscle is able to draw back the apex and even the whole of the tongue. Because this muscle is also paired, one-sided activity can produce side-to-side movement of the tongue.

Intrinsic muscles of the tongue

Transverse muscle (musculus transversus linguae) originates from both sides of the septum and extends to the mucosa of the margin and dorsum of the tongue. The posterior fibers are also joined to the muscles of the gullet.

Vertical muscle (musculus verticalis linguae) arises with its fibers perpendicular to the transverse muscles, while the fibers of the inferior and superior longitudinal muscles *(M longitudinalis inferior* and *superior)* run from front to back and thus perpendicular to the genioglossus and hyoglossus muscles.

When the longitudinal muscles and transverse muscles of the tongue are contracted, the vertical muscles are relaxed and the tongue becomes short and high. If the longitudinal muscles and the vertical muscles are stretched as the transverse muscles relax, the tongue becomes short and low.

The *interaction of all the muscles* produces the complex tongue movements during speech. The extremely active deformability of the tongue also means that all areas of the oral cavity and vestibule can be reached, which ensures self-cleaning of the dentition. Even in resting phases, with the mouth closed, the tongue exerts gentle, constant pressure on the rows of teeth, which have to be kept in equilibrium by pressure from the lips and cheeks. This equilibrium of muscle tone helps to create and maintain the correct jaw shape.

During *chewing*, the tongue turns the food over on the rough pressure and fricative field of the palate while mixing saliva in with the food. The food particles dissolved in saliva are pressed into the taste papillae, which is how the taste stimuli are sensed. In addition, the tongue continually pushes the food between the teeth on the working side and checks the food for inedible fragments (eg, fishbones, bone splinters).

The *swallowing process* involves bringing the mandible into a stable position by habitual intercuspation. The hyoid and floor of the mouth are raised so that the tongue is able to push the food over the palate into the gullet. This is done by the movable soft palate falling downward, allowing the food to be guided backward toward the esophagus.

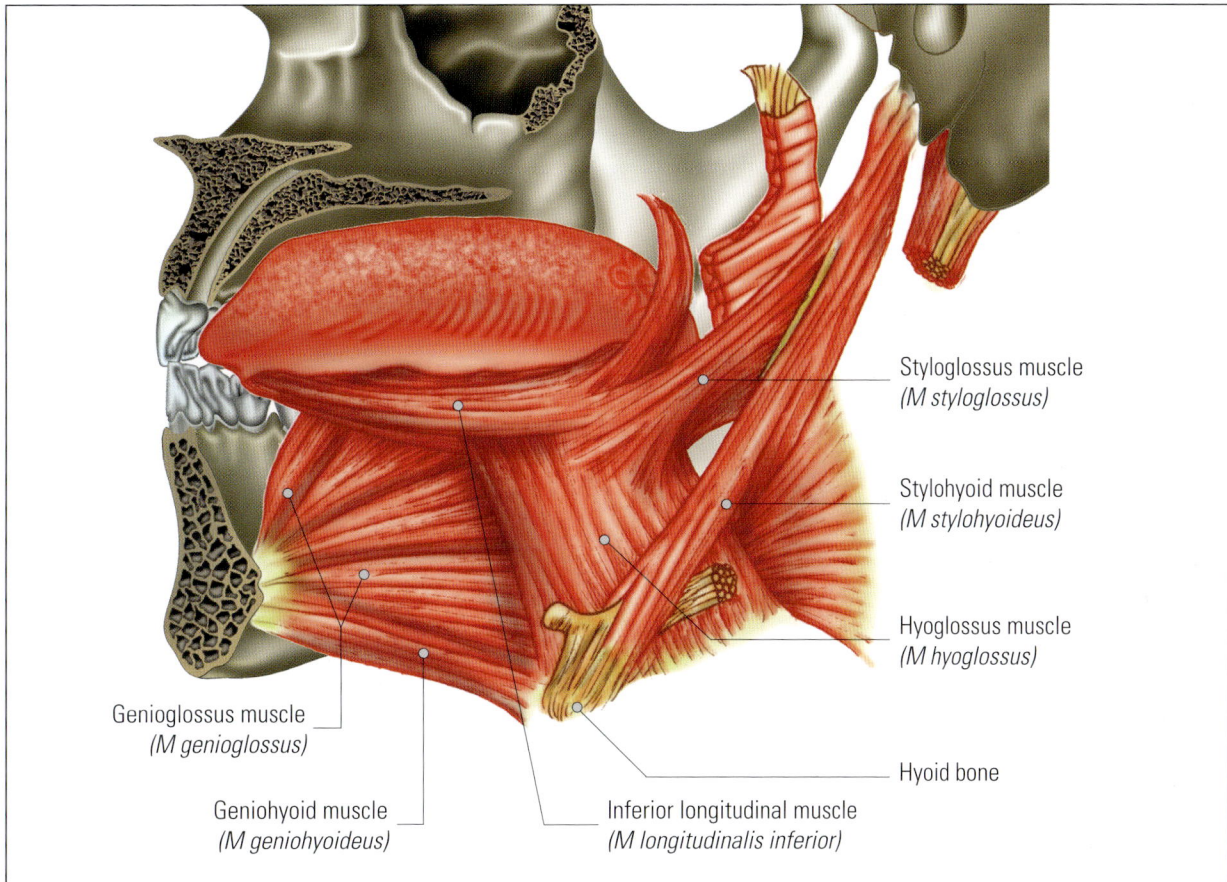

Fig 6-51 Diagram of the extrinsic muscles of the tongue, originating from the mandible, the hyoid bone, and the styloid process.

Styloglossus muscle
(M styloglossus)

Stylohyoid muscle
(M stylohyoideus)

Hyoglossus muscle
(M hyoglossus)

Hyoid bone

Inferior longitudinal muscle
(M longitudinalis inferior)

Geniohyoid muscle
(M geniohyoideus)

Genioglossus muscle
(M genioglossus)

Physiology of Mandibular Movement

Mandibular Movement

The positional changes of the mandible in comparison with the maxilla can be observed and measured at three places (Fig 7-1): between the condyle and the articular fossa, between the jawbones, and between the occlusal surfaces of the teeth.

Only the mandibular movements with tooth contact, ie, occlusal displacements, are of interest to the dental technician. The changes of position between condyle and condylar path can be measured, and thus the inclinations of the condylar path can be determined. The positional changes between the jaws are recorded when the jaw relation is being determined. The complex mandibular movements are attributed to two types of movement of the joint: *(1)* rotary or hinge movement and *(2)* translatory or sliding movement.

The temporomandibular joint (TMJ) is both a pivot (rotary) and a sliding joint, which permits the following three basic mandibular movements: opening and closing movement, forward and backward movement, and lateral movement.

Opening and closing movement (depression and elevation or abduction and adduction) can be interpreted as pure hinge movement. This kind of hinge action is possible up to an opening movement of approximately 10 mm when the mandible is pushed

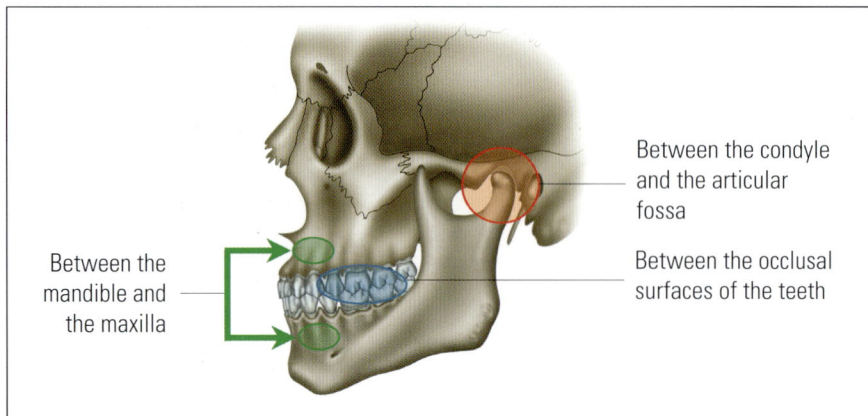

Fig 7-1 The change in the position of the jaws in mandibular movements can be observed at three places.

Between the condyle and the articular fossa

Between the occlusal surfaces of the teeth

Between the mandible and the maxilla

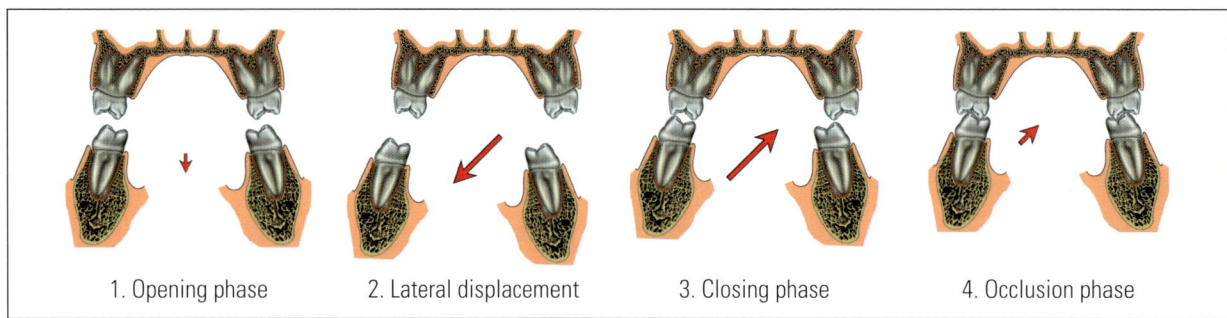

| 1. Opening phase | 2. Lateral displacement | 3. Closing phase | 4. Occlusion phase |

Fig 7-2 Movement phases of a masticatory cycle.

backward at the same time. For wider opening, the condyle slides forward and downward (ventral-caudal direction) on the condylar path.

Forward and backward movement (protrusion and retrusion) happens as a simultaneous sliding movement of both condyles on the particular condylar paths downward and forward.

Lateral movement (laterotrusion and mediotrusion) can happen when one condyle slides downward and forward on its condylar path while the opposing condyle rotates around a vertical axis in its articular fossa.

The *translating condyle* (mediotrusive, nonworking-side, balancing, idling, or orbiting condyle) denotes the condyle sliding downward and forward during lateral movement; the side of the jaw of the translating condyle is correspondingly known as the *translation* or *mediotrusive side* or the *nonworking or balancing side* because the teeth are taken out of contact on that side.

The *rotating condyle* (laterotrusive, working-side condyle) is the condyle that turns. It is found on the side toward which the mandible is being moved; this side is known as the *active or working side* (laterotrusive side) because here the teeth remain in full contact and perform masticatory activity.

The mandibular movements are performed in accordance with the function of the masticatory system during speaking, chewing, or swallowing and are therefore known as *functional movements*. A distinction is made between free movements without tooth contact and movements with tooth contact, the so-called articulatory movements. During speaking, the mandibular movements happen both with and without tooth contact; when swallowing and grinding up food in the final phase, occlusal contacts are required.

The *masticatory process* goes through specific, habitual movement cycles that can be divided into

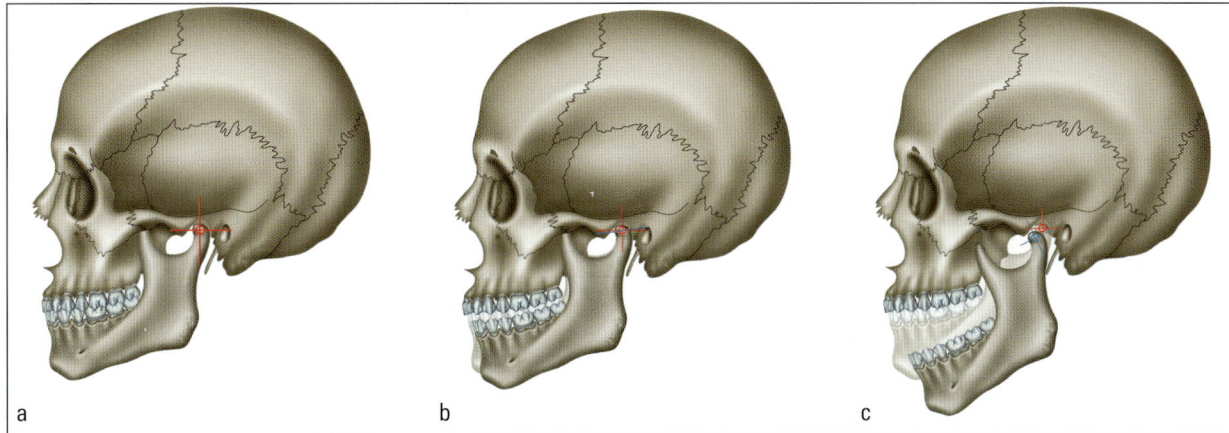

Fig 7-3 Opening movement of the mandible. *(a)* In centric occlusion, the teeth are in uniform contact on all sides with the antagonists; the mandible is at its closest to the maxilla, and the condyle lies deep in the articular fossa. *(b)* From centric occlusion, an opening movement of approximately 10 mm can be made as a pure hinge movement. For wider jaw opening, a gliding movement downward and forward is added to the pure hinge movement. *(c)* For maximum opening movement, the condyle now slides downward and forward as far as the horizontal surface of the articular tuberosity. This movement is enforced by the lateral pterygoid muscle.

phases. The sequence of movements depends on the consistency of the food and varies considerably among individuals, but it does follow a set principle. This means that food is crushed not by a "chopping" action (simply opening and closing the rows of teeth) but by occlusal surfaces grinding as they push against each other. To do this, the mandible must be brought into a slightly lateral position from where the teeth slide back into terminal occlusion, with a grinding effect.

Movement phases of a masticatory cycle run smoothly into each other (Fig 7-2):

1. *Opening phase:* Starts with lowering of the mandible to take in the food.
2. *Lateral displacement (or protrusive movement):* The mandible slides to the chewing side to grasp the food.
3. *Closing phase:* The mandible is raised until it approaches cusp-to-cusp contact so that the food is crushed but not ground up.
4. *Occlusion phase:* The mandible slides out of the lateral position and into terminal occlusion, during which the food is made smaller by a constant increase in the force applied until maximal intercuspation of the teeth is achieved. Now the mandible is guided not merely by joints and muscles but by the occlusal pattern of the teeth.

Mandibular Border Movements

In *centric occlusion*, the teeth are in uniform contact on all sides with the antagonists; in this position, the periodontal tissues are centrically loaded (Fig 7-3a). The mandible is at its closest to the maxilla in this position. The condyle of the mandible lies without pressure deep in the articular fossa. Centric occlusion is normally adopted as a reflex to a wide opening position, so that this position can also be regarded as the habitual occlusion or intercuspation. An opening movement of approximately 10 mm can be made out of centric occlusion as a pure hinge movement (Fig 7-3b). However, the mandible has to be forcibly held back to do this. For wider jaw opening, the mandibular condyle slides forward and downward on the oblique condylar path; thus, a gliding movement is added to the pure hinge movement.

For *maximum opening movement*, the condyle now slides as far downward and forward as necessary until it comes to rest on the horizontal surface of the articular tuberosity (Fig 7-3c). The condyle is thus slid out of the articular fossa. So that the joint is not dislocated, any further movement is prevented by the articular ligaments. This

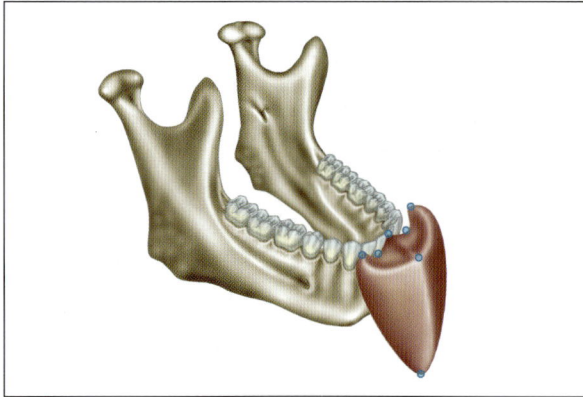

Fig 7-4 The movement paths can be combined to form a three-dimensional border movement envelope.

special movement is enforced by the lateral pterygoid muscle, which, with a few muscle fibers, attaches to the articular disc and draws it forward. The joint capsule itself can be stretched so that it is also involved in this movement without being abnormally stretched.

A particular problem when analyzing mandibular movements is that functional movements cannot be exactly reproduced. It is assumed that all functional movements lie within a range of border movements. The border movements are therefore mapped in all three planes so that the whole range of functional movements can be outlined. The inferior incisive point and the midpoints of the condyles are chosen as measuring points for tracing this pattern of border movements. The maximum movement paths of the points are thus transferred to the median or sagittal plane, frontal plane, and horizontal plane. When these are combined, the result is an envelope of border movements in space, within which all mandibular movements take place (Fig 7-4). The border movement of the mandible in each of these planes is described below.

Sagittal plane: Movements out of centric occlusion are possible, both as movements with tooth contact and as free mandibular movements. This yields reproducible limit positions, including the following (Fig 7-5):

1. Centric occlusion
2. Retroposition
3. Maximum protrusion of the mandible
4. Endpoint of pure hinge movement
5. Maximum opening point
6. Rest position

The lines connecting the limit points correspond to the possible border movement paths.

Frontal plane: Plotting of mandibular movement shows a border movement that is reflected on the line of the sagittal limit points. From centric occlusion, the mandible drops and moves over the occlusal contact out to the right or left limit position and from there in an even curve to the maximum opening point.

Horizontal plane: Movement of the mandible creates a rhomboid, symmetric movement path of the mandibular incisive point, which in principle can be reproduced at each centric stop in the contact area of the antagonists (Fig 7-6). The movement path arises from mapping of the interocclusal record and here corresponds to the Gothic arch or needlepoint tracing (Fig 7-7).

The *needlepoint* or Gothic arch is based on the tracing of protrusive and lateral movements during interocclusal record registration. For this purpose, a tracer should be attached centrally to a baseplate, then used to track the horizontal border movements on a registration plate in the opposing jaw.

Posselt's diagram can be used for two-dimensional plotting of the pattern of border movements of the mandibular incisive point in the sagittal, horizontal, and frontal planes. The record of the area covered by the border movements created by joining the limit points of free mandibular movements in all planes of space can be referred to as *Posselt's envelope*. All mandibular movements take place within that space.

Fig 7-5 Border movements of the mandible in the sagittal plane.

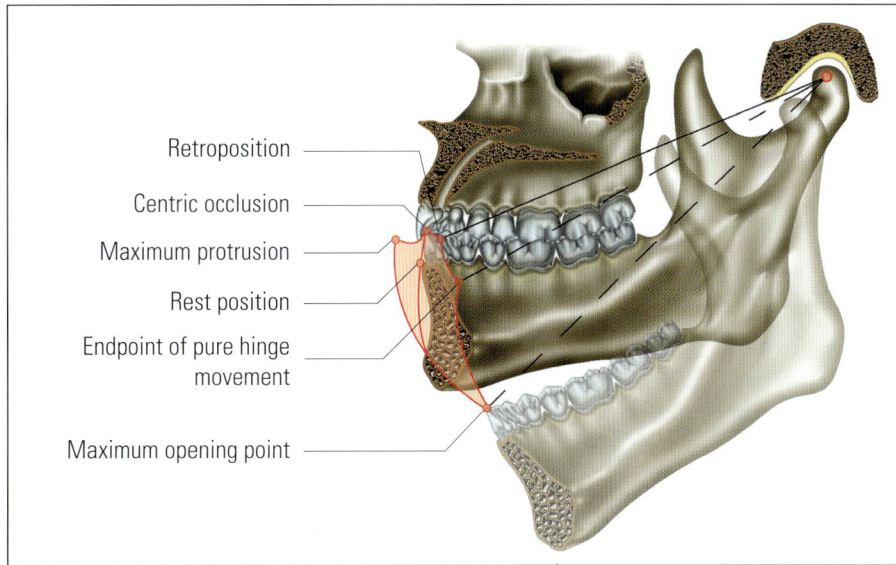

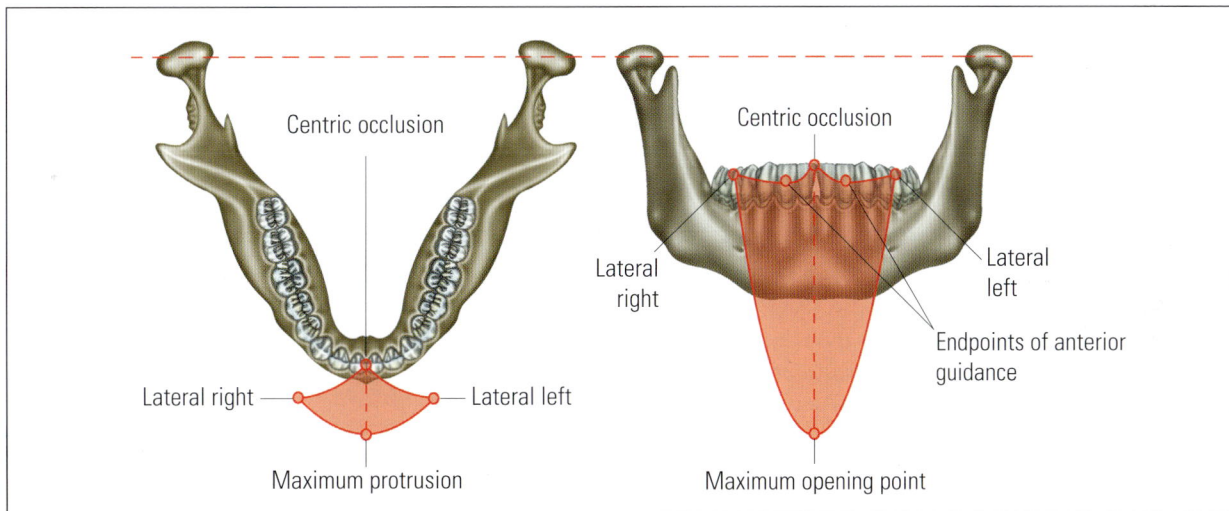

Retroposition

Centric occlusion

Maximum protrusion

Rest position

Endpoint of pure hinge movement

Maximum opening point

Fig 7-6 Border movements of the mandible in the horizontal and transverse planes.

Centric occlusion

Lateral right

Lateral left

Maximum protrusion

Centric occlusion

Lateral right

Lateral left

Endpoints of anterior guidance

Maximum opening point

Fig 7-7 The movement path of the mandibular incisive point in the horizontal plane emerges from a tracing of the interocclusal record as a Gothic arch or needlepoint tracing.

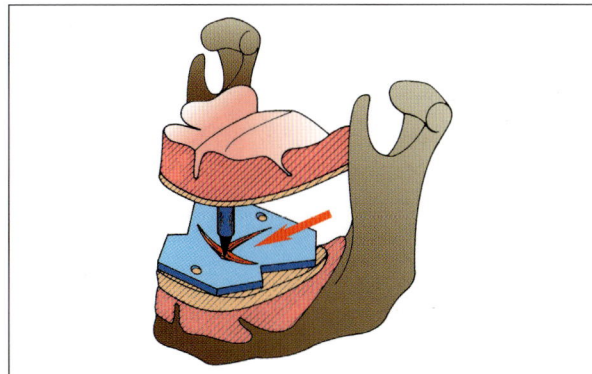

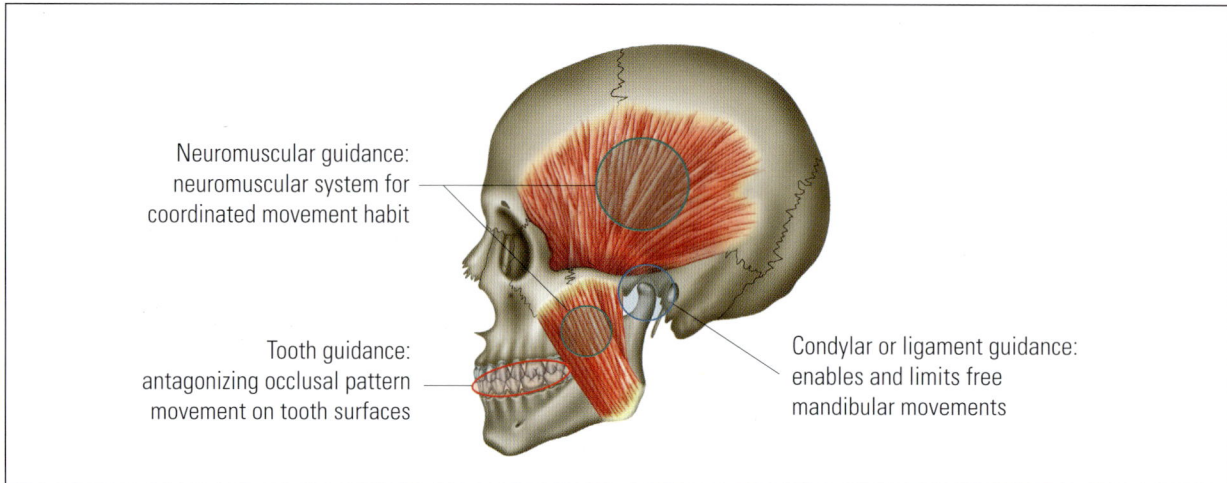

Fig 7-8 Mandibular movements are determined by three guidance factors.

Guidance Factors in Mandibular Movement

Mandibular movements are determined by three guidance factors (Fig 7-8):

1. *Condylar (TMJ or ligament) guidance* is the limitation of movement by the TMJ. The condyle is guided both on the condylar path and by the articular disc. The joint capsule and articular ligaments limit these movements. It is mainly the free mandibular movements that are limited by the capsule and ligaments.
2. *Tooth guidance* arises from the spatial arrangement of antagonizing occlusal patterns; in this case, movement is performed along the occlusal tooth surfaces as effective chewing movements.
3. *Neuromuscular guidance* takes place via the active neuromuscular system of the masticatory muscles. This guidance produces a coordinated movement habit in fixed patterns.

Function of condylar guidance

In a technical articulator device for imitating mandibular movement, neither ligament guidance nor neuromuscular guidance can be mimicked. The parts of the articulator can only be moved against each other via rigid condylar guidance; this is why precise analysis of condylar guidance is necessary. The most common form of movement in the TMJ is rotary sliding: rotation with simultaneous translation. Real mandibular movements take place around three spatial axes, in which the condyles of the TMJ form the centers of rotation (Figs 7-9 and 7-10).

In a *pure opening movement*, there is one rotation point in each condyle, through which a hinge axis can be placed that can be projected onto the external skin at each condyle. Other rotation axes are necessary in lateral movements. When the nonworking condyle slides forward, downward, and inward on its condylar path during lateral movement (Fig 7-11), the working condyle on the opposite side must rotate around several axes that are perpendicular to each other (see Fig 7-10):

1. *Hinge axis*: Because a lateral movement is only possible when a slight opening movement takes place, the rotating (working) condyle turns around the hinge axis.
2. *Vertical axis*: Because the nonworking condyle describes a section of a circular arc *forward and inward* on the condylar path, the rotating condyle has to turn around a vertical axis.
3. *Sagittal axis*: Because the nonworking condyle slides downward and forward on the condylar path, the rotating condyle has to turn around a horizontal-sagittal axis.

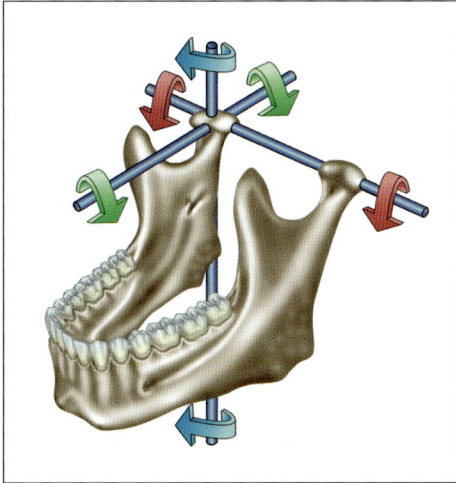

Fig 7-9 Rotation axes of the mandible.

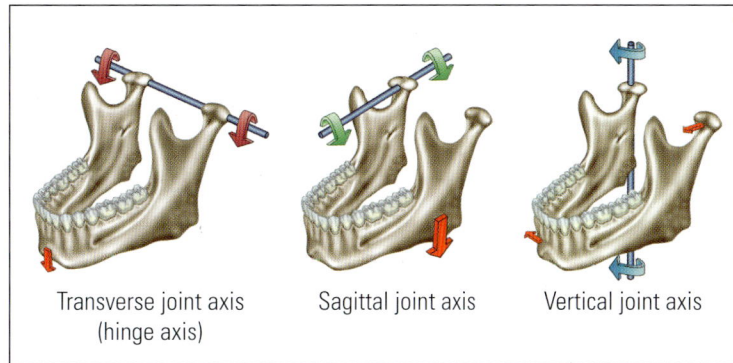

Transverse joint axis (hinge axis)   Sagittal joint axis   Vertical joint axis

Fig 7-10 The movement of the condyles in the articular surfaces is a combination of rotation with simultaneous translation. Three rotation axes can be constructed at the condyles to accomplish the movements.

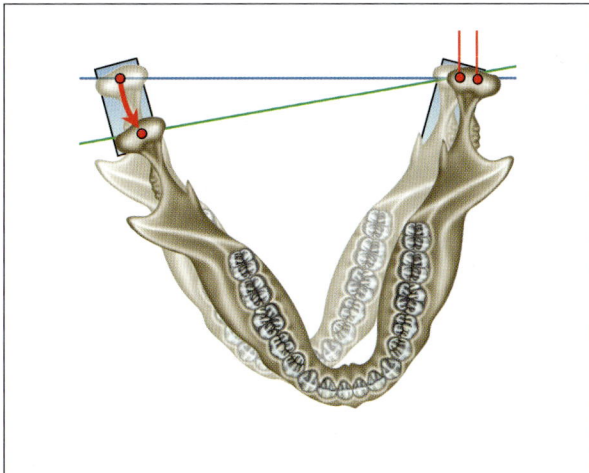

Fig 7-11 In lateral movement of the mandible, the nonworking condyle slides downward, forward, and inward on the condylar path; it describes a flattened circular path. The working condyle slides outward by the Bennett movement.

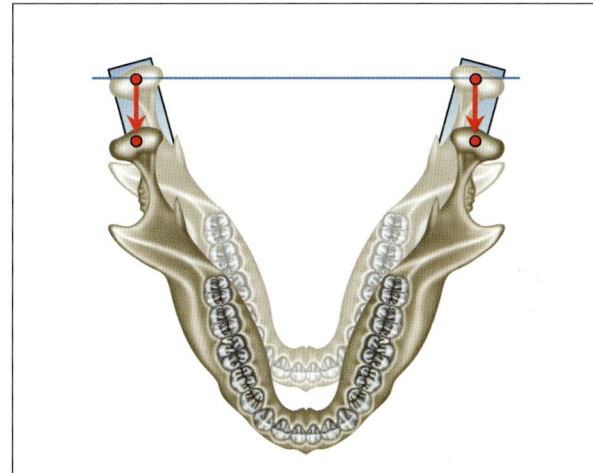

Fig 7-12 In a protrusive movement, both condyles slide downward and forward on the condylar paths. When this movement path is plotted, two lines running parallel to each other are produced (parallels to the median plane).

When the *condyles* slide forward during forward (protrusive) movement, they move in line with the sagittal condylar path inclination downward as far as the articular tubercle, which means the mandible has to drop down in the dorsal area (Fig 7-12). If the mouth remains closed, the incisors come into contact but the posterior teeth do not touch.

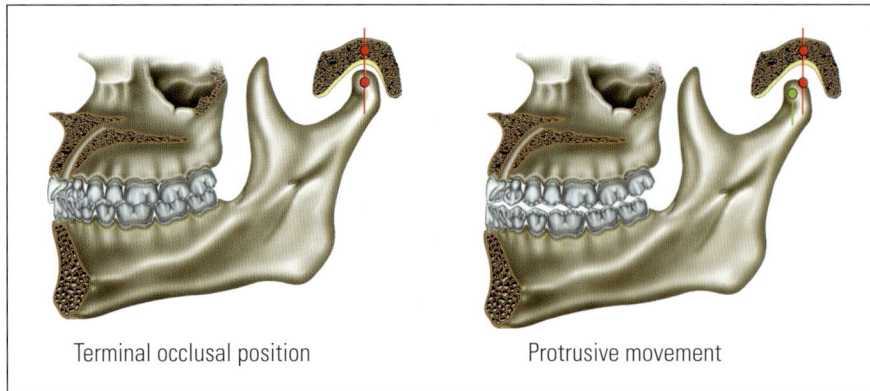

Fig 7-13 Illustrative diagram of Christensen's phenomenon. In protrusive movement to bite food, the condyles slide downward and forward on the condylar paths and the mandibular body is depressed in the dorsal area. The posterior teeth come out of contact, while the incisors have "biting off" (incision) contact.

Terminal occlusal position

Protrusive movement

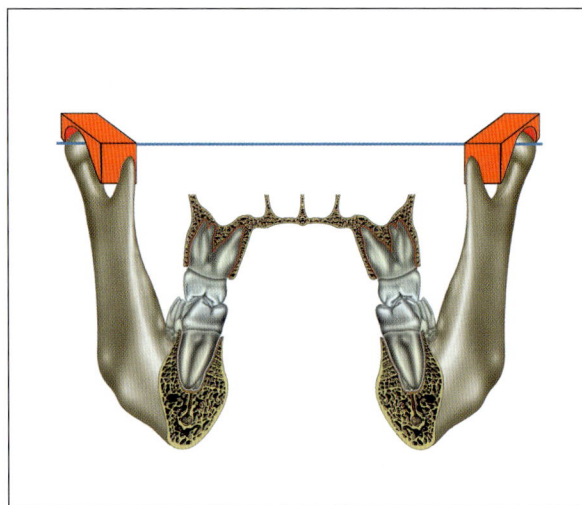

Fig 7-14 Transverse Christensen's phenomenon: During lateral movements of the mandible, the sagittal inclination of the condylar path leads to separation of the posterior rows of teeth when one condyle slides downward and forward on the condylar path. This condyle is the nonworking condyle; the working condyle is on the other side.

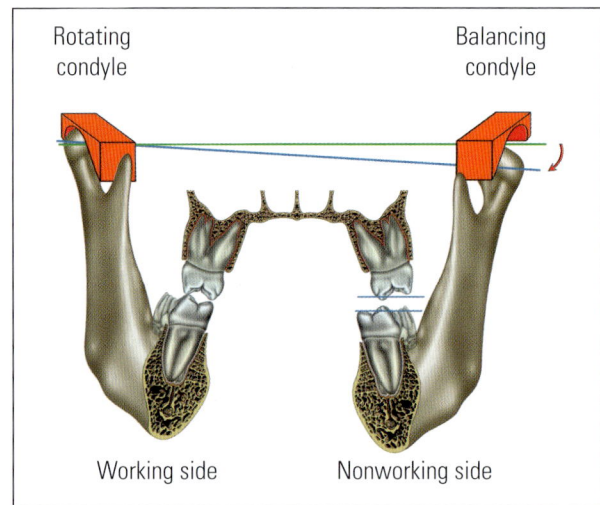

Rotating condyle

Balancing condyle

Working side

Nonworking side

Fig 7-15 The balancing or nonworking condyle is found on the nonworking side (mediotrusive side); the opposite side is referred to as the *working side* (laterotrusive side); here the posterior teeth are firmly pressed together. This is how Christensen's phenomenon operates: separation of the teeth on the nonworking side but full contact on the working side.

Christensen's phenomenon

While intraorally measuring condylar paths for complete dentures, Danish dentist Carl Christensen (1857–1921) observed a separation in coplanar occlusion rims and steep condylar paths. The phenomenon by which localized gaps appear between the rows of teeth during lateral or protrusive movements while partial functional contacts are maintained is named after him: Christensen's phenomenon (Fig 7-13). This phenomenon denotes the functional separation into working side and

nonworking side, or selective tooth contact. In a fully dentate dentition, this is a necessary step to avoid premature contacts with unused teeth, which can lead to periodontal damage.

Sagittal Christensen's phenomenon denotes the separation in the area of the posterior teeth during protrusive movement when both condyles slide downward and forward and the mandible is depressed dorsally (see Fig 7-13).

Transverse Christensen's phenomenon arises during lateral movement when the nonworking condyle slides downward and forward onto the

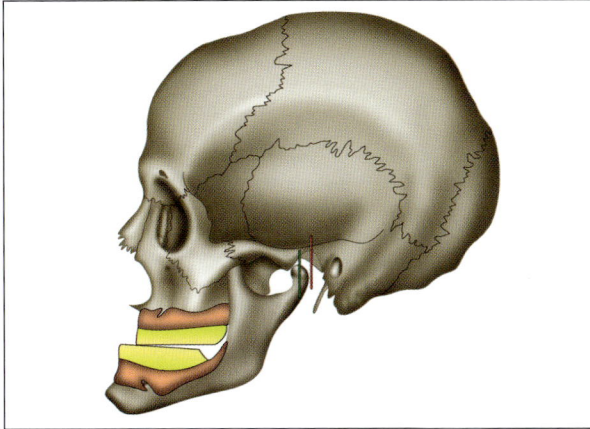

Fig 7-16 Christensen observed that coplanar occlusion rims aligned with the occlusal plane are separated in the molar region during protrusion of the mandible, while contact is maintained in the incisor area. If the difference in position is to be eliminated with occlusion rims, these need to be shaped in curves that correspond to the course of the occlusal curves but are slightly more arched.

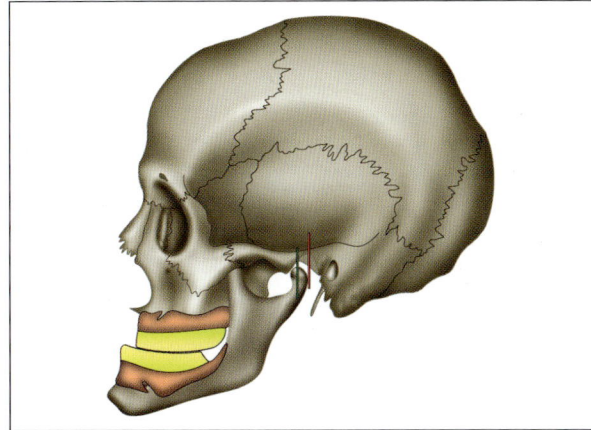

Fig 7-17 These arched curves are intended to compensate for the separation of the occlusion rims in the molar area and are therefore known as *compensatory curves*. The artificial teeth of complete dentures also lie within such compensatory curves, their curvature depending on the condylar path inclinations and the cusp inclinations of the posterior teeth.

articular tubercle, the mandible is depressed on one side, and, on that side, the teeth come out of contact (Figs 7-14 and 7-15); meanwhile, on the laterotrusive side, the working condyle slides backward and outward in keeping with Bennett (lateral) movement, and full functional tooth contact is achieved.

If the difference in position is to be eliminated in the case of occlusion rims, these need to be shaped in curves that correspond to the course of the occlusal curves but are slightly more arched (Figs 7-16). These curves then compensate for the separation of the occlusion rims in the molar area and are therefore referred to as *compensatory curves* (Fig 7-17).

Bennett Movement

The sideways movement of the mandible is mainly enforced by the lateral pterygoid muscle, which runs from the neck of the mandible to the lateral lamella of the wing of the sphenoid bone. The mandible will not only rotate around the working condyle (rotating condyle) during a lateral movement, but it is additionally moved to the side as a whole by the musculature. This lateral move-

ment of the whole mandible is known as *Bennett movement* (Fig 7-18). This sideways shift is generally no greater than 2 mm. Bennett movement is measured between the resting position and the displacement after a completed lateral movement of the mandible, in which the rotating condyle can perform different movements. Bennett movement can follow a uniform course, or it may be more pronounced at the start of the mandibular movement. A distinction is made between the initial and the integrated Bennett movement (Fig 7-19).

Progressive side shift (ie, integrated or distributed Bennett movement) means that the rotating condyle is displaced out of the resting position to the side by about 2 mm, which takes place steadily during lateral movement of the mandible.

Immediate side shift (initial Bennett movement) means that both condyles are displaced to the side at the start of lateral movement of the mandible; ie, the whole mandible performs a sideways movement running parallel to the hinge axis before the nonworking condyle moves forward, downward, and inward.

This side shift can only be performed with difficulty as an isolated movement, and it may then be interpreted as evidence of joint damage, eg, capsule or ligament strain.

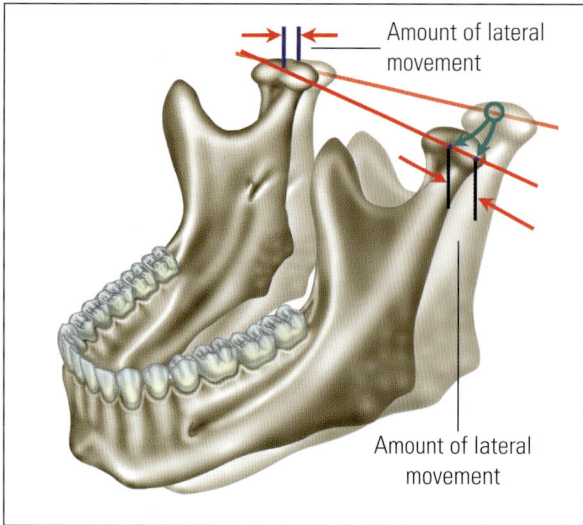

Fig 7-18 Diagram of Bennett movement. Bennett movement is the sideways spatial displacement of the working condyle during lateral movement of the mandible. It is measured between the resting position and the displacement after the lateral mandibular movement. It is approximately 2 mm and is enforced by the function of the lateral pterygoid muscle. As a result of sideways shift of the mandible, the amount of movement of the balancing condyle is also greater.

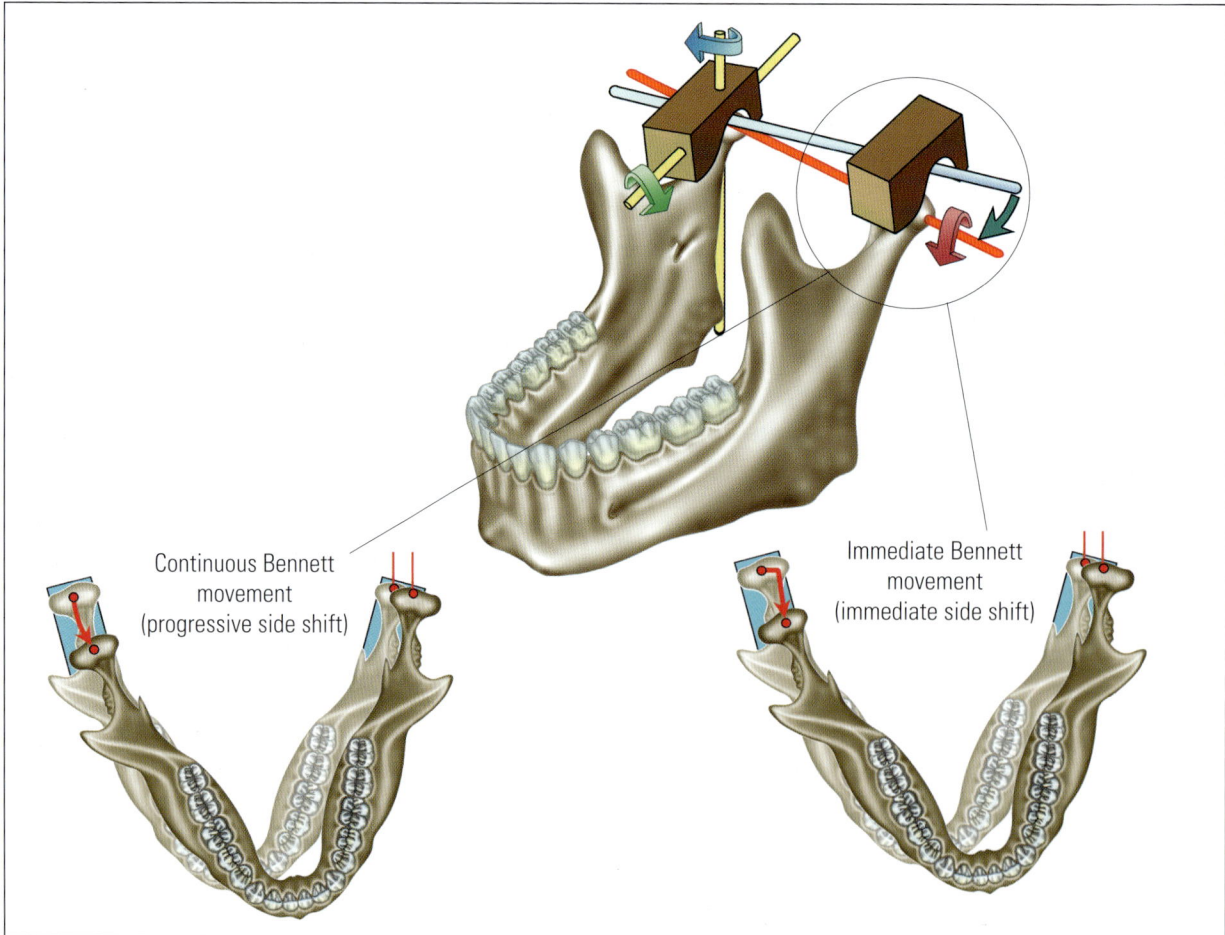

Fig 7-19 Bennett movement. A distinction is made between initial Bennett movement, which appears as a side shift of both condyles immediately at the start of lateral movement (immediate side shift), and integrated Bennett movement, which occurs continuously during lateral movement (progressive side shift).

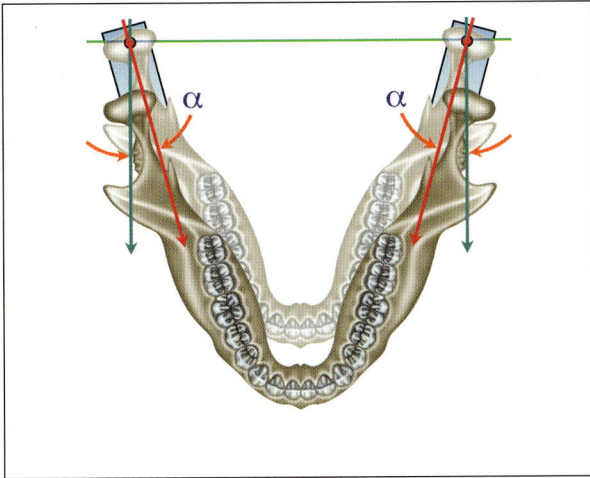

Fig 7-20 When the movement path of the nonworking condyle is plotted and connected to the movement path from the protrusive movement, the two movement paths enclose the individual Bennett angle between 0 and 20 degrees. The Bennett angle (α), measured in the horizontal plane, is an angle between the movement paths of the condyle during protrusive movement and during lateral movement.

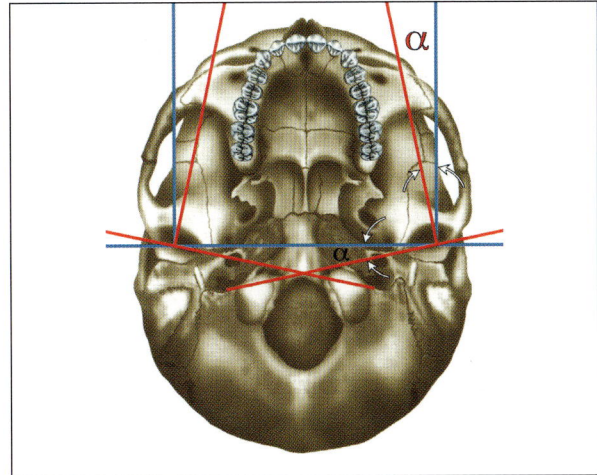

Fig 7-21 Assuming that joint parts are differentiated as passive elements of mandibular guidance, it may be assumed that the Bennett angle can be reproduced on the articular surfaces of the base of the skull. The transverse axes through the articular fossae *(red)* ought to enclose this angle for the idealized hinge axis *(blue)*. In an articulator, the Bennett angle is actually considered as rotation against the hinge axis.

Bennett movement takes place in the simplest case as a linear side shift of the working condyle. In many cases, the condyle is displaced in a particular spatial direction. The spatial side shift is described as follows:

- *Laterotrusion* is the linear sideways shift of the working condyle to the laterotrusive side.
- *Lateroretrusion* is the spatial shift of the working condyle to the side and *backward*.
- *Lateroprotrusion* is the spatial shift of the working condyle to the side and *forward*.
- *Laterodetrusion* is the spatial shift of the working condyle to the side and *downward*.
- *Laterosurtrusion* is the spatial shift of the working condyle to the side and *upward*.

The size of the Bennett movement can be measured directly or expressed indirectly via movement tracings based on the Bennett angle.

The *Bennett angle* is an angle between the movement paths of the condyle during protrusive and lateral movement of the mandible, measured in the horizontal plane. In a protrusive movement, both condyles slide downward and forward on the condylar paths. When this movement path is plotted, two lines emerge that are roughly paral-

lel to each other (parallels to the median plane) (see Fig 7-12). When the movement path of the nonworking condyle is plotted and connected to the movement path from the protrusive movement, the two movement paths enclose the individual's Bennett angle between 0 and 20 degrees (Fig 7-20). However, the Bennett angle is not the same on each side in humans.

What is the connection between Bennett movement and the Bennett angle? If, during a lateral movement of the mandible, the working condyle were only to complete a rotation around its vertical axis, a Bennett angle of approximately 6 degrees could be measured. Lateral displacement of the Bennett movement will result in an average Bennett angle of about 15 degrees.

Study of the TMJ revealed that the transverse axes of the condyles are not aligned but are rather at an angle to each other and meet at a point in front of the occipital foramen; the same is true of the transverse axes of the articular fossae. Because the condylar paths have differentiated according to the forms of mandibular movement based on the relationship between form and function, it ought to be possible to reproduce the Bennett angle on the articular surfaces of the base of the skull (Fig 7-21). If, for an idealized hinge axis, the transverse axes are drawn through the articular fossae and meet in front of the occipital foramen, this produces an angle between the idealized hinge axis and the transverse axes that roughly corresponds to the Bennett angle. Within the same angle, it can be seen that the hinge axes of the two condyles differ from an idealized, common hinge axis.

Tooth Guidance (Occlusion)

Occlusion (Latin, *occludere* = to close; closure of the teeth) generally denotes each contact between the teeth of the maxilla and the teeth of the mandible in a dentition. The status of tooth contacts in occlusion is covered by various terms intended to describe the diversity of possible mandibular positions in which tooth contact takes place. There are also terms used to describe the tooth contacts that deviate from normal. The following paragraphs outline the distinctions among terms.

Centric occlusion or *terminal occlusion* refers to closure of the dentition in which all the teeth are loaded centrally in respect of their periodontal tissue and the teeth are positioned with maximum multipoint contact (maximal intercuspation) in the sagittal and transverse directions (Fig 7-22). The condyles lie in a pressure-free centric position in terms of their articular fossae, approximately 1.0 to 1.5 mm in front of the rearmost position possible. As the dentition grows, the occluding masticatory surfaces become arranged so that the periodontal tissues are loaded exactly centrally and the masticatory force is directed onto the middle of the periodontal tissue.

Centric occlusion describes the correct physiologic loading state of the teeth involved and the TMJs. By contrast, the term **harmonious occlusion** denotes the state of idealized closure of the dentition in which all coordinating tissues of the masticatory system are harmoniously matched and absorb the load from masticatory force without interference in the periodontium, the joints, or the musculature. In harmonious occlusion, a maximum of masticatory work is performed with a minimum of muscular force.

Maximal intercuspation (or *intercuspal position*) is the smooth interlocking (intercusping) position of cusp and fossa with maximum multipoint con-

tact of the antagonizing cusps. In a normal dentition, the anatomical surfaces of the teeth, especially the oblique surfaces of the cusps, permit only one final position in which uniform contact on all sides exists (Fig 7-23). In centric occlusion, the teeth of a normal dentition are supposed to fit together in maximal intercuspation so that the transfer of forces runs axially in the teeth involved and the periodontal tissues are centrically loaded. The following paragraphs describe the relationship between tooth guidance and neuromuscular guidance and its corresponding terms.

Habitual intercuspation (or *habitual occlusion*) denotes the closure position of the teeth adopted as a result of habit, in which the reflex is to guide the teeth out of a wide opening movement into static occlusion. Ideally, maximal intercuspation would thus be achieved. The system of muscles and nerves is programmed to this centric position of the dentition. This is because a specific individual movement habit also develops during growth of the dentition, which then continues to progress in a reflex fashion and is based on occlusion of the two jaws. This is why centric occlusion with maximal intercuspation and habitual intercuspation are the same thing in a normal occlusion.

Physiologic rest position is the neutral position of the mandible in relation to the maxilla (unconscious maintenance of space between the jaws) adopted by reflex and held by the resting tension of the muscles, without any tooth contact (Fig 7-24). In this neuromuscular resting position of the mandible, all the muscles of mastication have a specific length. In the relaxed state, the mandible opens out of centric occlusion in a pure hinge movement of a few millimeters and is suspended in muscular guidance; the lips lie together without pressure. In this habitual position, the teeth have what is known as **freeway space**, the amount of which can fluctuate with the circadian rhythm. The physiologic rest position can be reproduced in edentulous patients and can be used to determine the occlusal height.

Static occlusion is the terminal occlusal position when there is full contact between mandibular and maxillary teeth in the resting position.

Dynamic occlusion or articulation denotes the tooth contacts during mandibular movements where the centric stops move out of the contact areas on the antagonizing triangular ridges of the cusps and on the tooth guidance paths (articula-

Fig 7-22 Centric occlusion denotes the position of dentate jaws in relation to each other, in which the teeth lie in maximal intercuspation in the sagittal (A) and transverse (B) directions and the periodontal tissues are loaded exactly in the middle (centrically). The condyles (C) of the mandible generally lie slightly in front of the rearmost position in the articular fossa, but they could be pulled back about 1.5 mm.

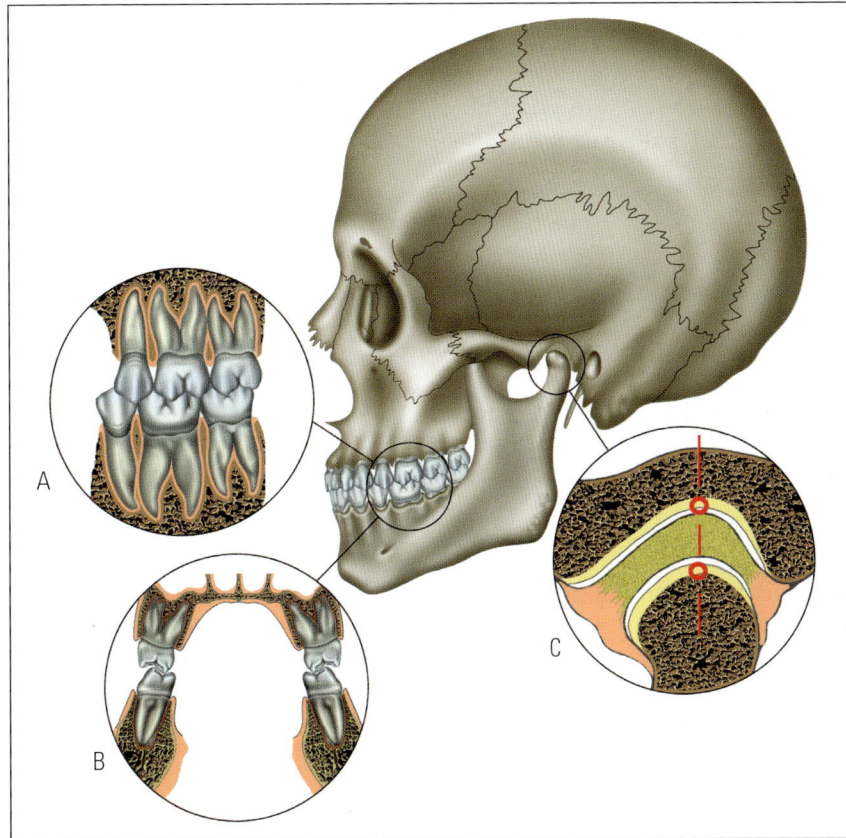

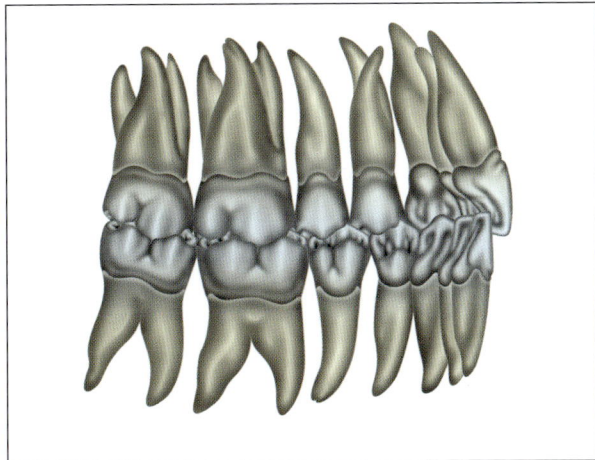

Fig 7-23 In a regular occlusion, simultaneous and smooth cusp-fossa occlusion occurs with maximal intercuspation. All the palatal cusps of the maxillary teeth fit into the areas of the central developmental grooves of the mandibular teeth, while the mandibular buccal cusps fit into the central developmental grooves of the maxillary teeth. In a normal occlusion, the maxillary anterior teeth interlock labially over and in front of the mandibular anterior teeth.

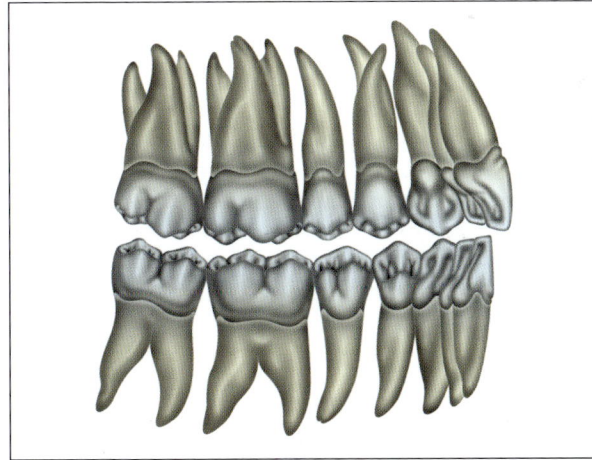

Fig 7-24 In a relaxed state, the teeth are not in occlusal contact but show an interocclusal gap (freeway space). In the lingual view, the rows of cusps can be seen arranged in the sagittal and transverse directions. When the teeth are brought together, the cusps fit together according to the two-cusp principle.

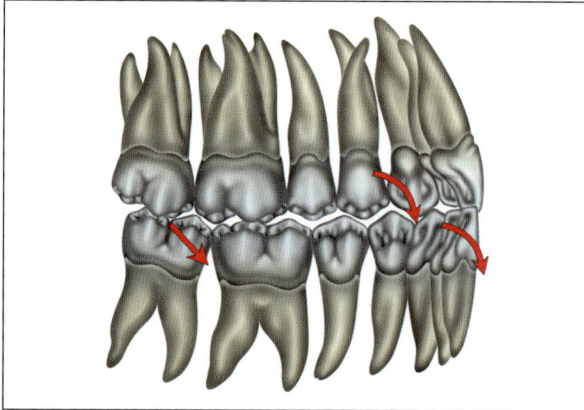

Fig 7-25 Anterior guidance takes place during mandibular movement ventrally (protrusion) and in lateral movement; the other teeth disocclude.

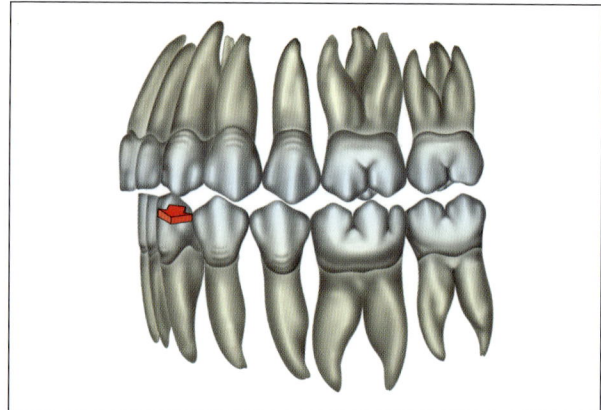

Fig 7-26 In canine guidance, dynamic occlusion contacts are only found between the maxillary and mandibular canines.

tion paths). The tooth contacts in dynamic occlusion occur during regular chewing movements and are therefore a particular focus of analysis. *Eccentric occlusion*, a term used to designate all tooth contacts deviating from maximal intercuspation, can be seen as a synonym for *dynamic occlusion*.

Dynamic Occlusion

In dynamic occlusion, different physiologic sliding movement situations arise within the dentition, and these are described by different concepts of occlusion.

Physiologically, dynamic occlusion means there are no pathologic changes to hard tissues, periodontal tissue, the TMJs, or masticatory musculature. It is characterized by mutual functioning of the anterior and posterior teeth; ie, there is an uninterrupted, progressive continuity of occlusal surfaces whereby harmonious jaw movements are undertaken by incisal or canine guidance.

A distinction is made between various occlusal concepts to describe **selective tooth contacts** of individual groups of teeth or parts of the dentition for preparing food in protrusive and lateral jaw movements. Because a mouthful of food is only ever processed on one side of the dentition, there needs to be a functional separation of the nonworking portions of the dentition to avoid inter-

ference with sliding on that side. To bite off food, the anterior teeth must form a selective "biting off" (incision) contact without the posterior teeth being caught in interfering sliding contacts. A distinction is made between anterior-supported, canine-supported, and balanced occlusion.

Anterior-supported occlusion (or *anterior guidance*) denotes the selective contact of anterior teeth during habitual mandibular movements in which all the other teeth are disoccluding (separating) (Fig 7-25).

Canine-supported occlusion (or *canine guidance*) is the selective tooth contact during habitual mandibular movements that leads to disocclusion of all the other teeth (Fig 7-26).

Balanced occlusion denotes contact between the rows of teeth during habitual mandibular movements; it can be either unilaterally balanced or bilaterally balanced occlusion.

Unilaterally balanced occlusion is guidance by a group of teeth in a natural, fully dentate dentition where the teeth on the working side enter into a smooth sliding contact while there is a gap between the rows of posterior teeth on the nonworking side (Fig 7-27).

Bilaterally balanced occlusion means sliding contact of all teeth on both the working side and the nonworking side during lateral mandibular movements (Fig 7-28). This form of occlusion is rarely found in a normal occlusal situation, mostly in a worn dentition. Bilaterally balanced occlusion is avoided in reconstruction of a permanent

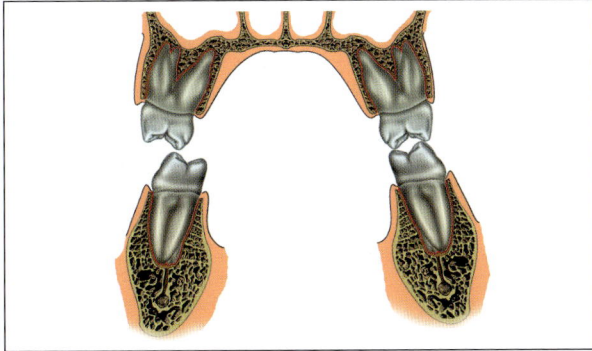

Fig 7-27 Unilaterally balanced occlusion means dynamic occlusion contacts on the working side (laterotrusive side) during lateral movements.

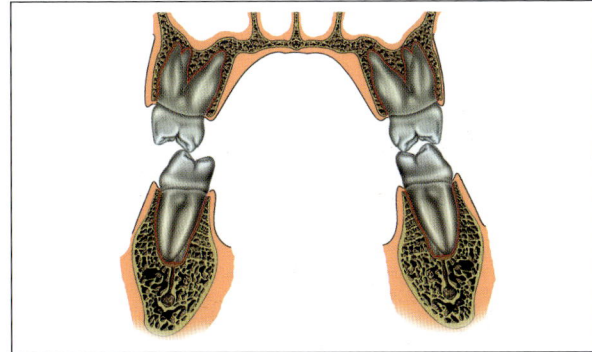

Fig 7-28 Bilaterally balanced occlusion denotes dynamic occlusion contacts on both the working side and the nonworking side.

restoration. However, it is required for mucosa-supported complete dentures for static reasons, in which case it is referred to as *fully balanced occlusion* or ***prosthetic occlusion***.

The transition of movement out of static into dynamic occlusion, with its selective tooth contacts, takes place in a horizontal movement field 0.5 to 1.0 mm wide, which is known as the ***occlusal field*** (or *occlusal area*). During lateral movements, there is tooth guidance without malocclusions or occlusal interferences. The occlusal field between habitual intercuspation and the rearmost contact position is known as ***long centric***.

A ***malocclusion*** denotes incorrect occlusion that is locally limited or more extensive and is caused by the malposition of individual teeth or groups of teeth, by shifts in occlusal position, by premature contacts of restorations, or by fillings. These malocclusions will become a ***traumatizing occlusion*** if faulty loading of individual teeth or groups of teeth takes place, which can cause changes in the stomatognathic system.

Occlusal interferences are disruptions of tooth contact that force the mandible into a slipping-off position. A distinction is drawn between premature contacts and obstacles to gliding during mandibular movements.

Centric occlusion is synonymous with a central, middle position of the jaws in relation to each other, from which any movement position of the mandible can be performed. When occluding teeth are absent, this central position must be rediscovered (Fig 7-29). The centric relation denotes the position of the mandible when both condyles

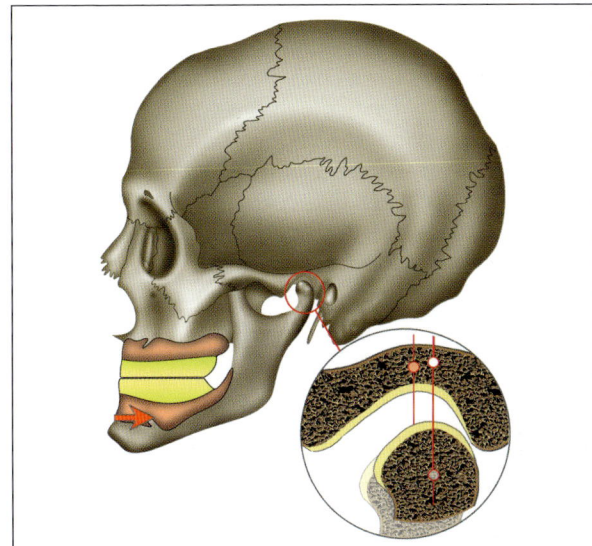

Fig 7-29 The central position of the edentulous jaws in relation to each other can be established if the condyles of the mandible are brought into the posterior position in the articular fossa. This is usually a forced position but is the only position that can be exactly reproduced in edentulous jaws.

of the TMJs rest in their superoposterior position in the articular fossae (retral contact position); the central relation is jaw- and joint-oriented. The mandible often has to be manipulated back into this position, which is why this position is of limited suitability for prosthetic rehabilitation work.

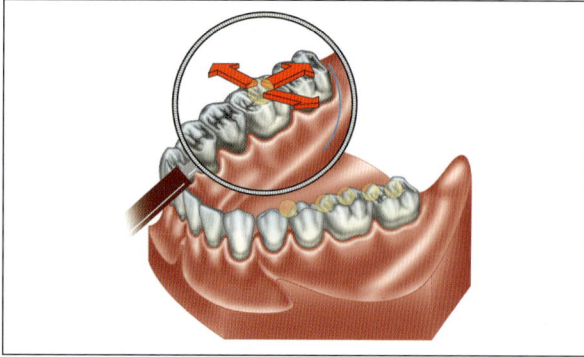

Fig 7-30 Centric stops in the contact fields depicted as circles.

Tooth Contacts During Mandibular Movement

When depicting the occlusal contact points in detail, it is essential to view these contacts in articulation or establish the paths they follow during mandibular movement. The articular movements of the centric stops run on precisely fixed occlusal guidance paths of their antagonists (Fig 7-30).

During **protrusive movement**, the working cusps with their centric stops slide out of their analogous contact areas, the approximal marginal ridges or central fossae, in the central developmental groove in a sagittal direction. The movement paths tend to point distally in the mandible and mesially in the maxilla.

In **lateral movements**, the movement paths must be regarded separately for the working and nonworking sides for both the maxilla and the mandible. On the **working side in the maxilla**, the centric stops of the antagonizing cusps slide out of the contact areas via the approximal furrows or the buccal notches of the molars in a vestibular direction (Fig 7-31). The occlusal guidance paths are the palatally directed oblique surfaces of the triangular ridges of the buccal cusps.

- The buccal cusps of the mandibular premolars and the mesiobuccal cusps of the mandibular molars slide in a vestibular direction in the approximal marginal ridges of the maxillary teeth; contact is not lost until there is a wide deflection of movement.
- The distobuccal cusps of the mandibular molars slide out of the central fossae along the main developmental groove on the triangular ridges of their antagonists in a vestibular direction.

On the **working side in the mandible**, the centric stops of the antagonizing cusps slide out of the contact areas, such as approximal furrows or the central fossae, in a lingual direction (Fig 7-32). The occlusal guidance paths in the mandible are on the buccal oblique surfaces of the triangular ridges of the lingual cusps.

- The palatal cusps of the maxillary premolars and the distopalatal cusps of the maxillary molars slide in the approximal marginal ridges of the mandibular teeth in a lingual direction; contact is not lost until there is a wide deflection of movement.
- The mesiopalatal cusps of the maxillary molars slide out of the central fossa along the main developmental groove on the triangular ridges of their antagonists in a lingual direction.

On the **nonworking side in the maxilla**, the centric stops slide out of the contact areas (approximal furrows, central fossae) in a lingual direction. The occlusal guidance paths in the maxilla are the buccally directed oblique surfaces of the triangular ridges of the maxillary palatal cusps. The lingual movement paths lose contact in regular intercuspal conditions, which is taken into account in permanent restoration work.

- The buccal centric stops of the mandibular premolars and the mesiobuccal cusps of the mandibular molars slide from the approximal marginal ridges of the maxillary antagonists on the cusp ridges to the cusp tips in a lingual direction.

Fig 7-31 *(a)* The combination of the movement paths from the contact fields shows that the movements in the maxilla have a tendency to the mesial. In protrusive movements, the centric stops run almost in the central developmental grooves of the antagonists. In the maxilla, the centric stops during lateral movements either run through the approximal furrows or the buccal notches of the molars in a vestibular direction or extend from the approximal furrows on the cusp ridges to the cusp tips in a lingual direction. *(b)* The working-side contacts are marked in *yellow*, while the cusps of the nonworking side *(blue)* remain without occlusal contact. *(c)* In protrusive movement, the cusps are taken out of occlusal contact. *(d)* The working-side contacts are again shown in *yellow* and the cusps of the nonworking side (without occlusal contact) in *blue*.

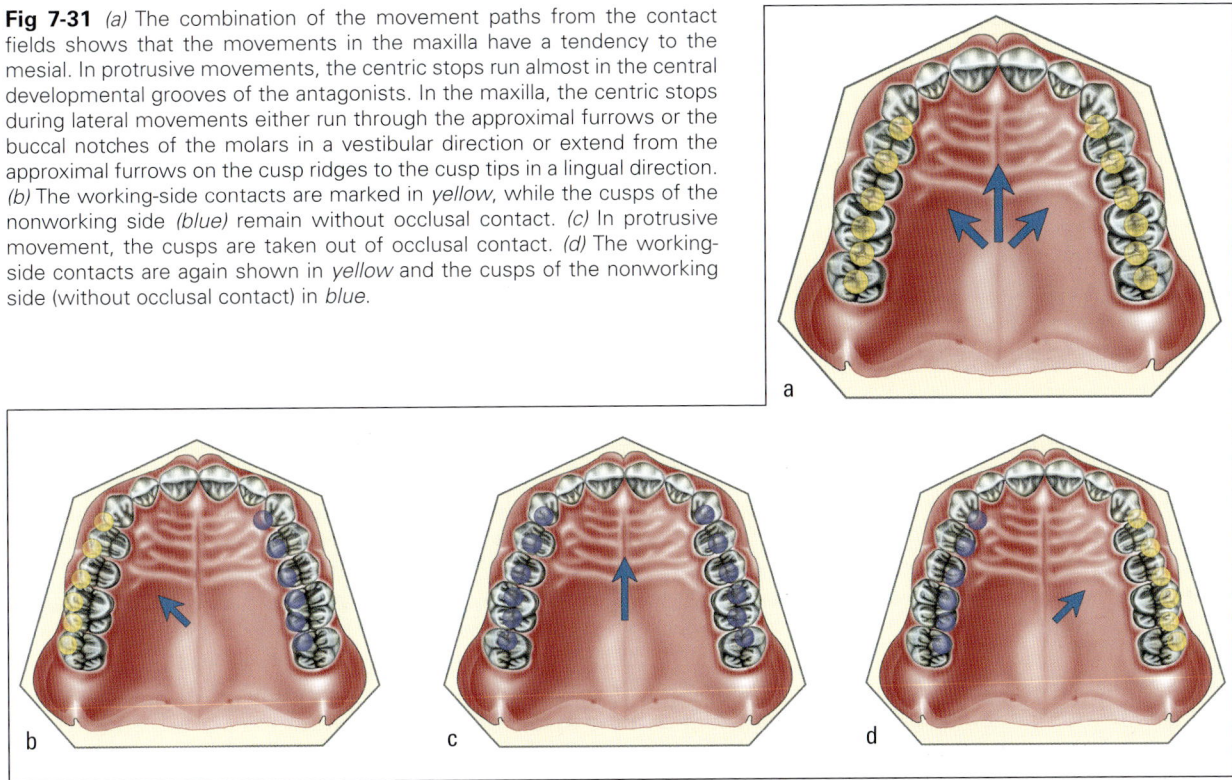

Fig 7-32 *(a to d)* The movement paths from the contact fields of the mandible in relation to mandibular movement show a pronounced form-and-function relationship. The antagonizing centric stops run out of the contact fields in the pits and furrows of the occlusal surfaces. Only the nonworking contacts would run over the cusp ridges or cusp tips. In canine guidance, contact areas of the other teeth are raised.

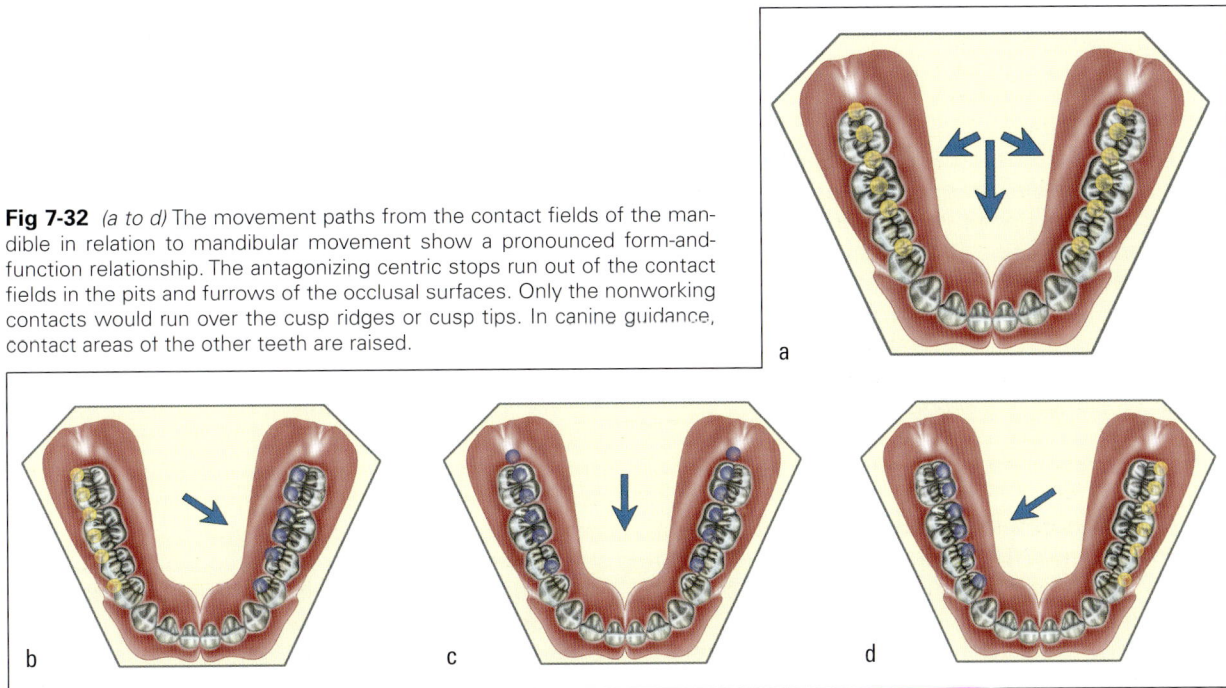

• The distobuccal cusps of the mandibular molars slide out of the central fossae on the mesial triangular ridges of the maxillary mesiopalatal molar cusps in a lingual direction.

On the **nonworking side in the mandible**, the centric stops slide out of the contact areas in a vestibular direction. The occlusal guidance paths in the mandible are the lingually directed oblique surfaces of the buccal cusps.

• The palatal cusps of the maxillary premolars and the distopalatal cusps of the maxillary molars slide from the approximal marginal ridges of the mandibular teeth along the mesial triangular ridges of the mesiobuccal mandibular cusps.
• The mesiobuccal cusps of the maxillary molars slide out of the central fossae on the mesial articulation surfaces of the distobuccal cusps of the mandibular molars.

In complete dentures, the stabilizing balancing contacts lie on the palatal cusps in the maxilla or on the vestibular cusps in the mandible. If guidance by a particular group of teeth (canine or anterior guidance) is being constructed, all the contact areas of the other teeth are raised.

Muscle Tissue

A **muscle** is an organ of movement made up of many muscle cells that uses its contractive ability to move the bones or, as a hollow muscle or sphincter muscle does, make cavities smaller and close openings. The individual muscle cells are joined together by connective tissue membranes or sheaths, which in turn merge to form tendons and are thus able to transfer forces (Fig 7-33).

Muscle tissue is a contractile tissue, which means that its cytoplasm (known as *sarcoplasm*) has special fibers (myofibrils) that are able to contract. Based on differences in structure and very different physiologic characteristics, three separate types of muscle tissue are described: smooth muscle tissue, cardiac muscle tissue, and striated muscle tissue.

Smooth muscle cells are oval or spindle-shaped cells 20 to 500 µm in length. These muscle cells have only one nucleus, which is always centrally located. In terms of microstructure, the myofibrils of the sarcoplasm run parallel to the long axis of the cell. Each smooth muscle cell is sheathed in a delicate membrane (sarcolemma) made up of reticulin fibers, while the ends of the cell merge into very fine tendons. This type of muscle tissue is only able to contract very slowly but displays excellent endurance. This is why smooth musculature is found in vessel walls, the intestinal walls, the airways, and other places where prolonged, rhythmic contractions are involved. This musculature is therefore also described as visceral musculature.

A typical form of work is the peristaltic movement in the digestive tract, which propels food forward in the intestinal tube. Smooth musculature may also form powerful rings of muscle (sphincter muscles) that serve as opening and closing muscles (eg, pyloric part of the stomach). Another special characteristic of the smooth musculature is that it is controlled by the autonomic nervous system, which means that it is not influenced voluntarily. Autonomic conduction pathways, which are activated by certain stimulating substances (epinephrine/adrenaline and acetylcholine), may thus be found in the muscle layers of the smooth musculature.

Cardiac musculature (myocardium) is a specific type of striated musculature that nevertheless bears strong similarities to smooth musculature. Different cells join together in the myocardium to form a network, and holes in the network are filled with loose connective tissue. The cell nuclei lie in the middle of the cells and are surrounded by transverse striated (striped) myofibrils. The individual muscle cells are meshed in what are known as *intercalated discs* and are cemented with intercellular substance, as if a kind of cell fusion were taking place. The myocardial cells are also enclosed by a sheath of reticulin fibers.

The conduction system of the cardiac musculature lies within a connective tissue sheath close to the lining membrane of the heart (endocardium). This autonomic control system produces a strong, rhythmic, and involuntary contraction of the cardiac musculature, but this contraction can also be influenced by the autonomic nervous system and by hormonal regulation.

Striated muscle cells are fibers measuring a few millimeters to 10 cm in length, with a great

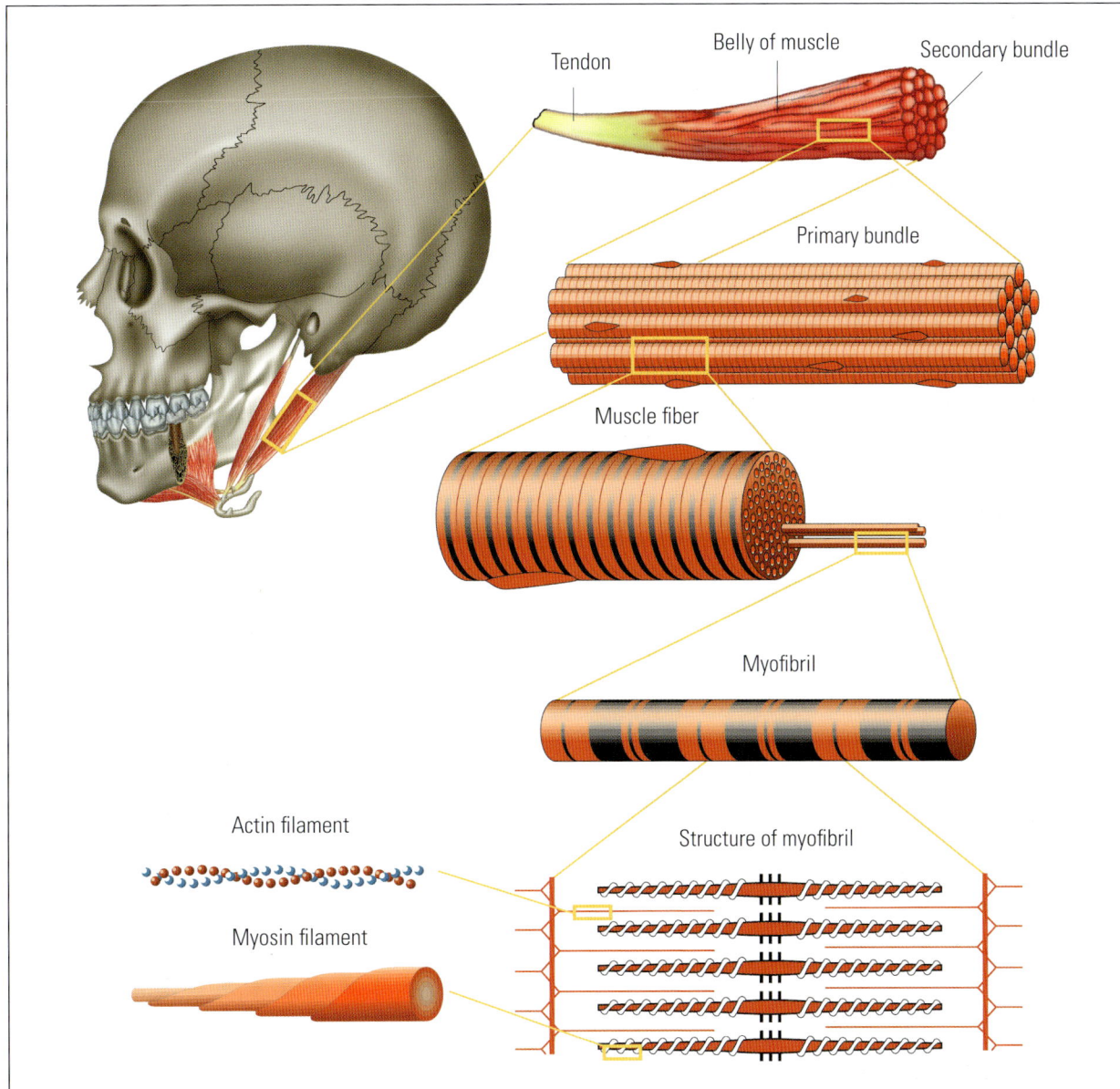

Fig 7-33 Diagram of the structure of a muscle.

number of cell nuclei at their periphery; as many as 100 nuclei may be found in one cell. The myofibrils lie in the middle of the cell and, as a result of their arrangement into light and dark segments, give the impression of crosswise stripes (transverse striation) (Fig 7-34).

The striated muscle fibers are also encased in a membrane (sarcolemma) made of ultrathin reticulin fibers, which again form tendons at the ends. Muscle fibers with varying proportions of sarcoplasm and mitochondria (sarcosomes) can be differentiated. Muscle fibers with a lot of sar-

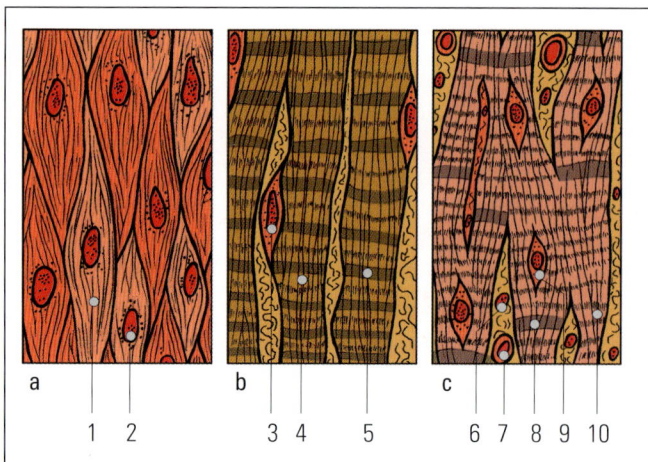

Fig 7-34 Longitudinal sections through muscle tissue. *(a)* Longitudinal striated musculature. 1, muscle cell with myofibrils; 2, muscle cell nucleus. *(b)* Transverse striated musculature. 3, cell nucleus lying in the sarcolemma; 4, muscle fiber with myofibrils; 5, transverse striation of anisotropic discs. *(c)* Cardiac musculature. 6, nucleus of a connective tissue cell; 7, blood capillary; 8, intercalated disc; 9, muscle cell nucleus; 10, cardiac muscle fiber with fine transverse striation.

coplasm but few mitochondria appear light in color and only work for a short time, but very quickly; muscle fibers with little sarcoplasm and a lot of mitochondria appear dark and, at a moderate contraction speed, can work for a relatively long time.

Skeletal musculature made up of striated muscle fibers is the main constituent of the active locomotor system. It is controlled by the somatic nervous system, so it is subject to a person's will. The striated muscle cells react rapidly but tire very quickly. They can be stimulated by electrical impulses and can be influenced by heat and cold. The masticatory musculature, as part of the active locomotor system, is made up of striated muscle fibers.

Muscle as a Motor Unit

Muscle contractions are triggered by nerve impulses. In the case of voluntary movements, the nerve impulses are transmitted by motor nerve pathways from the cerebral cortex via the spinal cord to the motor end plates on the individual muscle fibers. The number of muscle fibers in a muscle may be as high as two million. Each muscle fiber can be stimulated independently and contract separately from the other fibers. All the muscle fibers can be stimulated at once by the nervous system, or only some of them can

be stimulated and a movement can be performed with graduated expenditure of energy. Destruction of nerve conduction results in paralysis of the muscle and inactivity atrophy; ie, the muscle shrinks or atrophies. Muscle mass will increase if put under heavy strain.

Skeletal muscles have a uniform structure: The ends of a muscle are referred to as the *insertion* and the *origin* (sites of attachment), while the actual muscle mass is known as the *belly (venter)*. The origin *(caput)* denotes the point where the muscle attaches to the passive locomotor system. Contraction of the muscle mass pulls the point of insertion and point of origin closer together so that the bones are moved, mostly via joints. However, there are also muscles in the locomotor system without a specific origin and insertion, eg, certain facial expression muscles. As a rule, the skeletal muscles always have corresponding antagonists that accomplish the same movement but in reverse. This is not actual antagonism but a functional interaction, even where the pull is in opposite directions, because this is the only way that coordinated movements can take place.

Muscle tone refers to the resting tension when a muscle is in its relaxed state. The tone ensures that certain permanent postures can be assumed, eg, that of the trunk when the body is erect. The tone of the masticatory musculature holds the mandible in the physiologic rest position.

Contraction of a muscle takes place through a very rapid succession of individual shortenings of

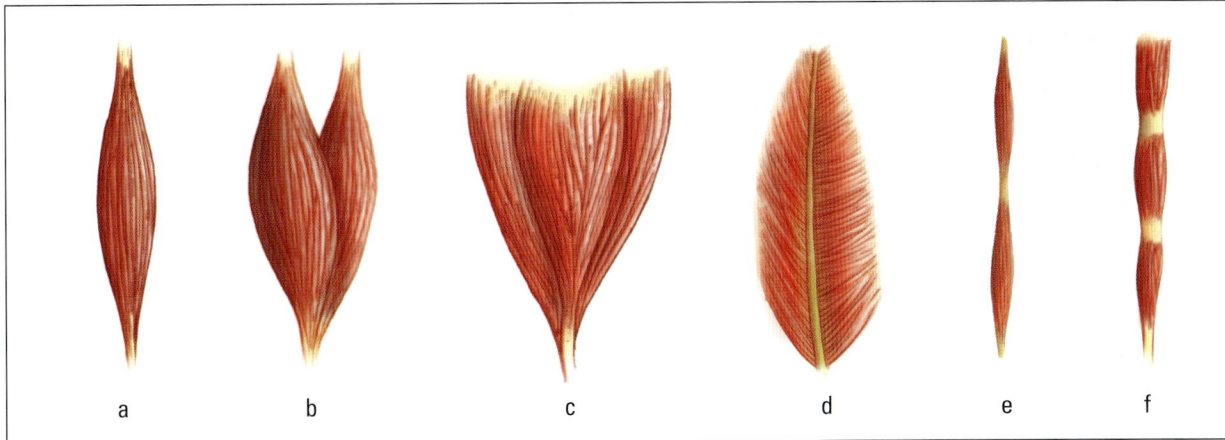

Fig 7-35 The relationship of the muscle to the tendon is dependent on the assigned functions. The following distinctions are made: *(a)* simple, spindle-shaped muscle; *(b)* two-headed muscle (eg, bicep); *(c)* three-headed muscle (eg, deltoid); *(d)* double-sided pennate muscle; *(e)* biventer muscle; *(f)* muscle with tendinous intersections (eg, rectus abdominis muscle).

the muscle fibers. To maintain continuous shortening, the nervous stimulation has to activate the muscle periodically; in other words, the muscle has to be switched on and off. In terms of frequency, the muscle starts to vibrate and thus produces a muscle tone of roughly 30 Hz.

Muscle power can be determined in relation to the cross-sectional area of the muscle: A muscle with a cross-sectional area of 1 cm^2 produces an absolute muscular power of about 100 N. Certain auxiliary organs, such as nerves and blood vessels, tendons and tendon sheaths, and bursae and fasciae belong to muscles.

Tendons are made up of white, shiny, parallel fibers of collagenous connective tissue with high tensile strength (50 N/mm^2). They emerge from the combination of sheaths of individual muscle fibers and generally attach in the periosteum of the bones. However, direct insertion of a tendon into the bone may also occur.

Tendon sheaths affix tendons to the bone or joints to safeguard the functioning of the tendons themselves. The tendon sheath secretes mucus—similar to synovial fluid in the joints—so that the tendon is able to glide back and forth smoothly.

Bursae are sacs or saclike cavities found around joints that act like a cushion of water; ie, they hold

pressure away from the bone to prevent bone destruction. Bursae are found wherever tendons pass close by the bone, especially at the joints.

Fasciae are sheaths of connective tissue around individual muscles or muscle groups. The fasciae form guiding sheaths and hold the muscles in the correct position in their relaxed state. When they are particularly sturdy and tendonlike, fasciae may also form points of origin and insertion for muscle fibers.

Muscles vary in shape; they can be short, long, wide, or flat (Fig 7-35). Skeletal muscles are classified according to their tendinous parts:

- Spindle-shaped muscles with a tendon of origin and insertion on a spindle-shaped belly; simple, two-headed (bicipital), three-headed (tricipital), or multitailed muscles are possible (see Figs 7-35a to 7-35c)
- Pennate (feathery) muscles with a central tendon from which the muscle fibers emanate on one or both sides (see Fig 7-35d)
- Fan-shaped muscles are multiserrated or multi-divided muscles
- Muscles with tendinous intersections, eg, biventer muscles (mylohyoid muscle) (see Figs 7-35e and 7-35f)

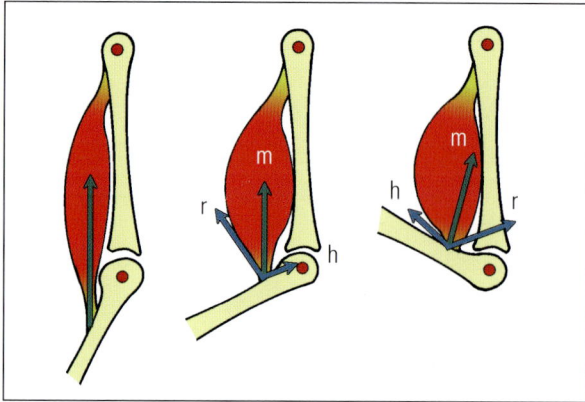

Fig 7-36 In each muscle, a distinction is made between a rotary action (r) and a hinge action (h). Where muscles and the bone to be moved are at right angles to each other, the rotary action is greatest, actually equal to the muscular traction (m). Given the different positions of the bones being moved, the hinge action brings either tractive forces or compressive forces to bear on the joint.

In each muscle, a distinction is made between a rotary action and a hinge action. Figure 7-36 illustrates this distinction and what kind of forces each action bears on the joint.

Muscles of Mandibular Movement

The *TMJs* and *teeth* are the rigid guide elements of mandibular movement; muscle guidance forms the third element. Muscles of mastication, as an active part of the locomotor system, move the mandible against the cranium and produce masticatory pressure. The TMJ is relatively elastic and unstable because of the intrinsic mobility and compressibility of tissue and the bisection of the joint by the disc. Tooth guidance functions within small deflections of movement (ie, only movements with tooth contact are maintained). All movements outside of tooth contact are mainly guided by the interaction of the different masticatory muscles. Each person develops a differentiated habit of masticatory movements for different food consistencies.

The *habitual movements* are matched to the shapes of the teeth and the form of the TMJ. Both tissue parts "imprint" themselves onto this movement habit, just as this habit is determined by the particular form of the other guidance factors. The process of differentiation follows the laws of form and function and is always changeable; ie, movement habits and the TMJ adapt to changes within

the dentition, whether due to tooth loss or prosthetic treatment. However, this means that faulty dentures can lead to pathologic changes in these guide elements.

The *masticatory musculature* does not include all the muscles involved in mandibular movement but only those that are excited by the mandibular branch of the trigeminal nerve and extend from the skull to the mandible. They form a functional unit that developed genetically from the branchial muscles (*branchial* = relating to fishes' gills). There are four pairs of muscles that originated from a common muscle mass and are still interconnected at their borders. The four paired masticatory muscles are the temporal muscle, the masseter muscle, and the medial and lateral pterygoid muscles (Fig 7-37).

A *theoretical classification of muscles* in relation to mandibular movement divides them into mouth-closing and mouth-opening muscles and those that pull forward and sideways. This classification names the main functions of these muscles and conceals the relationship whereby mandibular movement is only performed by the combined activity of the different groups of muscles. For instance, all the muscles of mandibular movement become active during highly discriminating tactile movements.

Mouth-closing muscles (masseter, medial pterygoid, temporal muscle) produce an average of 700 N and a maximum of 1,250 N of masticatory pressure in the molar region. In the incisal area, masticatory pressure is approximately 400 N because of the unfavorable leverage conditions. Where a denture is not supported by the

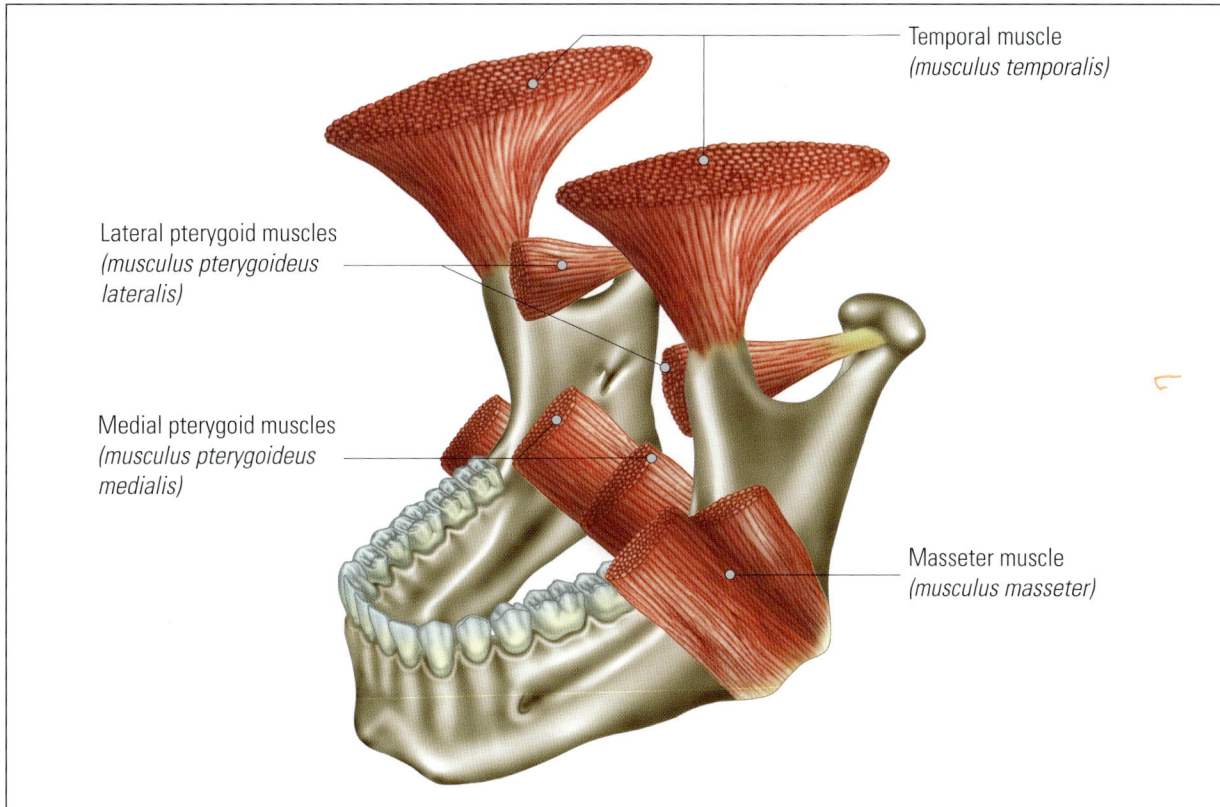

Temporal muscle
(musculus temporalis)

Lateral pterygoid muscles
(musculus pterygoideus
lateralis)

Medial pterygoid muscles
(musculus pterygoideus
medialis)

Masseter muscle
(musculus masseter)

Fig 7-37 Muscles of mandibular movement.

periodontium, the average masticatory pressure is about 100 N.

Mouth closing (elevation; raising the mandible) is performed by the masseter muscles, medial pterygoid muscles, and the vertical fibers of the temporal muscles; the suprahyoid muscles prevent closing from occurring too quickly or from being uncontrolled.

Mouth-opening muscles are muscles of the floor of the mouth, namely the mylohyoid, geniohyoid, and digastric muscles as well as the suprahyoid and infrahyoid muscles. **Sideways and forward movement** is performed by several muscles.

Mouth opening (depression; lowering the mandible) is performed by the geniohyoid and mylohyoid muscles, the anterior bellies of the digastric muscles, and parts of the lateral pterygoid muscles. In this movement, the hyoid is fixed by the infrahyoid muscles.

Forward movements of the mandible (protrusion) are effected by the lateral pterygoid muscles, the transverse fibers of the medial pterygoid muscles and masseter muscles, as well as the fibers of the temporal muscles that run forward.

Sideways movements (laterotrusion; grinding movements) are firstly performed by the muscles on the opposite side, with support from the backward-running fibers of the temporal muscle on the laterotrusive side. When the mandible is sliding into centric occlusion from the lateral position, all the muscles on the laterotrusive side come into action, so that the mandible is also pulled forward from a slightly retruded position.

The mandible is pulled backward (retrusion) by the horizontal fibers of the temporal muscles and the infrahyoid muscles, the hyoid bone being fixed by the infrahyoid muscles.

Figure 7-38 illustrates the direction of movement of the masticatory muscles.

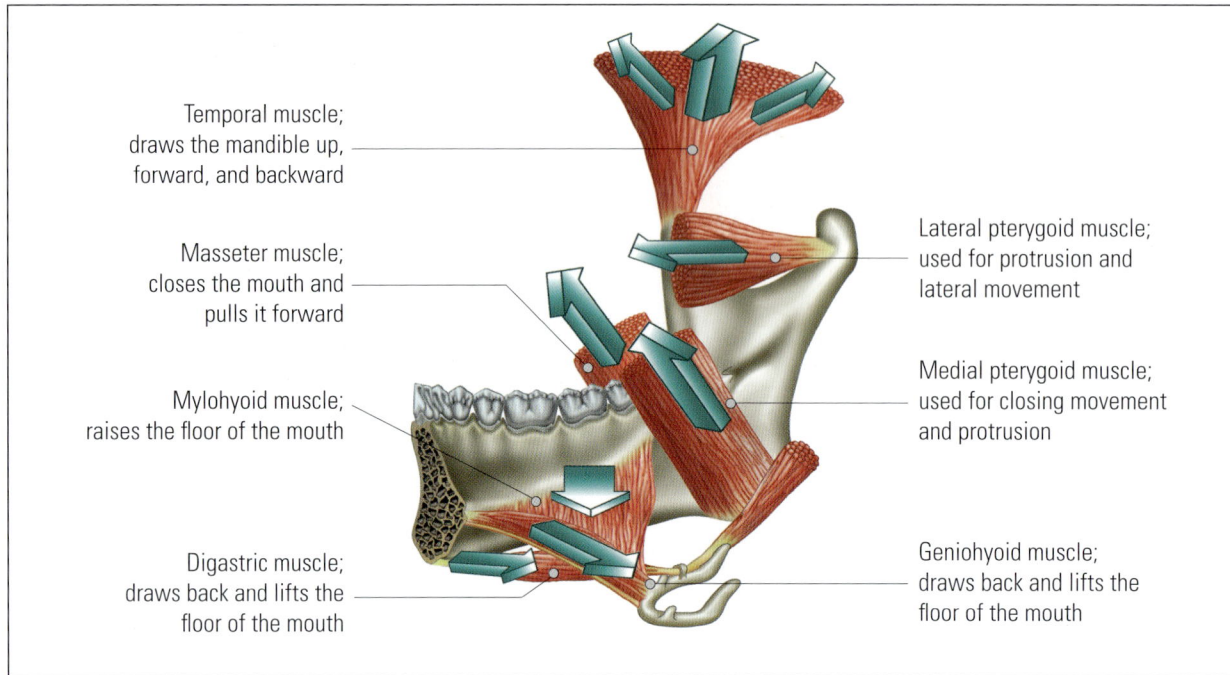

Temporal muscle; draws the mandible up, forward, and backward

Masseter muscle; closes the mouth and pulls it forward

Mylohyoid muscle; raises the floor of the mouth

Digastric muscle; draws back and lifts the floor of the mouth

Lateral pterygoid muscle; used for protrusion and lateral movement

Medial pterygoid muscle; used for closing movement and protrusion

Geniohyoid muscle; draws back and lifts the floor of the mouth

Fig 7-38 Direction of movement of the masticatory muscles.

Masticatory Muscles

The **temporal muscle** *(musculus temporalis)* is the strongest mouth-closing muscle. Its origin is in the whole temporal fossa, which is almost completely filled. It is made up of a fan-shaped muscle bundle, whose fibers combine to form a very sturdy tendon that runs within the zygoma to the muscular process of the ramus of the mandible. The muscle insertion is actually the whole anterior edge of the ramus of the mandible. The individual bundles of fibers of the fan of muscle partly run in opposite directions.

The fibers running backward draw the mandible backward, while the fibers running vertically work as true mouth-closing muscles; those running obliquely forward are also able to pull the mandible forward. After tooth loss, when this muscle is no longer fully stressed, the muscle mass atrophies and the temporal fossae become sunken. In older people, this reinforces the impression of aging.

The **lateral pterygoid muscle** *(musculus pterygoideus lateralis)* is the muscle that is involved in all movements of the mandible. It comprises two muscle bundles, the upper head of which has its origin on the external surface of the lateral lamina of the pterygoid process of the sphenoid bone *(lamina lateralis processus pterygoidei)*. The lower head of the muscle originates rather deeper at the infratemporal surface of the sphenoid *(facies infratemporalis ossis sphenoidalis)*. The upper muscle bundle runs backward to the capsule of the TMJ and into the articular disc, suggesting that the disc developed from the tendon of this muscle. The lower bundle converges toward the pterygoid fossa of the neck of the mandible below the condyle.

The lateral pterygoid muscle pulls the condyle and the articular disc forward. When the muscles contract on both sides, the mandible moves forward. When it contracts on one side, a lateral movement is performed. The lateral pterygoid muscles are always involved in jaw opening.

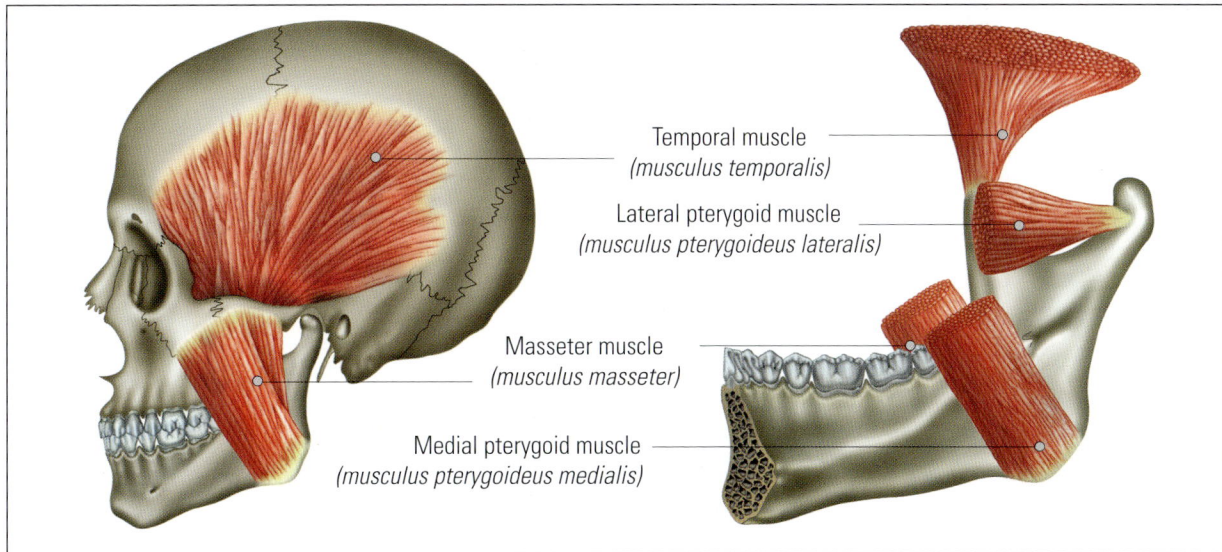

Fig 7-39 Lateral view of masticatory muscles.

The **masseter muscle** *(musculus masseter)* has its origin at the zygoma and the zygomatic arch and its insertion at the mandibular angle, externally at the masseteric tuberosities *(tuberositates massetericae)*. The muscle is divided into a sturdy, superficial part *(pars superficialis)* and a deeper-lying part *(pars profunda)*. The fibers of the superficial part run from the zygoma, coming obliquely downward and backward to the vertical edge of the ramus at the mandibular angle. The fibers of the deeper part run almost perpendicular from the zygoma to the inferior edge of the mandibular body.

The **masseter** is a powerful mouth-closing muscle that lies along the surface of the side of the face. The two muscle bundles cross over and form a pocket that is open posteriorly. The direction of pull of both bundles produces a rocking movement around the first molar.

The **medial pterygoid muscle** *(musculus pterygoideus medialis)* originates in the pterygoid fossa of the pterygoid process of the sphenoid *(fossa pterygoidea)* at the internal lamina of this process and runs obliquely downward and backward to the mandibular angle, inward to the pterygoid tuberosities. A few fibers also have their origin at the infratemporal surface of the maxilla. As these sites of origin lie closer together than the sites of insertion on the mandible, the muscle rather fans out toward the mandibular angle.

The medial pterygoid muscle runs parallel to the masseter and therefore also has the same direction of pull as a mouth-closing muscle. It raises the mandible and, like the superficial part of the masseter, may be involved in protrusive movements.

The masseter and the medial pterygoid muscle form a loop around the mandibular angle in which the mandible lies. The muscle bundle of the masseter is directed upward and outward from the mandibular angle, while that of the medial pterygoid is directed upward and inward. These two pull components—those directed outward and those directed inward—balance each other out during simultaneous contraction, which is why these two muscles can be seen as synergistic (acting together).

During lateral movements, both muscles may also become active. When the jaw is moved to the right, the medial pterygoid muscle and the masseter muscle on the left become active; lateral movement will be supported by the fibers running obliquely forward and upward from the mandibular angle to their origin.

Figures 7-39 and 7-40 illustrate the masticatory muscles from different views.

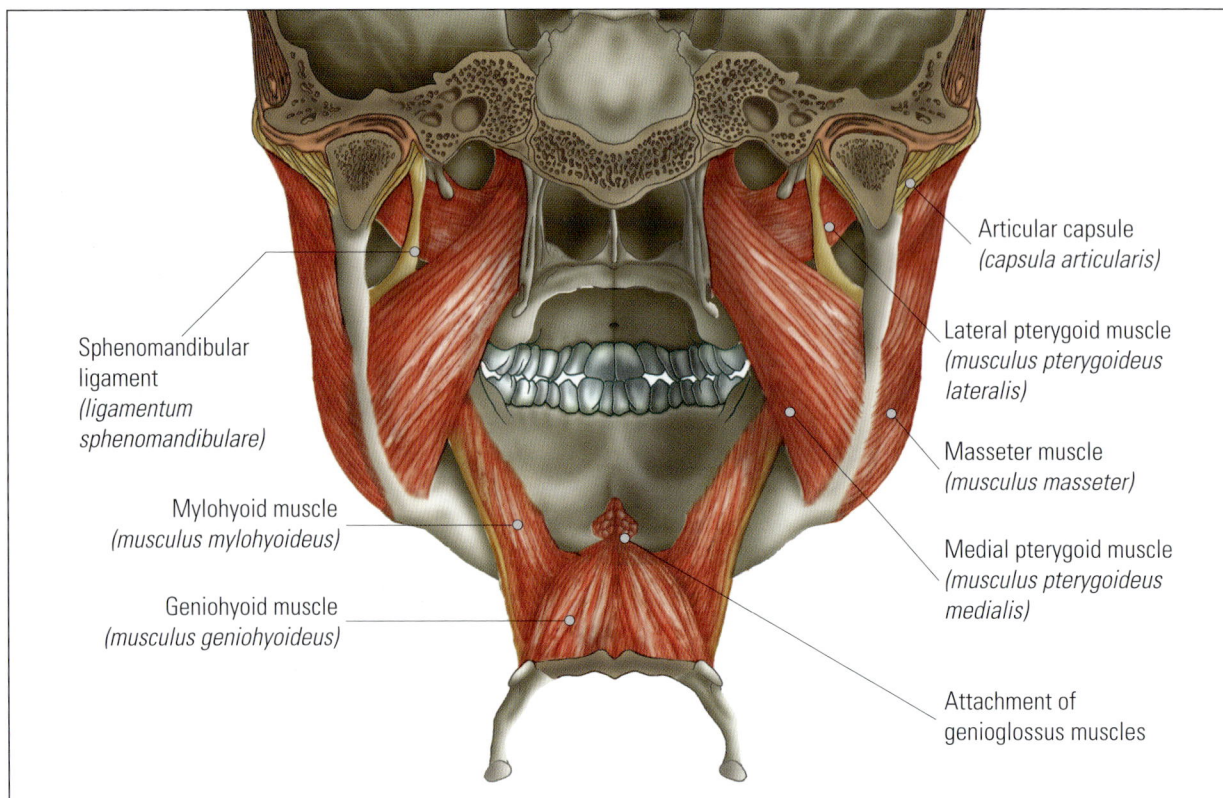

Fig 7-40 Posterior view of masticatory muscles.

Muscle Groups of the Hyoid Bone

Several functional groups of muscles attach to the hyoid; these are involved in both jaw movement and the swallowing process. According to the theoretical classification, they can be characterized as mouth-opening muscles. A distinction is made between the suprahyoid muscles (above the hyoid) and the infrahyoid muscles (below the hyoid).

Suprahyoid muscles (musculi suprahyoidei) form a functional group of muscles that are all fixed above the hyoid bone (Figs 7-41 and 7-42). They form the floor of the mouth and are not part of the actual masticatory musculature but act as mouth-opening muscles. During swallowing, they pull the hyoid with the larynx up and forward and raise the floor of the mouth and tongue. In the

process, the mandible is fixed in terminal occlusion by the masticatory muscles. The following paragraphs outline these muscles in detail.

The **digastric muscle** *(musculus biventer or musculus digastricus)* has its origin at the inferior edge of the mandible in the digastric fossa. This first belly of the muscle *(venter anterior)* lies under the floor of the mouth and joins at the hyoid to form a round intermediate tendon, which is able to slide back and forth here in a fibrous loop. From there, the second belly *(venter posterior)* runs at an obtuse angle downward and upward to the digastric sulcus of the mastoid process on the temporal bone *(sulcus digastricus processus mastoideus)*. When both bellies of the muscle contract, the hyoid is moved upward and forward. With the hyoid fixed, the mandible is opened. The bellies of the muscle are able to contract separately from each other.

Fig 7-41 Suprahyoid muscles.

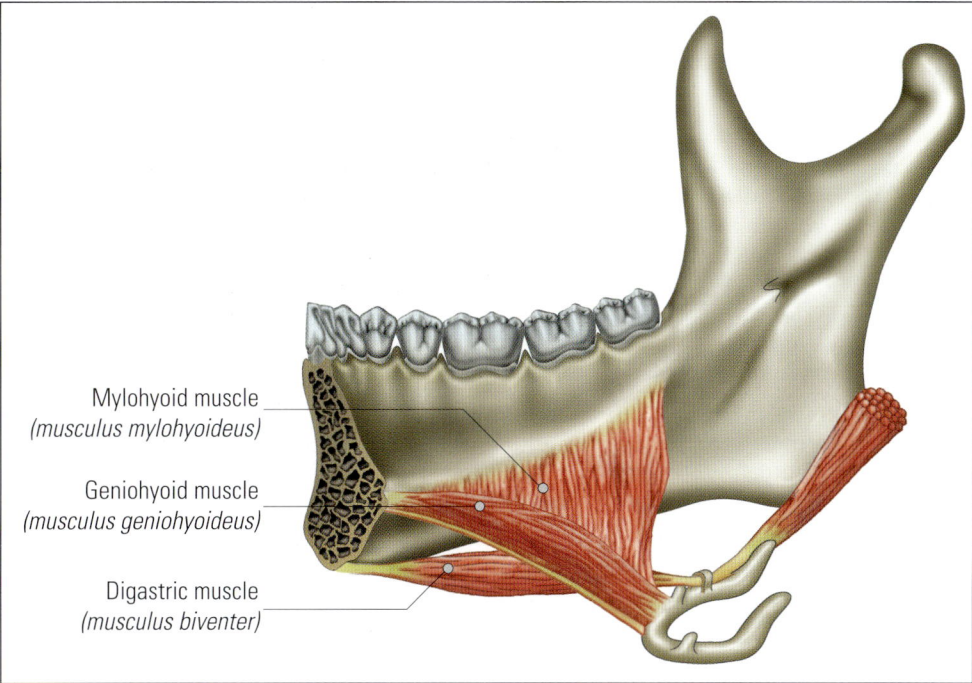

Mylohyoid muscle
(musculus mylohyoideus)

Geniohyoid muscle
(musculus geniohyoideus)

Digastric muscle
(musculus biventer)

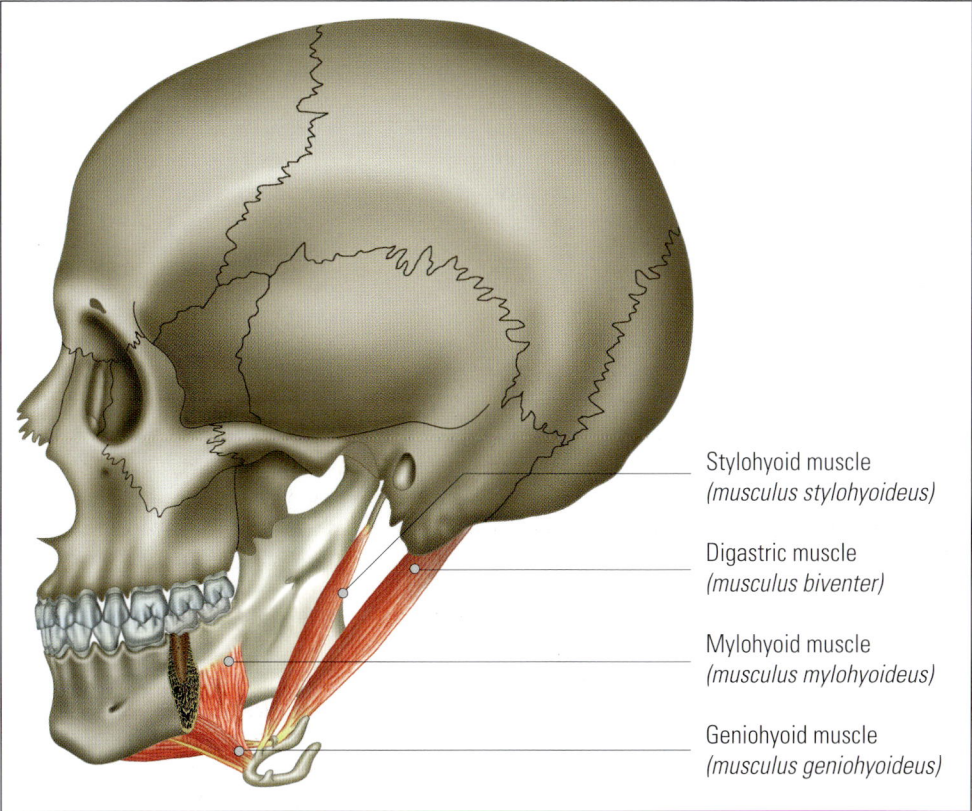

Stylohyoid muscle
(musculus stylohyoideus)

Digastric muscle
(musculus biventer)

Mylohyoid muscle
(musculus mylohyoideus)

Geniohyoid muscle
(musculus geniohyoideus)

Fig 7-42 Suprahyoid muscles on the skull.

227

The **mylohyoid muscle** *(musculus mylohyoideus)* is known as the muscle of the floor of the mouth and, together with the muscle on the opposite side and the connecting fused tendon, as the *diaphragma oris*. This paired muscle originates at the mylohyoid line on the interior of the mandible. This line of origin extends dorsally to the anterior edge of the medial pterygoid muscle. The mylohyoid muscle attaches in the middle of the hyoid body and, with the muscle bundle on the opposite side, forms a raphe that extends from the middle of the hyoid to the symphysis of the mandible *(raphe mylohyoidea)*. When this muscle is in its resting position, the hyoid lies roughly level with the mandibular angle. However, the mylohyoid line lies much higher dorsally so that posteriorly both muscle bundles are at sharp angles to each other. On contraction, they pull the floor of the mouth and the hyoid upward to support swallowing, because raising the floor of the mouth presses the tongue against the palate.

The **geniohyoid muscle** *(musculus geniohyoideus)* originates at the inferior mental spines on the interior of the mandible *(spina mentalis mandibulae)* and, as a thick muscle bundle, runs to the superior edge of the body of the hyoid *(corpus ossis hyoidei)*. When the hyoid is fixed in its position by the middle constrictor muscle of the pharynx and the infrahyoid muscles, the geniohyoid muscle is able to draw the mandible back. In centric occlusion, this muscle pulls the hyoid upward and forward, which supports the swallowing process. The geniohyoid muscle lies on the mylohyoid muscle.

The **stylohyoid muscle** *(musculus stylohyoideus)* originates on the dorsal side of the styloid process of the temporal bone *(processus styloideus)*, divides into two bellies, and attaches to the body of the hyoid and the greater horn of the hyoid; it encloses the intermediate tendon of the digastric muscle. It draws the hyoid upward and backward.

The **infrahyoid muscles** *(musculi infrahyoidei)* form a functional group of muscles that are all fixed below the hyoid bone. They fix the hyoid and prevent it from rising when the mouth is opened. There are four muscles in this muscle group:

1. The **sternohyoid muscle** *(musculus sternohyoideus)* has its origin on the sternum and its insertion on the body of the hyoid.
2. The **sternothyroid muscle** *(musculus sternothyroideus)* has its origin on the sternum and its insertion on the oblique line of the thyroid cartilage.
3. The **thyrohyoid muscle** *(musculus thyreohyoideus)* runs from the oblique line of the thyroid cartilage to the body and greater horn of the hyoid.
4. The **omohyoid muscle** *(musculus omohyoideus)* has its origin at the superior border of the clavicle and its insertion on the body of the hyoid.

Perioral Muscles of Facial Expression

The **muscles of facial expression** (also known as "mimic muscles") do not run from one bone over a joint to another bone but often only attach to the skin, without an intermediate tendon. The facial expression muscles move the facial skin and give the face its expressiveness. The numerous furrows, dimples, and creases that are produced by these muscles are an expression of a person's mood. The facial expression muscles are mainly arranged around the orifices of the mouth, nose, and eyes, as well as the ears, because the position and shape of these openings in the face determine the particular expressive quality of the face.

The **perioral muscles of facial expression** are the muscles of the mouth and cheek area that belong to what are known as the *accessory masticatory muscles* and play an important role in eating (Fig 7-43). They form the bulk of the muscular basis of the external wall of the vestibule of the mouth (cheeks and lips), while their sites of origin influence the position of denture borders (Figs 7-44 to 7-46). Furthermore, the movement of the facial expression muscles can jeopardize the retention of a complete denture but also stabilize it. To make use of this stabilizing force, the denture base must make allowance for the position and path of the muscles at rest and during activity.

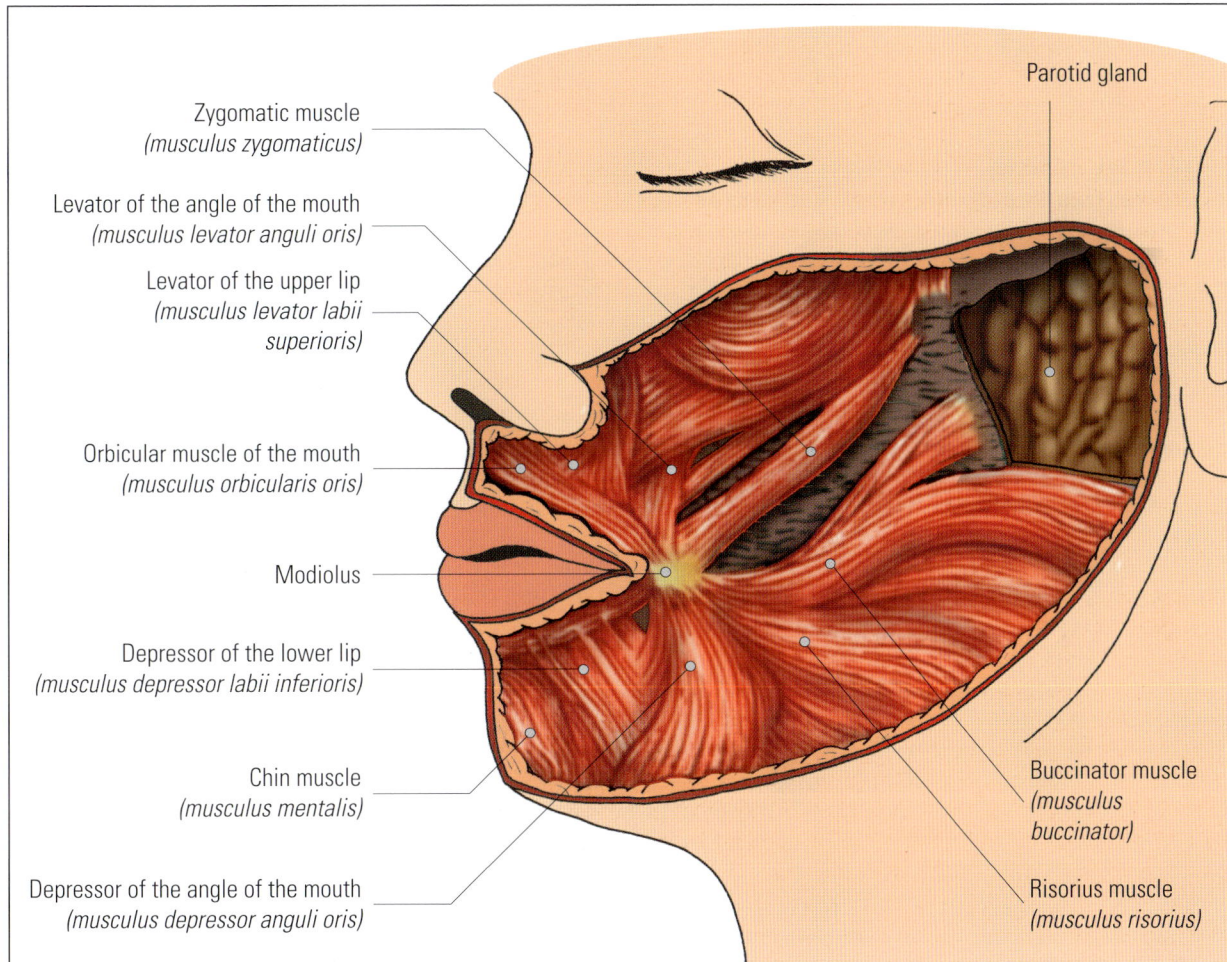

Zygomatic muscle
(musculus zygomaticus)

Levator of the angle of the mouth
(musculus levator anguli oris)

Levator of the upper lip
(musculus levator labii
superioris)

Orbicular muscle of the mouth
(musculus orbicularis oris)

Modiolus

Depressor of the lower lip
(musculus depressor labii inferioris)

Chin muscle
(musculus mentalis)

Depressor of the angle of the mouth
(musculus depressor anguli oris)

Parotid gland

Buccinator muscle
(musculus
buccinator)

Risorius muscle
(musculus risorius)

Fig 7-43 Perioral muscles of facial expression.

In *advanced age*, the muscles of facial expression atrophy so that they lie more or less loosely against the teeth. In the area of the posterior teeth, there is a risk that patients will bite their cheek. This can be counteracted when shaping the denture borders, while supporting the stability of the denture at the same time.

The *external surfaces of the denture body* are shaped so that they grip the muscles. In the anterior area, lip shields for the orbicular muscle of the mouth are prepared; the border of the denture should be chamfered cervically above the vestibular fornix so that the orbicular muscle is firmly engaged to stabilize the denture.

In the *posterior area*, buccinator supports are created and the muscular tracts are redrawn on the ligaments of the cheek. The denture border is shortened in keeping with the oblique line (buccinator attachment) and widened horizontally into the cheek. As a result, the cheek lies on the border and presses the denture onto the jaw, while at the same time the cheek is pushed away from the teeth so the patient will not bite it.

The *path of the muscular tracts*, starting from the modiolus in the angle of the mouth, can be utilized when shaping the denture body to make it grip the muscles (Fig 7-47). The denture acrylic resin must not be shaped too thickly in the labial vestibule because this will widen the vestibular fornix as if the patient had a roll of cotton wool there, drawing the red of the lips inward (see Fig 7-45).

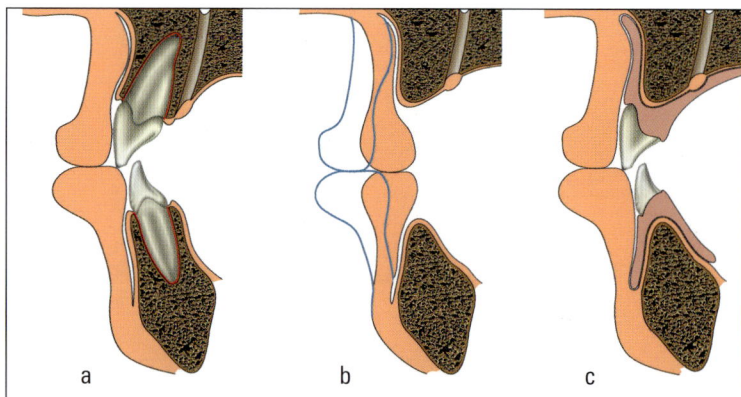

Fig 7-44 In the normal occlusion, the anterior teeth are inclined in a labial direction. In a fully dentate jaw (a), the lips retain their natural fullness because of support from the maxillary incisors. When the alveolar ridges shrink during tooth loss (b), the mouth sinks in markedly and the fullness of the lips is lost. The anterior teeth must be restored to their original position (c) so that the natural lip position is re-created. The correct position of the anterior teeth and hence the correct lip position also have functional significance for articulation of speech.

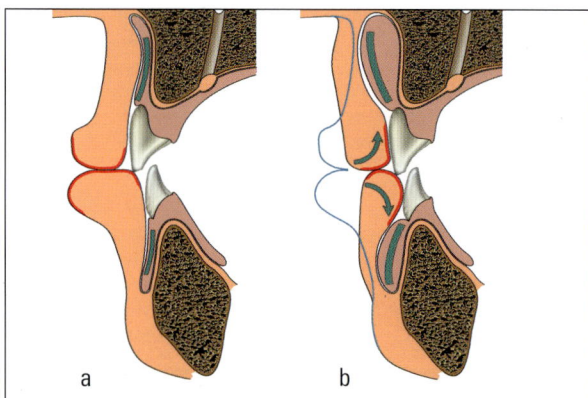

Fig 7-45 If a denture base is placed between the alveolar ridge and the lips, the labial vestibule is widened. The fullness of the lips is not recovered if the base thickness compensates for the extent of alveolar ridge shrinkage. (a) With correct tooth positioning, the amount of lip redness displayed appears normal. (b) If the denture base and denture body are padded vestibularly to fill the labial vestibule and smooth out creases around the mouth while the teeth are positioned in the middle of the alveolar ridge for stability reasons, the redness of the lips is drawn inward, and the orifice of the mouth becomes very narrow and sunken.

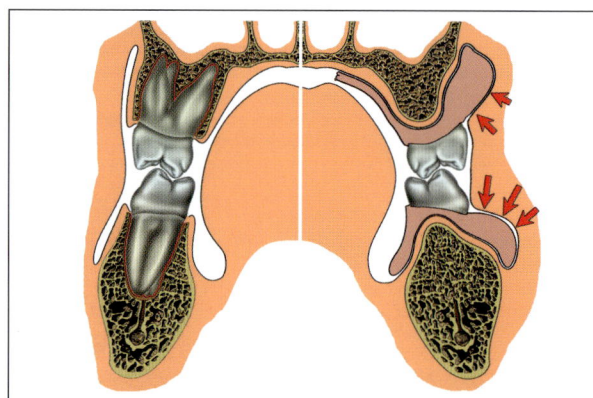

Fig 7-46 In the lateral vestibular area, the buccinator can be used to stabilize a complete denture base. To do this, the denture border is extended into the buccal cavity so that the muscle bundles of the cheek are able to lie on these convexities. In the maxilla, this so-called buccinator support starts above the vestibular fornix. In the mandible, the denture border is extended beyond the oblique line in a vestibular direction in order to shape a buccinator support. An accurate impression is always a necessary basis for creating this accessory retention aid.

The **anterior teeth** should stand within the vertical anterior dental arch so that the incisors fill out the upper lip with their labial surface and can support the lower lip with their incisal edges.

In the maxilla, the buccal vestibular space should be shaped thinly because the masseter presses the buccinator into the vestibule here. One way of gaining an overview of the large number of muscles of facial expression is to start from a distinctive point and look at the muscles grouped around that point.

In this model, the corner of the mouth (labial commissure) should be chosen as the orientation point for the following reasons: Starting from the corner of the mouth, antagonistic muscle groups can be described, which provides a certain overview. Around the corner of the mouth, six essential, partly antagonistic muscles of the perioral region come together in the modiolus.

The **modiolus** is a small aponeurosis (a tendinous plate) into which most of the muscles of facial expression attach (Fig 7-48). Consequently, the corner of the mouth is particularly mobile, which should be taken into account when shaping the denture. As a result of the position of the mandibular anterior teeth, the modiolus may help

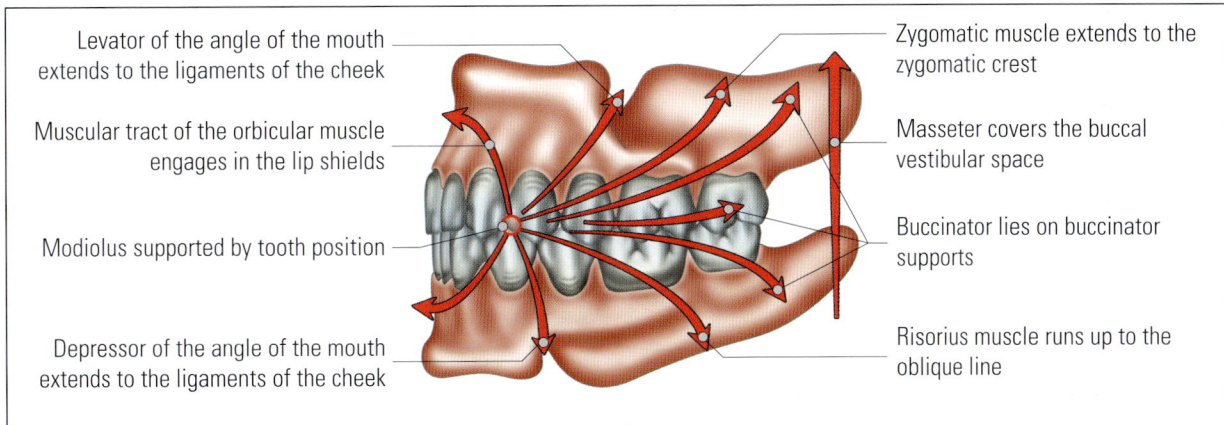

Levator of the angle of the mouth extends to the ligaments of the cheek

Muscular tract of the orbicular muscle engages in the lip shields

Modiolus supported by tooth position

Depressor of the angle of the mouth extends to the ligaments of the cheek

Zygomatic muscle extends to the zygomatic crest

Masseter covers the buccal vestibular space

Buccinator lies on buccinator supports

Risorius muscle runs up to the oblique line

Fig 7-47 The perioral muscular tracts must be taken into account when shaping denture bodies. The external surfaces of the denture body can be shaped so that they grip the muscles; lip shields can be fashioned for the orbicular muscle in the anterior area, and buccinator supports can be created in the area of the posterior teeth.

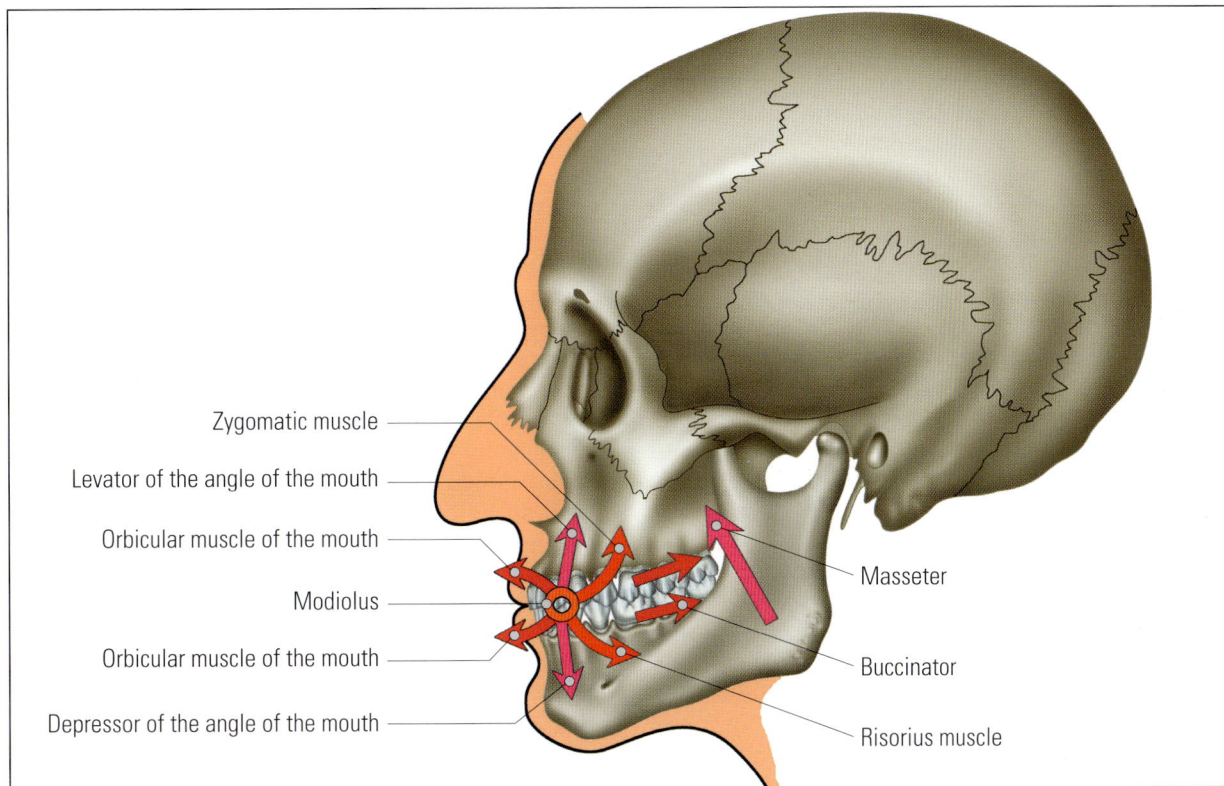

Zygomatic muscle

Levator of the angle of the mouth

Orbicular muscle of the mouth

Modiolus

Orbicular muscle of the mouth

Depressor of the angle of the mouth

Masseter

Buccinator

Risorius muscle

Fig 7-48 The modiolus brings together several muscles in the region of the angle of the mouth. This area is influenced by the position of the canines. If the canine is too lingual or if the occlusal height is too small, saliva will pool at the corners of the mouth.

to stabilize a mandibular denture if it lies higher than the mandibular anterior teeth and is able to press onto the incisal edges. Therefore, the man-dibular incisors should never stand higher than the lip closure line.

The **arch width** of the mandibular anterior teeth must also be kept in correct proportion because, if it is too wide in the canine area, the denture may be lifted by muscular activity (eg, that of the levator muscle of the angle of the mouth).

First antagonistic muscle pair

The first antagonistic muscle pair in the angle of the mouth comprises the orbicular muscle of the mouth and the buccinator muscle as well as their accessory muscles. They form the muscular basis of the lips and cheeks. The fibers of these two muscles cross at the modiolus.

The **orbicular muscle of the mouth** *(musculus orbicularis oris)* is the whole muscular mass lying around the orifice of the mouth, which can be regarded as the closing muscle of the mouth. Only a small part of the fibers contained in this muscle follow a wholly orbicular (ring-shaped) course; instead, the orbicular muscle is made up of fibers from adjacent muscles that radiate in from the upper and lower lips or the cheeks.

As a whole, the fibers following a circular path bring about closure of the orifice of the mouth. If the peripheral fibers are mainly activated, the orifice is narrowed in a circular fashion and the lips are pursed. Activation of the central fibers presses the lips together until the redness of the lips disappears (ie, slides inward). When contracted, the orbicular muscle lies firmly against the incisors and narrows the anterior part of the oral vestibule.

Because the orbicular muscle itself does not have an origin in the skull, it is held by various muscles. For instance, the muscle fibers of the masseter radiate in from the side over the modiolus. From above, the two incisive muscles run into the upper lip. These two muscles have their origin in the skull and therefore give the orbicular muscle support.

The **superior incisive muscle** *(musculus incisivi superioris)* has its origin at the alveolar mounds of the incisors and ideally extends to the angle of the mouth. The **posterior incisive muscle** *(musculus incisivi inferioris)* has its origin at the alveolar mounds of the canine and the first premolars and extends to the upper lip and the angle of the mouth. When contracted, these muscles give the mouth a round shape, eg, when whistling or forming the sounds "oh" and "you".

The **buccinator muscle** *(musculus buccinator)* forms the anterior region of the cheek and can be seen as an antagonist of the orbicular muscle. Its origin is on the outer surface of the alveolar process of the maxilla. In the mandible, its path of insertion corresponds to the oblique line as far as the *crista buccinatoria (crus laterale* of the *trigonum retromolare)* and up to the pterygomandibular raphe *(plica pterygomandibularis)*. This raphe forms the boundary between the buccinator and the muscles of the throat.

The fibers of the buccinator initially run forward in a horizontal direction and converge on the angle of the mouth, where they cross and extend into the lips: the lower fibers run into the upper lip, the upper fibers into the lower lip, and the middle fibers directly to the angle of the mouth. The buccinator is perforated by the duct of the parotid gland (Stensen duct), whose opening in the oral vestibule is located at the maxillary second molar. The buccinator is the only muscle of facial expression to be covered by a fascia, which gives way to the tendinous plate of the modiolus. The fascia increases the strength and elasticity of the muscle and the cheek.

When **activated**, the **buccinator** brings about shortening of the cheek in a sagittal direction, which narrows the vestibule while widening the orifice of the mouth. The activity of this muscular foundation of the cheek works in a twofold way as an antagonist for the tongue: During chewing, the food is pressed back between the masticatory surfaces by the buccinator. On the other hand, the tissue tension while at rest maintains a balance against the pressure of the tongue, as a result of which shaping of the dentition takes place. During sucking (drinking), the buccinator forms the cylinder wall to which the tongue acts as a "suction valve." The buccinator is particularly important when playing wind instruments, which is where it derives its name (Latin, *bucinator* = trumpeter).

The **risorius muscle** *(musculus risorius;* Latin, *risus* = laughter; therefore, also called "laughing muscle")* is a small muscle that runs parallel to the buccinator; it is usually poorly developed and only present on one side or entirely absent. Its fibers overlie the buccinator or are interwoven with the fibers of the buccinator. The risorius muscle originates in the fascia of the masseter muscle. It produces the dimple in the cheek by contracting and drawing the skin of the cheek toward the angle of the mouth and pulling the angle of the mouth backward. It has no significance in prosthetic work.

The external surface of denture bodies is shaped to grip the muscles, which involves fashioning lip shields for the orbicular muscle in the anterior area, starting from the modiolus. In the area of the posterior teeth, buccinator supports can be created; the muscular tracts are redrawn on the ligaments of the cheek. The areas in need of reduction should be heeded.

Second antagonistic muscle pair

The second antagonistic pair of facial expression muscles comprises the levator muscle and the depressor muscle of the angle of the mouth with their accessory muscles.

The *levator muscle of the angle of the mouth* (*musculus levator anguli oris;* also known as *musculus caninus*) starts wide and flat in the canine fossa below the infraorbital foramen and extends downward and forward to the angle of the mouth, where a few fibers attach and others pass into the orbicular muscle to the lower lip. Downward to the oral vestibule, a few fibers reach into the ligaments of the cheek and are responsible for their mobility. The muscular activity of this muscle will appear in the functional impression: It raises the angle of the mouth and releases the canine (baring the teeth).

The *zygomatic muscle* (*musculus zygomaticus*) lifts the angle of the mouth and draws it upward and outward. It originates at the external surface of the temporal process of the zygomatic bone, hence above the masseter attachment in front of the zygomatic arch. It covers the superoanterior edge of the masseter, where it extends downward and obliquely forward to the angle of the mouth and radiates into the upper lip with a few fibers. Its muscular activity draws the angle of the mouth upward as an expression of pleasure and laughter; therefore, it, not the risorius muscle, ought to be called the "laughter muscle." Its activity is also reflected in the functional impression because it tightens the upper and lower lips.

The *levator muscle of the upper lip* (*musculus levator labii superioris;* also *musculus quadratus labii superioris*) is another accessory muscle that lifts the angle of the mouth forward but has no influence on the retention of a complete denture. This multiheaded muscle can be divided into three parts:

1. The *caput angulare* originates as the medial part on the frontal process of the maxilla and a small part at the nasal wing; it runs vertically downward into the upper lip and into the nasolabial sulcus and, when activated, pulls up the upper lip and the nasal wing.
2. The *caput infraorbitale* has its origin at the edge of the infraorbital foramen and converges downward toward the upper lip and raises the lip.
3. The *caput zygomaticum* has its origin on the facial surface of the zygoma and radiates medially downward into the upper lip and nasolabial sulcus in order to raise this area.

The *depressor muscle of the angle of the mouth* (*musculus depressor anguli oris;* or *musculus triangularis*) is the antagonist for the levator of the angle of the mouth, the zygomatic muscle, and the upper lip levator. Its origin is at the lateral edge of the mandible between the canine and the second premolar, and with its converging fibers it runs obliquely upward and forward to the angle of the mouth, the fibers passing into the orbicular muscle. It draws the angle of the mouth downward as an expression of sadness, depression, and pessimism and thereby also has an effect on the nasolabial sulcus.

A denture must not be developed too much in this cheek area, and the dental arch must remain narrow enough because the muscle lies very close to the rows of teeth here.

The *depressor muscle of the lower lip* (*musculus depressor labii inferioris*) is the first accessory muscle, originating below the mental foramen but above the attachment of the depressor muscle of the angle of the mouth on the mandibular body. Its fibers lie below those of the depressor of the angle of the mouth, where they run upward and forward to the lower lip to draw it downward; it has no prosthetic significance.

The *chin muscle* (*musculus mentalis*) is the second accessory muscle, and it limits the scope for extension of the mandibular denture border because, when active, it narrows the mandibular vestibular fornix; if severe resorption of the mandibular bone has taken place, it can produce

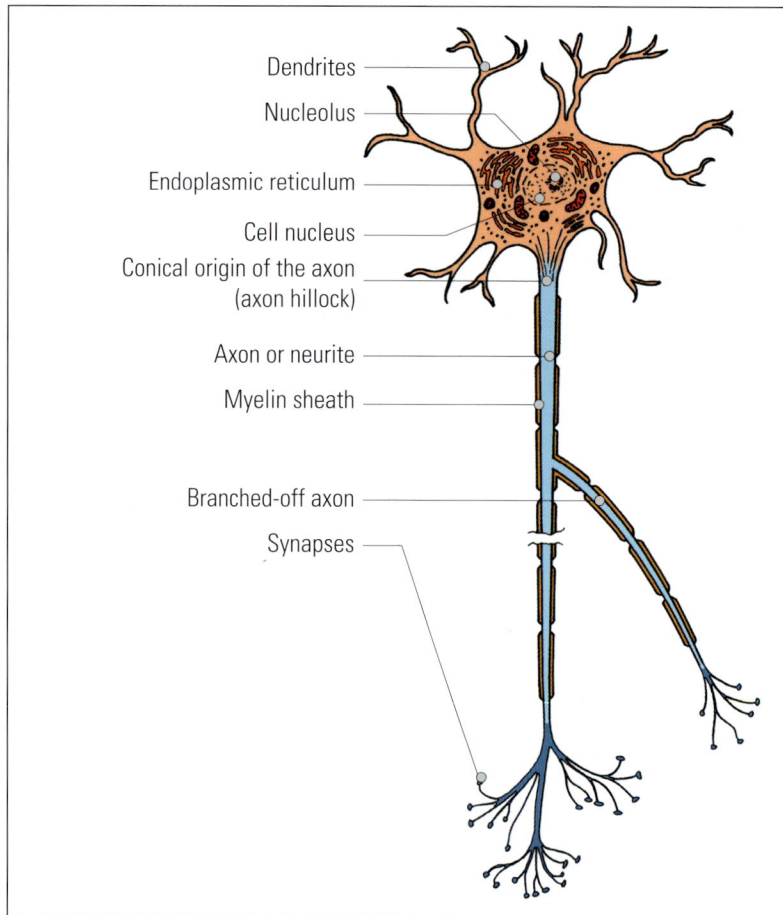

Fig 7-49 Diagram of a nerve cell (neuron) consisting of the cell body with the cell processes.

Dendrites

Nucleolus

Endoplasmic reticulum

Cell nucleus

Conical origin of the axon (axon hillock)

Axon or neurite

Myelin sheath

Branched-off axon

Synapses

pressure points at the denture border. Its origin is at the alveolar eminences of the mandibular incisors, where the inferior incisive muscles also originate. It runs downward to the chin and raises it by muscular action, but when strongly contracted it can raise the lower lip or the orifice of the mouth to create a pout.

Nerve Tissue

The ability to react to external stimuli is a basic characteristic of living tissue. In single-celled organisms, all the stages of receiving, transmitting, processing, and responding to stimuli take place in a single cell. In more highly developed, multicellular animals, the stimulus is transmitted by special conductive tissues—the nerves. Receiv-

ing, conducting, and processing stimuli enables living beings to orient themselves in their surroundings and to act and react independently.

Ganglia (singular: ganglion) are the groups and knots of nerve cells known as *ganglion cells*. They make up the nervous system with one center for processing stimuli, namely the brain and the spinal cord. The size of nerve cells varies from 4 to 120 µm, excluding the processes located on the cells. Adult nerve cells have lost their ability to divide in favor of very pronounced differentiation; in other words, dead nerve cells are not replaced. There are around 14 billion nerve cells in the cerebral cortex, which are already preformed at birth.

Nerve cells (neurocytes) have various long extensions or processes. Processes that direct the stimulus away from the nerve cell are called *neurites* and can be very long (up to 1 m). Other processes that receive the stimulus from other nerve

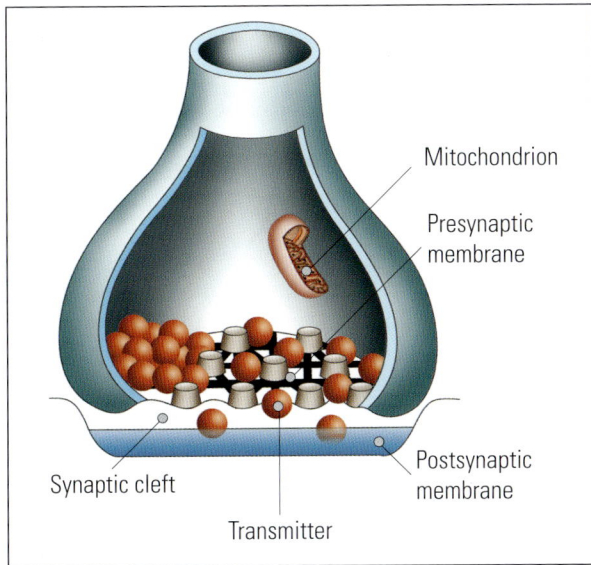

Fig 7-50 Schematic diagram of a synapse. The axon ends in a conical swelling (bouton) that lies against a membrane of the downstream neuron. This is where transmission of chemical transmitters (acetylcholine, norepinephrine/noradrenaline, dopamine) takes place, which are synthesized in the boutons. The clear, round vesicles are seen as carriers of transmitter substances. The vesicles lie in front of the presynaptic membrane and are thrust into the synaptic cleft to transmit an impulse, where they diffuse through the postsynaptic membrane into the receiving neuron.

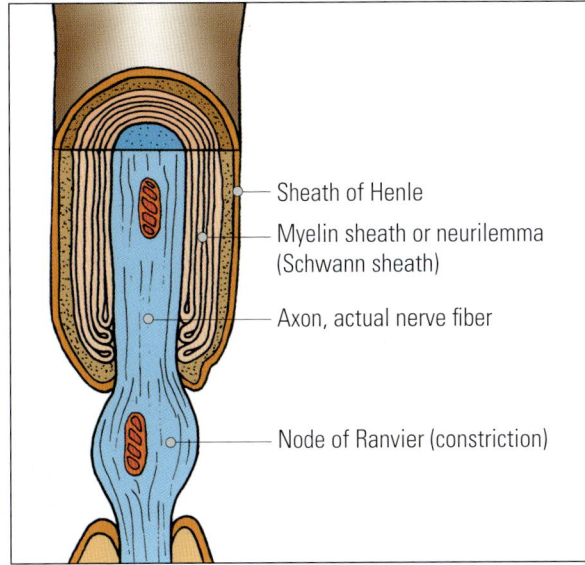

Fig 7-51 Diagram of a peripheral nerve fiber with myelin sheath.

cells are very short and are called *dendrites*. A nerve cell with its processes is referred to as a *neuron* and is the smallest unit in the nervous system (Fig 7-49). The nerve fibers are the processes that emanate from the nerve cells.

Synapses are the contact points between the extensions of different nerve cells (Fig 7-50). The nerve fibers touch in the synapses but do not merge into each other. The transmission of nerve impulses by contact takes place by means of chemical transmitters: epinephrine (adrenaline) and acetylcholine.

Nerve cells have a strong tendency to form processes and synapses but also the ability to break down synapses. The nerve cells retain this ability for life; in other words, the connection of nerve cells among themselves remains variable, changeable, and expandable throughout life. In addition to the number of nerve cells in the brain, the number of synaptic connections between the nerve cells in particular accounts for the functional capacity of the brain.

Structure of nerve fibers

Neurites and dendrites have a similar cellular structure (Fig 7-51), which can be broken down as follows:

- The **axon** or **axis cylinder** emerges directly from the nerve cells and lies in the middle of a nerve fiber. The axon is made up of neurofibrils.
- The **neurilemma** (Schwann sheath) forms the covering around the axon. This outer membrane is enveloped around fatlike substances containing phosphorus, namely myelin. The outer covering has regular constrictions where the neurilemma has direct contact with the axon. These constrictions are known as *nodes of Ranvier*.
- The **sheath of Henle** (endoneurium) is the outer covering around a nerve fiber; it is made up of connective tissue fibers with blood vessels.

Reception of stimuli happens by means of the special senses: the sense of sight and hearing, the sense of smell and taste, the sense of balance and touch, and the sense of temperature and pain. The nerve impulse is the signal that is conducted by the nerve fiber. The conduction speed, depending on the diameter of the fiber, is between 2 m/s for a fiber thickness of 1 µm and 120 m/s for a 20-µm-thick fiber.

When a nerve cell is in a resting state, there is electrical tension (voltage) between the nerve fiber and the neurilemma. As a result of stimulation, the outer covering loses its positive charge compared with the nerve fiber and becomes slightly negatively charged. Sodium ions then flow into the inside of the cell and positively charge the cell briefly. From the stimulated site, the impulse spreads to both sides and jumps from one node of Ranvier to another.

A nerve can be stimulated mechanically, chemically, thermally, or electrically. The stimulus must have a specific strength in order to cross the stimulus threshold so that the nerve is excited to the maximum. Because nerves are always combined to form bundles, the strength of sensation depends on how many nerve fibers are stimulated and conducting an impulse. After an impulse has been conducted, there is a resting pause of about 0.4 thousandths of a second. The nerve impulse is conducted until it is passed on to another nerve cell via the synapse or is delivered to a motor end plate of a muscle cell or another organ cell.

Nervous Control

Two nervous systems are involved in nervous control: the somatic nervous system and the autonomic nervous system. Both systems have the spinal cord (medulla spinalis) and the brain (cerebrum) at their center. The peripheral pathways, which are the neurites (nerve fibers) of the nerve cells, run from the centers outward. If these neurites conduct an impulse from the periphery to the center, they are esthesodic fibers (ie, they convey sensory impulses). If an impulse is transmitted from the center to the effector organ, they are fibers that stimulate movement.

Somatic Nervous System

The processing of stimuli by conscious action is the characteristic of the somatic nervous system. Stimuli from the outside world received by sensory organs are responded to with deliberate reactions.

The **spinal cord** is the first and primary center of the somatic and the autonomic nervous systems. It lies in a canal formed by the spinal column and is encased in a very firm covering. The spinal cord is able to respond to certain stimuli itself in the form of rapid but unconscious reflexes.

A **reflex** is the simplest form of response to a stimulus by the central nervous system. In this process, there are reflex arcs (or paths) that comprise at least two neurons (nerve cells with processes). The reflex arc also includes afferent conduction toward the receptor and efferent conduction away to the effector organ. A distinction can be drawn between innate and conditioned reflexes. People possess innate (or inborn) reflexes from birth; in medical examinations, these reflexes can provide information about the state of health of the spinal cord.

Conditioned reflexes are learned sequences of movement. Conditioned reflexes are triggered by unconnected impressions that are linked to each other by frequent associations. Reflexes can be influenced by medicines or by a person's will.

The Brain

The brain (cerebrum) is the more highly developed center of the nervous system (Figs 7-52 and 7-53). It lies in the cranial vault and is made up of five segments, divided according to their form and development:

1. Cerebrum or endbrain (telencephalon)
2. Midbrain (mesencephalon)
3. Interbrain (diencephalon)
4. Cerebellum
5. Medulla oblongata (myelencephalon)

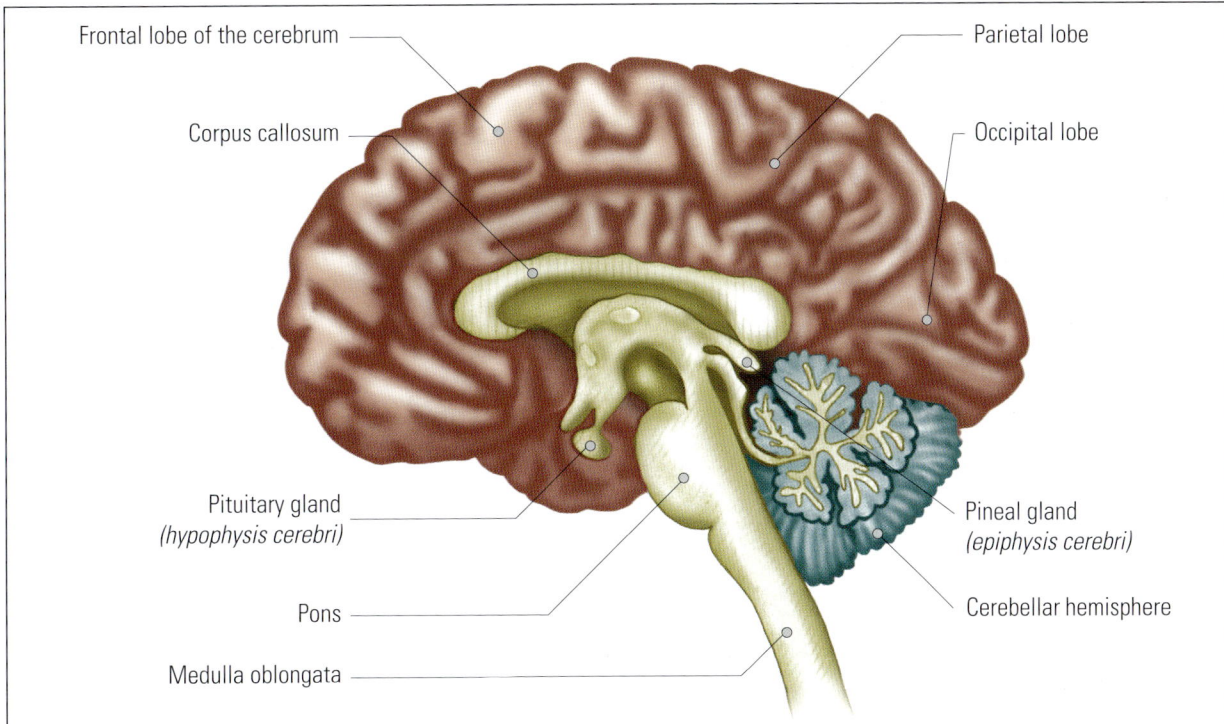

Fig 7-52 Sagittal section of the parts of the brain, based on the developmental structure.

Frontal lobe of the cerebrum

Corpus callosum

Parietal lobe

Occipital lobe

Pituitary gland
(hypophysis cerebri)

Pineal gland
(epiphysis cerebri)

Pons

Cerebellar hemisphere

Medulla oblongata

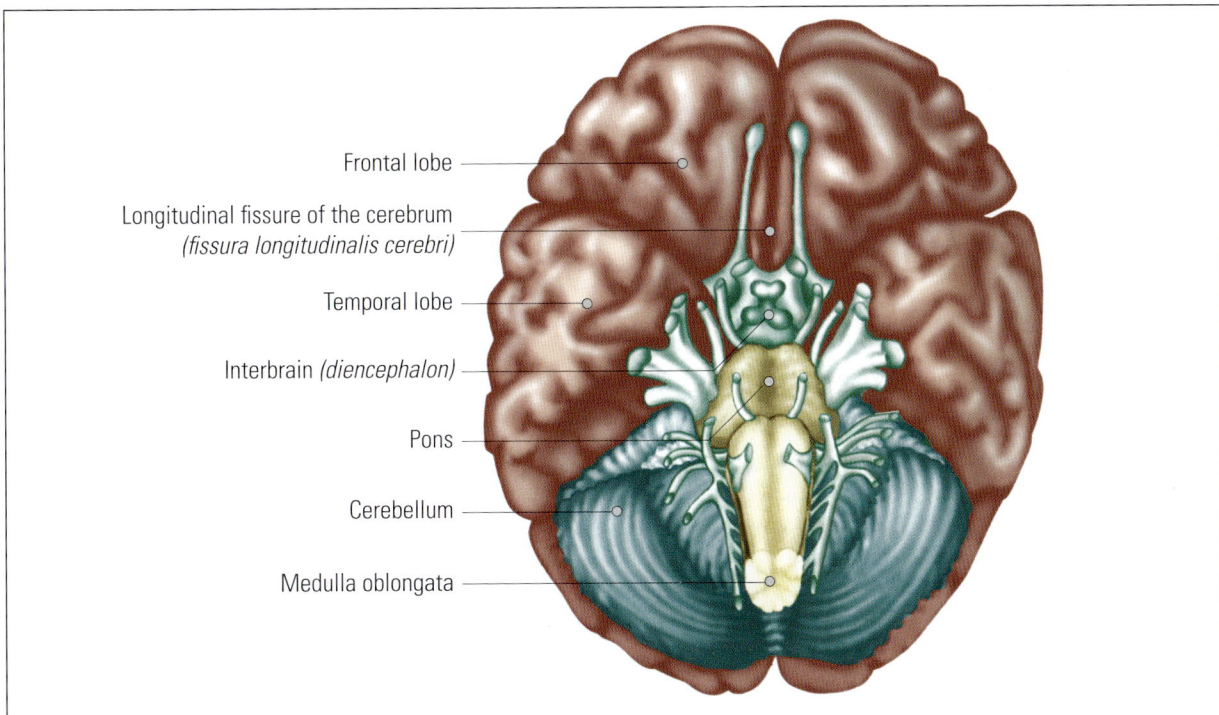

Fig 7-53 The differentiated sections of the cerebrum, viewed from the base.

Frontal lobe

Longitudinal fissure of the cerebrum
(fissura longitudinalis cerebri)

Temporal lobe

Interbrain (diencephalon)

Pons

Cerebellum

Medulla oblongata

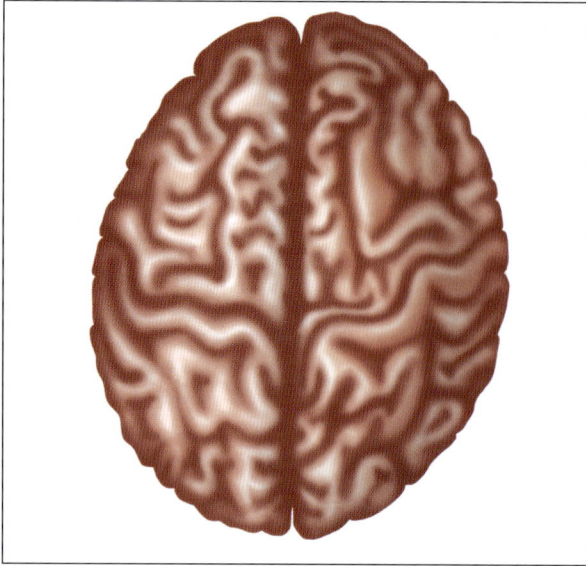

Fig 7-54 The brain seen from above shows the symmetric division into the left and right hemispheres. The distinctive sulci (furrows) can also be seen. The sulci separate different bulges in the coating layer (gyri), where it is suspected that specific centers of brain function are located. This view of the brain shows the broad cerebrum in the human being, which covers all the other parts of the brain.

The first three parts together form the *brainstem*, which is structured like the spinal cord and contains the cell bodies of the cranial nerves as well as the centers for respiration and circulation.

The *cerebrum* or *endbrain* contains the stem ganglia; the two halves (hemispheres) of the brain with their cortices, which are linked by the *corpus callosum*; and the olfactory brain *(rhinencephalon)*. Its purpose is to connect deeper-lying parts of the nervous system so that, as all sections of the nervous system interact, special brain functions of thinking, willing, and feeling can be achieved. In other words, the purpose of the cerebrum is to create consciousness.

The cerebrum weighs up to 1,400 g in adults and is made up of the two hemispheres whose surfaces are between 4.5 and 5.0 mm thick and consist of gray matter (Fig 7-54). This surface is known as the *cortex*. The cortical layer is shaped by numerous furrows (sulci) and convolutions (gyri) so that this layer can have a surface area of around 2,200 cm². The number of convolutions is not a direct indication of the functional capacity of the brain.

In the cortical layer, the ganglion cells are concentrated as gray matter, while the white medullary substance, made up of afferent and efferent nerve fibers, is surrounded by the cortical layer. The contact surfaces between the gray and white brain matter are enlarged as a result of the deep furrowing of the cortex.

Almost 200 centers of sensory perception and response to stimuli can be identified on the cortical layer, and these are described as the visual, tactile, speech, and motor centers. The individual cortical centers differ in their fibrous and cellular structure so that six or seven layers of cortex can be found.

Topographically, the *midbrain (mesencephalon)* can be precisely identified, but it does not have a precise function of its own. However, it does regulate motor functions of posture and position in humans. It coordinates the instructions from the higher centers of the brain within the motor system.

The *interbrain* lies between the two hemispheres and is composed of the thalamus, the hypothalamus, and the extrapyramidal system. The interbrain *(diencephalon)* is an important relay center for nearly all stimuli from the skin, eyes, and ears as well as other parts of the brain.

As the main mass in the diencephalon, the *thalamus* is an independent coordinating center in which all sensory pathways from the spinal cord are "switched over" to the cerebral cortex. It is here that feelings of pleasure, dislike, pain, and fear are triggered and conducted to the cerebrum.

The *hypothalamus* is the center of the autonomic nervous system and, with the adjacent pituitary gland (or *hypophysis*), controls the endocrine system. The hypothalamus regulates body temperature, water and sugar balance, fat and mineral metabolism, and especially sleeping and waking states. The extrapyramidal system regulates the voluntary actions by controlling muscle tone.

The *cerebellum* is a segment of the brain lying in the dorsal part of the cranium. It is the integrating organ for programming and coordinating the movement of striated muscles and for maintaining muscle tone and balance.

The *medulla oblongata (myelencephalon)* is an extremely complicated part of the central nervous system. The control centers for waking functions are located here; these centers protect the other

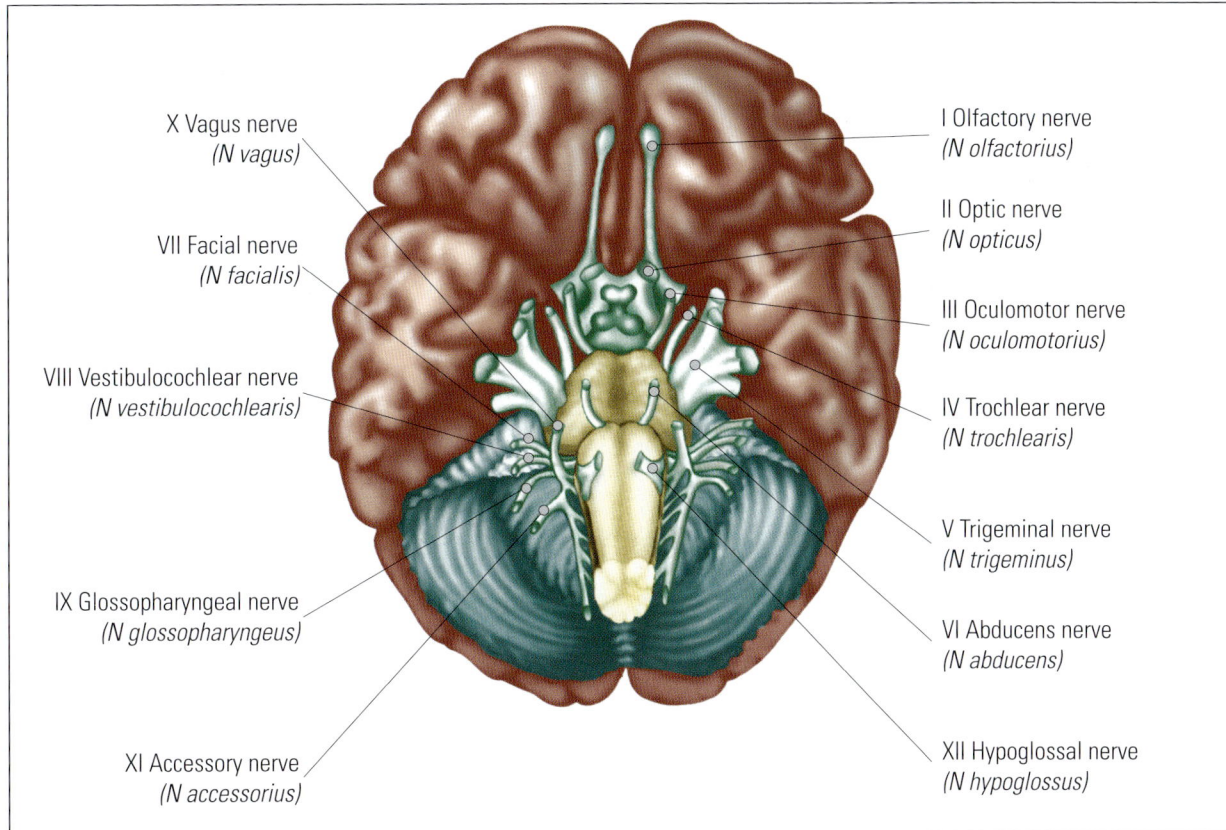

Fig 7-55 The cranial nerves at the base of the brain.

parts of the brain against overstimulation. This is where vital control centers (eg, for respiration or cardiac activity) and reflex control centers (eg, vomiting, swallowing) are located.

Cranial nerves

Cranial nerves are found paired as ganglia in the medulla oblongata at the base of the brain (Fig 7-55). Pairs of cranial nerves already leave the brain while inside the cranial cavity. The cranial nerves are numbered in Roman numerals in the order they exit from the brain from front to back.

The cranial nerves can be divided into three groups, classified according to their function:

1. Sensory nerves (I, II, VIII, IX)
2. Nerves responsible for eye movement (III, IV, VI)
3. Pharyngeal arch nerves (V, VII, IX, X, XI)

I. Olfactory nerve (nerve of smell, *nervus olfactorius*; also known as *fila olfactoria*): Consists of processes of the olfactory epithelium of the nasal mucosa and extends to the olfactory bulb as a protuberance of the forebrain *(proencephalon)*; it is not regarded as a true cranial nerve.

II. Optic nerve (*N opticus*; also known as *fasciculus opticus*): A protuberance of the diencephalon as a fiber tract at the rear of the eyeball; it is encased in meninges and is hence part of the brain. With its terminal branches, it supplies the retina of the eye.

III. Oculomotor nerve (*N oculomotorius*): A cranial nerve emerging from the midbrain whose fibers mainly supply the eye muscles; the parasympathetic fibers control narrowing of the pupils.

IV. Trochlear nerve (*N trochlearis*): A nerve emerging dorsally from the midbrain that supplies the outer muscles of the eye.

V. Trigeminal nerve (N trigeminus; see detailed description later in this chapter).

VI. Abducens nerve (N abducens): A motor nerve that supplies the outer muscles of the eye.

VII. Facial nerve (N facialis): Responsible for supplying the muscles of facial expression, parts of the sense of taste, the salivary glands of the mandible, and the lacrimal glands.

VIII. Vestibulocochlear nerve (N vestibulocochlearis): A sensory nerve arising in the pons of the myelencephalon responsible for supplying the organ of balance and the cochlea in the ear.

IX. Glossopharyngeal nerve (N glossopharyngeus): The main nerve of taste for the tongue; responsible for movement of the esophagus and for the parotid gland.

X. Vagus nerve (N vagus): Supplies the muscles of the larynx and is responsible for the digestive tract as far as the curvature of the large intestine.

XI. Accessory nerve (N accessorius): A motor cranial nerve that supplies the sternocleidomastoid muscle in the neck and functions as a supplementary nerve to cranial nerve X.

XII. Hypoglossal nerve (N hypoglossus): runs as a motor nerve from the medulla oblongata to the tongue and ensures tongue movement.

Autonomic Nervous System

The nervous control of the human body, independently regulating vital functions such as respiration, metabolism, and digestion, is largely not subject to our will. There is a close functional connection between the autonomic and somatic nervous systems. The center of the autonomic nervous system mainly lies in the diencephalon and the medulla oblongata. In the autonomic nervous system, two antagonistic regulatory divisions can be distinguished: the sympathetic nervous system and the parasympathetic nervous system.

The **sympathetic nervous system** causes an increase in activity in the organs it supplies, activating the organs to maximum performance (eg, the heart and circulation) by the formation of epinephrine (adrenaline) and norepinephrine (noradrenaline). The sympathetic nervous system is therefore also known as the *adrenergic system*.

The **parasympathetic nervous system** diminishes latent vitality but increases all processes that are important to recovery and restoration of the body's reserves; one of its functions is to stimulate bowel activity and the storage of food.

Hormonal Control

In addition to the nervous system, a second regulatory system keeps the body's activities harmoniously in balance: hormones (Fig 7-56).

Hormones are formed in the body and intervene in the enzyme balance of the cells in a regulatory way. They control growth, metabolism, and reproduction. Hormones are chemical substances that are extremely effective even in very small quantities, being able to exert a stimulating or inhibiting effect in the appropriate organs or cells. They appear to be ubiquitous, at least in more highly developed mammals, because the active substances in these animals are also effective in humans. This offers various possibilities of dealing with disturbed hormonal control: transplantation of the appropriate hormonal organs; direct administration of animal hormones to counteract inadequate function (hypoactivity, hypofunction); or use of antagonistic substances to restrict the hormonal effect in the case of excessive function (hyperactivity, hyperfunction).

The regulation of the body's functions by hormones is relatively slow and widely diversified; they are able to act on several bodily functions at once. The hormones and other active substances reach the cells and organs with the bloodstream; the stimulating effect produced by hormones is thus dependent on the speed of blood flow and always lasts several seconds.

The **stimulating effect** of hormonal control can be equated with the stimulation by nerves. This is because chemical substances (often the very same hormones) are released at the synapses and motor end plates of the nerves. The subsequent conduction of nerve impulses is simply a special type of hormonal control. The hormones and the active substances of this regulatory system are produced in the endocrine glands (Fig 7-57), which secrete their hormones into the bloodstream.

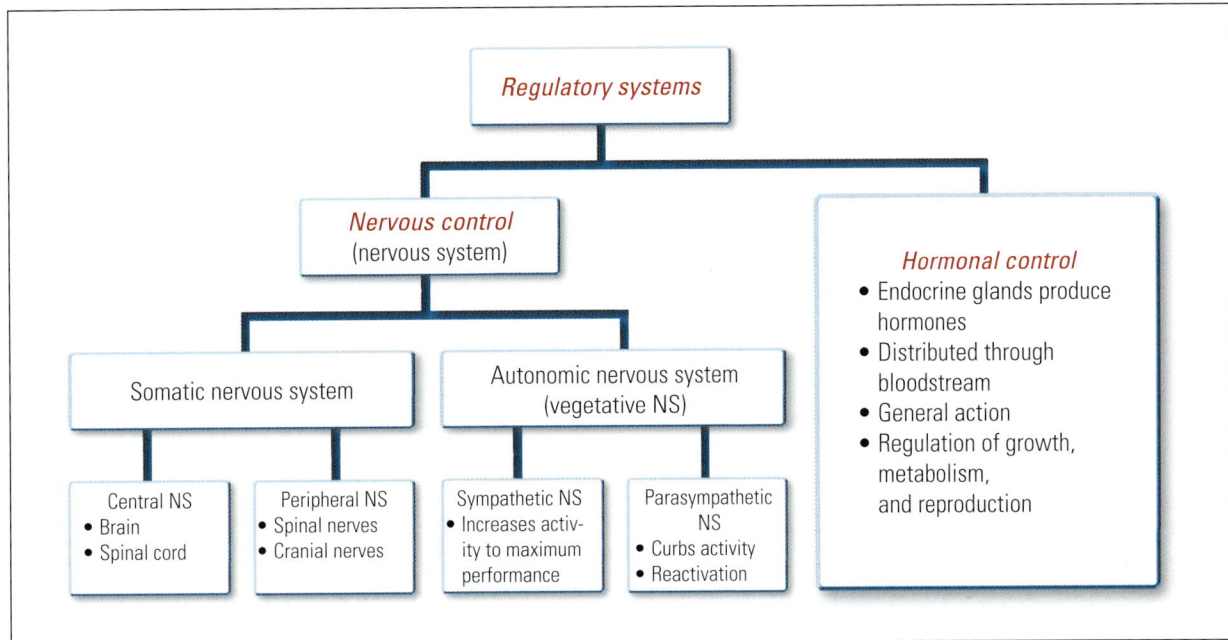

Fig 7-56 Regulatory systems of the body. NS, nervous system.

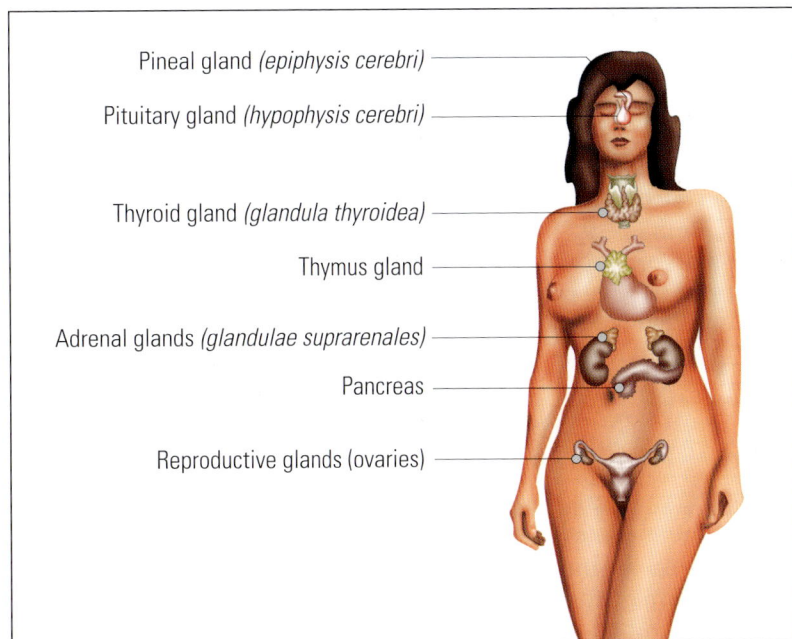

Pineal gland *(epiphysis cerebri)*

Pituitary gland *(hypophysis cerebri)*

Thyroid gland *(glandula thyroidea)*

Thymus gland

Adrenal glands *(glandulae suprarenales)*

Pancreas

Reproductive glands (ovaries)

Fig 7-57 The location of the endocrine hormonal glands.

These endocrine glands include the following:

- The **pineal gland** *(epiphysis)* sits in the diencephalon; its active substance is melatonin, and it regulates sexual maturity. Disturbances inhibit sexual maturation or lead to premature development.
- The **pituitary gland** *(hypophysis)* regulates hormonal control. Disturbances lead to dwarfism, obesity, and genital underdevelopment.
- The **thyroid gland** *(glandula thyroidea)* regulates the metabolic processes by increasing the uptake of oxygen in the cells. Disturbances lead to distinctive metabolic disorders, cretinism, and Graves disease.
- The **thymus gland** lies in front of the pericardium and is a lymphatic organ. Its active substance has a growth-regulating effect; it inhibits the development of the sexual organs and monitors the immune system. Disturbances lead to an increased tendency to infection; hyperactivity of the thymus prevents sexual maturation.
- The **adrenal glands** *(glandulae suprarenalis)* lie on the kidneys and produce epinephrine (adrenaline) and norepinephrine (noradrenaline) to regulate the metabolism. Disturbances lead to excessive pigmentation of the skin (Addison disease or bronzed skin), a fall in blood sugar, muscle weakness, and sluggish thinking.
- The **islets of Langerhans** in the pancreas produce active substances to regulate the sugar content of the blood. Disturbances lead to diabetes, imbalance in blood sugar levels, and even diabetic coma.
- The **reproductive glands** are the male testes and the female ovaries.

Trigeminal Nerve

The nerve supply to the oral cavity, masticatory muscles, and parts of the face is provided by the three-part nerve, the **trigeminal nerve**. This paired nerve emerges from the medulla oblongata and is the fifth cranial nerve. It carries sensory fibers (sensory root, *radix sensoria, portio major*) to the facial skin, the mucous membranes of the mouth, the nasal cavity, and the paranasal sinuses, as well as sensory fibers to the conjunctiva of the eye and to the lacrimal glands. In addition, sensory nerves of taste from the anterior area of the tongue to the brain are carried in the trigeminal nerve. The trigeminal nerve also carries motor fibers (motor root, *radix motoria, portio minor*) to the muscles of mastication and thereby regulates the movement of the mandible.

The trigeminal nerve consists of three branches that pass through separate openings in the middle cranial fossa into the adjacent cavities of the facial skeleton, where they again divide into three terminal branches (Fig 7-58). The root cells of the nerve form a powerful ganglion (*ganglion semilunare*, trigeminal ganglion, gasserian ganglion) in the middle cranial fossa in front of the apex of the petrous bone, where the ganglia create an impression in the bone (trigeminal impression).

The **ophthalmic branch** *(nervus ophthalmicus)* is the first division of the trigeminal nerve, which enters the orbit through the superior orbital fissure. It only carries sensory fibers and divides into three terminal branches with the following names and areas of distribution:

1. The **lacrimal nerve** *(nervus lacrimalis)* runs laterally to the lacrimal gland, the corner of the eye, and the eyelids.
2. The **frontal nerve** *(nervus frontalis)* runs from the superior edge of the orbit over the forehead to the crown of the head; consequently, it supplies the skin of the root of the nose, the forehead, and the upper eyelid.
3. The **nasociliary nerve** *(nervus nasociliaris)* runs centrally to the inner corner of the eye, the outer skin of the nose as far as the tip of the nose, and to the upper nasal mucosa.

The **maxillary branch** *(nervus maxillaris)* is the second division of the trigeminal nerve. It enters the pterygopalatine fossa through the foramen rotundum and carries sensory fibers (Fig 7-59); it divides into three terminal branches with the following names and areas of distribution:

1. The **zygomatic nerve** *(nervus zygomaticus)* runs from the inferior orbital fissure into the side wall of the orbit to reach the skin of the cheek and the temple area through bony channels in the zygomatic bone.
2. The **infraorbital nerve** *(nervus infraorbitalis)* runs straight and forward from the foramen rotundum to the infraorbital groove and into the

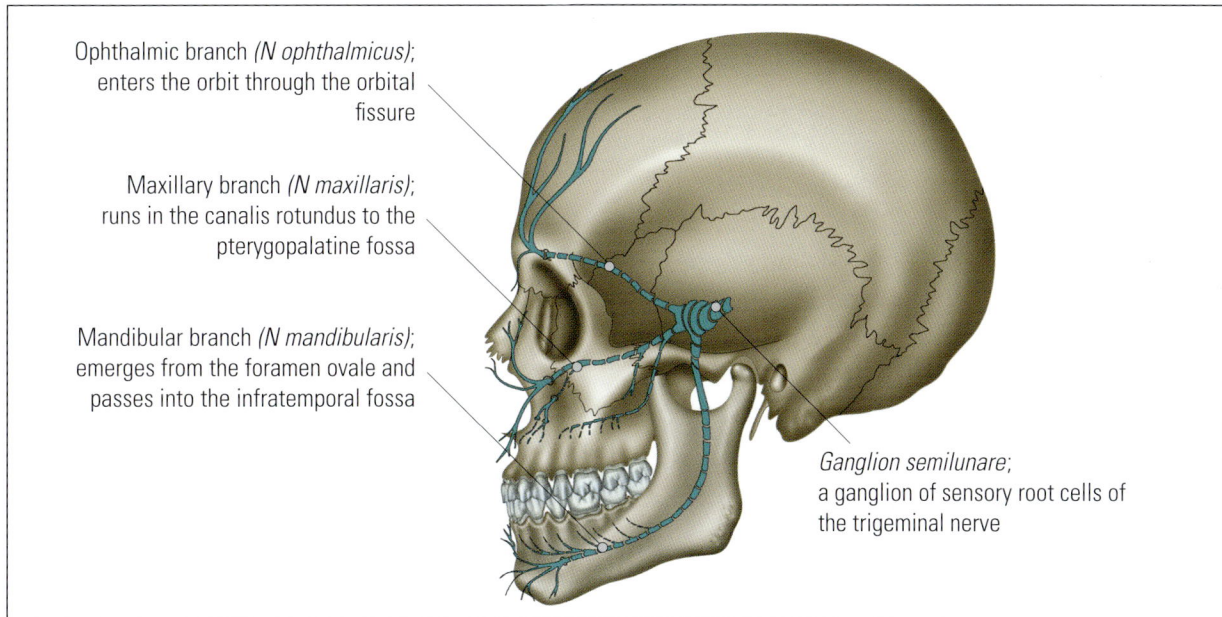

Fig 7-58 The three divisions of the trigeminal nerve.

Ophthalmic branch *(N ophthalmicus)*; enters the orbit through the orbital fissure

Maxillary branch *(N maxillaris)*; runs in the canalis rotundus to the pterygopalatine fossa

Mandibular branch *(N mandibularis)*; emerges from the foramen ovale and passes into the infratemporal fossa

Ganglion semilunare; a ganglion of sensory root cells of the trigeminal nerve

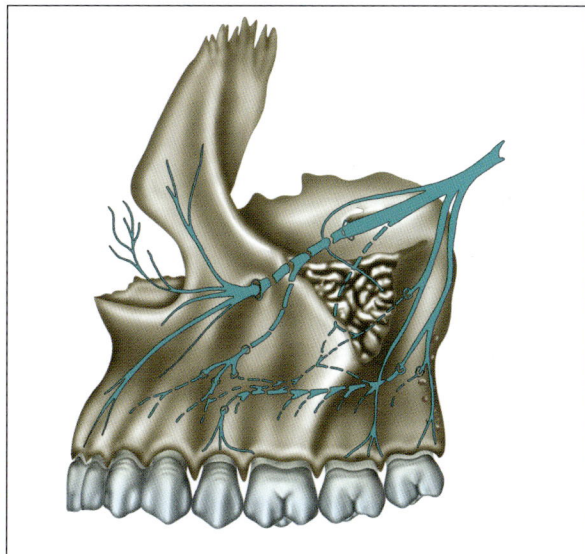

Fig 7-59 The maxillary branch only carries sensory fibers. Its area of innervation is the dura mater; the skin of the lower eyelid, cheek, upper lip, and wing of the nose; the mucosa of the nasal cavity, palate, upper lip, and maxillary sinuses; and the maxillary teeth.

infraorbital canal, to exit at the infraorbital foramen. Before it enters the infraorbital groove, a few fibers branch off to enter the infratemporal surface in the body of the maxilla, where they supply the posterior teeth and the gingiva. In the floor of the groove and the canal, a few fibers of the nerve pass through to the premolars and the anterior teeth of the maxilla. After exiting from the infraorbital foramen, the nerves run to the conjunctiva, the upper lip, and the wing of the nose.

3. The **pterygopalatine nerve** (or sphenopalatine branch) passes through the sphenopalatine foramen into the nasal cavity and runs through

243

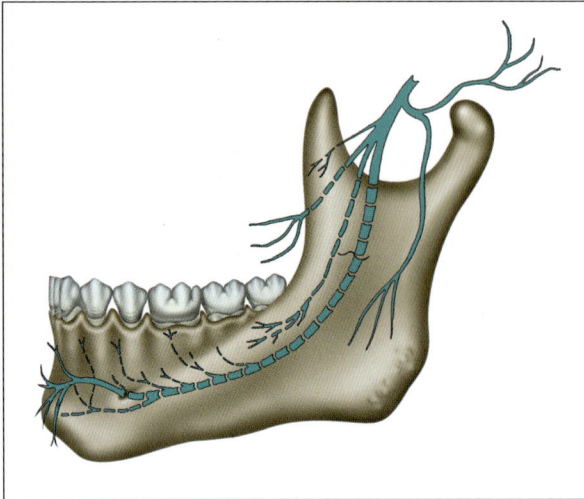

Fig 7-60 The mandibular branch is a mixed nerve with a sensory part and a motor part. It supplies the dura mater; the skin of the chin, lower lip, lower areas of the cheek, and anterior part of the external ear and the temple; the mucosa of the cheek, floor of the mouth, and anterior area of the tongue; the mandibular teeth; and the TMJs. The motor part supplies portions of the muscles of mastication.

the greater and lesser palatine foramina to the palate. It supplies the nasal mucosa and the mucous membrane of the palate as far as the anterior area.

The **mandibular branch** (nervus mandibularis) is the third division of the trigeminal nerve, which enters through the foramen ovale into the infratemporal fossa. It is the thickest of the three trigeminal divisions and contains, as well as a proportion of sensory fibers, all the motor fibers of the trigeminal nerve with which the individual masticatory muscles are supplied (Fig 7-60).

The nerves are named after these muscles of mastication:

• **Lateral pterygoid nerve** (nervus pterygoideus lateralis) for the lateral pterygoid muscle
• **Medial pterygoid nerve** (nervus pterygoideus medialis) for the medial pterygoid muscle
• **Temporal nerve** (nervus temporalis) for the temporal muscle
• **Masseteric nerve** (nervus massetericus) for the masseter muscle

The sensory fibers are divided into three terminal branches:

1. The **auriculotemporal nerve** (nervus auriculotemporalis) supplies the parotid gland.
2. The **inferior alveolar nerve** (nervus alveolaris inferior) supplies the mandibular teeth, the gingiva, and the skin of the chin and lower lip; passes through the mandibular foramen into the mandibular canal; and partly emerges again at the mental foramen.
3. The **lingual nerve** (nervus lingualis) runs to the lateral margin and anterior part of the tongue with a few taste fibers, to the sublingual salivary gland, to the oropharyngeal isthmus with the tonsils, to the mucosa of the floor of the mouth, and to the gingiva.

8

Articulators

Analysis of the guidance parameters for mandibular movement shows how the movement capabilities of the temporomandibular joint (TMJ), the neuromuscular system, and the shape and arrangement of the teeth relate to each other. All the parts of the system are in harmony. The shape and arrangement of the occlusal surfaces must be related to the TMJ for a properly functioning denture.

To produce a denture that takes account of the special function of the TMJ or mandibular movements, a device is required that can simulate the movements of the joint and the mandible. Occlusal surfaces are created in this device by replicating mandibular movement while constantly checking the occlusion. As the occlusal surfaces become more accurate and more functional, the individual mandibular movements of the patient can be better replicated.

Mechanical articulator devices reproduce the centric occlusal position or jaw relationship and the movement function with tooth contact (ie, articulation). That is why these devices are commonly called *articulators*. However, the function of the neuromuscular system cannot be replicated by a mechanical device.

Articulator Components

Despite all the special structural features of the different devices, the basic components of any articulator are the same (Fig 8-1). Each device has an upper part (arm or member) and a lower part (arm or member), and each part has a removable model holder. The upper part of the device is connected movably to the lower part by means of a simulated joint, which is arranged as a condylar roller or a condylar housing (casing or box). The

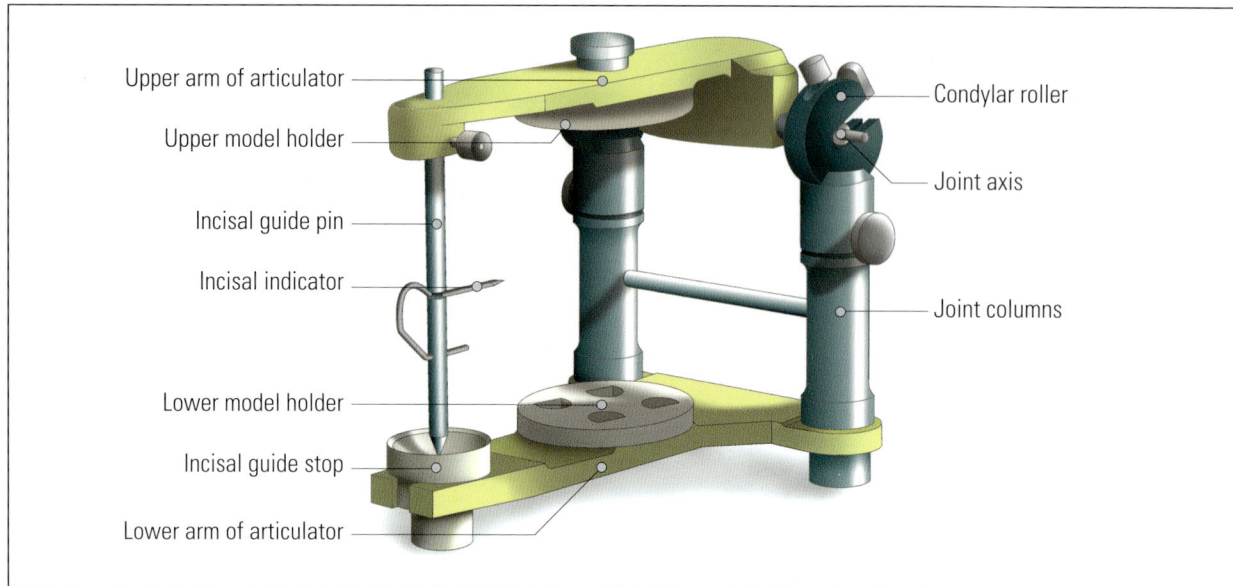

Fig 8-1 Components of an articulator.

joints are fixed to the joint columns (or condylar supports); in many articulators, the joints can be variably moved on these joint columns (eg, to measure the Bennett angle, condylar inclination, or intercondylar distance).

In most articulators, the incisal guide pin is fitted to the upper arm, while the incisal guide stop with the adjustable or exchangeable incisal guide table is fixed to the lower arm. The guide pin and guide table can also be interchanged. The incisal guide table represents tooth guidance in an articulator by enabling the upper part of the device to be guided against the lower part via articular guidance and the incisal guide table. In average-value articulators, the incisal guide pin carries an incisal indicator that denotes the mandibular incisal point or the occlusal plane.

Articulators can be classified according to the following:

- Reference planes for model adjustment
- Nature of the joint and movement simulation
- Range of anatomical values used

Reference Planes for Model Adjustment

The working models (maxilla and mandible) have to be adjusted in the articulators so that the movement paths of the device are congruent with the occlusal guidance paths of the rows of teeth being depicted.

It must therefore be possible to transfer to the articulator the geometric reference points and planes of the skull or masticatory system as well as their spatial relationships to the dentition. The reference planes are the Camper plane, the hinge-axis orbital plane, and the midface horizontal plane, and each plane has corresponding reference points (Fig 8-2). The reference planes are used not only for arbitrary (average-value) methods but also for individual, custom measurements.

The *Camper plane* runs from the superior edges of the outer orifices of the ears to the subnasal

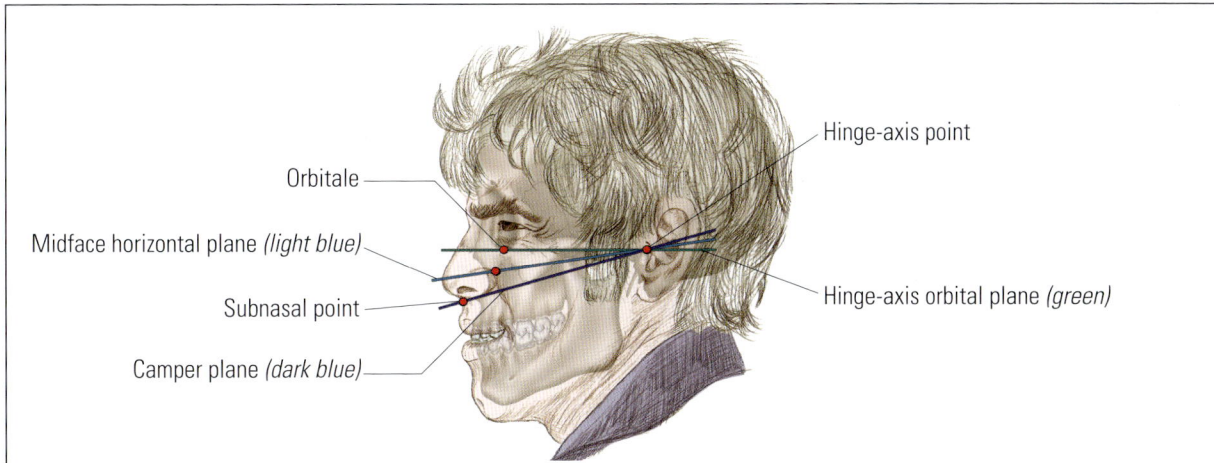

Fig 8-2 Reference planes for model adjustment.

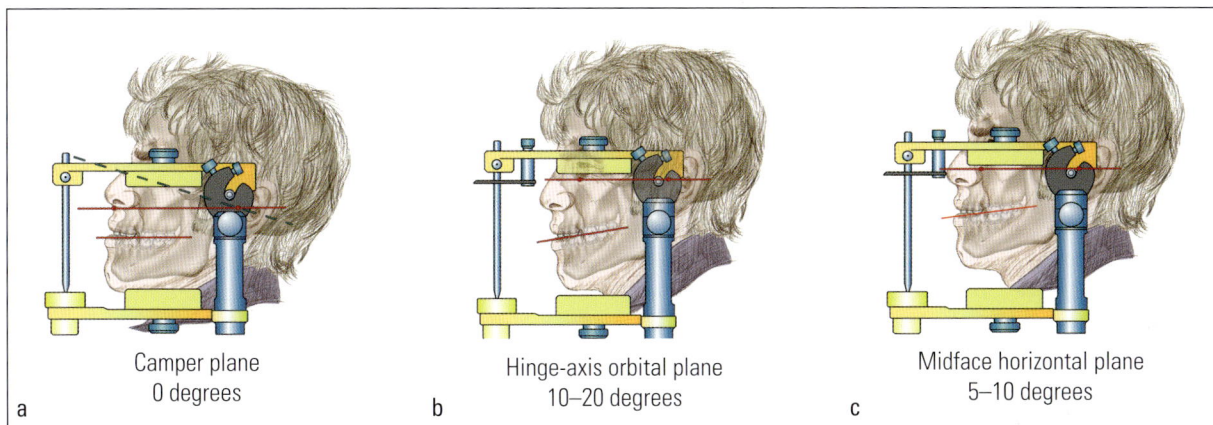

Fig 8-3 (a to c) Inclination of the occlusal plane based on the reference plane used.

point and, in articulators, lies parallel to the upper and lower arm (Fig 8-3a); the occlusal plane lies midway between the model holders parallel to the Camper plane. The models are aligned with the occlusal plane and then lie parallel to the table plane. Even when joint-related adjustment of the models is carried out using individual transfer methods, the occlusal plane as a parallel to the Camper plane is the reference plane for reconstruction of the occlusal field.

The *hinge-axis orbital plane* runs from the hinge-axis point to the main orbital point and, in the appropriate articulators, also lies parallel to

the upper and lower arms. The occlusal plane and hence the models are inclined at an individual angle (approximately 10 to 20 degrees) (Fig 8-3b). In addition to the hinge-axis orbital plane, the Frankfort plane and the auriculo-infraorbital plane are used as corresponding reference planes.

The *midface horizontal plane* or patient horizontal plane lies between the hinge-axis orbital plane and the Camper plane. It is referenced on the articulator and runs through the hinge-axis points and a reference point approximately 43 mm above the mandibular incisal point (Fig 8-3c).

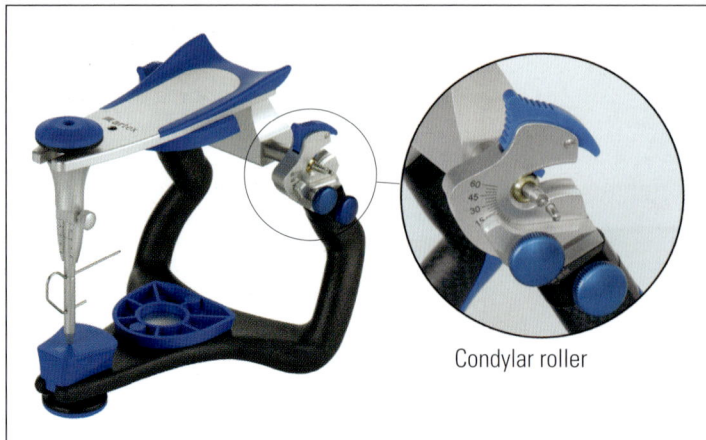

Fig 8-4 In a nonarcon articulator, the condylar rollers with the articular surfaces are located on the lower arm of the articulator and the condylar balls on the upper arm. Movement of the condylar balls is performed in the opposite direction to the natural model. (Courtesy of AmannGirrbach.)

Condylar roller

Replication of Joints and Movements

In the natural masticatory system, the mandible moves in condylar, tooth, and neuromuscular guidance against the fixed maxilla; however, the conventional design of articulators only allows the upper arm to be moved in relation to the fixed mandibular model holder, imitating only condylar and tooth guidance. This means that relative movements with calculable variations are possible.

The **conventional design** of articulators only permits movement of the upper arm in relation to the fixed mandibular model holder. This mechanical simplification allows better handling and produces movements of the rows of teeth that are analogous but opposite to those of the natural dentition.

Condylar guidance is produced by mechanical replication with mainly linear forms of the condylar path, where neuromuscular guidance to Bennett movement is simulated by adjustable Bennett angles.

Joint geometry is also replicated differently in different articulators; a distinction is made between arcon and non-arcon articulators in terms of joint replication. The term *arcon* is formed from the words *articulation* and *condyle*.

Nonarcon articulators are devices in which the articular surfaces and condyles are transposed in comparison with the natural dentition: The con-dylar rollers (with condylar path) are located on the lower arm of the articulator and the condylar balls or spheres (condyles) on the upper arm. As a result, the condylar balls move in the opposite direction to the condyles in the human skull (Fig 8-4).

A **condylar ball** is an artificial, spherical condyle as a simplified replication of the articular condyle of the mandible *(caput mandibulae)*. In addition, the condyles may be shaped as rollers or double spheres based on the shape of the condylar path.

In nonarcon articulators, a **condylar roller** represents a closed simulation of the articular surface of the TMJ on the lower arm of the device, in which the condylar ball fixed to the upper arm is accurately guided. With some condylar rollers, both the horizontal condylar inclination and the Bennett angle are adjustable; the condylar inclination is altered by twisting the roller, and the Bennett angle is changed by pivoting around a vertical axis.

Movement errors arise because, during movements of the maxilla, the condylar ball moves upward and backward instead of downward and forward. As a result, the gap between the condylar ball and the maxillary teeth is altered. In the natural masticatory system, the condyles as rotation centers are always at a constant distance from the mandibular teeth. However, if the joint parts are transposed in comparison with the anatomical model, the distance between the mandibular teeth and the rotation center changes during protrusive and lateral movements (Fig 8-5).

Fig 8-5 For reasons of technical simplification, the upper models are moved relative to the lower models in articulators. This design difference and the relative movement of the jaws do not cause any movement errors. In the natural masticatory system, the distances from the mandibular condyle to any desired occlusal points are always the same. *(a and b)* With nonarcon articulators, the distances of the mandibular teeth from the rotation center change with every movement under tooth contact. *(c and d)* With an arcon articulator, the distances of the mandibular teeth from the rotation center do not change.

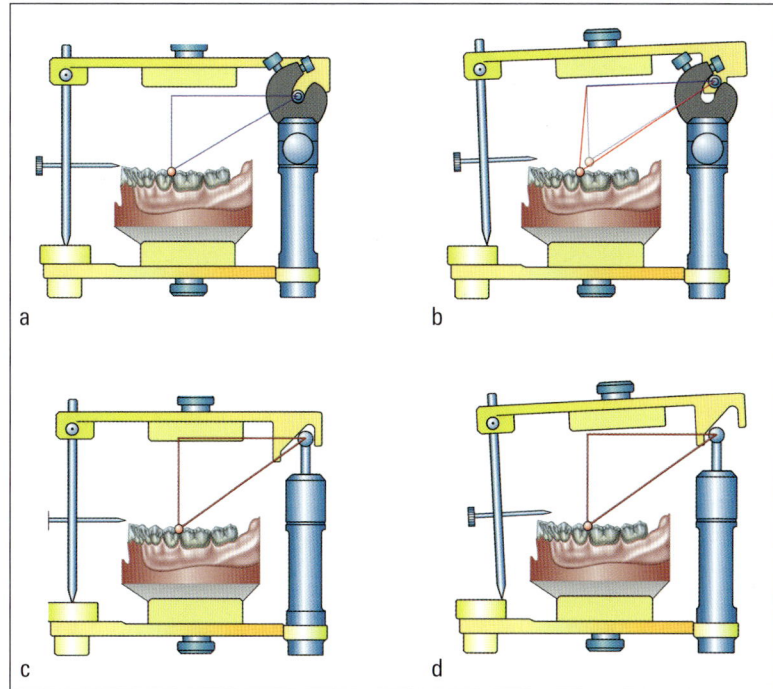

Fig 8-6 Arcon articulators, corresponding to the natural model, have the condylar housing with the articular surface on the upper arm of the device and the condylar ball on the lower arm. As a result, movement is performed as in the natural TMJ. The articular surfaces follow curved paths and can be adjusted in terms of horizontal inclination and in the range of the Bennett angle. (Courtesy of AmannGirrbach.)

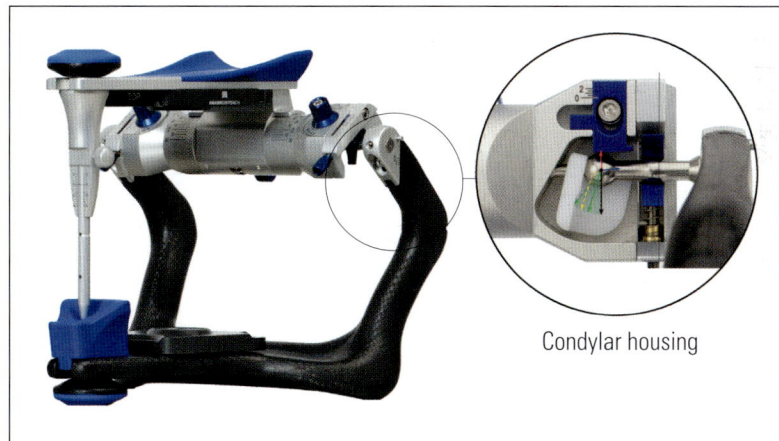

Condylar housing

Arcon articulators are average-value or fully adjustable devices in which the articular surfaces and condyles are arranged in accordance with the natural model: The condylar ball (condyle) is located on the lower arm, and the condylar housing (with condylar path) is fixed to the upper part of the articulator (Fig 8-6). This design corresponds to anatomical reality and allows movements in roughly the same direction as in the masticatory organ. The mandibular movements are performed as relative movements because the upper arm (the maxilla) is moved relative to the lower arm (mandible). No movement errors caused by displacement of the rotation center compared with the mandibular teeth will occur during lateral movements (see Fig 8-5).

Condylar housings (casings or boxes) are the articular surfaces open at the bottom and located on the top part of an arcon articulator. The condyle on the lower arm of the articulator slides downward and forward on the articular surface when TMJ movements are being simulated, which corresponds to the natural pattern of movement. The condylar housing can be adjusted in accordance with the angle of the condylar path. In order to simulate Bennett movement, the condylar paths are differently shaped in the condylar housing. The articular surface can be rotated and adjusted around a vertical axis corresponding to the Bennett angle, and exchangeable inserts with curved movement paths are provided to simulate different courses of Bennett movement (see Fig 8-6). Some articulators have exchangeable condylar path inserts for individually milled condylar paths.

The condylar housing open at the bottom can be closed with a pivoting locking device on some articulators to hold the condyle on the articular surface during simulation of lateral or protrusive movements.

Anatomical Values Used

The possibilities and limitations of movement replication with mechanical articulators depend on the aforementioned joint replication and furthermore on the use of anatomical geometric values of the masticatory system. Accordingly, all articulators can be classified as fixed-value, semi-adjustable, or fully adjustable devices. The values that can be individually measured and variably applied are the following:

- Horizontal condylar inclination
- Bennett angle (Bennett paths)
- Bonwill triangle, Balkwill angle, and incisal point
- Relationship between the joints and the occlusal field

Fixed-value articulators are all devices in which the geometric values used are incorporated in a nonadjustable way. These devices can be differentiated according to the range of values they use.

A **fixator** (occlusion holder) is a device or plaster block on which two models are mounted in a fixed occlusal situation (Fig 8-7). The models can be separated to carry out dental laboratory work. Fixators are mainly used to fix orthodontic models according to a construction bite position (Fig 8-8). The maxillary and mandibular models are fixed in the sagittal, vertical, and horizontal planes at a distance determined by the construction bite so that maxillomandibular appliances can be fabricated. In a fixator or a plaster base, occlusal surfaces or a denture can be reconstructed according to the terminal occlusal position. The mandibular movements are not taken into account initially with this technique; the occlusal surfaces have to be more or less roughly reground in the patient's mouth. Such fabrication methods are outdated and are only rarely used today. A variety of fixators are used for preparing indirect relinings to hold the dental arch of the denture being worked against the model.

An **occluder** is the simplest device with which centric occlusion can be reproduced (Fig 8-9). Occluders are devices in which maxillary and mandibular models can be moved against each other via a simple hinge joint. Sliding movements cannot be replicated.

A distinction is made between occluders with and without occlusal height fixation. Occluders with a locking screw for occlusal height can fix the vertical distance between the jaws. Occluders without a locking screw for occlusal height can only be used for dentate models in which the occlusal height is established by opposing groups of teeth. Occluders are entirely unsuitable for individual shaping of occlusal surfaces.

Average-value cranial devices are occluders with mechanisms for incorporating so-called average-value *calottes* (a device for holding a plate to which teeth can be formed). This average-value calotte is arched in the same way as the curves of occlusion would be if TMJs had average inclinations and angles. These devices cannot be used to simulate any of the articulation movements (lateral or protrusive) performed by TMJs. However, once the occlusal surfaces have been reconstructed, the models can be moved back and forth on these occlusal surfaces while the upper base holder is loosened. Nevertheless, these are not genuine jaw movements because an essential guidance element, namely the TMJ, is absent.

It is assumed that the movements of the mandible follow specific paths, guided by the TMJ, so

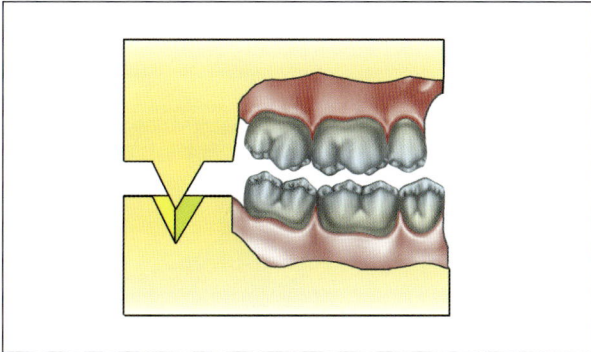

Fig 8-7 The plaster fixator is the simplest but also the least adequate means of fixing two rows of teeth against each other in terminal occlusion. Simple models with a wax occlusion prepared in thermoplastic impression material were mainly combined in a plaster fixator to fabricate single crowns.

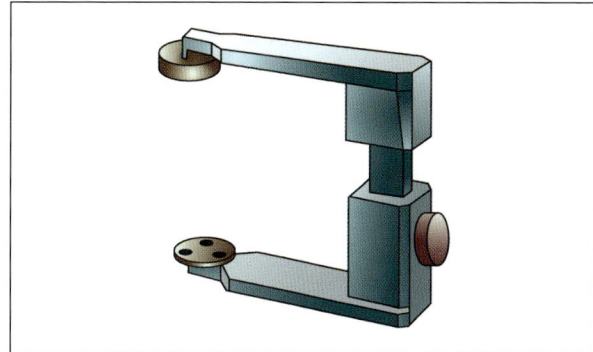

Fig 8-8 *Fixator* denotes an occlusion holder for fixing orthodontic models based on a construction bite position. The maxillary and mandibular models are fixed in the sagittal, vertical, and horizontal planes at the distance predetermined by the construction bite so that maxillomandibular appliances can be produced.

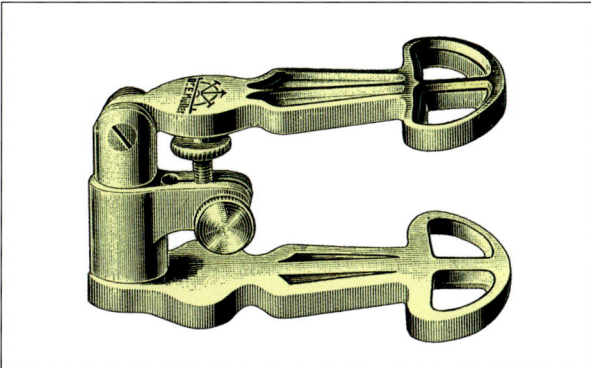

Fig 8-9 An occluder is a mechanical articulator with which the terminal occlusal position can be reproduced. Occluders contain a simple hinge joint that is not intended to imitate any joint movements, but the models can be quickly separated and brought together for the working position. Occluders without an adjusting screw to set the occlusal height can only be used for models that contain opposing groups of teeth so that the occlusal height is fixed. (Illustration circa 1925.)

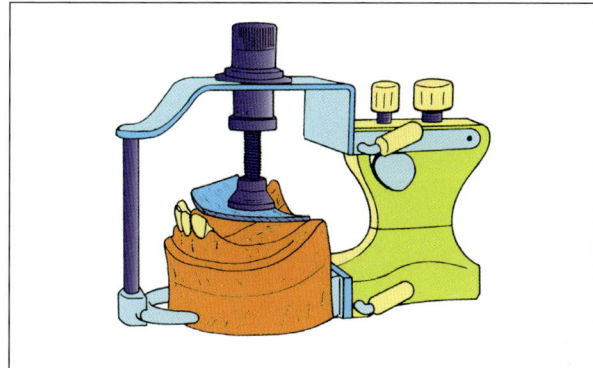

Fig 8-10 Another type of occluder enables approximately joint-related occlusal fields to be created though the clamping of a calotte. This calotte is constructed on the basis of average condylar paths. Joint-related jaw movements cannot be performed with these devices.

that very specific occlusion curves and shapes of occlusal surfaces develop or are ground in. In this state, the mandible is guided no longer by the TMJ alone but primarily by the occlusal pattern of the teeth. Changes to the occlusal surfaces, particularly in elderly people, will involve a change to the TMJ, which will display signs of wear and no longer guarantee accurate guidance of the mandible. That is why occlusion curves are set up on the basis of calottes, which present the average values for the condylar path inclinations (Fig 8-10). Thus, a "chewing path" is created that di-

rects the mandibular movements and hence the TMJ.

This method, in which curves of occlusion are preset, may be described as chewing path–based generation of the occlusal field. With these devices, a chewing path based on average values is generated that enforces a mandibular movement with tooth contact but does not necessarily coincide with TMJ guidance. The natural TMJs have to be adjusted to this occlusal guidance (ie, altered).

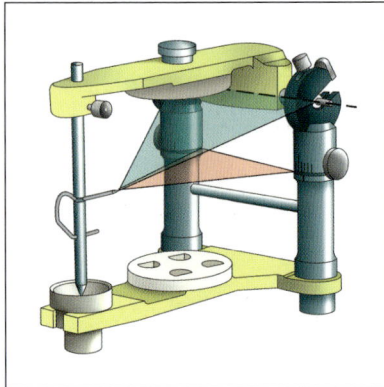

Fig 8-11 Average-value articulators are constructed according to statistical average values: a condylar inclination of approximately 30 to 34 degrees; a Bennett angle of approximately 15 to 20 degrees; the intercondylar distance, position of the occlusal plane, and incisal point determined according to the Bonwill triangle; and the occlusal plane at an angle of approximately 22 degrees to the Bonwill triangle. The devices contain markings or calibration keys for mounting the models.

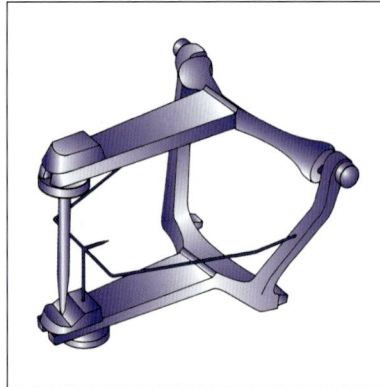

Fig 8-12 The Heilborn articulator is a simple arcon average-value articulator with fixed condylar inclinations (approximately 30 degrees), no Bennett angle, and an incisal guidance of approximately 15 degrees. A wire holder fixes the occlusal plane and the incisal point. In principle, jaw movements can be simulated, but only as a rough approximation. The models are aligned in accordance with the Bonwill triangle.

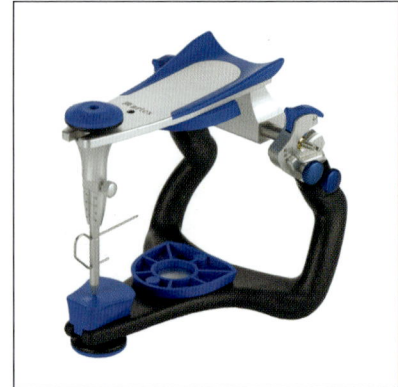

Fig 8-13 The average-value nonarcon articulator in the Artex range (AmannGirrbach) has a curved condylar path. The standard device is oriented to the Bonwill triangle and shows the occlusal plane; the Bennett angle is adjustable between 0 and 20 degrees, and the sagittal condylar path is in the range of 15 to 60 degrees. The exchangeable guide tables have an inclination of 10 to 20 degrees.

Average-Value Articulators

Average-value articulators are fixed-value devices whose overall size is defined by the average Bonwill triangle (approximately 11-cm side length) and an average Balkwill angle (approximately 22 degrees). The Camper plane is the reference plane. The horizontal condylar inclinations are generally at an angle of 30 to 34 degrees to the occlusal plane. A Bennett angle of 0 to 20 degrees is also firmly set (Figs 8-11 to 8-13).

The **relationship of the occlusal plane** to the joints corresponds to average values in fixed-value articulators; it is determined by the Bonwill triangle and the average Balkwill angle and identified with markings. The distances of the joints from each other and from the mandibular incisal point are measured according to the average values of the Bonwill triangle. The overall height and hence the Balkwill angle can be changed in some devices simply by altering the distance from the joints to the occlusal plane (eg, with spacer discs).

Average-value articulators enable the basic mandibular movements to be performed with tooth contact: protrusive excursions and lateral movements as well as opening and closing in a narrowly limited opening range. The movements are guided by straight condylar paths and the incisal guide table with average-value inclination, as the upper arm of the device is supported against the lower arm on the incisal guide table via the vertical guide pin. Anterior guidance and the two articular points give rise to three-point support of the upper arm of the articulator. These three guide areas (condylar paths and incisal guide table) establish the movement paths of the models or of the rows of teeth against each other.

System errors occur as a result of the shape, position, and inclinations of the condylar paths and the position of the models in relation to the joint axis. The setting of the angles of inclination of the condylar path, the Bennett angle, and incisal guidance is not based on precise measurement of the patient's TMJs but rather lies within a rough range of values. Occlusal guidance that only roughly approximates the real TMJ guidance is generated based on average values.

In contrast to the shape of the anatomical path, the condylar paths in average-value articulators

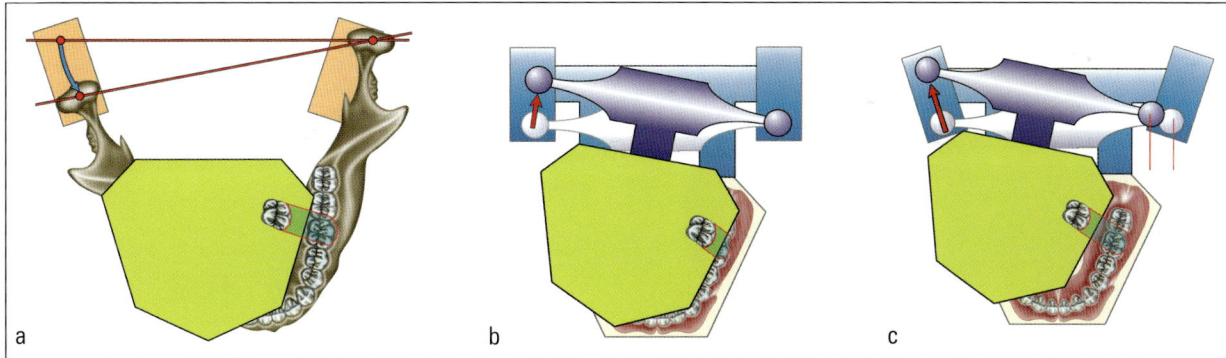

Fig 8-14 *(a)* During lateral movements of the mandible, the nonworking condyle follows a circular path that is flattened or deformed by the individual Bennett movement. *(b)* If the Bennett movement is not simulated in an articulator, the movement paths of the centric stops vary markedly from the real movement. *(c)* Bennett movement can be reproduced as a first approximation by setting a Bennett angle in the articulator.

are mainly depicted as straight. The natural joint, however, has a curved path. Therefore, the curved movement path of the condyle is reproduced inadequately in the mechanical device. If the Bennett movement is not simulated in an articulator, noticeable deviations from real movement will arise in the occlusal movement paths. In average-value articulators, the position of the orthodontic models at the articular points can only be set as an average, possibly with a calibration key. The position of the occlusal plane is set as a fixed value. The incisal point and the occlusal plane of the models are aligned with the occlusal plane markings on the average-value articulator by visual judgment or with a calibration key.

Semi-Adjustable Average-Value Articulators

An attempt is made with these devices to optimize the simulation of movements achieved with average-value articulators. These devices can be adjusted to different reference planes. The *fixed geometric values* are the following:

• *Intercondylar distance:* The gap between the two condyles is fixed.
• *Condylar guidance:* The condylar path is preset as straight or curved.
• *Bennett movement:* The paths are straight.

The following are *variable values* on semi-adjustable articulators:

• Sagittal condylar inclination, right and left
• Bennett angle, right and left
• Anterior guidance by variable horizontal inclination of the guide table
• Position of the occlusal plane at the hinge axis, determined by transferring models using facebows

Semi-adjustable average-value articulators require clinical identification of the joint values and the joint-related position of the occlusal plane.

As a result of the *Bennett side shift*, the arched movement curve of the balancing mandibular condyle in the anatomical system flattens out slightly (Fig 8-14). In the device, the condyle slides on a straight, rigid condylar path guidance. If the Bennett movement follows a straight course in an articulator, the endpoint of the Bennett movement is actually the same as in the natural case. However, because the balancing mandibular condyle does not describe a circular arc but rather follows a straight path, variations in the paths are unavoidable in the occlusal field. This is why some semi-adjustable articulators are fitted with curved condylar inserts.

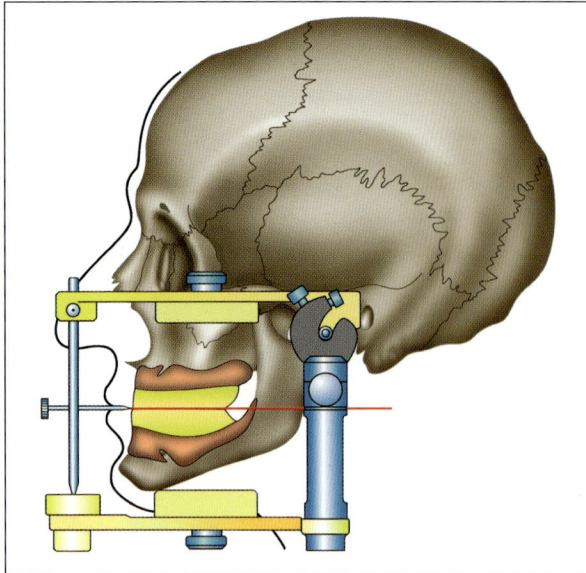

Fig 8-15 In average-value articulators, the occlusal plane in the interocclusal record is aligned with the occlusal plane markings and the incisal point on the articulator. As a result, a first approximation of the position of the jaws in relation to the articular points is achieved. This average-value method has some calculable system errors that must be corrected on the finished product, eg, by grinding in occlusal patterns in the mouth.

Errors of Technique with Average-Value Articulators

The quality of a mechanical articulator must be measured by what system errors occur and the seriousness of the individual errors. The best and most expensive equipment will not achieve the desired results if it is operated incorrectly or carelessly. Any system errors will be compounded by operating errors.

The *geometric arrangement* of the occlusal pattern at the articular surfaces is an important measure with which the movement paths of the centric stops in their contact areas are determined. If the anatomical system is transferred to a mechanical system, special attention must be paid to accurate measurement and transfer of these geometric values. If the opposing occlusal pattern with different geometric values is mounted in an articulator, the centric stops are unable to follow the same movement paths as in the anatomical system.

The *positional relationship* between occlusal patterns and articular surfaces is established by an average-value method with statistical averages, dispensing with accurate measuring (Fig 8-15). The mandibular incisal point, based on the average Bonwill triangle, is shown as a marking in the articulator by the incisal indicator, which is moved by the vertical support pin. The dorsal markings are found on the joint columns of the lower arm of the device; as a result, the occlusal plane is fixed. If transfer errors are made when models are being mounted in an average-value articulator, it is no longer possible to fabricate a denture fit for function.

The *following errors* can occur when aligning the models in an average-value articulator (Fig 8-16):

- Articulator marks are not placed in the neutral position:
  - Vertical support pin is not firmly seated on the upper arm.
  - Incisal guide table is not in the neutral position.
  - Support pin does not rest midway on the guide table.
  - Joints are not in the starting position.
  - Model holder is not firmly screwed in place.
- The occlusal plane of the models does not run parallel to the occlusal plane marking on the articulator.
- The incisal point of the models (interocclusal record) is not lined up with the appropriate marking on the device.

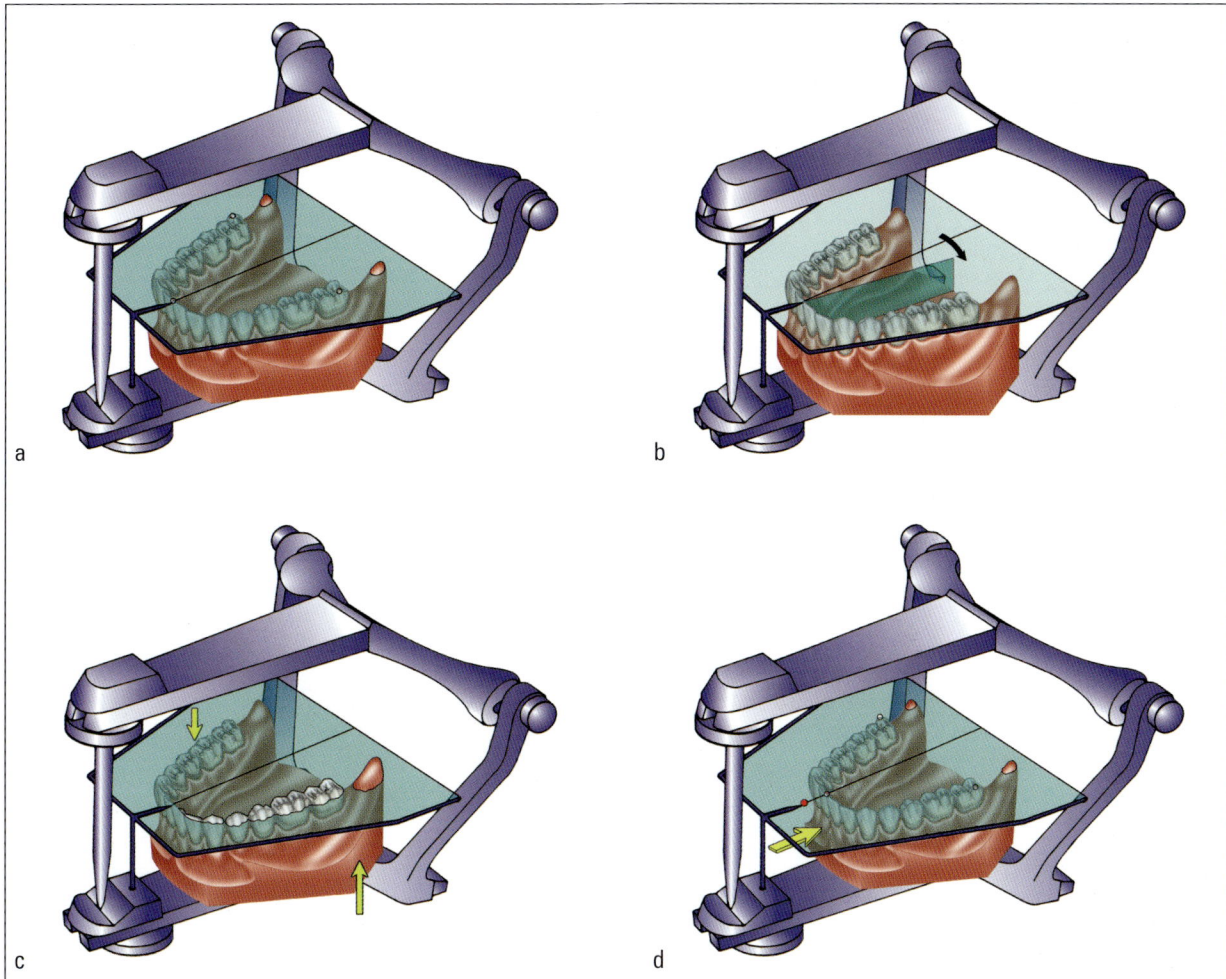

Fig 8-16 A striking error of technique when using articulators is to not align the models accurately in the correct position in relation to the articulator joints. *(a)* In average-value devices, the occlusal plane of the models must coincide; ie, the incisal points of the articulator and the model must be lined up. The occlusal plane marking on the device bisects the height of the retromolar triangle. *(b)* Twisting the model in the horizontal plane is a common error, which often goes unnoticed when the models lie at the incisal point and at the correct height. *(c)* Tilting of the occlusal plane often happens when edentulous jaw models are being mounted because accurate marking of half the height of the triangle has been omitted. *(d)* If the model is shifted dorsally, ie, the incisal point is not lined up, the movement radius of the occlusal points is altered.

• The middle of the models and the middle of the articulator are not lined up (the models are twisted). It makes sense to mount the models in two phases; first the mandibular model is aligned, and only after a thorough check is the maxillary model placed in the correct position in relation to the other.

Calibration keys are accessories for average-value mounting in average-value articulators (Fig 8-17). These accessories can be used to position the mandibular model correctly in relation to the articulator joints according to average values. To do this, defined fixed points on the models are lined up with markings on the calibration key. In

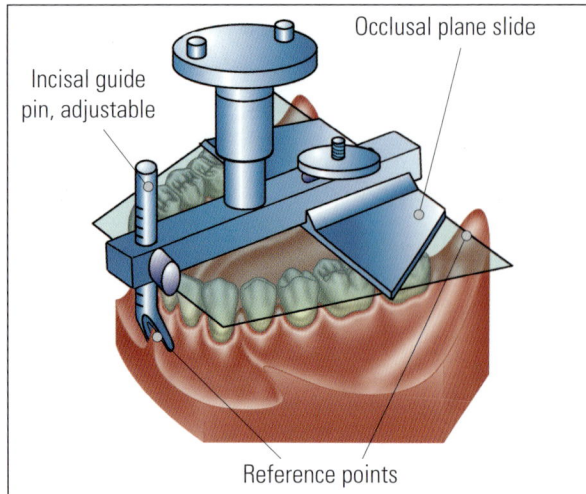

Fig 8-17 For average-value mounting of models in average-value articulators, manufacturers provide calibration keys with which the models are accurately placed and fixed on preset marker points (reference points). These marker points are set by the manufacturer and can be adjusted to the position of the occlusal plane. In this case, the incisal guide pin (symphyseal fork) must be placed immediately next to the labial frenum in the vestibular fornix, while the occlusal plane slide (measuring wedge) is set at half the height of the retromolar triangle or the distobuccal cusps of the mandibular second molar.

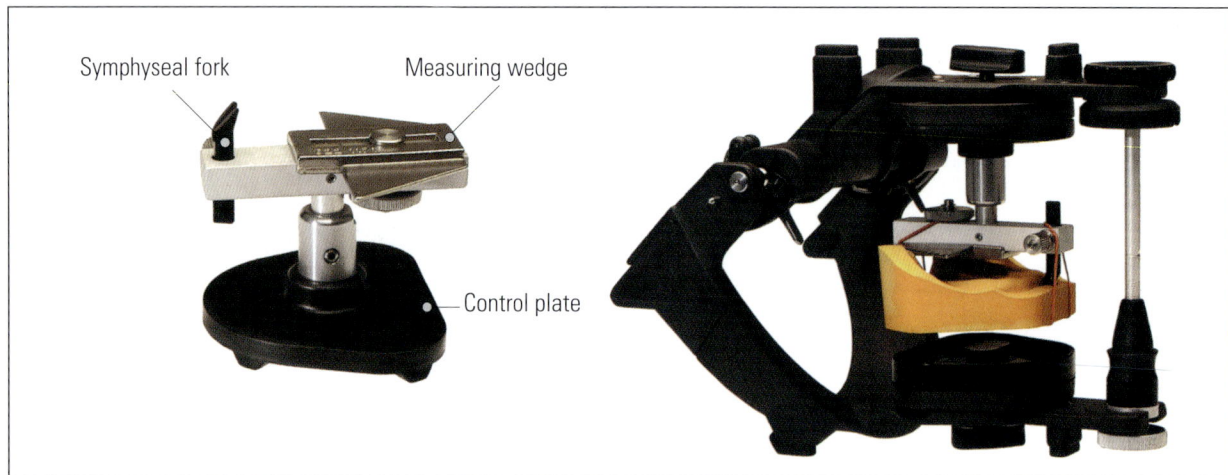

Fig 8-18 The calibration key to the PROTAR (KaVo) is magnetically retained in the articulator with the control plate.

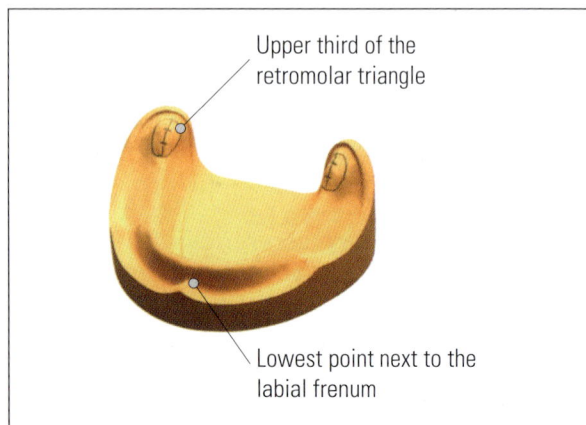

Fig 8-19 The articulator system from KaVo provides a mounting aid for the PROTAR articulator for average-value alignment of edentulous and dentate models. In relation to the Bonwill triangle, the models are aligned with the occlusal plane of the device based on average values. The mandibular incisal point or the lowest point next to the labial frenum is used as an anterior reference point on the models; the posterior reference points are the upper third of the retromolar triangles or the distobuccal cusps of the mandibular second molars.

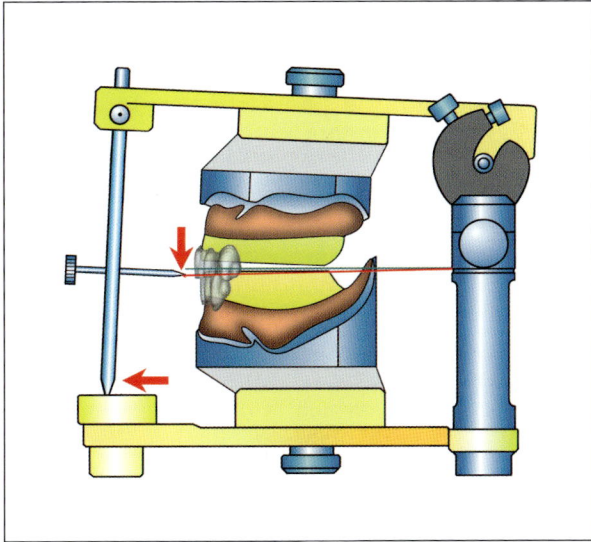

Fig 8-20 Changing the occlusal height in the average-value articulator is a gross error of technique. This means the incisal guide pin is lengthened and the upper arm of the articulator is raised. The position of the occlusal plane in the articulator is tilted because the incisal indicator tilts downward. In addition, the incisal guide pin is misaligned in the anterior guide table.

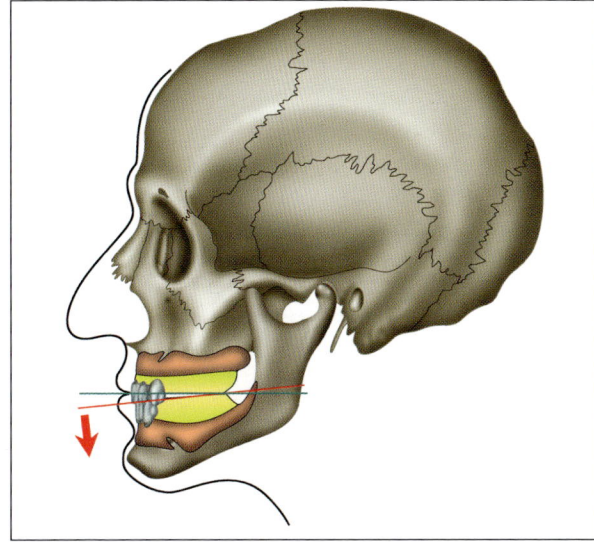

Fig 8-21 If, after the occlusal height has been increased, the tooth position is constructed in relation to the articulator occlusal plane, the occlusal plane is displaced in comparison with the natural model. An error of technique is now added to the system error of the average-value method. In the natural system, the occlusal plane moves downward by the amount of the occlusal height increase. The maxillary anterior teeth appear too long, and the attempted dynamic occlusal contacts are completely lost. Therefore, changing the occlusal height is a gross error when using average-value articulators.

most cases, the mandibular incisal point and the retromolar triangle are used as fixed points (Figs 8-18 and 8-19). A vertically movable incisal guide pin is placed into the vestibular fornix at the mandibular incisal point (mainly labial frenum), while a horizontal slide should be placed onto the occlusal plane marking of the retromolar triangle (usually upper third of the triangle). Errors arise if these fixed points are not adhered to.

Setting the occlusal height too high is a basic error. With every articulator there is a possibility of pushing the vertical support pin against the upper arm of the device to enlarge or reduce the working space. Before the models are mounted, it is important to check whether the support pin is fixed at the neutral height. If the working space is too small, this can be remedied by moving the support pin and the incisal guide table before

mounting. Changing the occlusal height after mounting, eg, increasing it for a complete denture, is a gross error (Figs 8-20 and 8-21). Changing the occlusal height in the articulator changes the vertical distance between the jaws while the position of the occlusal plane in the articulator remains unchanged. In the anatomical system, however, the occlusal plane is shifted by exactly half the amount of the occlusal height increase, and therefore the distance of the occlusal plane to the joints is also shifted.

A similar error is to ignore the occlusal plane (eg, when setting up teeth). This will change the positional relationship of the occlusal plane to the joints in the anatomical system, which also occurs if the height of the occlusal plane was not maintained on one side and the occlusal plane was tilted.

Fully Adjustable Articulators

Using these articulators, it is possible to mimic the individual movements of dynamic occlusion as far as possible, provided all the relevant geometric values have been determined following special registration and model transfer methods. Devices of this kind might also be referred to as *simulators of masticatory movement*. The variations from the actual movement paths are so minimal that they can be disregarded in practice.

The **reference plane** for fully adjustable articulators is preferably the hinge-axis orbital plane (auriculo-infraorbital plane, Frankfort plane); the Camper plane and the midface horizontal or patient horizontal plane also act as reference planes for some articulators. The devices are supplied in arcon or nonarcon versions.

Precise mounting of models requires time-consuming registration methods. All the values must be measured and transferred individually. Discrepancies between the individual and the simulated movement paths are usually due to handling and measuring errors.

When using a **fully adjustable articulator** (or individually adjustable articulator), it must be possible to perform all the movements out of centric occlusion that are possible for the patient while maintaining tooth contact. Therefore, articulators must meet the following conditions:

- *Individually adjustable values* for:
  - Sagittal condylar path inclination, left and right
  - Bennett angle, separately left and right
  - Shaping of individual incisal guidance or variably adjustable incisal guide table
  - Intercondylar distance
- Position of the occlusal plane relative to joint axis or cranium, ie, the exact position of the occlusal field in relation to the hinge axis in all spatial directions
- Specially shaped condyles and condylar paths
- Distraction adjustment for relieving compressed TMJs
- Exact replication of the individual Bennett movement
- Analogous movement directions
- Adequate working space for working models

System Errors

In an articulator, the primary aim is to simulate mandibular movements with tooth contact. Open mandibular movements are of minor importance in denture fabrication, namely when shaping the denture base: The denture base must not impinge on muscle attachments and ligaments that tighten during open mandibular movement. This movement of muscle attachments and ligaments cannot be reproduced with the articulator.

Intercondylar distance is the distance between the two condyles, which is only individually adjustable with very elaborate devices. However, the distances between the joints differ considerably from patient to patient. The intercondylar distance of articulators is based on the side length of the Bonwill triangle as a fixed value (Fig 8-22). This can result in substantial shifts in the occlusal field, because different movement curves of the centric stops can arise during lateral movements, depending on the difference from the individual case.

Condylar path inclinations in the sagittal direction can be accurately adjusted on nearly all articulators. However, it is more difficult to replicate the precise Bennett movement. If the Bennett movement is imitated by setting the condylar paths in the horizontal plane more toward the middle, the Bennett movement occurs as a pure axial shift, whereas in the anatomical case it follows a curved path or may even run dorsally to cranially or ventrally to caudally with the condyle in a resting position (Fig 8-23).

If the **Bennett movement** is incorrect, tooth contacts will also occur on the nonworking side during lateral movement, even though none are present in the articulator because they have not been incorporated. In a complete denture, for instance, it is exactly these balancing contacts still present in the articulator that are missing.

Functions of the articular disc and the joint capsule and naturally the neuromuscular system can only be mimicked indirectly or very inadequately. The neuromuscular system is the system unit of nerves and muscles, or in a wider sense, the movement habit. Thus, denture reconstructions are only ever checked in a "gentle" sliding state, never under masticatory loading.

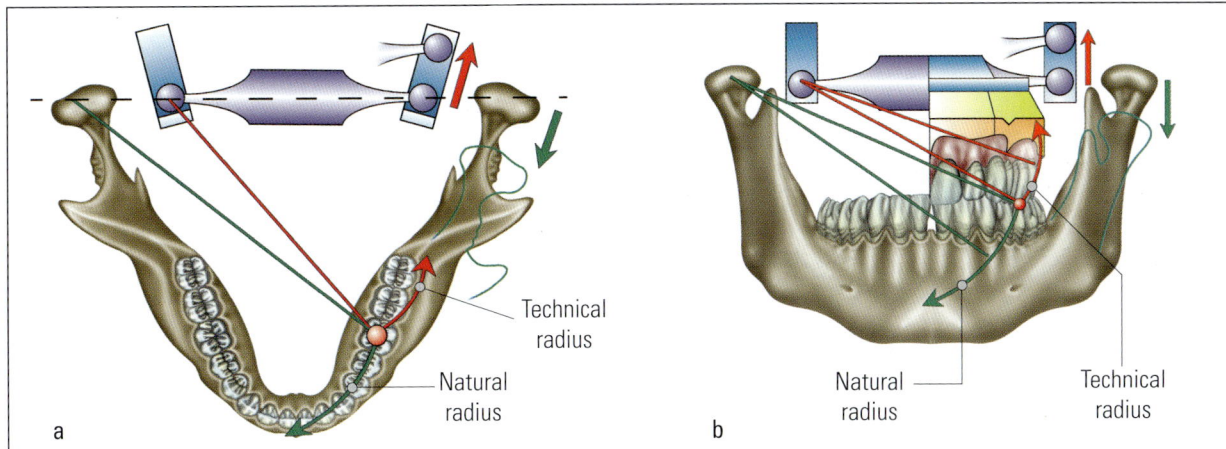

Fig 8-22 *(a and b)* One system error with articulators is the fixed intercondylar distance. The rotation radii of the centric stops in the occlusal field vary to the same extent as the variation in intercondylar distance between the articulator and the natural system.

Fig 8-23 In the natural joint, the upper joint cavity curves in an S-shape from the depth of the fossa downward and forward to the articular condyle; the articular disc sits on the condyle like a cap and forms the roughly "circular" lower joint cavity. This particular movement path of the condyle is imitated differently in technical devices. The simple technical simulation of the condylar path is linear, but curved condylar paths are becoming more and more established. The function of the articular disc cannot be simulated. In modern, fully adjustable articulators, the condylar casings are equipped with curved condylar paths, which are shaped in line with the natural model. Nonarcon average-value articulators may also have curved guidance surfaces.

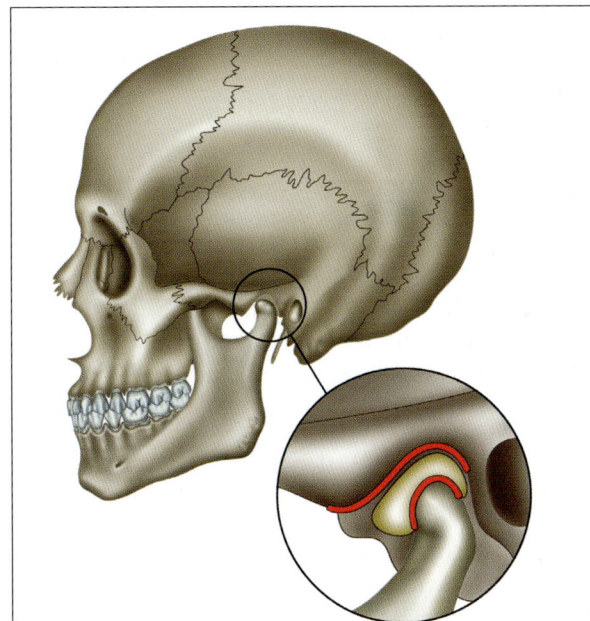

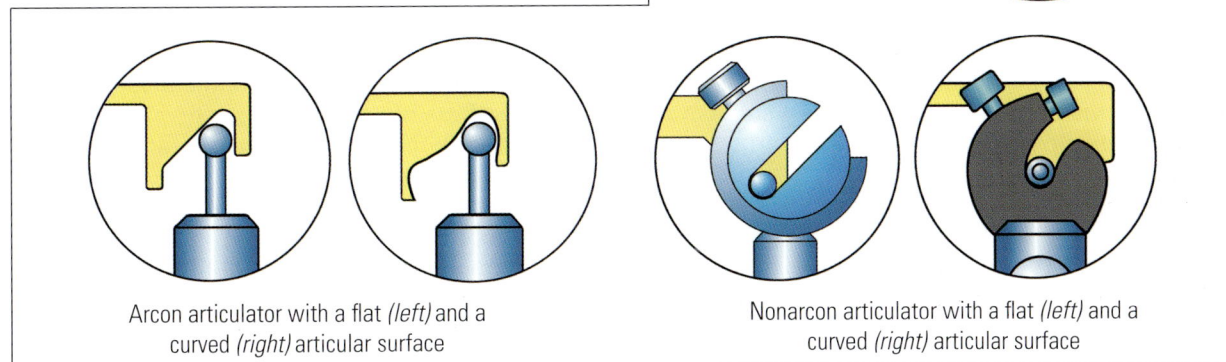

Arcon articulator with a flat *(left)* and a curved *(right)* articular surface

Nonarcon articulator with a flat *(left)* and a curved *(right)* articular surface

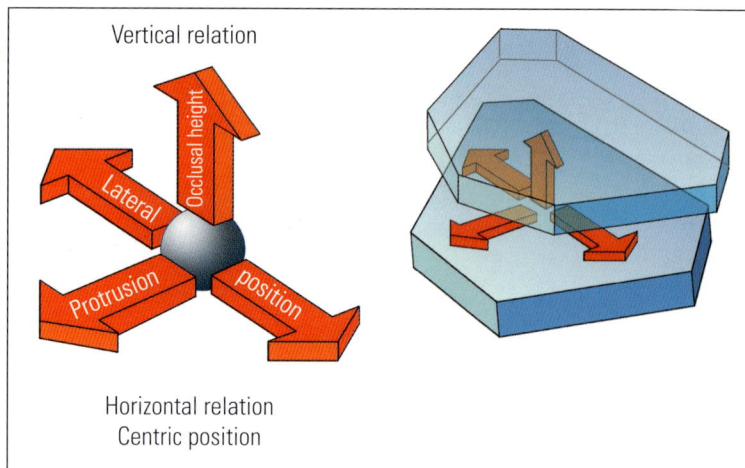

Jaw Relation Registration

The **jaw relation** is any position that the movable mandible can adopt relative to the fixed maxilla. In definition terms, *jaw relation* in a healthy occlusal system means the constantly reproducible, centric position of the mandible where the condyles are located deep in the mandibular fossae without pressure or tension and where maximal intercuspation and centric loading of the teeth exist. Jaw relation registration is intended to rediscover this centric occlusion or habitual intercuspation position.

In a fully dentate, normal dentition, the position of the mandible relative to the maxilla is clearly fixed by the occlusal pattern of the teeth, the TMJs, and the musculature. In a reduced residual dentition, the situation of opposing teeth may be so impaired that a definite centric position cannot be established with the models in the way it can with fully dentate models. In **edentulous jaws**, the centric occlusion position cannot be established with models alone. It has to be reconstructed by suitable methods.

Relation of the mandible to the maxilla can be determined in three dimensions. The central position analogous to centric occlusion is established by the occlusal height (vertical relation) and by the centric position (horizontal relation), which corresponds to the physiologic hinge-axis position (Fig 8-24). To reconstruct this occlusal position, baseplates are fabricated and then used in different types of jaw relation registration. The recording takes place in two phases: establishing the vertical relation and establishing the horizontal relation.

The **vertical relation** (occlusal height) can be determined on the basis of the interrelations among four variables:

1. Adoption of the physiologic rest position as the neuromuscular position of the mandible. In the relaxed state, there is a very small distance between the rows of teeth, which is adopted by the resting muscular tension.
2. Smallest speaking distance resulting from pronunciation of consonants or series of numbers.
3. Statistical mean in edentulous jaws: 38 to 42 mm distance from the mandibular to the maxillary vestibular fornix.
4. Establishment of harmonious facial proportions according to the golden ratio; the distance from the tip of the nose to the upper lip and from the upper lip to the tip of the chin is set at a length ratio of 3:5. The facial proportions can also be determined by average-value measurements of cranial dimensions (craniometry), whereby the distances between the forehead point, root of the nose, subnasal point, and tip of the chin are equal.

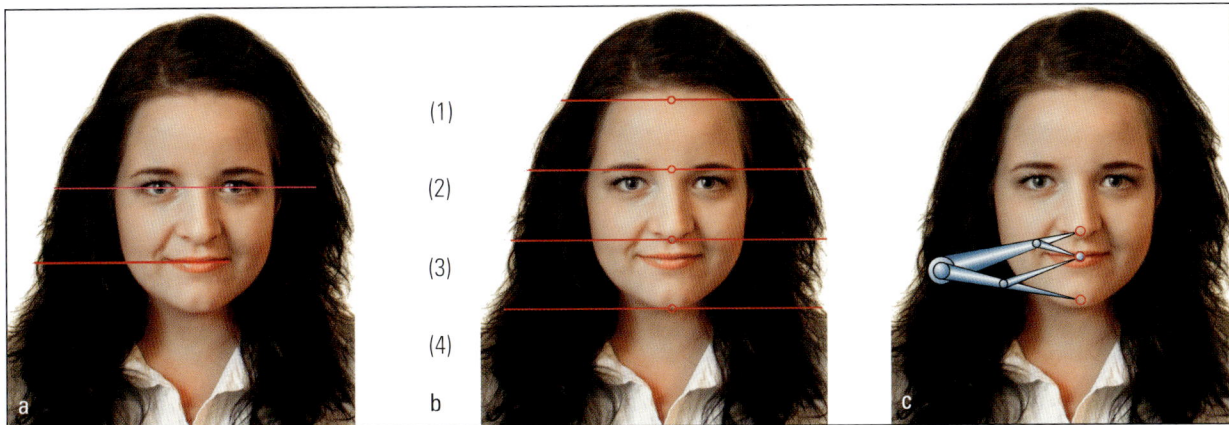

Fig 8-25 *(a)* For interocclusal record registration, the occlusion rims are aligned horizontally and parallel to the interpupillary line, which runs through both pupils. *(b)* To determine the vertical relation (occlusal height), a craniometric method can be used in which the face is divided symmetrically into three sections: The distance from the forehead point (1) to the root of the nose (2) is equal to the distance from the root of the nose to the subnasal point (3) and between the subnasal point and the tip of the chin (4). *(c)* However, dividers can also be used to measure the vertical maxillomandibular distance, determining the distance from the tip of the nose to the upper lip to the chin according to the golden ratio.

The **horizontal relation** or physiologic hinge-axis position is determined by the following methods:

- Adopting the most retruded mandibular position by:
  - Guiding it back by hand.
  - Getting the patient to swallow.
  - Having the patient touch the superior dorsal edge of the plate with the tip of the tongue. A wax ball can be placed exactly in the middle at the edge of the vibrating line on the baseplate, which the patient then has to touch with the tongue. As a result, the mandible is forcibly pulled back. In most cases, this is a forced position in which the condyles are in contact with the dorsal limit of the joint, hence about 1 mm behind the normal position. These methods are used for edentulous jaws.
- Gothic arch tracing (intraoral support pin registration) in which a centrally attached tracing stylus (or pin) records the horizontal mandibular movement on a tracing plate. Only this method yields the physiologic hinge-axis position.
- Electronic registration methods.

Centric records are used to transfer the physiologic hinge-axis position or centric position of the mandible relative to the maxilla onto the model situation; they are used to code the models for mounting in an articulator. A centric record can be prepared as a wax squash bite, with occlusal plates made of thermoplastic acrylic, silicone, or composite impression materials.

Hand-guided occlusal registration involves recording the jaw relation with wax occlusion rims, usually for edentulous jaws in which the mandible is guided into the centric position by hand. Occlusal height and horizontal occlusal position can be located by the aforementioned methods. In addition, the occlusal plane and fullness of the lips are established, and other orientation marks for the artificial teeth are traced.

Figures 8-25 to 8-31 illustrate various considerations for jaw relation registration.

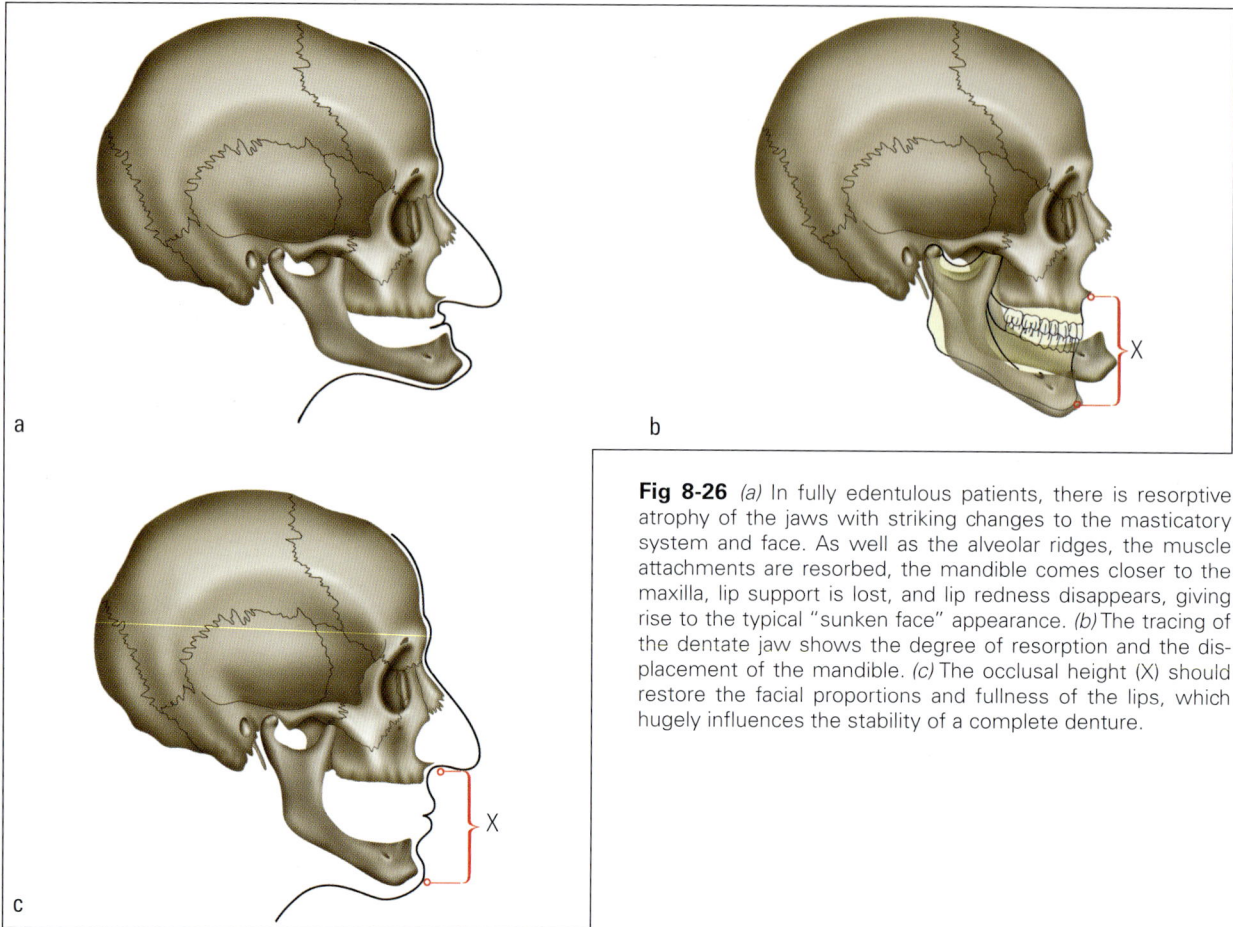

Fig 8-26 *(a)* In fully edentulous patients, there is resorptive atrophy of the jaws with striking changes to the masticatory system and face. As well as the alveolar ridges, the muscle attachments are resorbed, the mandible comes closer to the maxilla, lip support is lost, and lip redness disappears, giving rise to the typical "sunken face" appearance. *(b)* The tracing of the dentate jaw shows the degree of resorption and the displacement of the mandible. *(c)* The occlusal height (X) should restore the facial proportions and fullness of the lips, which hugely influences the stability of a complete denture.

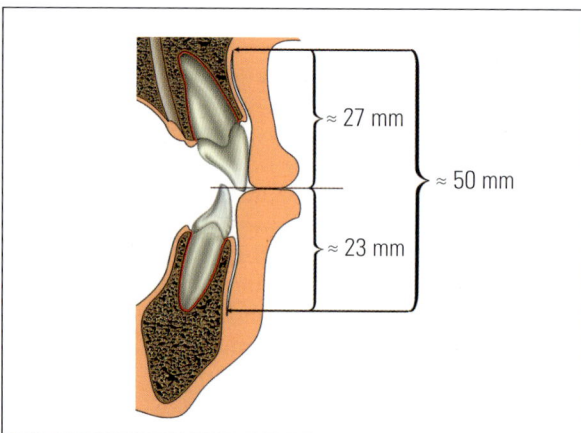

Fig 8-27 The vertical relation of the jaws in the natural dentition can be determined by the distance between the vestibular fornices. The lowest points in the fornices next to the labial frenum are taken as the measuring points. The average distance in a fully dentate mouth is about 50 mm.

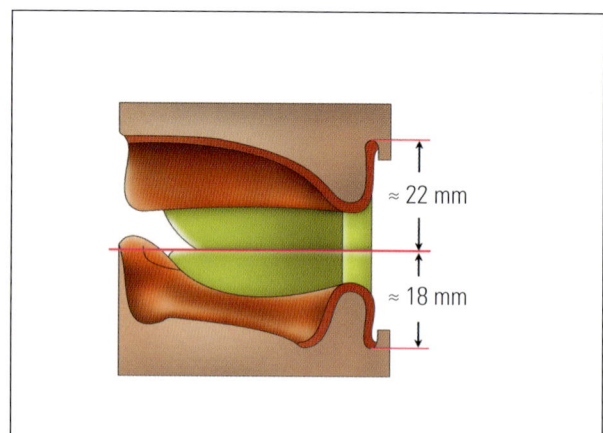

Fig 8-28 During jaw relation registration in edentulous jaws, the occlusal height is lowered by about 10 mm so that the mandibular occlusion rim is 18 to 20 mm and the maxillary occlusion rim 20 to 22 mm high from the lowest point in the fornix to the occlusal plane.

Fig 8-29 The positional stability of a denture is dependent on the state of shrinkage of the edentulous jaws. If artificial teeth are set up in the same position as in the natural dentition, the denture body will vary in height, depending on the level of shrinkage. The denture body acts as a lever arm. If the alveolar ridges are severely atrophied, the lever arm is longer because of the height of the denture body, and the denture is unstable. The occlusal height of a denture thus has a direct influence on denture stability.

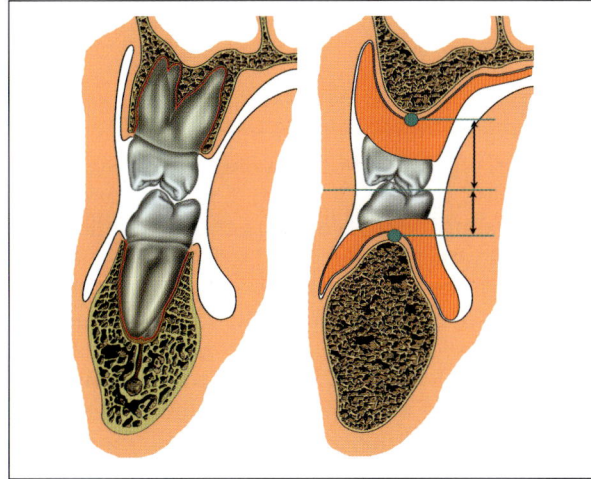

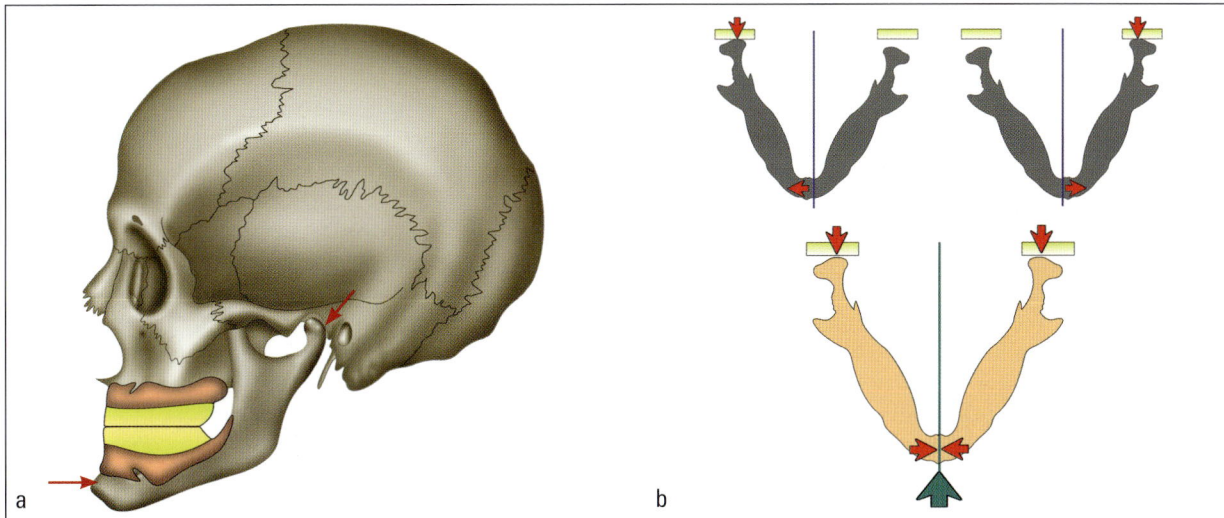

Fig 8-30 *(a and b)* The horizontal relation of the mandible can be established when both condyles are brought into the most retruded position. Then lateral misalignment or protrusive errors will not arise. In this method, the condyles are located at the posterior border of the fossa and the mandible lies behind the normal position by a certain amount. This jaw relation position is not the physiologic hinge-axis position, but it is reproducible at any time.

Fig 8-31 To bring the mandible into centric relation, namely both condyles in the most retruded position, a wax ball can be affixed to the dorsal edge of the plate in the maxilla, which the patient has to touch with the tip of the tongue. The mandible is pulled into the most retruded position by the activity of the muscles of the floor of the mouth and the tongue.

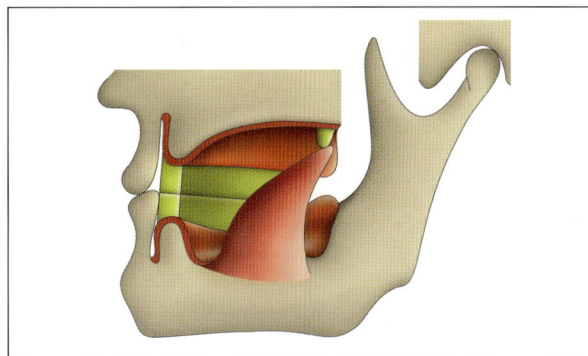

Gothic Arch Tracing

The centric position is established with a **Gothic arch tracing** (intraoral interocclusal record registration) by a method developed by Gysi, McGrane, and Gerber. This arch is formed when the horizontal border movements of the mandible are traced. A tracing stylus is attached to a baseplate and inscribes the horizontal mandibular movements on the tracing plate of the other baseplate. The advantage of this method is that it cancels out all uncontrollable occlusal contacts and reduces them to a central point. At the same time, a relaxed neuromuscular resting position can be adopted in which the joints are relieved of any loading.

For **practical purposes**, well-adhering baseplates are prepared (for edentulous jaws, on functional models). After a preliminary interocclusal record registration, to establish the correct occlusal height, the maxillary occlusion rim is shortened by about 5 mm, and the maxillary tracing plate is waxed on. The lower stylus holder is placed on the mandibular occlusion rim so that the stylus is exactly in the midpoint of the baseplate. The registration kit should be attached exactly centrally over the jaws so that tilting of the mandible is ruled out and the TMJs are able to balance each other (Figs 8-32 and 8-33). Both plates, the maxillary as well as the mandibular, have side grooves that must be extended in the occlusion rims. This provides retention for the subsequent encoding.

The **baseplates** are inserted into the mouth to check whether the stylus has the correct occlusal height setting. It can be reset, if necessary. On the tracing plate, a thin layer of wax (or color layer) can be applied in the contact area of the stylus, into which the stylus traces the mandibular movements. The patient makes protrusive, retrusive, and lateral movements several times, whereby the protrusive excursions create sagittal lines and the lateral movements create arcuate, transverse lines that produce the Gothic arch.

The apex of the Gothic arch indicates the most retruded contact position. In healthy TMJ conditions, the centric occlusion position lies about 1 to 2 mm behind the apex of the Gothic arch. Once protrusive and lateral movements have been performed several times, a perforated Perspex disc is screwed onto the tracing plate over the resulting Gothic arch, with the drill hole over the apex of the Gothic arch. The mandible is now directed until the stylus engages in the drill hole. This means the centric occlusion position has been found, and the baseplates are "encoded" (with impression plaster).

The **centric occlusion** is found, and the degree of possible backward movement during lateral excursions is determined. The condyles rest in the "zenith" of the mandibular fossae without pressure or tension, if the mandible is not tilted dorsally or laterally. The different shapes of the Gothic arch provide information about pathologic forms of movement, joint damage, or muscle spasms but are not diagnostically conclusive. Only the centric occlusion can clearly be established.

Electronic pantography denotes a computer-assisted registration method for the habitual intercuspation position and all mandibular movements in the patient. With a special registration kit (pantograph), the movement of the mandibular incisal point relative to the movement pattern of the condyles of both TMJs is plotted by the computer. The technical procedure involves fixing the registration kit to the patient's maxillary and mandibular teeth so that the relative movement of the mandible is plotted. At the same time, the exact position of the mandibular incisal point relative to the rotation center on the condyles is measured with a facebow and stored on the computer. To transfer the values to the articulator, the models of the occlusal situation are mounted in the articulator with a facebow. The registration kit is fixed on the models as previously in the patient, and the position of the mandibular incisal point relative to the rotation center of the articulator is measured. The computer plots the difference in the values on the patient and on the articulator; transfer and measuring errors are registered by the computer and compensated for mathematically.

Based on the situation of the models in the articulator, the computer calculates the shape of the condylar paths (with the condylar path inclination and Bennett angle) and the anterior guidance path and has these movement paths milled into acrylic blocks in the milling machine. These blocks are then clamped into the articulator.

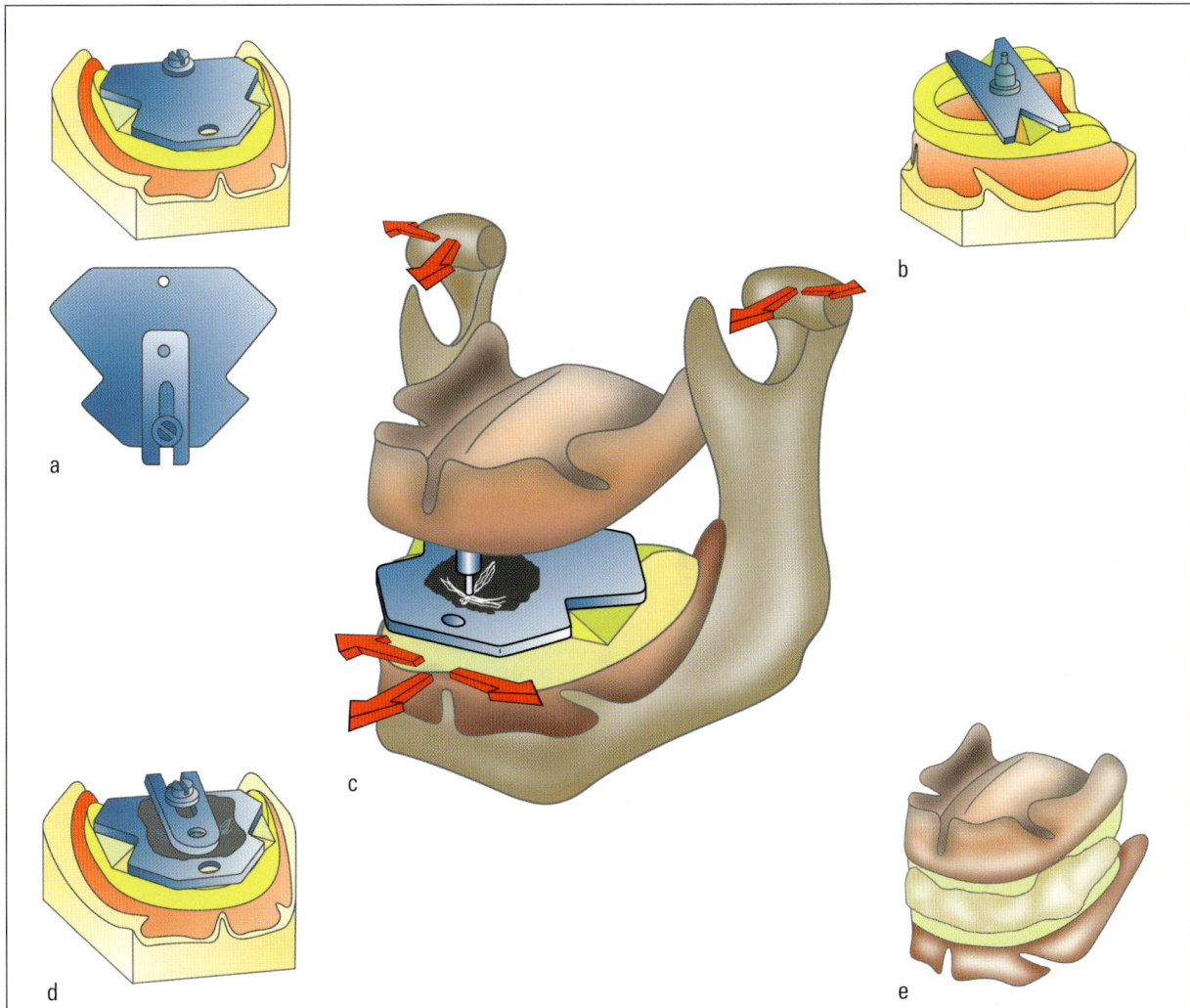

Fig 8-32 *(a to e)* In Gothic arch tracing, the registration kit is attached centrally over the jaws so that tilting is ruled out. During mandibular movement, the tracing stylus *(b)* inscribes the Gothic arch *(c)* on the tracing plate *(a)*. A perforated Perspex disc *(d)* is fixed over the intersection of the traced lines. The tracing stylus engages in the hole in the disc, and the mandible is fixed in centric occlusion. The baseplates are then fixed with impression plaster *(e)*.

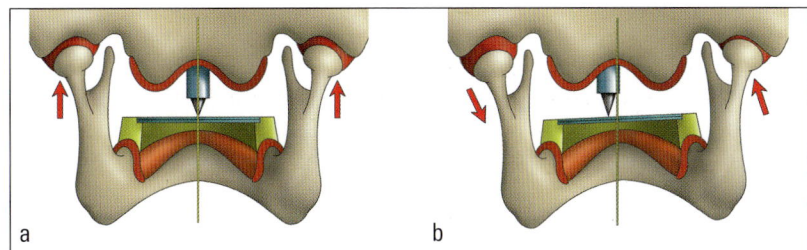

Fig 8-33 The tracing stylus is attached centrally *(a)* to prevent the baseplates from tilting and to load the joints evenly. If the stylus is displaced sideways, the mandible will be tilted *(b)*.

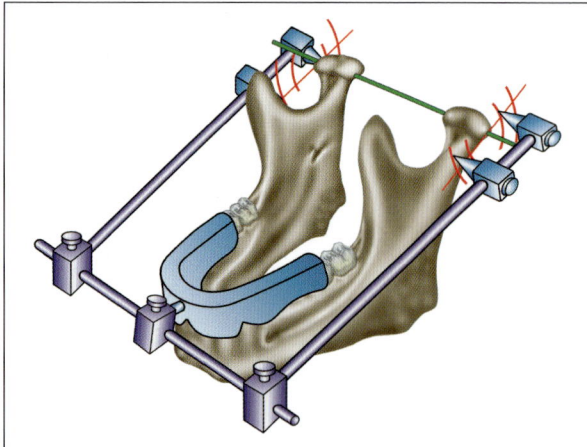

Fig 8-34 The axis locator is fixed to the mandibular dentition via a bite fork. The two tracing arms carry the adjustable tracing needles. The measuring needle is aligned over the assumed hinge-axis point. During several mandibular hinge movements, the measuring needle traces concentric lines of varying size whose midpoint is the hinge-axis point.

Facebow Technique

How well movement is duplicated in articulators depends directly on the precise positioning of the occlusal field relative to the joint axis and equally on precise setting of the joint values in relation to this positioning. Models can be mounted in an articulator as follows:

- As a rough approximation according to average values for the Bonwill triangle and the Balkwill angle, thereby producing an average-value occlusal field of minimal functional value. Mounting in fixed-value articulators is done by visual judgment or with a calibration key.
- Cranium- or joint-oriented mounting with a tracing arch (facebow or transfer arch) in semi-adjustable or fully adjustable devices, where models are mounted in alignment with defined reference planes and an individual occlusal field can be reconstructed.

For **cranium-oriented mounting** of models, a facebow is used that carries a bite fork for the maxillary dentition. The facebow is oriented toward the hinge axis and one other reference point. As a result, a spatial relationship can be created between the maxillary teeth, the hinge axis, and a reference plane.

The **reference planes** used are the Camper plane, the hinge-axis orbital plane (auriculo-infraorbital plane), and the midface horizontal plane. The fact that the alignment of these reference planes is parallel to the upper arm of the articulator means that the orientation of the occlusal plane in the articulator will vary. All the reference planes are oriented toward the hinge axis and only differ in their anterior reference point. The accuracy of this method relies on precise localization of the hinge-axis points and the reference point for the reference plane. The anatomical hinge axis can be determined by individual axis localization. As a rule, however, an arbitrary (average-value) hinge axis is adopted.

Individual axis localization is done with an axis locator, eg, the Almore facebow, which is fixed onto the mandible to locate the hinge axis. On a transverse fixing rod, the U-shaped arch carries a bite fork in the form of an impression tray for fitting onto the mandibular teeth (Fig 8-34). The side tracing arms can be lengthened or shortened and rotated around the transverse fixing rod. The tracing needles for fixing the hinge-axis point can in turn be adjusted on the side tracing arms.

Axis localization is based on the principle of amplitude: The tracing needles trace varying amplitudes depending on the distance from the rotation center. To this end, tracing flags are positioned over the suspected axis points (eg, by placing graph paper that sticks to the skin). The mandible then performs hinge movements, and the tracing needles trace circular movements. The needle is pushed nearer and nearer to the rotation center until it rotates over the center during hinge movements. The rotation centers are

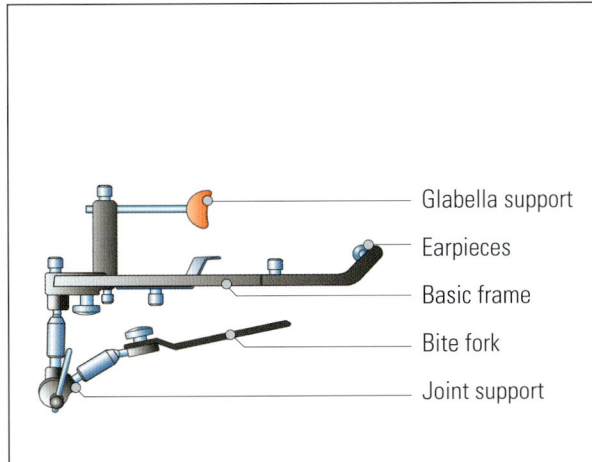

Fig 8-35 In an arbitrary facebow, the earpieces, the adjustable joint support with the bite fork, and the adjustable glabella support are mounted onto the variable basic frame.

Glabella support
Earpieces
Basic frame
Bite fork
Joint support

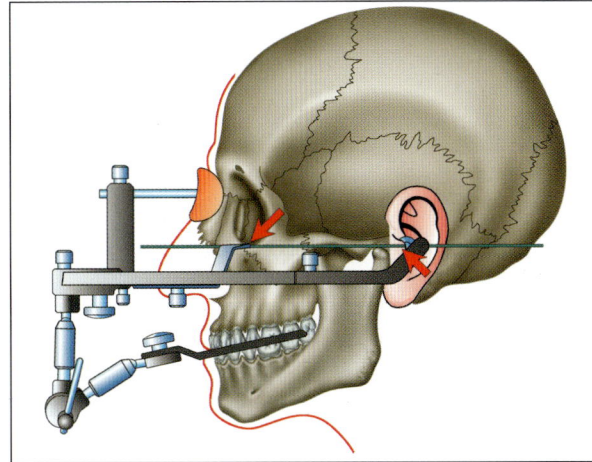

Fig 8-36 Precise joint-oriented alignment of the models in the articulator is possible with a facebow. To do this, the facebow is placed with the earpieces inserted into the external auditory canals and thus aligned with the condylar points; the nasion adapter is placed on the bridge of the nose, and another pin is aligned with the orbitale. The occlusal surfaces of the maxillary teeth are traced on the bite fork. Using the joint support, the bite fork can be firmly adjusted with the facebow in the correct position.

marked on the skin, and the individual hinge axis is thus located.

In a normal clinical case, an arbitrary (average-value) quick tracing arch will be used. The hinge axis is not localized individually but as an average value marked on the tragus-canthus plane as lying 12 mm before the tragus, or it is located in relation to the opening of the external auditory canal *(porus acusticus externus)*.

The **arbitrary facebow** comprises a width-adjustable basic device with **earpieces** mounted onto its side tracing arms. The transverse fixing rod carries the **joint support** adjustable in three directions, with which the bite fork can be fitted onto the maxillary teeth. In addition, the adjustable **glabella support** (nasion adapter) is attached to the transverse fixing rod for alignment with the reference point of the reference plane (Fig 8-35).

The **earpieces** of the arbitrary facebow are inserted into the external auditory canal, and the glabella support is placed on the bridge of the nose so that the facebow lies parallel to the chosen reference plane. The bite fork is fixed to the maxillary dentition with silicone impression material and connected to the facebow via the

joint support in its individual position (Fig 8-36). For cranium-oriented mounting of the maxillary model, the adjusted facebow is aligned with the reference points in the articulator and the maxillary model is set in plaster.

Mounting Models in the Articulator

Models are mounted with a facebow in two stages: The maxillary model is first inserted, then the mandibular model is mounted over a centric record.

To transfer the maxillary model position, telescopic legs can be attached to the facebow to set up the arch precisely in relation to the hinge-axis points of the articulator. The earpieces are placed onto the condylar casing, and the length of the telescopic legs is adjusted to align the facebow with the top part of the articulator. Depending on the reference plane chosen, the orientation of the occlusal plane is variably steep.

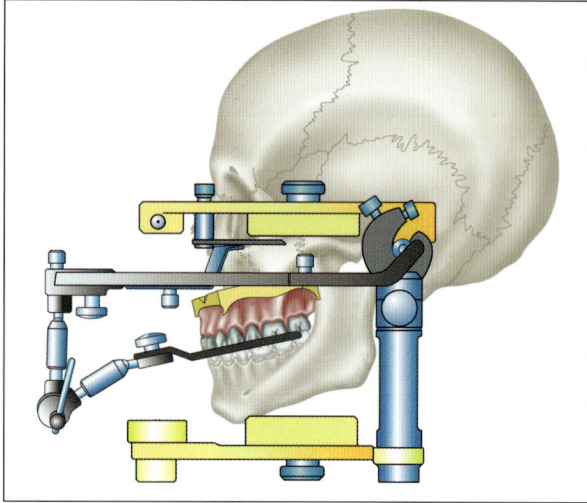

Fig 8-37 To align the models, the facebow is set to the joint axis in the articulator and aligned with the third fixed point (orbitale). This establishes the precise position of the occlusal field relative to the joints. The maxillary model is placed into the bite fork and plastered in place on the maxillary model holder of the articulator. The second stage is to mount the mandibular model in the device.

The position of the maxillary model can also be transferred with a transfer jig or transfer stand. With some articulators, this accessory can be inserted instead of the incisal guide plate in a firmly defined position and is designed to receive the joint support. The joint support is clamped into the transfer jig with the bite fork and is then in the correct position inside the articulator. The facebow stays with the dentist for further use.

Once the bite fork (whether with a facebow or a transfer jig) is set up in the articulator, the maxillary model fits into the bite fork. So that the bite fork is not displaced by the weight of the model, it has to be supported from below, either with a plaster block or a so-called forked bracket. If the maxillary model is fixed in such a way, it is set in plaster in the maxillary model holder. Then the mandibular model can be combined with the maxillary model by means of a centric record and also plastered in place (Fig 8-37).

To minimize error, the models are mounted by the split-model method (magnetic base system) (Fig 8-38). To do this, the model bases are split into a primary and a secondary base and fitted with wedge-shaped retention depressions and a magnetic connector. The split-model is used to check the correct occlusal position with the aid of several centric records (Fig 8-39).

Both split-models are mounted in the articulator in two stages, as described above. Then the retention magnet in the maxillary model is tem-porarily removed, and a second centric record is placed between the rows of teeth. When the upper arm of the articulator is closed, the slightest discrepancies between the masticatory organ and the articulator become noticeable from the gap between the maxillary model and base. This check must be repeated with different centric records. When there are discrepancies, the mandibular model is removed and reset with the correct record. As well as this check function, the split-model method allows the model to be rapidly removed from and inserted into the articulator.

The joint values are set either individually or based on average values, depending on the options offered by the articulator used.

In the ***average-value method***, the joint values must be selected in relation to the reference plane that was used for mounting the models. If the hinge-axis orbital plane was used, the occlusal plane is inclined at a relatively steep angle; if the midface horizontal plane was adopted, the occlusal plane is gently inclined; with the Camper plane, the occlusal plane is horizontal.

The sagittal inclination of the condylar paths varies in relation to the reference plane (Fig 8-40):

- Camper plane: approximately 30 to 40 degrees
- Hinge-axis orbital plane: approximately 45 to 55 degrees
- Midface horizontal plane: approximately 35 to 45 degrees

Fig 8-38 *(a and b)* The models are fixed in the articulator with a magnetic base (split-model) system. The system makes it easy to remove the models and is able to highlight errors of centric registration.

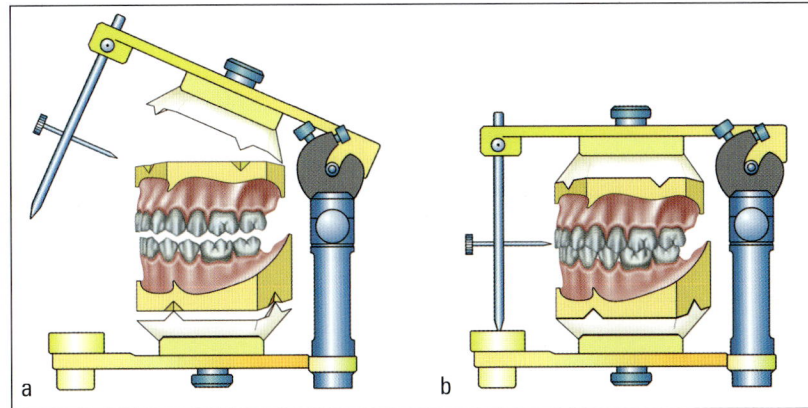

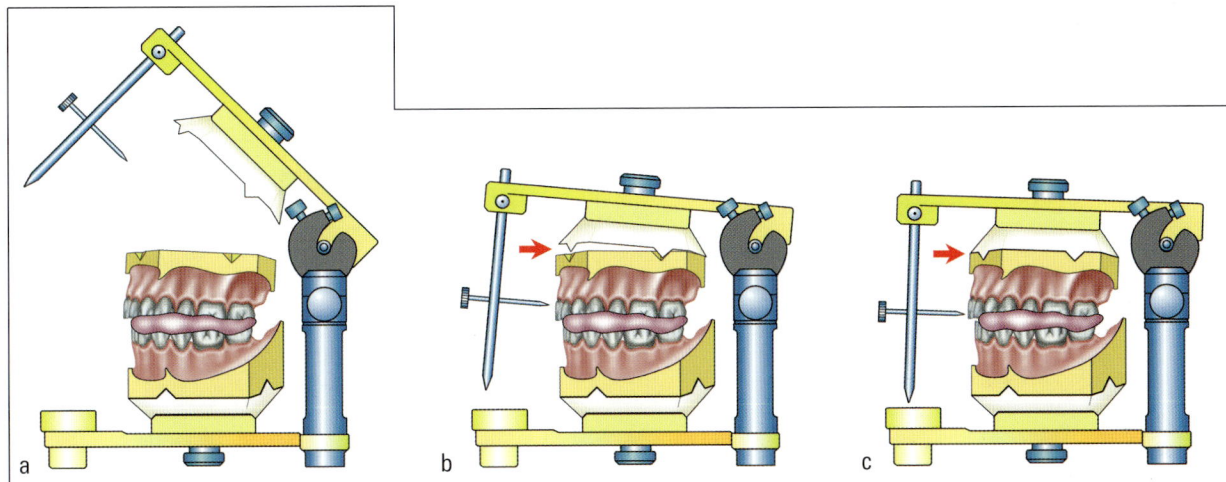

Fig 8-39 The centric check is done with split-models: *(a)* After insertion in the articulator, the maxillary model is separated from the split-model (the magnetic connection is removed). The maxillary model is placed onto the mandibular model with another centric record. *(b)* If there are discrepancies in the centric position, there is a gap between the split-model base and the model. *(c)* If there is agreement between the centric records, no gap appears between the model and the split-model base.

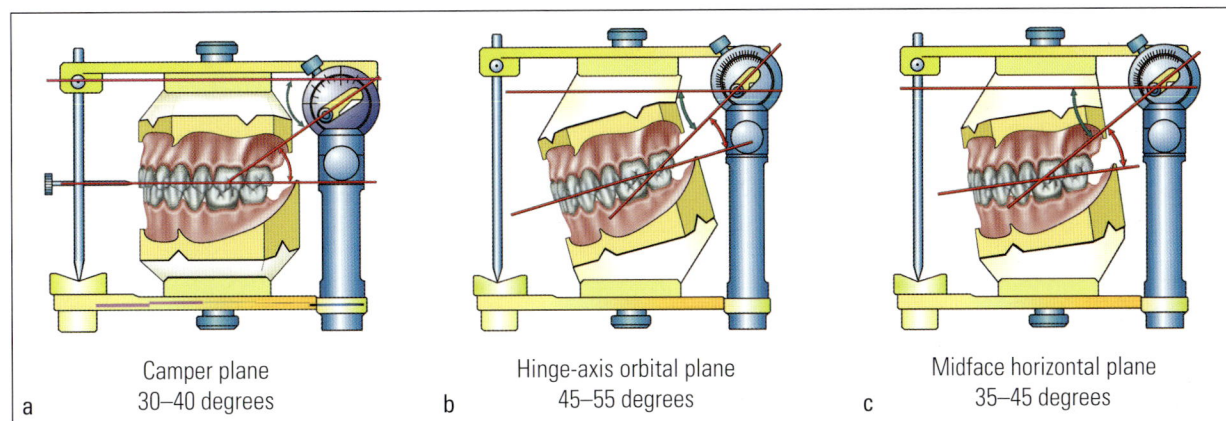

Camper plane
30–40 degrees

Hinge-axis orbital plane
45–55 degrees

Midface horizontal plane
35–45 degrees

Fig 8-40 *(a to c)* The reference plane according to which the models were placed in the articulator determines the angle at which the sagittal inclination of the condylar paths is set. The inclinations of anterior guidance should be selected on the basis of these values.

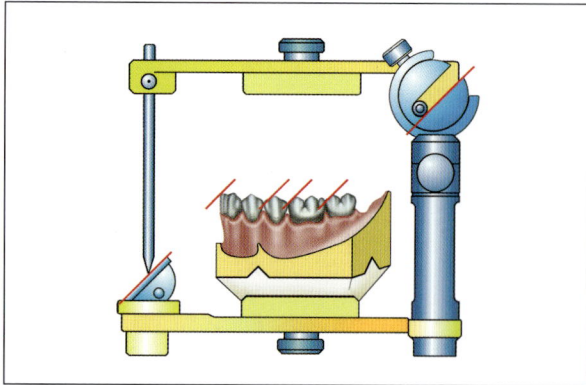

Fig 8-41 A steep condylar path together with similar incisal guidance is bound to mean a steep occlusal curve, which is associated with a severe vertical overlap of the incisors and steep cusp surfaces.

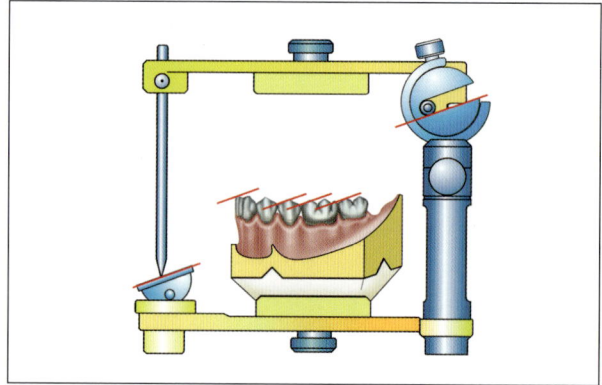

Fig 8-42 A flat occlusal curve arises when there is a small condylar inclination with flat incisal guidance. The incisal vertical overlap is small, and the cusp surfaces are flat.

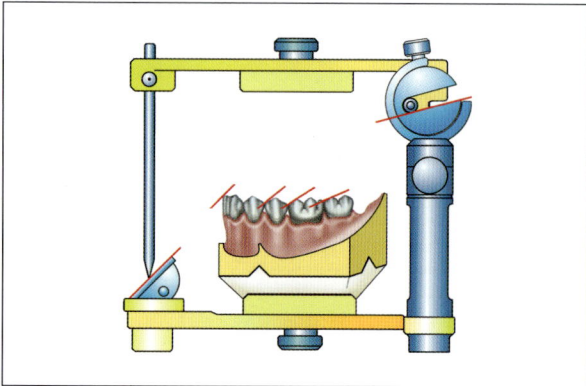

Fig 8-43 With a very flat condylar path inclination, a steep occlusal curve can be produced by setting a very steep incisal guidance. As a result, precise canine guidance can be produced as a "protective occlusion."

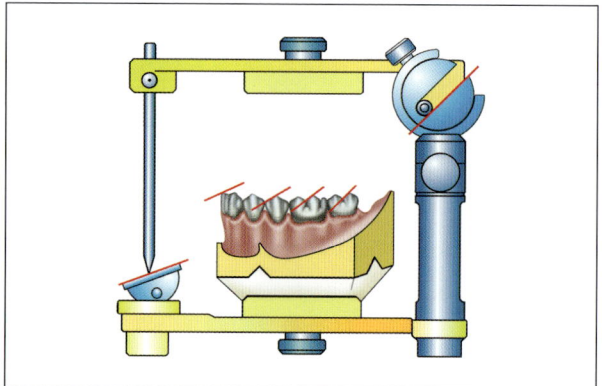

Fig 8-44 Combining a steep condylar path with flat incisal guidance produces a small incisal vertical overlap with a relatively steep occlusal curve in the area of the posterior teeth.

The inclinations of the incisal guide plate should be selected on the basis of these values. The entirety of the occlusal surfaces, which together with the articular surfaces form the mechanical guidance of the mandible, is reduced in an articulator to the incisal guide pin that rests on an incisal guide plate. This incisal guide plate represents the whole of the occlusal field. Thus, it is clear that the inclination of the incisal guide plate has the same influence on shaping the inclinations of the occlusal surfaces as it does on shaping the inclination of the condylar paths. If

anterior guidance is very steep, precise canine guidance can be produced. The vertical incisal guide pin must remain in contact with the guide plate during a whole movement stroke; if the tracing stylus lifts up, there is an occlusal disturbance present. In the case of complete dentures, the aim should be all-over sliding contact of the teeth in lateral and protrusive movements to support stability, whereas contacts on the nonworking side are undesirable with a fixed denture.

Figures 8-41 to 8-48 illustrate various considerations for mounting models in the articulator.

Fig 8-45 The facebow of the Artex articulator system (AmannGirrbach) on a patient. The earpieces are placed in the external auditory canals, and the nosepiece is fixed so that the facebow frame is aligned with the mid-face horizontal plane. The bite fork is joined to the face-bow frame via the three-dimensional joint support and fixes the positional relationship of the maxillary teeth to the joint points. (Courtesy of AmannGirrbach.)

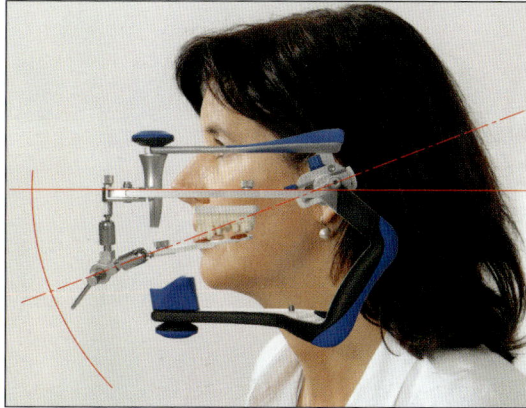

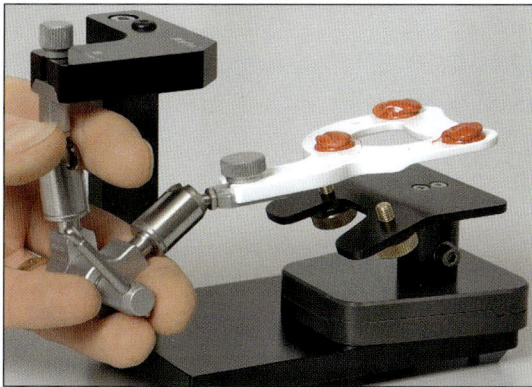

Fig 8-46 The three-dimensional joint support with bite fork is placed in a transfer stand and lies in a defined position over the transfer table, which has been adjusted to the mandibular model holder of the Artex articulator. (Courtesy of AmannGirrbach.)

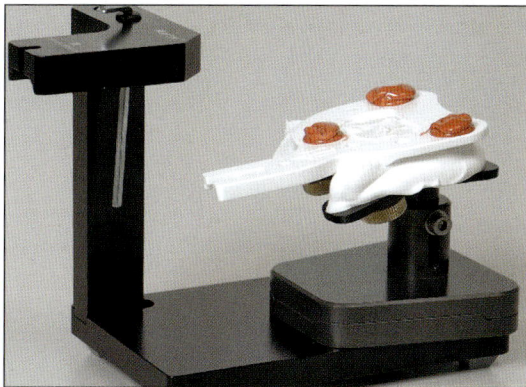

Fig 8-47 The bite fork is immovably fixed onto the transfer table with plaster. (Courtesy of AmannGirrbach.)

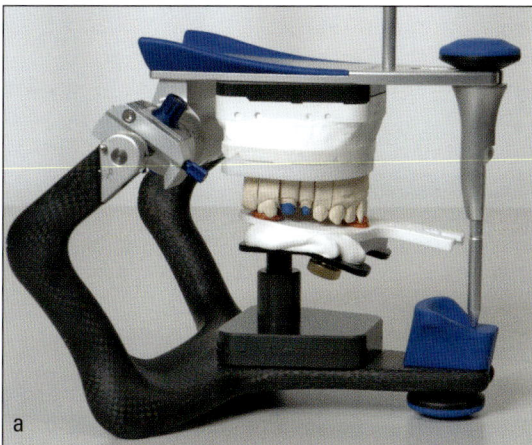

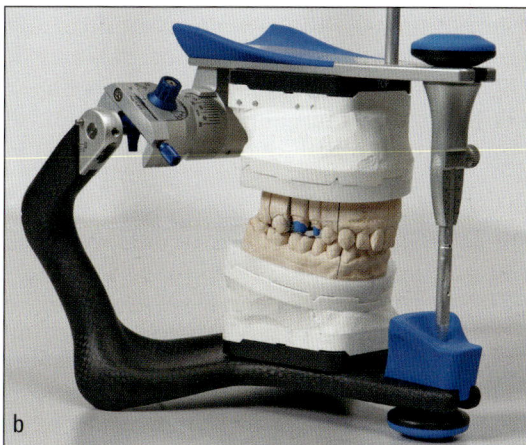

Fig 8-48 *(a)* The transfer table can be precisely placed onto the mandibular model holder of the articulator so that mounting of the maxillary model can take place. The maxillary dentition is now in the joint-oriented position in the articulator. *(b)* The mandibular model can also be fixed with squash bites to the maxillary model and inserted with plaster. (Courtesy of AmannGirrbach.)

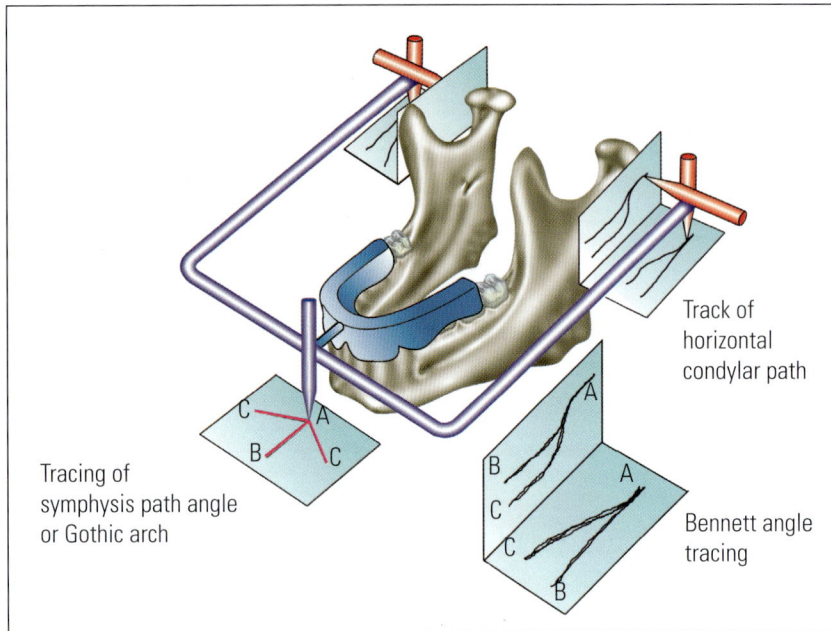

Fig 8-49 The principle of spatial tracing of the condylar paths and extraoral needlepoint registration with a tracing arch rigidly fixed to the mandible. From A to B is the tracing of the condylar movement path in protrusion of the mandible. From A to C is the tracing of the condylar movement path in laterotrusion of the mandible. It is noticeable that the tracing of the horizontal condylar path is flatter in protrusive movement than in lateral movement.

Determining Joint Values

The condylar paths are set in fully adjustable articulators after the tracks of the condylar paths have been traced and measured or by using eccentric positional records (interocclusal records).

The **interocclusal record method** exploits the Christensen phenomenon, such that the rows of teeth open on the mediotrusive side and hence space is left for the material of the positional record. The following positions of the jaws in relation to each other are established:

- Centric occlusion using the centric record, where the rows of teeth are about 3 mm apart
- Protrusive position using a protrusive record; in protrusion, the posterior teeth open and provide space for the record
- Lateral positions using laterotrusive records to the right and left on the mediotrusive side

The **positional records** are made of a tough elastic material, either silicone or wax reinforced with metal chips or textile inserts. With the facebow, the models are first inserted into the articulator in centric occlusion. The condylar paths are brought into an average inclination or into the neutral position, and the locks are loosened. The models are then pushed into the protrusive position and fixed with the interocclusal record. The joints can then be set to the sagittal condylar path inclination and locked.

To **set the Bennett angle**, the models are fixed one after another in the lateral positions with the interocclusal records; the condylar path of the nonworking condyle, which follows the movement of the upper arm of the articulator, is then adjusted to the Bennett angle. This setting of the condylar inclinations must be repeated and checked several times. The protrusive record is used as the interocclusal record, which must be correct after settings have been made with the lateral occlusions.

The **advantage of the interocclusal record method** is that it compensates for system errors in the arbitrary facebow technique. The interocclusal record method does not produce individual joint values but rather articulator settings for mandibular movements within a range of border move-

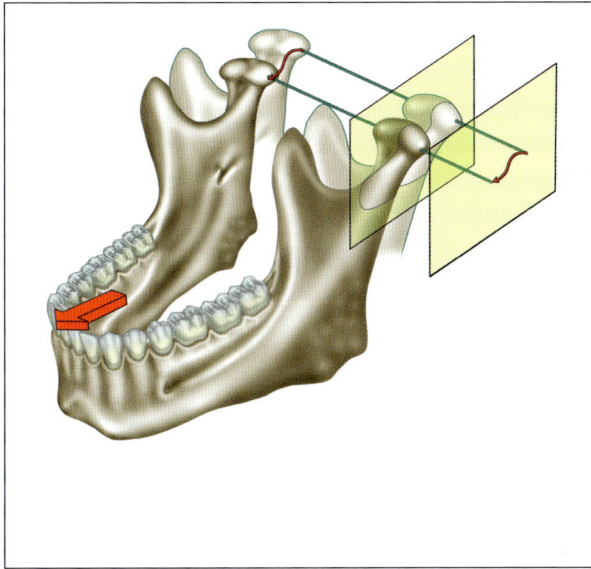

Fig 8-50 The S-shaped, curved track of the condylar path is traced in protrusive movement. The horizontal condylar path inclination to a reference plane can be determined with this tracing. The tracing is done using flags that are located at a distance from the movement plane.

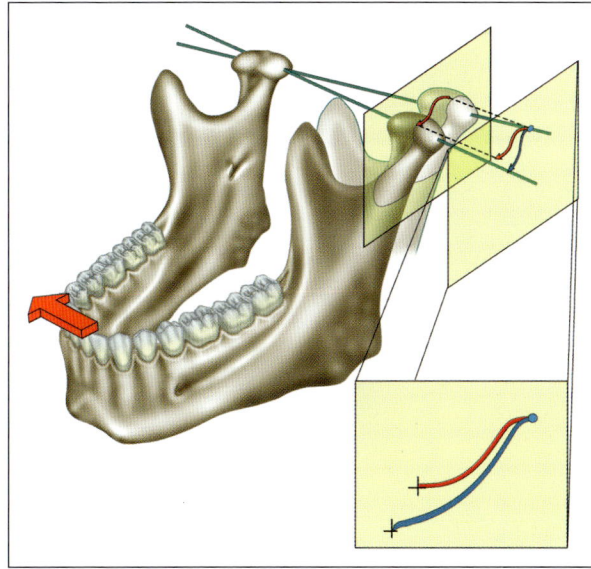

Fig 8-51 The tracing of the horizontal condylar path is steeper and longer in lateral movement and encloses the Fischer angle. The divergence in the tracing is a projection error caused by the gap between the movement plane and the tracing plane.

ments that is defined by the interocclusal records. It is assumed that tooth guidance and condylar guidance exactly correspond mechanically.

Individual registration of the joint values is done via extraoral, spatial tracing of the condylar movement paths with a tracing arch that is rigidly fixed to the mandibular dentition (Fig 8-49). The tracing arch corresponds to the axis locator (Almore facebow), whose tracers are oriented to the hinge-axis position. Vertical and horizontal tracing flags are arranged over the hinge-axis position. The vertical flags are used to trace the sagittal condylar path inclinations and are precisely aligned with a reference plane.

The horizontal flags are used for tracing the Bennett angle and are fixed roughly in the sagittal condylar path inclination. The flags can be fixed in the correct position with a headband. During mandibular movements, the tracing needles, which can be pressed on by elastic force, trace the condylar movement paths onto the tracing flags. In protrusive movements, the **protrusion paths** are produced on the vertical tracing flags as S-shaped curved lines (shape of sagittal condylar path) (Fig 8-50); on the horizontal flags, the

protrusion paths are produced as straight lines running forward.

During lateral movements, the **mediotrusion paths** are produced on the horizontal tracing flags; with the forward-running protrusion paths, these mediotrusion paths enclose the Bennett angle. Mediotrusion paths are also traced on the vertical flags. However, these patterns of sagittal condylar paths traced during lateral movements are steeper and longer than those resulting from pure protrusive movement (Fig 8-51).

The **Fischer angle** denotes the angle between the tracings of the sagittal condylar path during protrusive movements (protrusion path) and during lateral movement (mediotrusion path) of up to 10 degrees. The track of movement of the non-working condyle is longer during lateral movements than during protrusive movements, and it deflects caudally. This difference in the movement paths arises from the tracing error of the registration kit, which tilts when tracing the lateral movement in the horizontal plane so that the tracing points on the flags deflect further caudally and forward.

Pathology of the Orofacial System

Pathology of the orofacial system concerns developmental anomalies and their consequences, disease processes, and the course of diseases. It involves investigating the causes (etiology), physical changes (pathologic anatomy), and origin (pathogenesis) of diseases as well as their clinical appearance (signs and symptoms).

The formation and development of the teeth from tooth germs through to eruption is a differentiated, complex process involving active cell structures. Disturbances may arise during the normal course of development. These tissue anomalies have an effect on the functional ability of the masticatory system and therefore must be remedied.

Dysgnathia is a collective term for various morphologic and functional anomalies. It refers to occlusal anomalies such as malposition of teeth, missing tooth germs, or excessive numbers of teeth as well as abnormal jaw development, joint damage, malocclusions, and other forms of systemic damage. These dysgnathic anomalies can be compared with the normal occlusion to determine whether orthodontic treatment is needed.

There is a sliding scale from extreme malformations to an optimal occlusion, from deviations not requiring treatment to severe deformities that necessitate intensive orthodontic treatment. As well as developmental anomalies, the masticatory system can be affected by a variety of diseases caused by external (exogenous) or internal (endogenous) factors, the most severe consequence of which would be tooth loss. Most tooth loss is due to tooth decay (caries) and diseases of the tooth bed (periodontal diseases) (Fig 9-1).

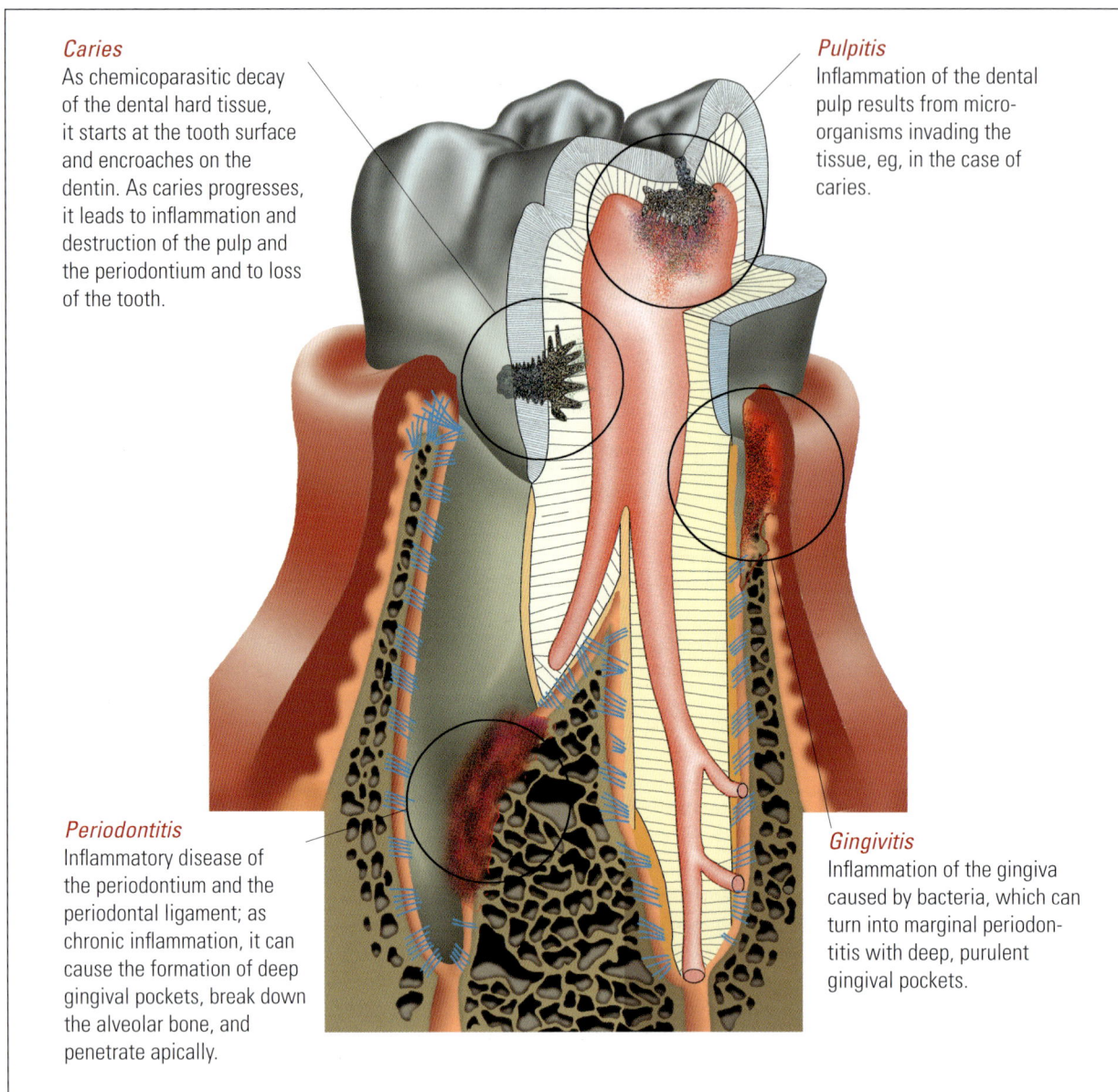

Caries
As chemicoparasitic decay of the dental hard tissue, it starts at the tooth surface and encroaches on the dentin. As caries progresses, it leads to inflammation and destruction of the pulp and the periodontium and to loss of the tooth.

Pulpitis
Inflammation of the dental pulp results from micro-organisms invading the tissue, eg, in the case of caries.

Periodontitis
Inflammatory disease of the periodontium and the periodontal ligament; as chronic inflammation, it can cause the formation of deep gingival pockets, break down the alveolar bone, and penetrate apically.

Gingivitis
Inflammation of the gingiva caused by bacteria, which can turn into marginal periodontitis with deep, purulent gingival pockets.

Fig 9-1 Diseases of the tooth and the periodontium.

Tooth decay is a chemicoparasitic process that, if left untreated, will progress and lead to destruction of the tooth. Acute or chronic decay of the dental hard tissue starts with demineralization of the enamel. Acid-forming bacteria in the soft deposits on the teeth first demineralize the dental hard substances, then other bacteria also break down the organic constituents.

Areas susceptible to caries are all the pits and fissures as well as unclean sites, such as the approximal and cervical areas. Caries does not occur on cusps and marginal ridges, which undergo self-cleaning because of the flow of food. The dental treatment of caries involves mechanically removing the diseased and softened dental hard tissue and replacing it with suitable filling material.

Periodontal diseases are all conditions affecting the tooth bed, especially the purulent, inflammatory processes that lead to reduction of the dental attachment apparatus (periodontium). A distinction is made between gingivitis, marginal periodontitis, and apical periodontal diseases resulting from pulp diseases (pulpitis).

Gingivitis is superficial inflammation of the gingiva with a variety of causes: bacterially induced marginal gingivitis caused by poor oral hygiene (simple gingivitis); necrotizing, ulcerative gingivitis caused by lowered resistance, smoking, and alcohol abuse (ulcerative gingivitis); and puberty gingivitis caused by poor oral hygiene and open mouth breathing.

Marginal periodontitis is an episodic, inflammatory condition of the marginal periodontium caused by bacterial deposits; it can affect the gingiva and the periodontal ligament. Chronic inflammation of the soft tissues, with gingiva that bleeds easily, gingival pockets that contain pus, and accretions on the root, causes the affected teeth to become loose and fall out. It arises from excessive stress on individual teeth, tartar build-up, vitamin C deficiency, metabolic diseases, and hormonal disturbances. To treat marginal periodontitis, causal factors are eliminated and gingival pockets surgically removed.

Pulpitis is inflammation of the dental pulp that may be caused by microbial invasion in the case of caries, by overheating when grinding the dental hard tissues, or by filling materials. This condition takes the form of closed pulpitis (pulp cavity is not open) or open pulpitis (pulp open to the oral cavity). In pulpitis, blood pools in the pulpal veins; if there are pus-forming (pyogenic) bacteria in the tissue, small abscesses will form, and the pus will penetrate the pulp tissue. Mild pulpitis can be fully cured if the causes of the condition are removed.

Developmental Anomalies of the Jaws

The *development of the jaw* starts around the end of the third week of embryonic life. The normal development process can be interrupted by malformations due to inhibitory factors, by which palatine tori do not develop fully and fail to fuse together in the midline.

Normal fusion advances like a zip fastener, closing from front to back as far as the uvula. If union of the palatine processes at the median palatine suture does not take place, this gives rise to a cleft palate extending from the incisive foramen to the uvula, which is also split. There are numerous degrees of severity, from a complete cleft through to a uvular cleft (Fig 9-2); clefts that only affect the soft palate may be referred to as *velar clefts*.

Forms of cleft lip, jaw, and palate

Cleft lip (cheiloschisis) denotes a split in the upper lip. This form can be surgically closed during the fourth to sixth month of life with a good functional and cosmetic outcome. Left-sided cleft lip is twice as common as right-sided, or the cleft may be bilateral (Fig 9-3); a cleft in the middle of the lip is very rarely seen.

Partial clefts of the lip, at their least pronounced, are evident as slight furrows in the red of the lips or as a small dent next to the philtrum. Cleft lip can be found in every possible combination with cleft palate.

Cleft jaw (gnathoschisis) denotes a split of the maxilla because the incisive bone has not grown together with the maxilla at the intermaxillary suture. It usually occurs in conjunction with other cleft deformities.

Isolated *cleft palate* (palatoschisis or uranoschisis) is a malformation of the hard and soft palate where the whole palatine vault is split along the median palatine suture.

Complete cleft (cheilognathopalatoschisis or cheilognathouranoschisis) is a cleft palate combined with bilateral cleft lip and jaw. This most severe form of cleft is twice as common in males as in females. The abnormality in development of the palate, jaw, and lips is usually accompanied by anomalies of the tooth germs in the region of the cleft. For instance, delayed growth or schizodontia (development of twin tooth forms) of the incisors may occur in both the primary and the permanent dentition. Frequently, individual teeth may be entirely absent, or several teeth may erupt.

In fact, anomalies of tooth formation often occur outside the cleft area as well. There is evidence that cleft formation and development of

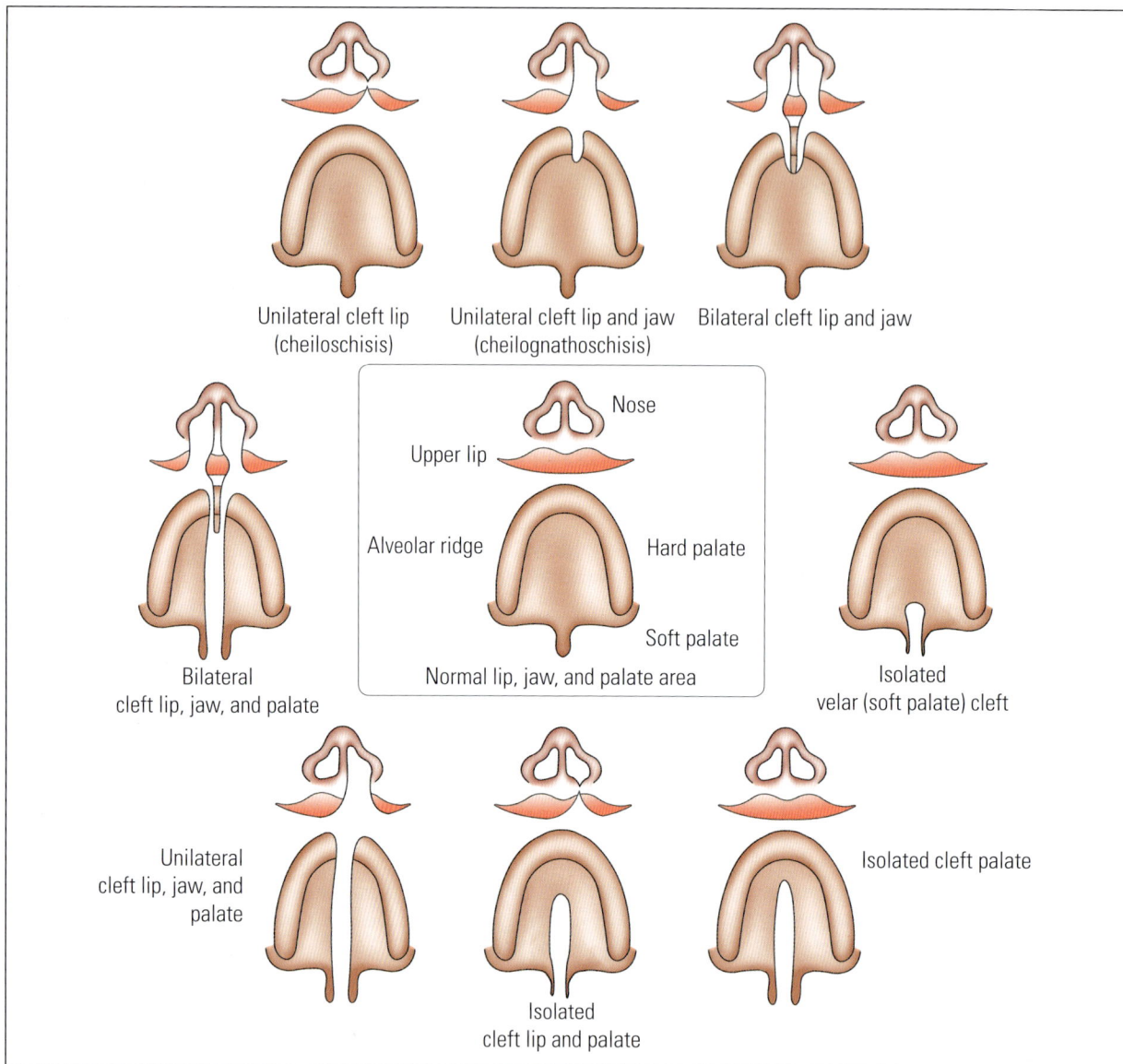

Fig 9-2 Classification of cleft lip, jaw, and palate.

the wrong number of teeth (too few or too many) have causes in common.

The **developmental anomaly** in the form of cleft lip, jaw, and palate leads to stunting of the maxilla, while the mandible grows to normal size. This creates an impression of prognathism and hence protrusion of the mandible. These complete clefts result from the combined effect of congenital and environmental factors or damage caused by

medication; they are therefore a multifactorial condition.

Developmental anomalies in the primary dentition

If there is no abnormality in the shape of a complete cleft, the primary dentition will develop nor-

Fig 9-3 The external features of a left-sided *(a)* and a bilateral *(b)* cleft lip. Various degrees of cleft jaw and cleft palate can be combined with cleft lip.

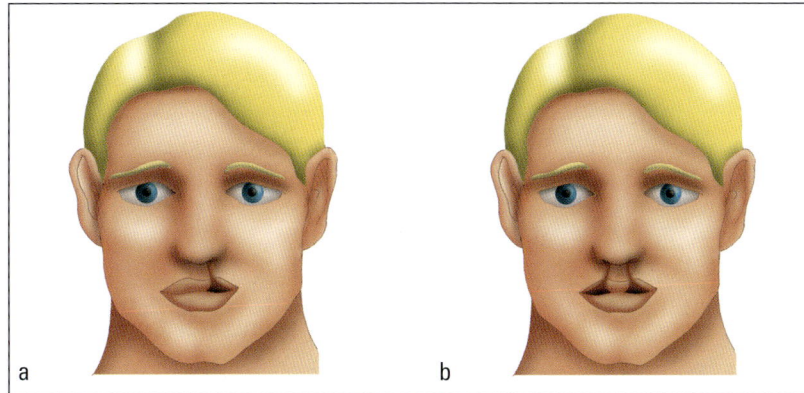

mally. Malposition of teeth is relatively rare and only slightly pronounced.

Typical anomalies in the immediate area of the mouth include the following:

- Tongue doubling, shortening (microglossia), absence (aglossia), or cleft
- Medial cleft of the mandible
- Duplication of the maxilla and the mandible (not viable)
- Underdevelopment of the mandible (hypoplasia)
- Crowding if a few primary teeth are duplicated
- Premature eruption of the primary teeth and permanent teeth; premature dentition (primary dentition complete after first year of life, permanent dentition complete after third year of life)

Facial clefts refer to various forms of malformation due to inhibited development, such as nasal, eyelid, forehead, lower lip, or tongue clefts, which are mostly associated with anomalies of tooth position and displacement of occlusal position. The oblique facial cleft (meloschisis) extends from the upper lip to the eye, while a transverse facial cleft (macrostomia) widens the oral orifice at the sides. Facial clefts can be remedied in several operations, the aim of which is to achieve normal anatomical forms with sufficiently esthetic conditions and to establish masticatory function and phonetics. In most cases, orthodontic treatments are required as well as the surgical procedures.

Developmental Anomalies in Individual Teeth

Developmental anomalies and structural defects (tooth dysplasias) are commonly found in individual teeth as a consequence of genetic or infectious factors, vitamin deficiency diseases (eg, rickets), or certain medications (eg, tetracycline or antibiotics). Because the development of the teeth takes place over very extended periods of time (from the fifth week of embryonic life through to the age of 16 years), during which time many events may intervene directly or indirectly in this process, the teeth often show traces of disorders and structural defects. The results are structural flaws, deviations in tooth size and shape, and abnormal numbers of teeth (Fig 9-4).

Dysplasias of dental hard tissue (defective development or underdevelopment) affecting dentin and enamel arise before eruption of the teeth and are relatively common. They are less frequent in the primary teeth than in the permanent dentition. Enamel hypoplasias disturb the tooth shape so that furrows, pits, convolutions, and jagged cusps are formed. These features are accompanied by discoloration of the enamel layers, such as whitish or yellowish spots.

Enamel hypoplasia is a disturbance of the cellular activity of ameloblasts. As the ameloblasts are unable to divide and therefore cannot be replaced, the degree of malformation depends on when the cells were damaged or killed.

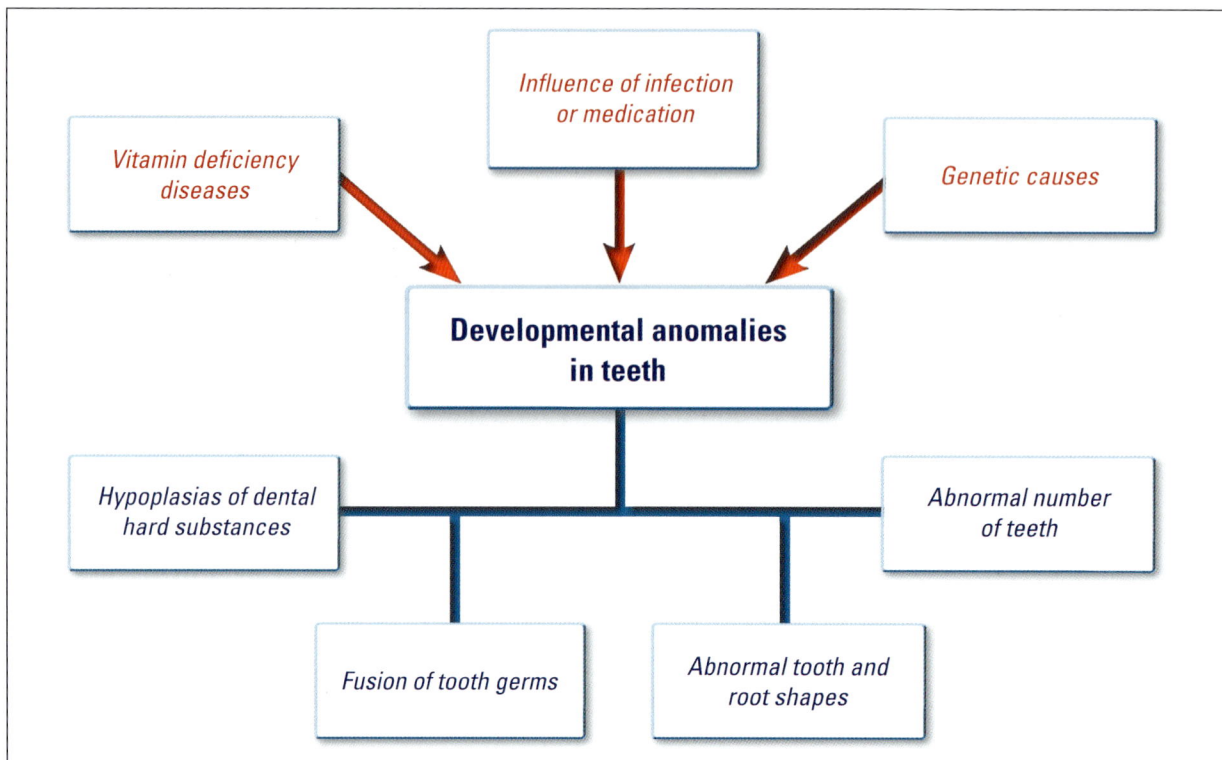

Fig 9-4 Developmental anomalies in individual teeth.

Damage to primary teeth, caused by the effects of impact during childhood or inflammation of the roots of the primary teeth, can lead to changes of shape and color in the enamel of the successional teeth. The enamel can be discolored by the effect of medications, or it may display other structural flaws.

Dentin hypoplasia, caused by defective functioning of the odontoblasts, is accompanied by enamel defects, is only visible under the microscope, and is not very noticeable because the odontoblasts can be replaced by other cells that form dental hard substance.

Abnormal root shapes result from the effects of trauma during eruption, which means that stunted or kinked roots may develop (Fig 9-5). Congenital dysplasias of the enamel and dentin are dominant hereditary conditions and also lead to conical or peg-shaped teeth. Such abnormal tooth shapes commonly occur as supernumerary teeth.

Congenital anomalies are more commonly found in the size and shape of the teeth. Distinct abnormalities of the tooth shape are evident on both the crown and the root.

Defects of the dental crown are manifest as conical canines, additional cusps on premolars and molars (Carabelli cusp), or stunted forms of the lateral incisors and third molars (less common on the second premolars). Additional roots on the premolars and molars are relatively common; shape anomalies of this kind are regularly found on third molars.

When tooth germs divide, the result is schizodontia of a tooth, where two identical teeth erupt. If division starts but is not completed, the result is doubling (gemination), where a far broader tooth with a distinct occlusal notch and only one pulp cavity is found. As well as abnormalities such as hypoplasia of the dental hard tissue or multiple structures, there can also be abnormalities in the number of teeth such as too many teeth (hyperdontia) or too few teeth (hypodontia).

If **tooth germs fuse**, teeth that have grown together will erupt. The fusion may be partial or

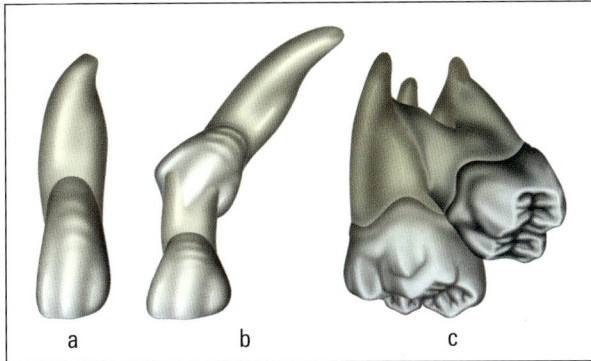

Fig 9-5 Abnormal tooth shapes as a result of exogenous (external) disturbances: *(a)* sickle-shaped teeth with stunted and kinked roots; *(b)* fusion of root and crown when tooth germs are displaced, here involving the canine; *(c)* tooth germs coalescing at the roots.

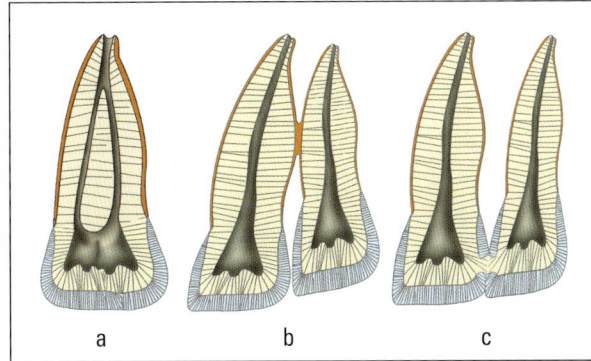

Fig 9-6 Developmental anomalies in teeth are evident in the form of double teeth and fusion of tooth germs: *(a)* pairing of tooth germs; *(b)* two germs coalesce in the cementum area; *(c)* two germs fused in the enamel area.

complete, with separate pulp chambers developing (Fig 9-6). Coalescence occurs in the root area of adjacent teeth as a result of fusion of the cementum.

Distinctive features that are characteristic of individual people can be identified in the structure of dental hard tissue because widened growth lines are formed as a result of the periodic process of enamel and dentin formation.

Forensic identification based on individual teeth is possible because childhood illnesses disrupt the normal variance, leaving lines of varying width and at varying distances in and on the teeth. A corpse or its remains can be identified by the individual, line-type disrupted patterns in the dental hard tissue. By means of forensic identification, it is possible, for instance, to tell whether several teeth-bearing jaw fragments or single teeth come from one or more people; equally, the age of a person can be roughly determined from the dental tissue structures.

Abnormal Tooth Numbers

The ***number of teeth*** changes depending on the course of exfoliation in that individual. Normally the primary dentition consists of 20 teeth, and the permanent dentition contains 32 teeth. However, the number of teeth present at any particular moment during exfoliation will not always correspond to the standard number. Part of an orthodontic examination is to establish whether any anomaly exists and its severity.

Supernumerary teeth (hyperdontia) can result from splitting of the tooth bud or the formation of a third tooth germ. Supernumerary structures are mainly found in the posterior region and at the end of the row of teeth, often combined with a complete cleft (lip, jaw, and palate). Frequently, they do not have regular tooth forms but have small, abnormally shaped crowns (*mesiodens* = conical form of crown and root). Supernumerary teeth in the posterior region are generally removed. Atypical supernumerary formations in the anterior region always have to be removed, and extraction must be followed by a jaw-regulating measure to close the spaces.

A distinction can be made between true and false hyperdontia as well as between true and false hypodontia. ***True hyperdontia*** refers to supernumerary formations, mainly as normal or abnormal tooth shapes in the permanent dentition (Fig 9-7). ***False hyperdontia*** means localized abnormalities of exfoliation when primary teeth have not yet been shed (a primary tooth persists) but the permanent teeth are already erupting (Fig 9-8); the permanent tooth usually erupts paraxially (not straight).

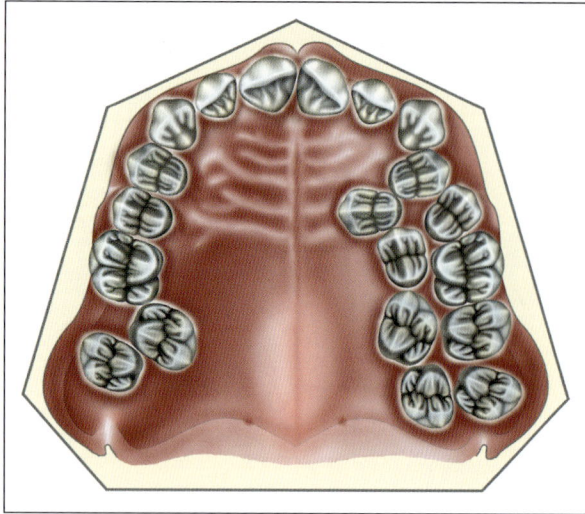

Fig 9-7 True hyperdontia results from excessive development. Duplication of tooth germs can lead to the formation of a second row of teeth next to the complete row. The obvious crowding can only be remedied by systematic extractions.

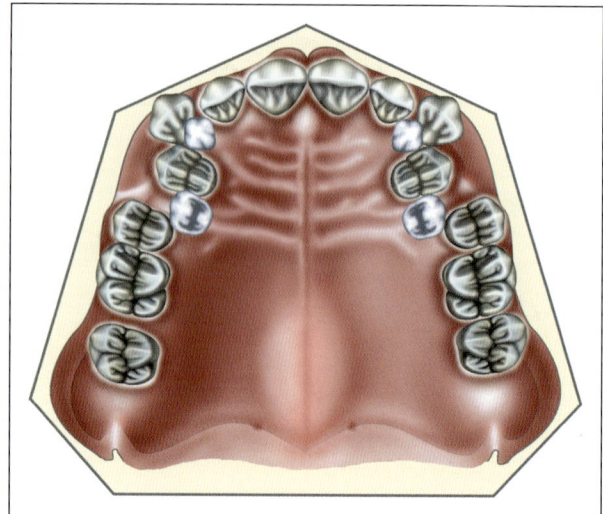

Fig 9-8 False hyperdontia exists when primary teeth persist, ie, they stay in the mixed dentition beyond the normal time, even though the permanent teeth have already erupted. This often displaces the permanent teeth, leading to a severely deformed dental arch.

True hypodontia denotes the loss of one or more teeth as a result of accident or disease; this term is also used to describe the state of dental aplasia. Whether or not a specific tooth is formed is decided during the embryonic period.

Dental aplasia refers to the failure of teeth to develop. This aplasia can be partial or complete. In complete aplasia, there are neither primary teeth nor permanent teeth present in one or both jaws; it is also possible that only the permanent teeth are absent. This condition is extremely rare and congenital. Partial aplasia is also genetically controlled and usually occurs symmetrically. It is most likely to affect the maxillary lateral incisors, the second premolars, and the third molars. Aplasia of the primary teeth is very rare.

In cases of **true hypodontia**, the decision must be made whether to achieve space closure by orthodontic measures or to leave the gap for later prosthetic treatment. Space closure is preferred if natural narrowing of the spaces has already started in a small, underdeveloped jaw. However, the space is kept open if the jaws are very large and other gaps exist, or if the outlook for tooth displacement does not appear very promising because the distance involved is too large.

False hypodontia can exist in the short term and temporarily during physiologic exfoliation. There can be a considerable difference between a patient's age and the stage of his or her occlusal development, which is why analysis of the absence of teeth needs to be confirmed with radiographs of the tooth germs. Premature loss of a primary tooth prior to eruption of its corresponding successional tooth can occur quite often. However, false hypodontia can also occur when primary teeth are shed at the normal time but there is a delay in eruption. False hypodontia may require treatment if space narrowing occurs or if jaw growth is inhibited, although jaw growth takes place independently of occlusal development. However, a space maintainer will become necessary because extreme space narrowing and hence displacement or disturbed tooth eruption can arise.

The **systematic extraction** of primary teeth for orthodontic planning requires precise analysis of the number of teeth. If premature loss of primary teeth is only unilateral, it may be worthwhile to extract the corresponding tooth on the opposite side to maintain the symmetry of the dental arch. Bilateral extraction of individual primary teeth

Fig 9-9 The preferred sites for caries are surfaces to which more plaque, bacteria, and cariogenic substrates (low–molecular weight carbohydrates) will adhere because of the tooth shape and the fact that self-cleaning is impeded.

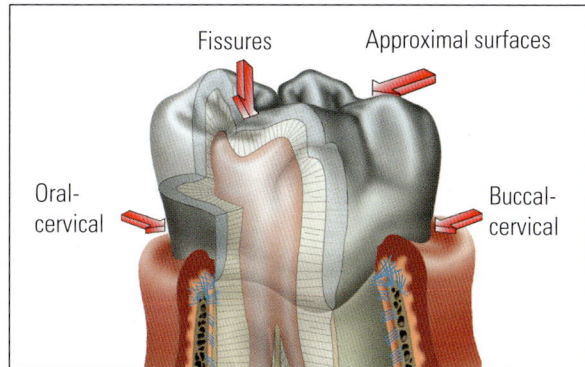

may also be considered if eruption of succession-al teeth is abnormal.

Inhibited development of the jaws and dental arches will occur if there is premature loss of primary teeth. This is because the tongue muscles lack the attachment surfaces for widening the dental arch. Unilateral primary tooth loss is therefore considered a localized abnormality of exfoliation from the orthodontic point of view.

Tooth Decay (Caries)

Caries is the most common dental disease. If the individual it affects is suitably predisposed, caries destroys the dental hard tissue by a chemicoparasitic process. Caries starts on the surface of the tooth, usually in the enamel of the dental crown (initial caries) or on the exposed cementum at the neck of the tooth (caries of cementum), and it goes on to attack the dentin.

The *caries lesion* initially takes the form of an opaque, chalky spot in the enamel; as demineralization progresses, the tooth surface becomes rougher. After destruction of the enamel layer, brown-colored cavities develop in the dentin. At this stage, cold, heat, or sweet foods will trigger a transitory throbbing pain. Progressive caries is first accompanied by infection, inflammation, and destruction of the pulp. Then the periodontal tissue is attacked, leading to loss of the affected tooth as a result of inflammatory processes.

Several factors encourage the *formation of caries*:

- Susceptibility of tissue to disease (tooth)
- Bacterial coating on the teeth (plaque)
- Consumption of cariogenic substrates (carbohydrates)
- Flow and composition of saliva
- Shape and position of teeth

The *chemical composition* of dental hard substances has an influence on the development of caries. The high fluoride content of enamel has an anticaries effect, whereas a high carbonate content in enamel encourages caries.

Plaque is a tough, matted, sticky coating on teeth made up of bacterial cells (streptococci are particularly cariogenic) and an intercellular matrix. Plaque forms on unclean areas of the tooth (preferred sites for caries), particularly in pits and fissures, the approximal surfaces, and in the cervical area (Fig 9-9). These sites are first colonized by aerobic microorganisms (which live in oxygen) and later by anaerobes (which do not require oxygen). Once plaque is fully developed, it can no longer be removed by self-cleaning mechanisms of the masticatory system. Plaque is mineralized into tartar (calculus) by constituents of saliva. Tartar forms close to the excretory ducts of the large salivary glands, ie, on the lingual surfaces of the anterior mandibular teeth and the buccal surfaces of the maxillary first molars.

The *fermentation* of carbohydrate food remnants (low–molecular weight carbohydrates, mono-

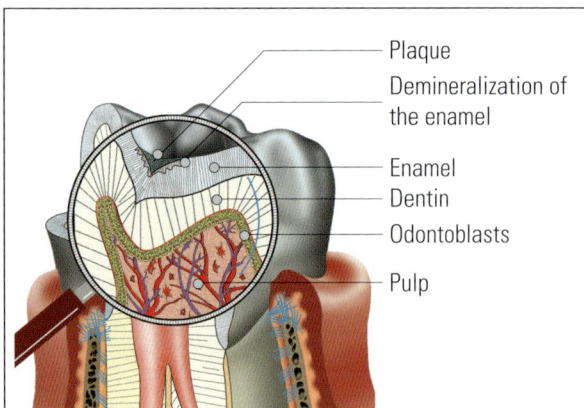

Fig 9-10 Plaque growth occurs at a preferred site for caries, usually with the production of lactic acid, whereby phosphate and calcium ions are released from the hydroxyapatite crystals. This initial lesion can be healed by suitable measures.

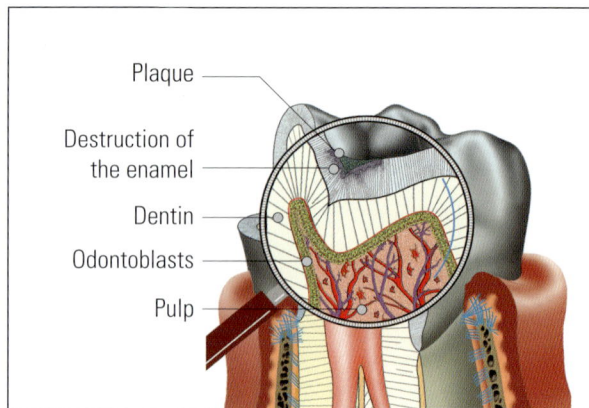

Fig 9-11 As the disease progresses, bacteria penetrate into the demineralization layer, and the ongoing production of lactic acid leads to accelerated destruction of the enamel. This results in a dark-colored hole that is now beyond healing.

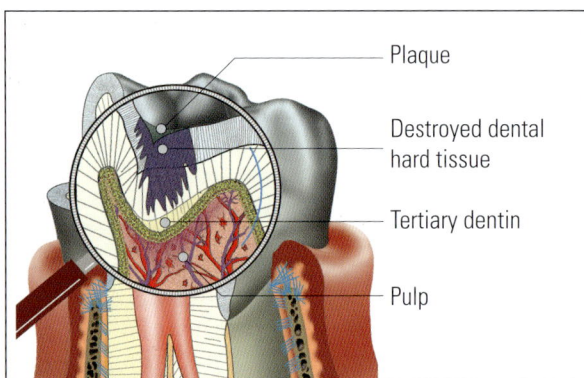

Fig 9-12 The caries attack has broken through the enamel layer and reached the dentin; the odontoblast processes in the dentin are destroyed. The odontoblasts form tertiary dentin to cover the wound in the dentin.

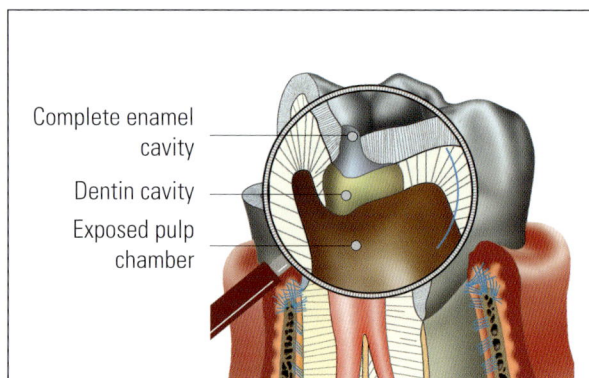

Fig 9-13 In the final stage, there is complete breakdown of the dental hard tissue, and the pulp is reached. The bacteria quickly penetrate the pulp tissue and infect the surrounding periodontium via the root canal.

saccharides) in plaque on the teeth acidifies the oral environment. This gives rise to lactic acid, which demineralizes the dental hard tissue while releasing salts (calcium and phosphate salts) (Fig 9-10). The tooth surface becomes rough and provides greater retention for food particles with increased fermentation. Bacteria are able to migrate into the loosened, demineralized tooth surface, where they then break down the organic supportive framework of the tooth (Figs 9-11 to 9-13).

Diet can encourage the formation and progression of caries lesions. Low–molecular weight car-

bohydrates such as sugar, glucose, and maltose allow caries to develop. By contrast, fatty foods (eg, cheese) have an anticaries effect because fat envelops the tooth material with a film. Saliva has a caries-preventive effect because of its rinsing function (quantity, viscosity) and its composition (sialic acid, pH).

Treatment of caries involves removing the diseased dental tissue, then restoring the original tooth shape by means of a dental filling, taking account of functional and cosmetic aspects. The following measures can be taken to prevent caries:

- Consuming a mixed diet rich in vitamins and mineral salts during the period of tooth development
- Eating foods that require chewing, which causes smoothing of the masticatory surface through abrasion and leads to self-cleaning because more saliva is secreted
- Early orthodontic measures for positional anomalies
- In certain circumstances, fluoride prophylaxis by the intake of suitable fluoride compounds (eg, drinking water containing low concentrations of fluoride)
- Coating the tooth surface with fluoride solutions, which means that poorly soluble hydroxyfluorapatite forms in the tooth enamel
- Careful dental hygiene
- Regular 6-month dental checkups
- Early filling even of small lesions

Erosion denotes the chemical dissolution of dental enamel without the involvement of microorganisms. It mainly happens on smooth tooth surfaces and is usually caused by acid vapors or consumption of acidic fruit juices or fizzy drinks.

Periodontal Diseases

The development and progression of inflammatory periodontal diseases are dependent on:

- Microorganisms in dental plaque
- Open caries lesions
- Ill-fitting crowns and filling margins
- Toothbrush trauma
- Effects of hormones and medicines
- Dietary habits
- Abnormalities of masticatory function

The inflammatory reaction and destruction of periodontal tissue depend on whether the patient's immune defense is rapid and effective. A poor immune response makes it easier for pathologic processes to take place.

Gingivitis is acute or chronic inflammation of the gingiva caused by plaque that only occurs around or in the vicinity of remaining teeth but does not occur in an edentulous mouth (Fig 9-14).

Simple marginal gingivitis can be found in nearly every adult. It can remain chronic in a mild form without periodontitis developing. Simple gingivitis is confined to the marginal periodontium above the alveolar bone, while the connective tissue adhesion of the attached gingiva remains intact.

Chronic gingivitis results from dental plaque or tartar accompanying poor oral hygiene. It is the most common painless disease of the gingiva, characterized by red and swollen mucosa that bleeds easily as well as bad breath; it can lead to periodontitis. The inflammation can be eliminated by regular oral hygiene and rinsing with astringent solutions. Chronic gingivitis may result from heavy metal poisoning (eg, with bismuth, lead, or mercury) and is characterized by a bluish-purple or bluish-gray gingival margin and even ulcerative mucosal changes.

Acute gingivitis in its simple form is mainly associated with febrile systemic diseases; it is characterized by small, painful mucosal swellings with a bright red border and sticky coating. It can develop into necrotizing gingivitis with a gray-brown mucosa and further into ulcerative or aphthous stomatitis.

In **hyperplastic gingivitis**, the gingival tissue proliferates in the interdental spaces and bleeds easily. This disease can be remedied by surgical resection of flaps of gingival tissue.

Periodontitis is inflammation of the tissues supporting the teeth in the region of the marginal periodontium. Chronic, profound marginal periodontitis denotes chronic inflammation of the tooth bed with inflamed gingiva that bleeds readily, pus-filled gingival pockets, and root plaque. This results in loosening of the teeth, and the affected teeth may fall out. Acute necrotizing gingivitis, excessive strain on individual teeth (grinding the teeth), tartar deposits, vitamin C deficiency, metabolic diseases, and hormonal disturbances lead to periodontitis.

The **metabolic products** of bacteria in plaque cause increased accumulation of neutrophilic granulocytes in the gingival margin, resulting in inflammatory reactions. The mobile microorganisms penetrate between the tooth and its junctional epithelium into the subgingival space so that a gingival pocket is formed. In the marginal periodontium, acute defensive reactions occur as defense cells collect there. The inflammatory

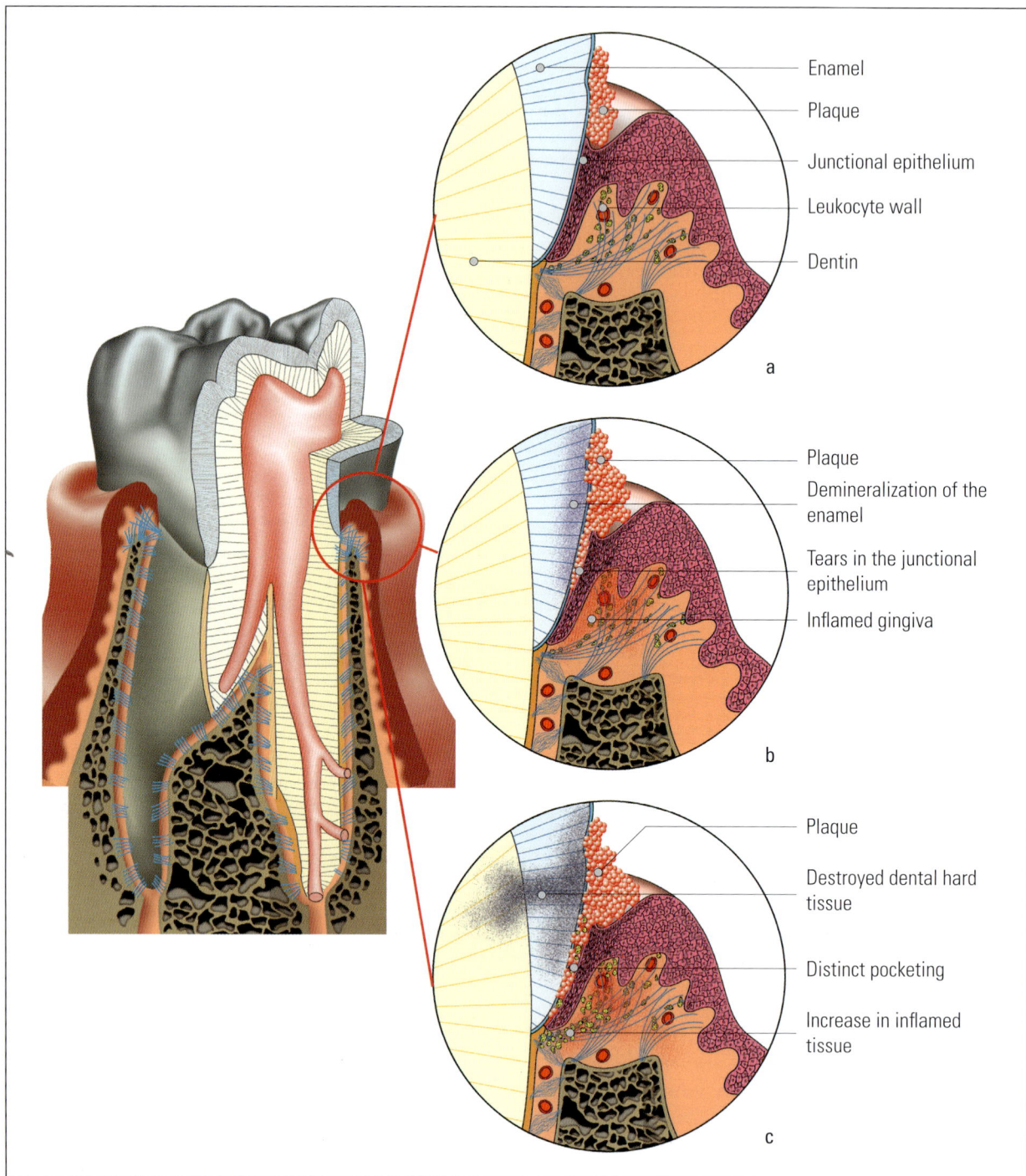

Enamel

Plaque

Junctional epithelium

Leukocyte wall

Dentin

a

Plaque

Demineralization of the enamel

Tears in the junctional epithelium

Inflamed gingiva

b

Plaque

Destroyed dental hard tissue

Distinct pocketing

Increase in inflamed tissue

c

Fig 9-14 The phases of gingivitis formation. *(a)* Clinically normal gingiva with supragingival plaque; only a few neutrophilic granulocytes leak through the junctional epithelium. *(b)* An initial lesion in the enamel under the plaque as well as tears in the area of the junctional epithelium with inflamed gingiva, through which the bacteria infiltrate. *(c)* Distinct pocketing with further destruction of the connective tissue and a massive flood of neutrophilic granulocytes to defend against the invading bacteria.

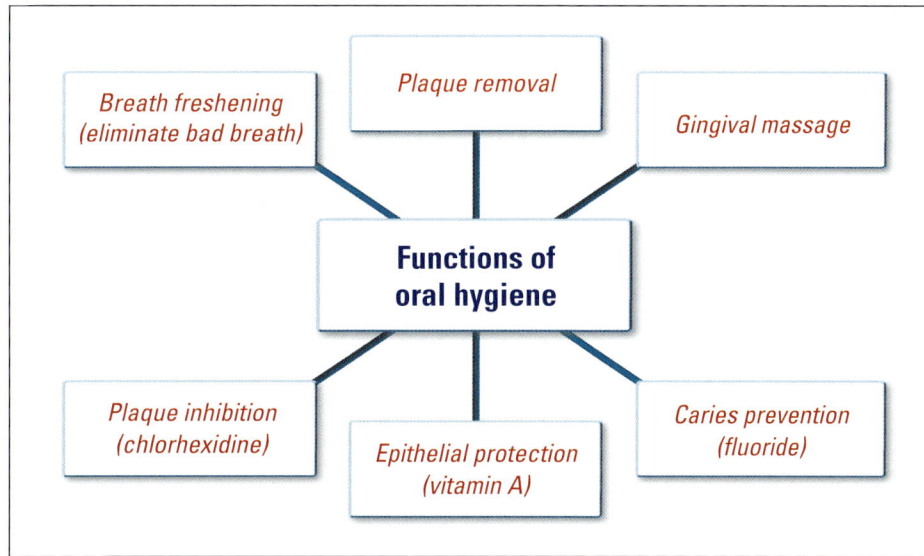

Fig 9-15 Functions of oral hygiene.

processes destroy the gingival collagen fibers, and the junctional epithelium becomes detached and transforms into pocket epithelium.

The ***treatment of marginal periodontitis*** first involves removing the inflammation-causing plaque and tartar and then surgically removing the gingival pockets. As well as inflammatory diseases of the tooth bed, fibrous gingival hyperplasia may occur, involving the formation of false pockets as a result of mechanical, chemical, or thermal injuries to the gingiva or occlusal overloading. In addition, there are noninflammatory forms of periodontal recession.

Acute apical periodontitis is a painless periodontal disease affecting teeth whose pulp is dead. It originates from the root apex and leads to purulent inflammation of the surrounding bony tissue.

Periodontosis, unlike periodontitis, progresses without inflammation and pocketing. It arises as atrophy (premature aging) of the tissue anchoring the teeth so that the tooth roots are partly exposed.

Oral Hygiene

Oral hygiene has the following functions (Fig 9-15):

- To remove plaque as a way of preventing caries, gingivitis, and periodontitis
- To remove nonbacterial deposits
- To massage the gingiva
- To freshen breath, eliminating bad breath
- To administer active substances such as:
  - Fluoride for caries prevention
  - Vitamin A to protect the epithelium
  - Chlorhexidine to prevent plaque

The ***toothbrush***, the most important oral hygiene tool, comprises a handle and a brush head that are separated by a neck. The handle is solid and long, tapering down to the head, and its surface is roughened to make it easier to hold. The bristles are inserted in tufts into the brush head and form the bristle array. Soft bacterial deposits (plaque) and food remnants are removed from

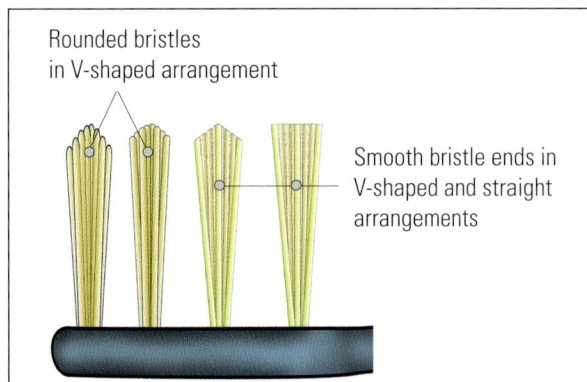

Rounded bristles
in V-shaped arrangement

Smooth bristle ends in
V-shaped and straight
arrangements

Fig 9-16 An ideal toothbrush has a short head holding multiple rows of even, homogenous, nonporous synthetic bristles with a smooth surface. The tufts may form a smooth or a V-shaped bristle array. The ends of the bristles are rounded. Nonrounded bristle ends are sharp-edged and can irritate the gums.

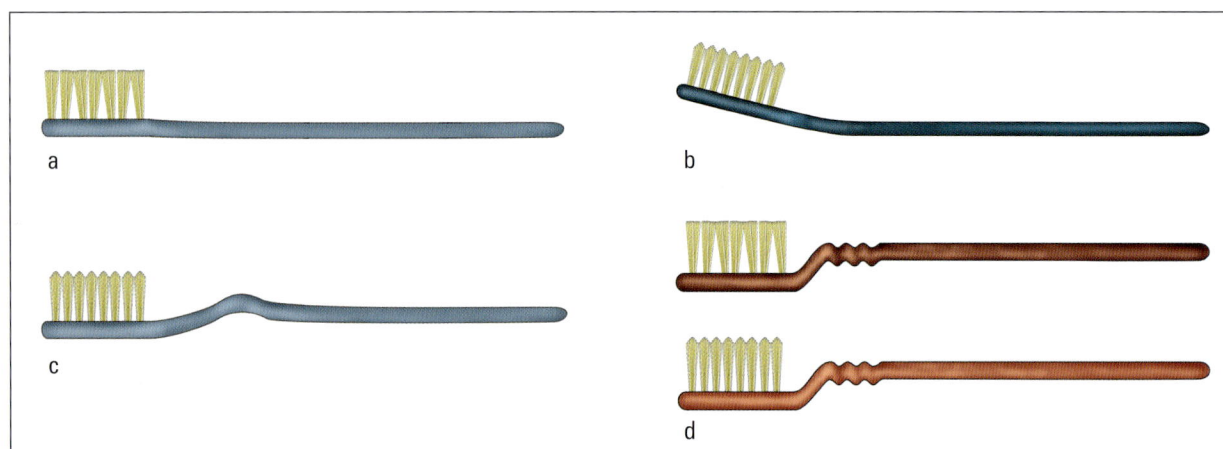

a

b

c

d

Fig 9-17 Toothbrushes differ in terms of their bristles and the design of their handles. *(a)* Toothbrush with a straight handle and a flat bristle array made up of rounded bristles. *(b)* Toothbrush with an angled handle and V-shaped tufts made up of rounded bristles. *(c)* Toothbrush with a contra-angled handle and a bristle array made up of V-shaped tufts. *(d)* Toothbrushes with an offset straight handle that is joined to the brush head by a flexible section; the bristle array of rounded bristles may be straight or V-shaped.

teeth and gingiva with the toothbrush. Toothbrushes have the following *quality characteristics* (Fig 9-16):

• Brush with a short head and multiple rows of bristles:
  – Length of bristle array: 20 to 30 mm
  – Width of bristle array: 7 to 11 mm
  – Bristle length: 10 to 12 mm
• Synthetic bristles (polyamide, polyurethane):
  – Are even, homogenous, and non-porous
  – Have a smooth surface
  – Are perfectly hygienic
  – Are unbreakable

  – Can be precisely manufactured in terms of density and hardness
• Have rounded bristle ends

Toothbrushes with a V-shaped tuft arrangement are rather unsuitable; a multitufted brush with thin synthetic filaments and a flat bristle array is better. Figure 9-17 illustrates various toothbrush designs.

Electric toothbrushes can be used as well as manual toothbrushes; they can perform rocking and swinging, forward and backward, as well as rotating movements. Electric toothbrushes are particularly suitable for patients lacking the necessary dexterity to use a manual toothbrush, including people who are bedridden or require nursing care, as well as children.

Jet irrigators are oral hygiene tools that rinse away food remnants but not plaque deposits. They can be recommended for patients with fixed orthodontic appliances or following orthodontic procedures. A jet of water that is not too powerful is directed vertically onto the gingiva, the interdental spaces, and the cervical area of the teeth. Chlorhexidine may be added to the irrigating water.

Toothpastes assist mechanical cleaning, make it easier to remove plaque, and deliver therapeutic ingredients. The cleaning is done by cleaning substances and surface-active materials, including the following:

- *Cleaning substances (polishing agents):* calcium carbonate, silicone dioxide, calcium phosphate, metaphosphates, aluminum hydroxide
- *Wetting and binding agents:* glycerin, sorbitol, propylene glycol, polyethylene glycol, methyl cellulose, alginate
- *Surface-active substances:* surfactants, tensides, amine fluorides
- *Preservatives:* alcohol, sodium benzoate, methyl paraben, p-hydroxybenzoic acid
- *Flavor additives:* menthol, peppermint oil, eucalyptus oil, aniseed oil, fruit flavoring
- *Colorings and pigments*
- *Medicinal additives:* fluorides, vitamin A, plant extracts
- *Desensitizing agents:* strontium chloride, potassium nitrate, formaldehyde
- *Tartar inhibitors:* etidronic acid

Strongly abrasive toothpastes can lead to loss of material from enamel, cementum, dentin, fillings, or gingival epithelium. After the teeth have been brushed, people should only rinse briefly with water to prolong the anticaries effect of the fluorides in the toothpaste.

Irrigating solutions for plaque prevention contain various ingredients that have an influence on plaque growth (chemical plaque control). They may contain the following active ingredients:

- Chlorhexidine (gluconate); side-effects include possible allergic reaction, reversible brown discoloration (of the mucosa, tongue, teeth, and filling margins), and taste irritation; only suitable for temporary use
- Hexetidine, sanguinarine, and cetyl pyridine chloride, which reduce plaque
- Tin fluoride; fluoride accumulates for caries prevention

Cleaning Techniques

Given the right cleaning materials (toothbrush and toothpaste) and appropriate brushing technique, it is possible to clean the teeth properly. A simple scrubbing technique will not achieve satisfactory cleaning and can cause damage to the gums and dental hard material (wedge-shaped defects). Therefore, a systematic approach to cleaning the teeth is essential.

Ideally one should start by brushing the buccal surface of the distalmost tooth in the maxilla so that the fluoride-containing toothpaste is able to flow downward and rinse around the mandibular teeth. The bristles should be placed at an angle to the tooth axis, pointing toward the gum line at the junction between the tooth and the gingiva, and the brush should be moved from the gingiva to the tooth in gentle circular movements (Figs 9-18 and 9-19). Gentle pressure should be applied without bending the bristles.

Cleaning is done tooth by tooth in a mesial direction over the midline of the maxilla and on to the opposite side as far as the distalmost molar. The oral surfaces of the teeth should also be cleaned with small rotating or horizontal movements. To do this, the brush head should lie parallel to the row of teeth. The toothbrush is only placed vertically in the oral area of the anterior teeth. It is impossible to reach the approximal tooth surfaces with a normal toothbrush.

Various oral hygiene aids are available for cleaning the interdental spaces. **Interdental brushes** are small, tapered, round brushes for cleaning between the teeth (Fig 9-20). The bristles stick out at the sides. Concave interdental tooth surfaces can be cleaned with interdental brushes, which can be inserted into the interdental space from a lateral cervical position and moved back and forth several times. The brushes can be wetted with an active substance such as chlorhexidine gluconate to prevent root caries.

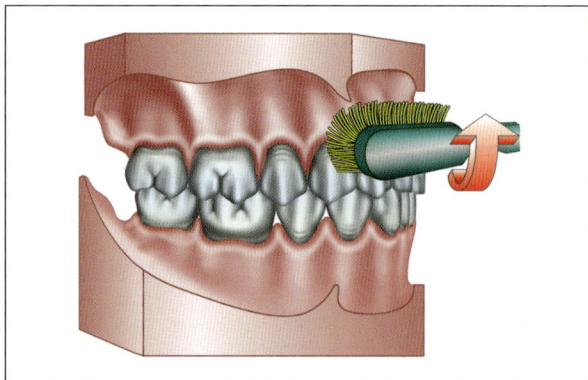

Fig 9-18 The toothbrush is guided from the gingiva toward the teeth, ie, from the vestibular fornix over the gingiva and the neck of the tooth toward the line of the closed occlusion.

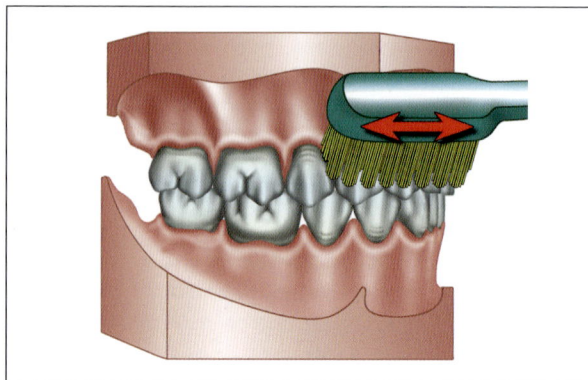

Fig 9-19 To massage the gingival margins, the brush is placed at a 45-degree angle to the gingiva and moved over this area with vibrating movements.

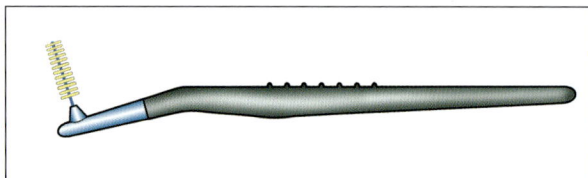

Fig 9-20 The interdental brush is a small, tapered, round brush for cleaning between the teeth, especially for exposed interdental spaces.

A *sulcus brush* has two rows of filaments and is used to clean the gingival sulcus.

Dental floss refers to synthetic threads of stretchy filaments on rolls. Dental floss is pulled through the contact points into the interdental spaces to remove any food remnants or bacterial deposits in the area of the interdental sulcus. A 30-cm-long thread should be wrapped around two fingers (eg, index fingers) and held taut. A floss tightening or holding device may also be used. The tightened thread is inserted into the approximal space with gentle sawing movements over the contact point. Deposits are removed from the surfaces with scraping movements. All the approximal surfaces of the dentition should be worked in the same way with a new section of floss.

Caries prevention by the use of fluoride demonstrably increases the caries resistance of dental enamel; regular use of fluorides results in pronounced caries reduction. As well as good oral hygiene and a dentally aware diet, the intake of fluoride is an essential form of caries prevention. Fluorides have the following effects:

- Formation of acid-resistant fluorapatite
- Remineralization in the presence of initial caries lesions
- Surface-active effect on dental enamel
- Inhibition of bacterial metabolism

The amount of fluorides consumed with food is not enough for a *caries-protective* effect, which is why various fluoridation measures have proved valuable, including the following:

- Fluoridation of drinking water as a long-term measure (Fig 9-21)
- Fluoridated table salt and milk
- Fluoride tablets
- Rinsing with solutions containing fluoride
- Use of toothpastes containing fluoride
- Brushing fluoride gels onto the teeth
- Fluoride solutions or fluoride varnishes

The regular topical application of low-dose fluorides has a stronger anticaries effect than irregular application of higher concentrations. Organic fluorides (eg, amine fluoride) have a greater caries-

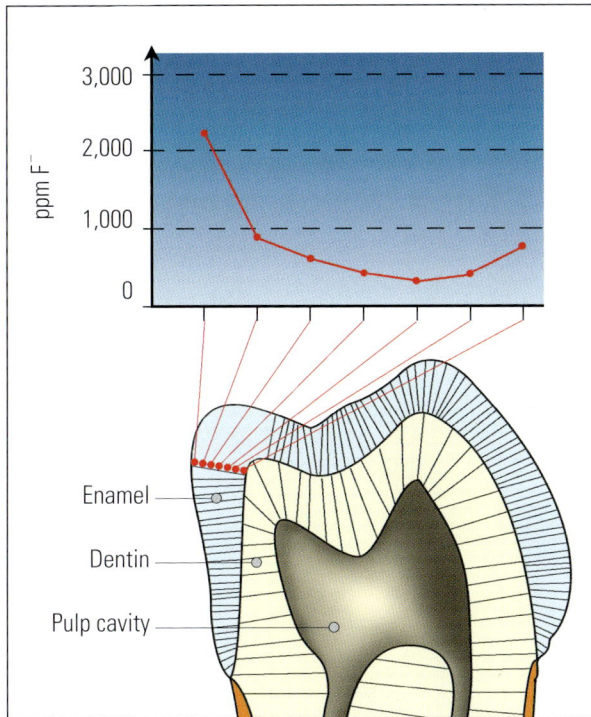

Fig 9-21 The fluoride concentration in the enamel of a patient who carries out oral hygiene using drinking water with a low fluoride content. The fluoride concentration is very high at the enamel surface, decreases inside the enamel, and increases again at the dentinoenamel junction.

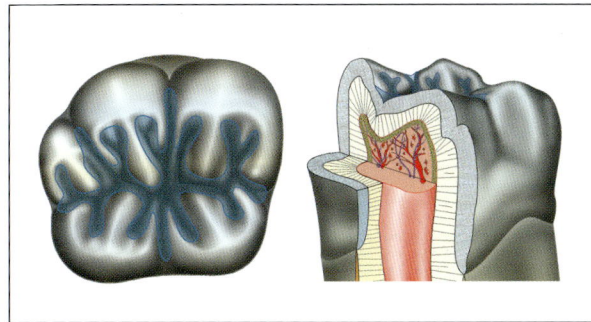

Fig 9-22 Pit and fissure sealing, as an anticaries measure, is performed on teeth that are impossible to clean with a toothbrush because of the depth of the fissures. So that plaque is unable to collect, the fissures can be covered with a composite that is bonded to the tooth surface by an acid-etching technique. This method is only used to seal fully erupted premolars and molars.

protective effect than inorganic fluorides (eg, sodium fluoride).

Pit and fissure sealing is a fluoridation measure to provide a tight and lasting fissure seal that is intended to prevent fissure caries entirely (Fig 9-22). Pit and fissure sealing involves an enamel-etching technique. The fissures can be mechanically cleaned with a nonfluoride cleaning paste and chemically cleansed with sodium hypochloride. The dry working area is conditioned with phosphoric acid and coated with liquid composite that is set with a halogen light. The sealing is checked by the dentist every 6 months and renewed if necessary.

Dental Services

Modern dentistry and dental technology services involve caring for patients throughout life, with dentists and technicians performing the following functions:

- Prophylaxis and prevention
- Basic dental treatment
- Oral rehabilitation by dental technology methods
- Aftercare

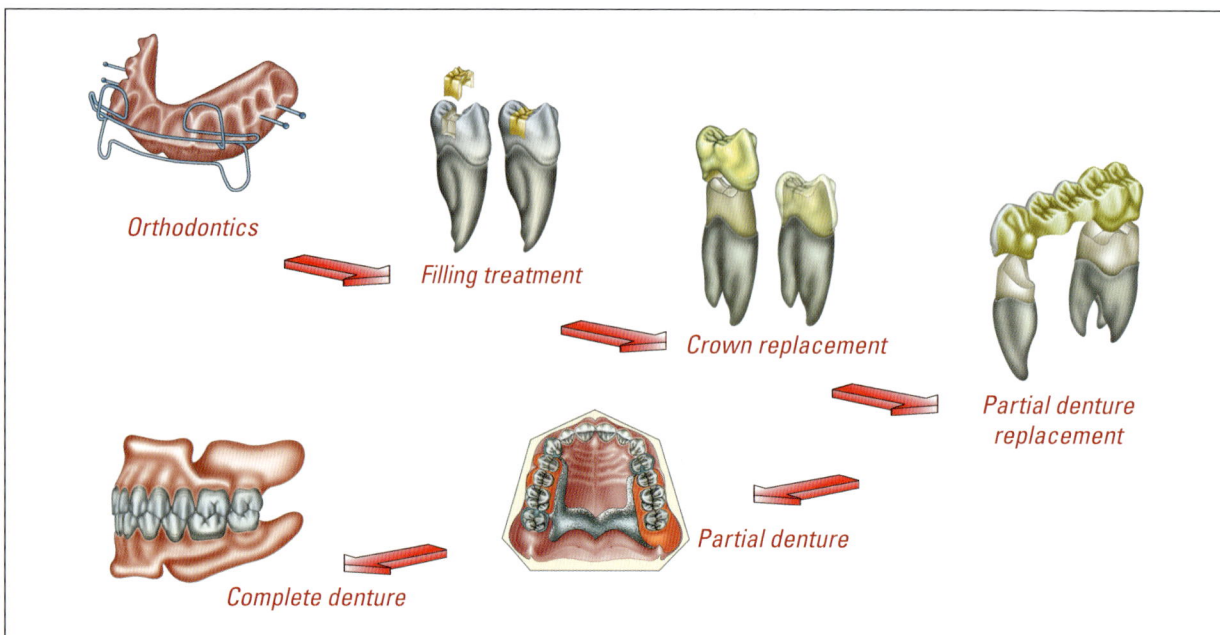

Fig 9-23 Nature of prosthodontic intervention with regard to the degree of dental destruction.

As well as medical prophylaxis of caries, periodontal disease, and gingivitis, **prophylaxis** also includes thorough oral hygiene measures, namely:

• Plaque removal
• Removal of nonbacterial deposits
• Gingival massage
• Fluoride treatment
• Motivating and instructing patients in oral hygiene

Prevention covers all the measures aimed at preventing and detecting diseases early. Disorders must first be prevented from developing, or damage must be detected at an early stage. Subsequent damage and chronic diseases can be avoided by early treatment. The area of dental prevention includes all the checkups performed on infants and schoolchildren before orthodontic measures are taken; prevention can sometimes include orthodontic treatment specifically aimed at dental prevention. Dental technicians are involved in the technical process of implementing orthodontic measures.

Basic dental treatment denotes all measures intended to restore and maintain dental health without prosthodontic methods. In the narrower sense, it means conservative dentistry, especially the treatment of carious, gingival, and periodontal diseases. Carious diseases are treated with fillings, which again involves dental technology.

Rehabilitation by dental technology methods involves the restoration of teeth altered by disease using conservative and prosthodontic measures and taking function into consideration. Dental technology measures are intended to arrest the pathologic changes; restore masticatory function, biostatics, and esthetics; and avoid future pathologic disorders.

The **types of prosthodontic measures** can be broken down according to the degree of dental destruction (Fig 9-23):

• **Pre-prosthetic measures:** orthodontics, splinting treatment; surgery, periodontology; implant dentistry; interim and immediate prosthetics.
• **Filling treatment:** restoration with plastic materials or inlays.

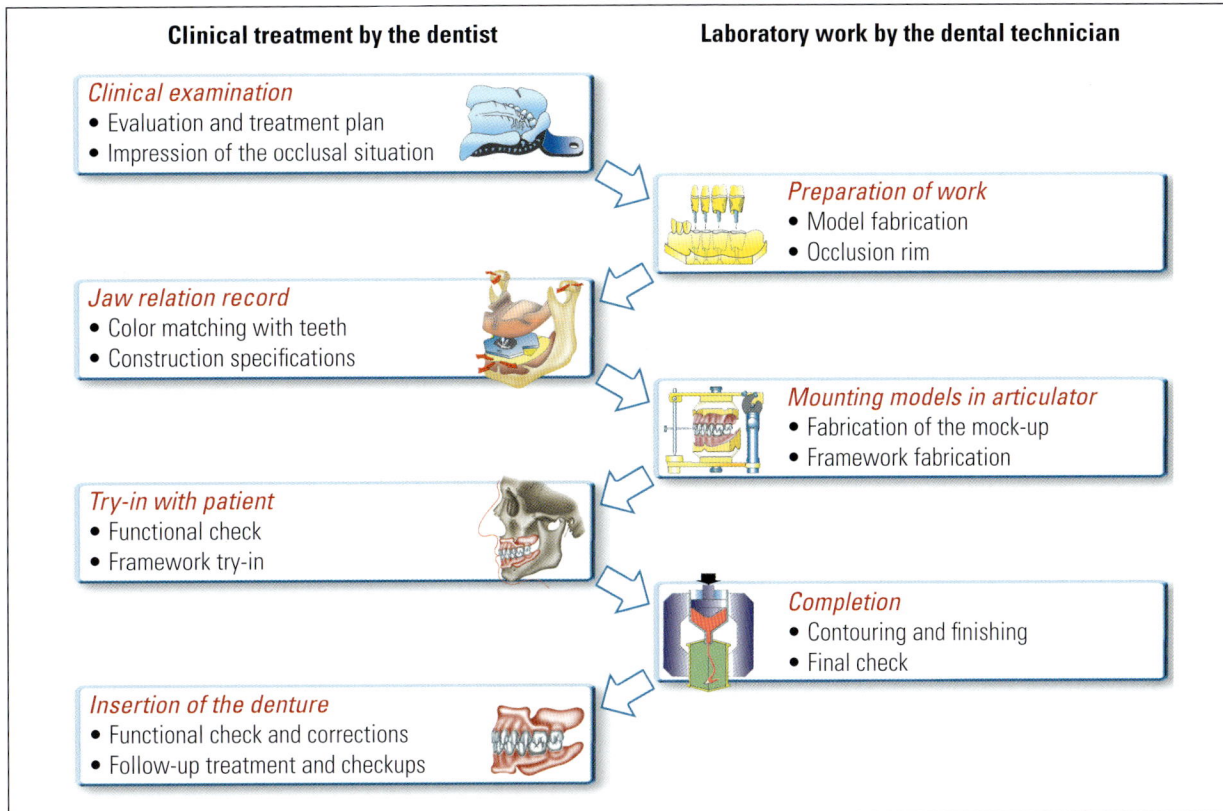

Fig 9-24 Principle of the cooperative relationship between the dentist and the dental technician.

- **Crown replacement:** partial crowns, full crowns, post crowns. This involves replacing lost dental tissue; complete replacement of function can be achieved for lifelong use.
- **Partial denture replacement** for fixed (or removable) dentures. This involves replacing dental tissue, missing teeth, and parts of the alveolar ridge; these measures do not entirely achieve complete replacement of function. Partial dentures can last up to 15 years.
- **Partial prosthetics** for removable tooth replacement. Teeth and parts of the alveolar ridge are replaced; only mediocre replacement of function or serviceability is achieved for a wearing period of about 5 years.
- **Complete dentures** for replacing all the teeth and the adjacent areas of the alveolar ridge; only limited replacement of function or serviceability is achieved for a wearing period of about 3 years.
- **Special prosthetics:** resection prosthetics and obturators.

Every prosthodontic form of replacement is the result of collaboration between the dentist and the dental technician. The sequence of treatment involved in the fabrication of prostheses thus alternates between clinical and laboratory working steps (Fig 9-24). An efficient collaborative relationship depends on both partners having comparable knowledge of their shared area of expertise so that understanding can be achieved.

In this context, the **shared expertise** of the dentist and the dental technician relates to:

- Anatomical and physiologic facts about the orofacial system
- Technical facts about dental materials; this aspect includes the chemistry and physics of such materials
- Techniques for processing materials
- Facts and interrelationships affecting the conditions of prosthetic design

Orthodontics

Orthodontics is the specialty involving the description and treatment of anomalies in the regular development of the masticatory system (Fig 10-1). Treatment relates to anomalies of tooth position, defective jaw development, and malocclusions, as well as abnormalities in the development of tooth germs and jaws. Maldevelopment of the dentition can be measured against statistical normal values of an optimal masticatory system. This normal dentition is a correct dentition in which the parts of the system have developed in a functional equilibrium during a process of differentiation. This process is genetically controlled, but it is supported by functional demands during chewing and altered by other influences. Therefore, the result is not always an optimal regular dentition; faulty development, referred to as *dysgnathia*, can arise.

The **functions** of orthodontics are to:

- Detect deviations from the normal course of development promptly
- Determine the extent of any faulty development
- Take suitable treatment measures
- Prevent further occlusal anomalies
- Prevent relapses after treatment is performed
- Improve masticatory and speech function
- Prevent periodontal damage and susceptibility to caries
- Improve the esthetic effect

295

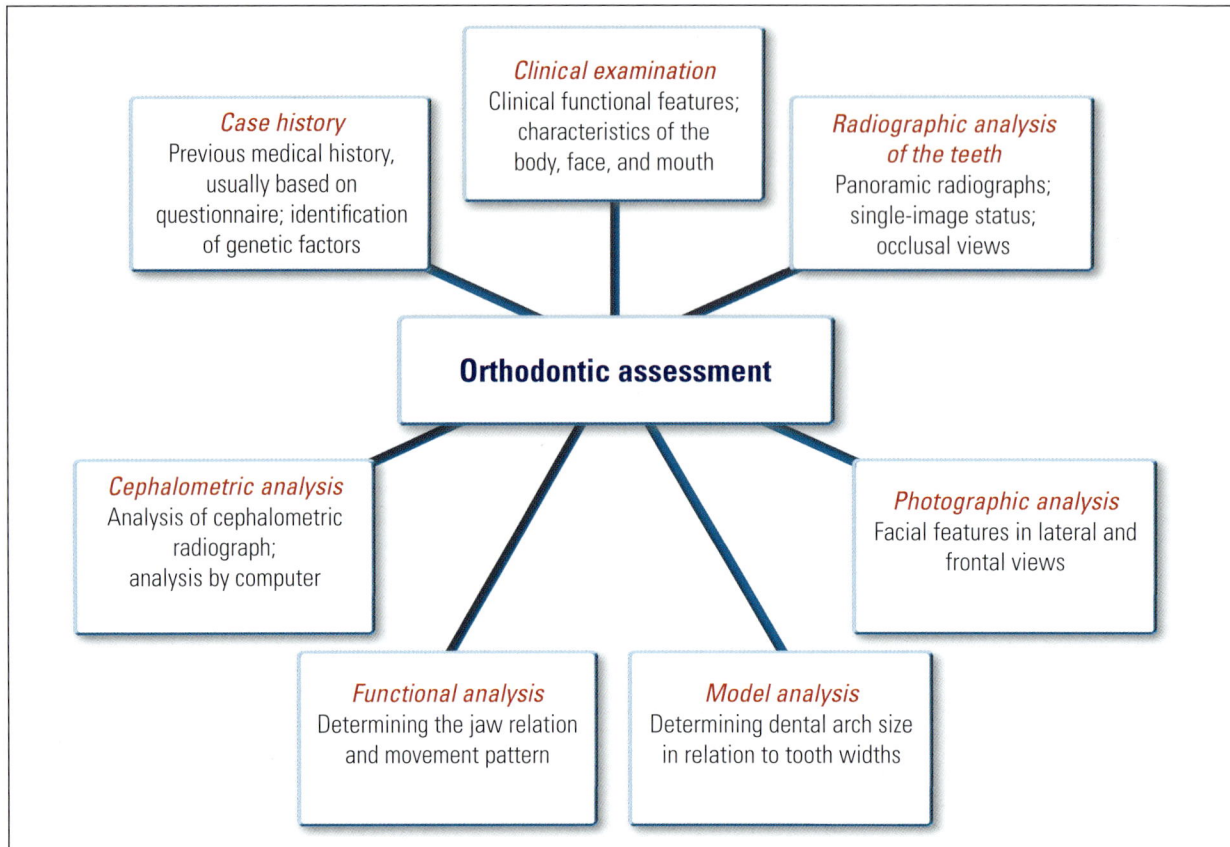

The diagram shows "Orthodontic assessment" in the center, connected to eight surrounding boxes:

Clinical examination
Clinical functional features; characteristics of the body, face, and mouth

Case history
Previous medical history, usually based on questionnaire; identification of genetic factors

Radiographic analysis of the teeth
Panoramic radiographs; single-image status; occlusal views

Cephalometric analysis
Analysis of cephalometric radiograph; analysis by computer

Photographic analysis
Facial features in lateral and frontal views

Functional analysis
Determining the jaw relation and movement pattern

Model analysis
Determining dental arch size in relation to tooth widths

Fig 10-1 The orthodontic assessment analyzes the extent of a maldevelopment of the dentition. The different areas of analysis record the deviations from regular development and give indications of the amount of treatment required.

The **aim of treatment** is to convert dysgnathias into regular dentitions and to compensate for malposition of individual teeth, deformed dental arches, or malocclusions without damaging the dentition.

Functional orthodontics involves using the functional processes during movement and loading of the masticatory system to develop the shape of the dental arches, the tooth positions, the jawbones, and the temporomandibular joints (TMJs) (Fig 10-2). Faulty development of the masticatory system is halted by orthodontic appliances and converted into regular development without the application of elastic components or external mechanical forces. The interaction between form and function is exploited to remedy

malfunctions and maldevelopment of the masticatory system.

In **functional orthodontics**, abnormal developments of the dentition are caught at the outset and treated by exploiting growth-related, functional forces. Normalization of the form is intended to rectify function, and the form is regulated by correction of the functional processes. The mechanical mode of action of functional orthodontic appliances is based on redirecting functional muscular forces and using them as remodeling stimuli. Physiologic tissue remodeling happens without active spring components or screws.

Orthodontic appliances (based on the principle of functional orthodontics) transfer the functional influences of the musculature acting in the mas-

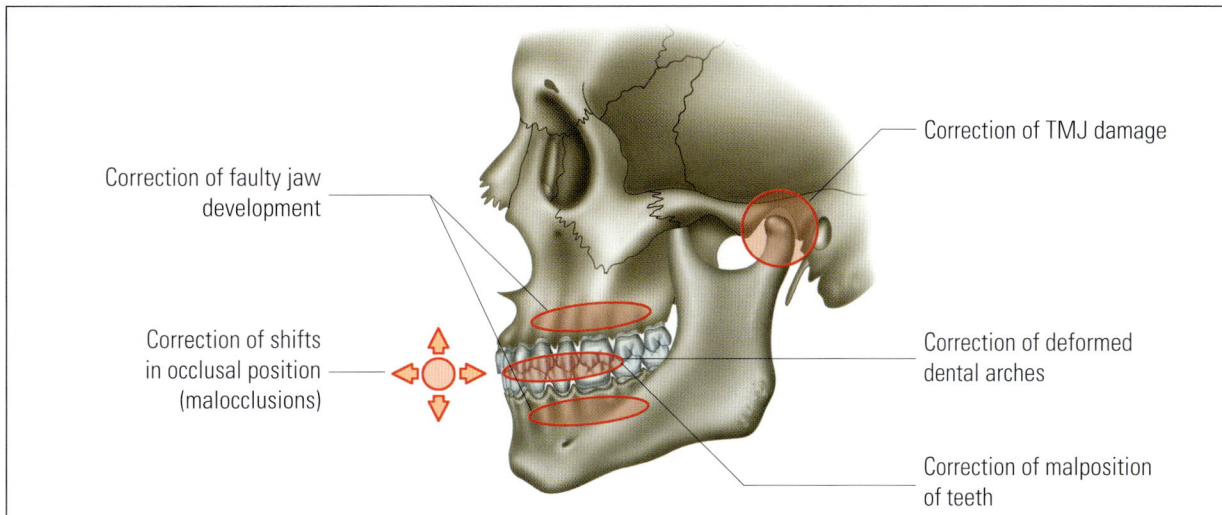

Fig 10-2 Orthodontic treatment relates to development of the form of the dental arches, the tooth positions, jawbones, and TMJs.

ticatory system to the teeth and parts of the jaw. This is done by converting vertical forces during biting into horizontal, intermittent stimuli to remodel the supportive tissue and at the same time alter the influences of the lips and tongue. The simplest principle of such an appliance is the inclined plane. Maldevelopment of form is usually accompanied by malfunction. However, isolated correction of one component (function) does not necessarily lead to correction of the other (form). In other words, achieving a change in functional processes by means of muscle training, in order to enforce changes of tooth position, will only be possible if dysfunction of the muscles was also a cause of the malposition. A variety of orthodontic treatment techniques have been established, reflecting the variety of therapeutic approaches in orthodontics.

Tooth displacement by orthodontic treatment techniques is achieved by application of force as remodeling processes are stimulated in the periodontal tissue, the alveolar jawbone, and the TMJ tissue.

Remodeling processes can be induced by functional stimuli, which originate from the muscles acting on the masticatory system. However, remodeling stimuli can also be initiated by continuous forces exerted by certain appliance designs.

The treatment methods differ in terms of how much they enable orthodontic remodeling stimuli to arise in tissue, and opinions differ on the feasibility and permissibility of certain types of appliances and techniques.

Orthodontic Model Analysis

Local occlusal deviations, malpositions of teeth, and anomalies in occlusal position can be identified directly in the patient or through the use of orthodontic models. These models are excellent aids to a thorough analysis of an occlusal anomaly and for planning purposes. As a means of measuring the shape of the dental arches and describing the deformations in the arches, these models are even better suited than examination of the patient.

There are several methods of model analysis with which a relationship between tooth width and dental arch dimensions can be mathematically recorded. A specific width and height of dental arch pertains to a particular width of incisors (Fig 10-3). In statistical records of normal dental arches, this ratio is summarized in formulae and tables. These analysis methods provide a good in-

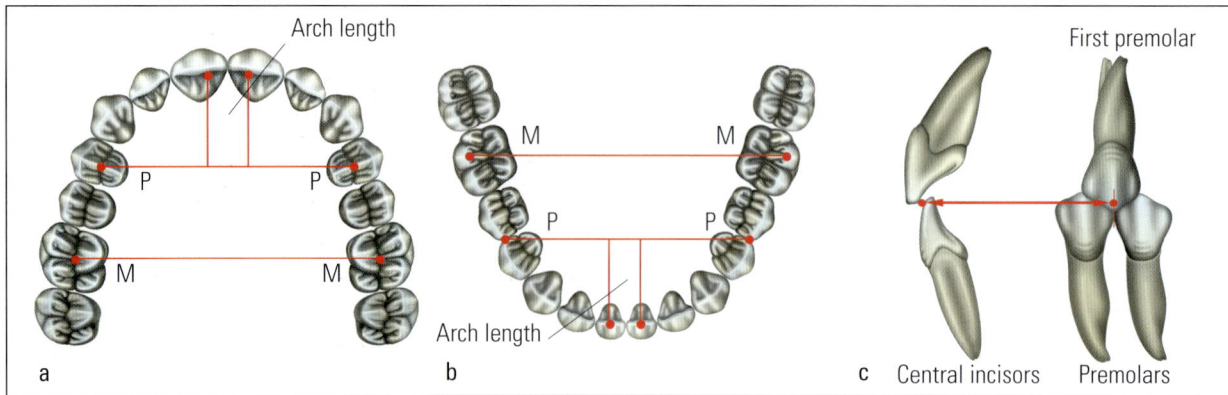

Fig 10-3 Orthodontic model analysis for technical measurement of the dental arch form produces a ratio between the sum of incisor widths and the dental arch width and length. Dental arch width is measured at corresponding measuring points between the premolars (P – P) and the molars (M – M). *(a)* Maxillary arch. *(b)* Mandibular arch. *(c)* Dental arch length.

dication of the dental arch widening or narrowing required.

Pont's index is the best-known method of model analysis, in which the sum of the width of all four maxillary incisors (sum of incisors = SI) indicates the ideal width of the dental arch at two points, namely at the first premolars and the first molars (see chapter 5).

To determine the anterior arch width, Pont's index uses the following equation:

$$\frac{SI \times 100}{80} = P - P$$

where *P* is the first premolar.

To measure the posterior arch width, Pont's index uses the following equation:

$$\frac{SI \times 100}{64} = M - M$$

where M is the first molar.

For the length of the dental arch, the vertical distance from the anterior arch width to the incisors is calculated as follows:

- Maxillary dental arch length = $\dfrac{SI \times 100}{160}$

- Mandibular dental arch length = $\dfrac{SI \times 100}{160} - 2$

It becomes clear that the position of the measuring points on the teeth must be precisely located for the measurement to be meaningful and especially verifiable. The sum of incisor widths is formed from the individual measurements of the mesiodistal distances between the approximal contacts in the four maxillary incisors. If the maxillary tooth widths cannot be measured because they have not all erupted, the widths of the mandibular incisors should be measured. Because there is a fixed size ratio between the mandibular and maxillary incisors, Pont's index can be calculated by means of this ratio. On average, the ratio of the maxillary incisor widths to the mandibular incisor widths is 4:3.

The **measuring points** for the anterior arch width on the maxillary first premolars lie in the middle of the central developmental groove. The measuring points for the posterior arch width on the maxillary first molars lie in the central fossa. In the mandible, the measuring points of the anterior arch width lie at the contact point between the first premolar and second premolar. The posterior arch width in the mandible runs between the central buccal cusps of the first molars. Orthodontic dividers can be used to measure the arch widths intraorally (Fig 10-4).

The **maxillary and mandibular dental arch lengths** run perpendicular to the anterior arch width to the occlusal contact points of the central incisors; this means they lie on the incisal edges

Fig 10-4 Orthodontic dividers are three-dimensional instruments for measuring the width and height of the palate. The curved tips of the dividers enable the arch widths to be measured from defined reference points, while palatal height can be read from a vertical sliding scale.

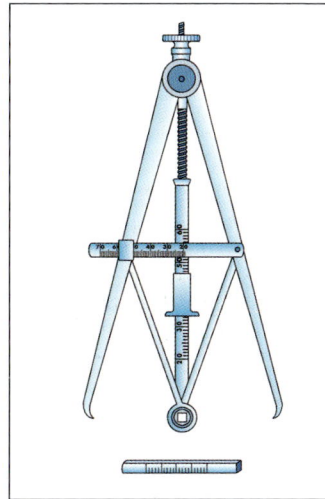

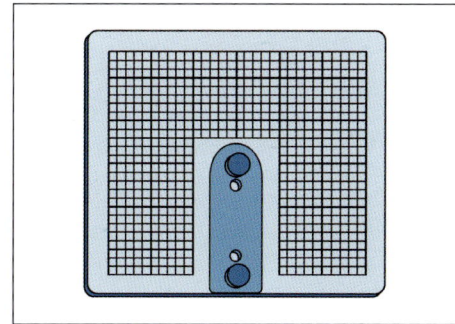

Fig 10-5 An orthodontic measuring sheet is available for practical model analysis. Its midline axis is placed onto the middle of the model being measured, and the corresponding measuring points are marked on the sheet.

Fig 10-6 (a and b) The millimeter grid on the orthodontic measuring sheet enables the malposition of individual teeth and any dental arch deformation to be measured and recorded.

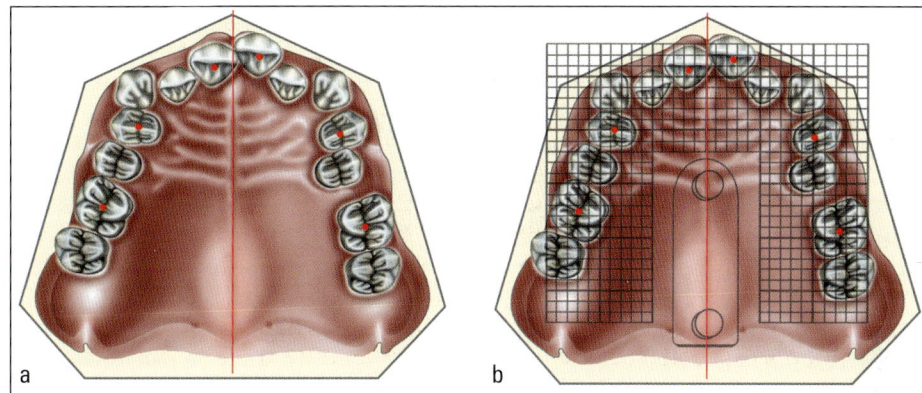

of the mandibular central incisors and on the palatal surfaces about 2 mm from the incisal edges of the maxillary central incisors.

For ***measuring orthodontic models***, a transparent sheet bearing a grid marked out in centimeters and millimeters is available. Pins are often placed at the midline, with which the measuring sheet can be fixed to the midline of the model (Fig 10-5). ***Measurement*** of the maxillary dental arch involves the ***following steps***:

1. Measure the incisor widths.
2. Calculate the anterior and posterior arch widths as well as the anterior arch length.
3. Establish and mark the middle of the model.
4. Place the measuring sheet with the midline mark over the middle of the model.

5. Lay the measuring sheet through the assumed anterior arch width.
6. Read off deviations from the actual values in two directions and note.

Asymmetries of the dental arches and migration of individual teeth are thus identified (Fig 10-6). The system error with this model analysis lies in the natural variance of individual dentitions and in the uncertainty of the position of the fixed points from which the deviations are determined. If the reference points (distal premolar or raphe-papillary transversal) are displaced, only relative deformations or displacements can be ascertained. Extraoral fixed points such as cranial reference lines, which are fixed in their direction and their distance from intraoral fixed points, allow more objective measurements to be made.

Remodeling Processes in Tooth Movement

It is possible to carry out orthodontically induced tooth movements because the dental attachment apparatus with all its tissue structures is capable of constantly renewing itself and adapting to functional changes. These tooth movements require accelerated, very active remodeling rates in the periodontal ligament and in the hard tissues, especially in the jawbone. In an analysis of remodeling processes, a distinction is made between physiologic tooth mobility, physiologic tooth migration, and therapeutic changes of tooth position.

Physiologic tooth mobility has the following advantages during normal masticatory function:

- The masticatory forces can be distributed to the rows of teeth.
- The blood supply is guaranteed via shifts in the volume of the network of vessels.
- The rate of renewal of the periodontal tissue is stimulated.

This tooth mobility will not result in any permanent change of tooth position.

Physiologic migration of teeth relates to changes in the position of individual teeth in the alveolar process, and it occurs in two directions:

- Mesially as physiologic mesial migration due to altered approximal contacts
- Occlusally during eruption phases or due to occlusal contacts altered by abrasion (see Fig 10-8)

Artificially produced tooth movements caused by orthodontic appliances are enforced by forces of differing strength. Changes of tooth position in all planes of space are possible. The tissue reactions at the cellular level are the same for both physiologic tooth migration and orthodontic tooth movements. These are complex, biologically controlled adaptive processes of the different cell structures:

- Bone renewal and bone resorption is carried out by osteoblasts, osteocytes, and osteoclasts.

- The periodontal ligament is remodeled by the activity of fibroblasts, as are the connective tissue fibers of the marginal periodontium.
- The cementum is broken down and built up by cementoblasts.

Mesial migration is driven by the permanent tensile forces of the circular ligamentous apparatus. These forces are still effective even if a tooth has been removed from the dentition; the adjacent teeth slowly tip into the gap.

Remodeling processes in mesial migration start with the resorption of all mesially located bone walls in the tooth sockets and with the laying down of bone mass on all distal alveolar walls (Fig 10-7). On the mesial walls, small bulges appear, with many osteoclasts particularly noticeable. Thin layers of bone are deposited on the distal walls. At the same time, remodeling processes take place in the periodontal ligament and the connective tissue of the marginal periodontium. The cementum shows new layers of cement on the distal walls with interposed fibrils for the fiber bundles of the periodontal ligament.

Increases in occlusal height to compensate for abraded chewing surfaces mainly occur due to bone substance being laid down in the depth of the alveolus or due to increases in the apical cementum (Fig 10-8). The driving force for an increase in occlusal height may be a combination of the tension from the fibers of the periodontal ligament and the lifting force of the hydrostatic vascular pressure in the periodontal space, which already raises the tooth out of the socket in normal circumstances.

Although *histologic reactions* are essentially the same in response to orthodontically controlled movements, the reactions are stronger depending on the distances of the movements and the degree of force. The following considerations are significant:

- Strength of the force and the lifting movement
- How long the force is applied
- Whether force is applied intermittently or continuously
- Whether tooth displacement, rotation, or tipping is being attempted

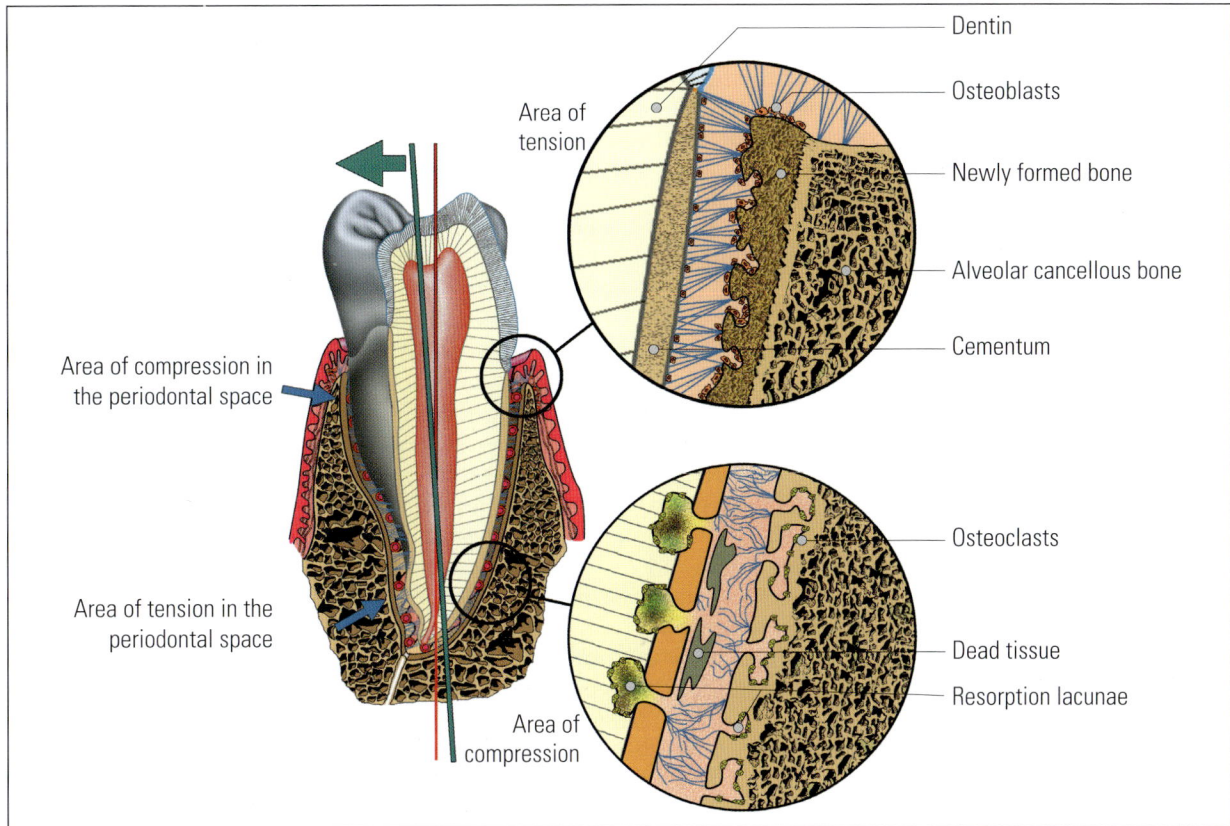

Dentin

Osteoblasts

Newly formed bone

Alveolar cancellous bone

Cementum

Area of tension

Area of compression in the periodontal space

Area of tension in the periodontal space

Osteoclasts

Dead tissue

Resorption lacunae

Area of compression

Fig 10-7 Schematic diagram of the remodeling processes during orthodontic tooth movements in the areas of compression and tension in the periodontal space.

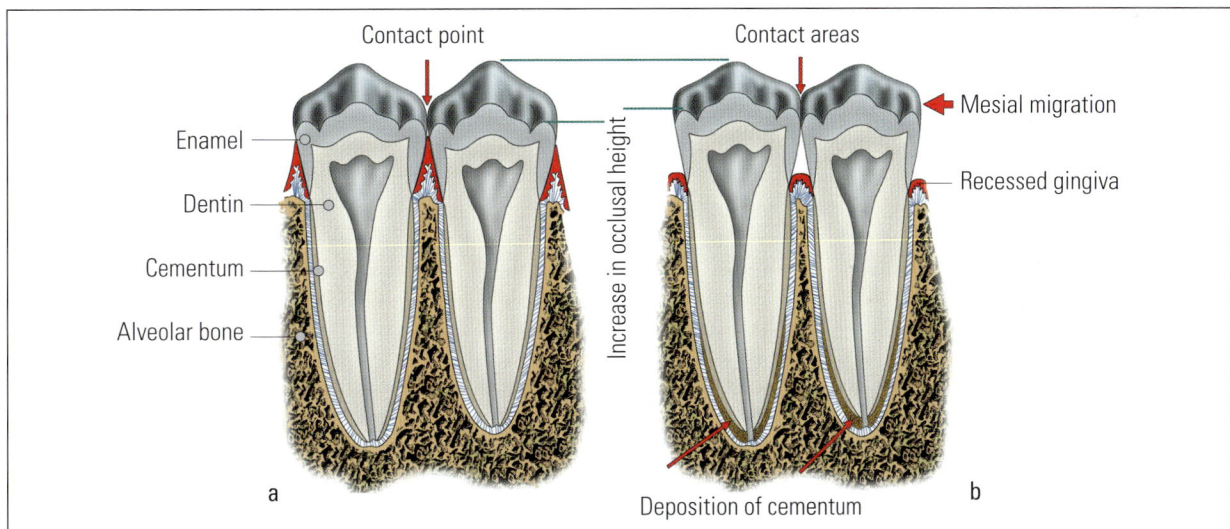

Contact point

Contact areas

Mesial migration

Enamel

Dentin

Cementum

Alveolar bone

Increase in occlusal height

Recessed gingiva

a

Deposition of cementum

b

Fig 10-8 Schematic diagram of the tooth attachment apparatus (mesiodistal sections) before (a) and after (b) decades of physiologic mesial migration due to altered approximal contacts and an increase in the vertical dimension (occlusal height) resulting from shortened crown height caused by abrasion. The apical cementum thickens as a result of deposition of cementum, so that the tooth root lengthens.

The force applied must not exceed a biologically tolerable degree if significant damage is to be avoided, such as permanent tooth loosening due to widening of the tooth socket, death of the periodontal ligament tissue, and resorption of tooth roots, which can lead to tooth loss. The biologically most favorable and hence orthodontically optimal force must not exceed the pressure of the capillary blood vessels and lies between 0.02 and 0.03 N/cm^2.

Levels of Biologic Intensity

With regard to the amount of force applied to achieve orthodontic tooth movements, four levels of biologic intensity are defined (Fig 10-9).

The *first level of biologic intensity* has no orthodontic effect. It applies to the operative forces during normal masticatory function and those of the dynamic equilibrium of the tongue, cheeks, and lips, which lead to physiologic structural adaptation.

The *second level of biologic intensity* arises from weak short-term pressures of 0.015 to 0.020 N/cm^2, which are not suitable for fully restricting the 0.1-mm periodontal space or stopping the blood flow. However, these forces can initiate orthodontically effective changes of position.

The *third level of biologic intensity* is achieved by medium-strength pressures of 0.02 to 0.05 N/cm^2. Capillary blood pressure is surpassed, but the tissue of the periodontal ligament is not fully constricted. These forces are too high for continuous use. Orthodontic appliances exerting this level of force have to be removed for a while after a wearing period of 8 to 12 hours. Otherwise, the fourth level of biologic intensity may ensue.

The *fourth level of biologic intensity* is achieved by forces that are even higher and are applied continuously. The cells in the areas of compression display irreversible damage after the force is applied for only 2 hours; changes in cellular tissue appear after only half an hour. The blood circulation is stopped, cell membranes rupture, cell nuclei disintegrate, and the cells start to die. After 2 days of continuous application of force, the tissue of the periodontal ligament is dead in the areas of compression. This extreme tissue reaction is seen only rarely in the areas of tension.

In the *area of compression*, the alveolar bone cannot be broken down by the dead cells of the periodontal ligament but is resorbed by the deeper-lying cancellous bone cells. Therefore, it takes about 3 weeks for the bone tissue and the dead cells from there to disintegrate. Orthodontic tooth movements are halted for that amount of time. Only afterward is new bone and periodontal ligament tissue formed, and the movement thrust can be reapplied. During such powerfully enforced changes of tooth position, resorptive processes also occur in the cementum of the area of compression, and these processes often spread to the dentin. Initially, only lateral parts of root walls are resorbed, but as the thrust continues, the root apex is resorbed and irreversible shortening of the root by several millimeters occurs. Under normal masticatory pressure, the shortened periodontium is permanently overloaded, the root continues to be resorbed, and the tooth is prematurely lost. Biologically favorable and hence orthodontically effective forces of the second level of biologic intensity promote tissue remodeling that does not leave any irreversible damage.

The *first tissue reactions* to the application of biologically tolerable force occur in the periodontal ligament as numerous fibroblasts develop. They cause alternating dissolution and formation of new connective tissue fibers. At the same time, bone resorption is stimulated in the areas of compression if the blood circulation is not constricted and cell activity remains intact. The first osteoclasts appear after only 24 hours.

In the *area of tension*, a layer of osteoblasts starts to form new bone layers after 2 to 4 days. In the process, the stretched straight fibers of the periodontal space are enclosed. Normally the cementum resists bone resorption in the area of compression; it only forms new cementum in the area of tension.

In the case of *rotating tooth movements*, remodeling processes of much greater magnitude are required in the fibrous system. If a tooth is rotated, the areas of tension are more extensive than the areas of compression. The bundles of fibers must be broken down and new bundles formed, which takes significantly more time than the formation of new alveolar bone. This results in loosening of the tooth, but this is clinically difficult to detect.

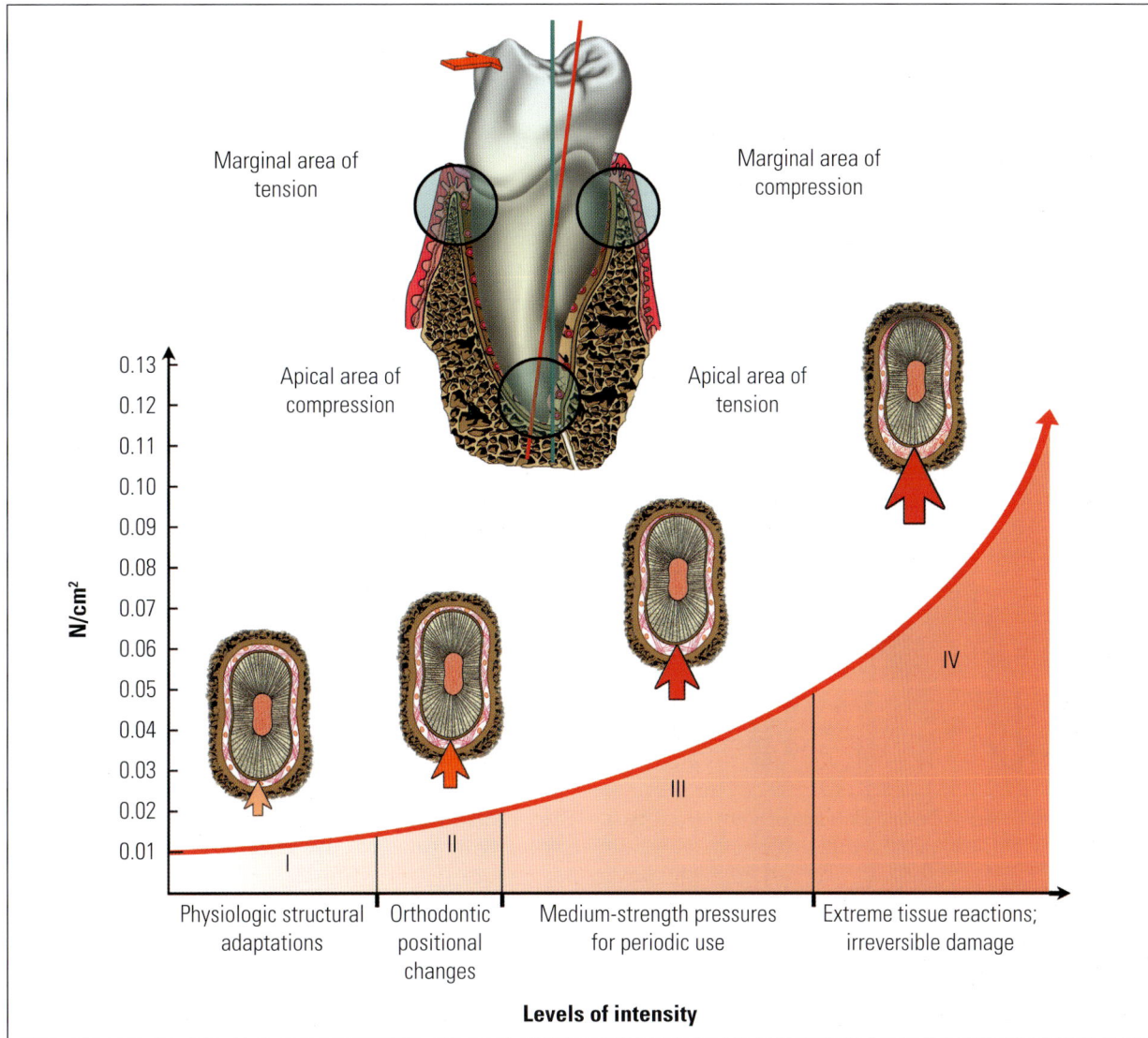

Fig 10-9 In relation to the force applied for orthodontically initiated tooth movement, levels of biologic intensity can be defined that stimulate specific tissue reactions. The tissue reactions are far more intensive in the areas of compression than in the areas of tension. The schematic cross section through the root of the tooth shows narrowing of the periodontal space dependent on the pressure applied.

Remodeling processes of the marginal fibrous systems need more than a year to reconstruct their functional processes. Sometimes reorientation is not achieved and the straightened tooth reverts to its initial position. When correcting severely rotated teeth, surgical resection of the fibrous systems of the marginal periodontium may become necessary so that the formation of new connective tissue structures is enforced and the tooth is prevented from rotating back again.

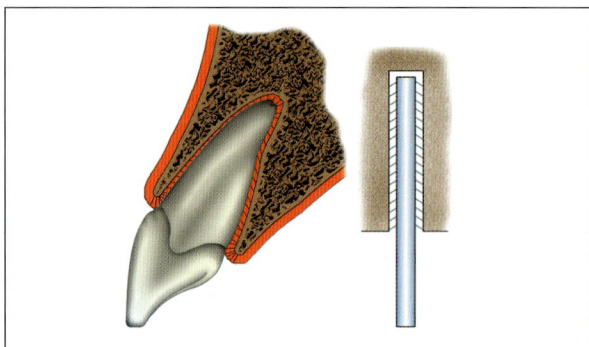

Fig 10-10 A tooth can be visualized as a rod that is elastically sunk into a base. Depending on the form and position of the application of force, a point of rotation arises in the area of elastic anchorage.

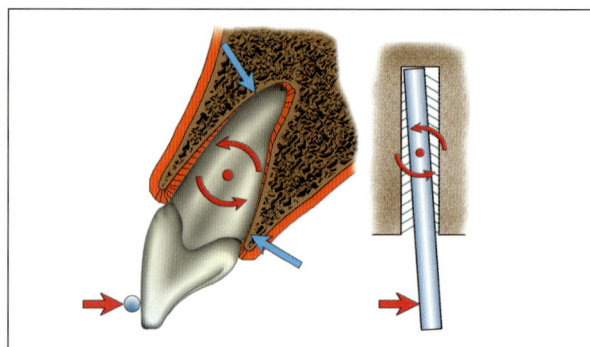

Fig 10-11 Single-point force application involves tipping of the tooth with a point of rotation in the coronal third of the tooth. Different areas of compression and tension arise in the periodontal space. The tooth can be tipped lingually or shifted.

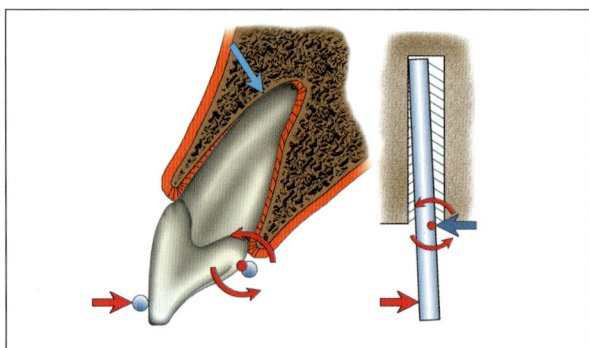

Fig 10-12 In the case of two-point force application (eg, by a labial bow and the lingual border of the plate of an appliance), the point of rotation lies at the fixed point of force application, and the areas of compression in the periodontal space are only apical on one side. The tooth is tipped lingually and not shifted.

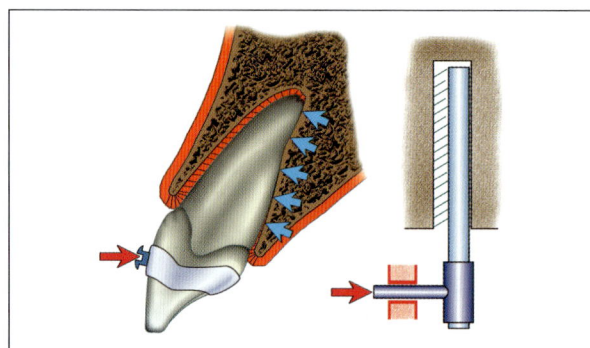

Fig 10-13 Multipoint application of force, as employed with fixed appliances, allows any desired tooth movements in all directions; the entire tooth has to participate in any movement caused by being bodily grasped. No point of rotation arises, and independent movements are prevented.

Transferring Forces for Tooth Movements

Forces are transferred to teeth by means of orthodontic appliances, and these forces are evident as tensile and compressive effects in the periodontium and produce the necessary remodeling stimuli. Every tooth movement causes areas of compression and tension in the periodontal ligament, the extent of which depends on the type of movement. Tipping movements produce neutral areas around the center of rotation in the middle of the root, while the pressure and tension peaks are found at the root apex and the alveolar margin. During a parallel shift of a tooth, the areas of compression and tension arise throughout the length of the root.

The *transfer of forces* to the teeth should initiate directed movement, which is why it is necessary to know precisely the effect of a force being exerted (Fig 10-10). Except in intrusion (sinking) or extrusion (lifting out) of a tooth, the forces for tooth movement will always act perpendicularly to the tooth axis. A force emanating from an orthodontic appliance to achieve rotation of a tooth will have to act differently on the tooth than a force intended to achieve parallel shift or tipping of teeth. A distinction is made between single-point, two-point, and multipoint application of force.

Fig 10-14 The shape of the root in cross section influences the pressure intensity and the size of the area that has to absorb the pressure. *(a)* In a rounded root, only small areas are loaded. *(b)* In a flattened root, larger areas are used for pressure absorption.

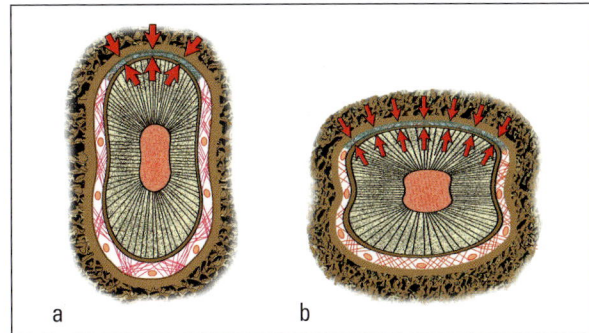

a　　　　　　　　　b

Single-point force application means the transfer of forces to teeth for guided orthodontic movements in which a force acts at a right angle to the tooth axis and produces tipping of the tooth (Fig 10-11). The connection between tooth and jawbone provided by the periodontal ligament does not act like a joint with a fixed point of rotation, but the position of the point of rotation can be variably influenced, depending on where the point of force application is located.

A **single-rooted tooth** with a conical root acts as a two-arm lever where the tipping axis lies roughly in the apical third of the tooth. However, the tipping axis is not fixed, and its position can change within the bottom half of the root as a result of the length of the coronal lever arm protruding out of the jaw and the position of the point of force application. Irrespective of the definitive position of the tipping axis in the apical half of the root, areas of compression arise in the periodontal space, around the apex of the root, and in the marginal area, with opposing areas of tension. The loaded areas increase in intensity with the distance from the point of rotation; the neutral area is located at the point of rotation itself. The loading strength is directly dependent on the magnitude of force applied and the position of the point of force application in relation to the point of rotation. The greater the force applied and the longer the lever arm (the more coronally the force is applied), the greater will be the compressive and tensile loading in the periodontal tissue.

Two-point force application or semirigid force application is a force couple with which eccentric tipping and rotations can be produced (Fig 10-12); a rotated tooth can also be regulated by such a couple. The tooth movement can be influenced by the precisely defined position of the tipping axis. All that is required is to fix—by means of an abutment—the point of rotation for the tooth movement relative to the application of force. If a clasp engages labially in the incisal third of the crown, a rigid abutment can serve as the point of rotation in the palatocervical position. In other words, a spring clasp presses from labially against the tooth, which is grasped on the rear by the appliance plate. Now the tooth is tipped over the border of the plate.

As a result, the position and intensity of the areas of tension and compression in the periodontium are altered. In fact, only one area of compression and tension arises in the apical region of the root.

Multipoint force application precludes any independent movement of a tooth. If the tooth is grasped bodily and the "grasping" device is moved, the whole tooth must adapt to this movement (Fig 10-13). This principle is put into practice with fixed appliances when the tooth being moved is bodily grasped by a broad metal band and this band is moved without distortion by a square arch. The tooth has to participate in any type of tipping, rotation, and parallel shift of that band. The attraction of multiband appliances actually lies in the possibility of successfully carrying out any chosen tooth movement by means of this principle of multipoint application of force.

The **forces for tooth movement** at first appear to originate from the appliance. They are absorbed by the teeth (Fig 10-14), passed on to the periodontal tissue, and from there transferred so that the remodeling stimuli can act on the bodies of the jaws, the sutures, and the TMJs. The appliance itself must be suitably supported to produce the necessary forces.

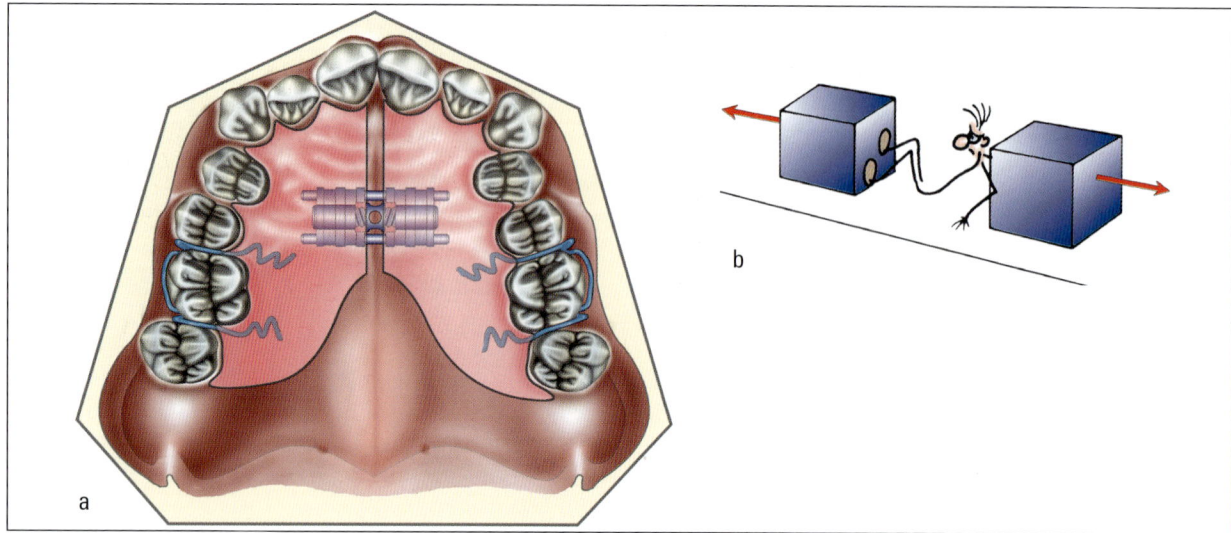

Fig 10-15 *(a and b)* Reciprocal anchorage with uniform distribution of forces arises between two equally sized partners that put up equal resistance. An allegorical depiction illustrates reciprocal anchorage: Two cubes of equal size move the same amount when the stick man braces himself between them.

Types of Anchorage for Force Distribution

When a tooth or group of teeth is moved by springs and bands, the appliance has to be supported on other teeth to exert the movement thrust. In the process, the same movement thrust acts on the abutment, which means the teeth to which the appliance is anchored are loaded and may also be moved. Depending on the nature of the fixation of appliances, the distribution of forces in the masticatory system being treated can vary widely. In relation to distribution of forces for orthodontic tooth movements, a distinction is made between the following **types of anchorage**:

- Reciprocal anchorage with uniform distribution of forces
- Stationary anchorage with unequal distribution of forces
- Maxillomandibular anchorage with maxillomandibular distribution of forces
- Extraoral anchorage with extraoral distribution of forces

Reciprocal anchorage offers uniform distribution of forces because the orthodontically exerted force lies between two equally strong partners that put up equal resistance (Fig 10-15). The anchor tooth is moved just like the tooth being corrected. An example is an active plate with a midline expansion screw. The plate will engage on insertion and exert the same pressure on both halves of the jaw and rows of teeth if there are teeth of the same size on both sides. If the gap between two incisors is to be closed with the aid of elastics, reciprocal anchorage exists and the teeth are moved equally toward each other because the same regulating force is exerted on both teeth.

Stationary anchorage arises if teeth or groups of teeth of unequal size are exposed to regulating pressure. An unequal distribution of forces is achieved because two unequally sized partners offer different amounts of resistance (Fig 10-16). The stronger components are not moved by the absorption of force, which means the stimulus remains below the relevant threshold and tissue remodeling does not ensue. There are smooth crossovers with reciprocal anchorage, because stationary and reciprocal anchorage can be combined in a single appliance. An expansion plate

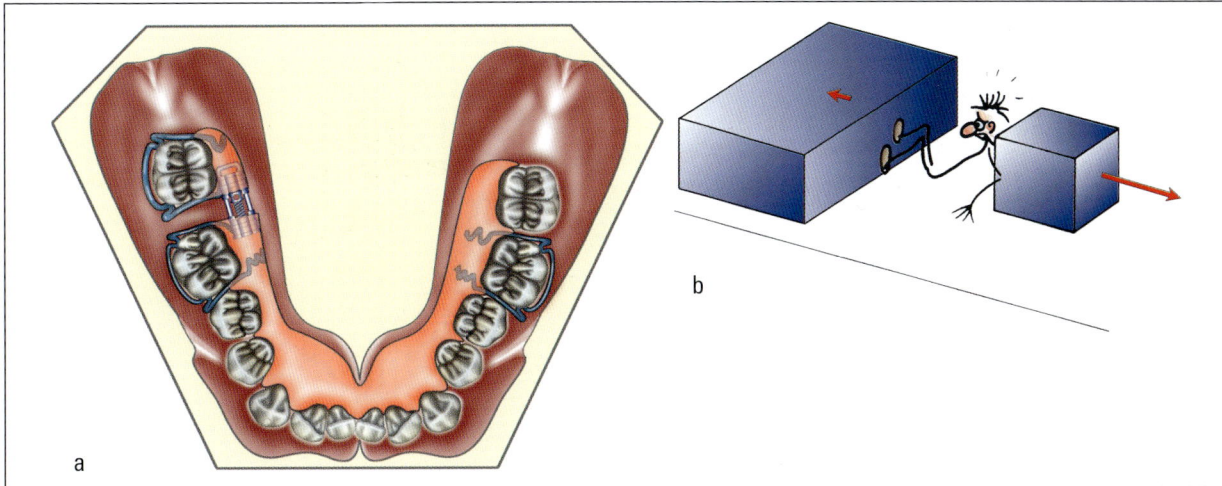

Fig 10-16 *(a and b)* Stationary anchorage with unequal distribution of forces arises between partners of unequal size that offer different amounts of resistance. In an active plate, which aims to move a distally migrated tooth back into the arch with a lag screw, pressure is also exerted on the row of teeth as the larger partner. However, the pressure is below the threshold to effect tissue remodeling. The allegorical image shows the stick man bracing himself between two blocks of different sizes, but he can only move the small cube.

acts reciprocally on both halves of the jaw, and with a mini-spring for single-tooth movement, the plate acts in a stationary fashion on the individual tooth; the spring force remains below-threshold for the teeth in the entire block. Using orthodontic implants or mini bone screws in the form of endosseous palatal implants results in anchorage for an orthodontic appliance that has full positional stability.

Maxillomandibular anchorage produces maxillomandibular distribution of forces between the mandibular and maxillary dental arches when, for example, disto-occlusion or mesiocclusion has to be rectified (Fig 10-17). An elastic module between a maxillary and a mandibular appliance is intended to pull the mandible in a distal direction. In this case, the maxilla is absolutely immovable so that a force from the maxilla is exerted on the mandible, enabling movement of the occlusal position. The most important maxillomandibular anchorage device is the activator, which as a passive appliance can produce maxillomandibular distribution of forces. Fixed hinges between the rows of teeth to remedy a disto-occlusion (Herbst appliance) are also classified as maxillomandibular anchorage.

Extraoral anchorage arises when orthodontic treatment is supported by bands or wire brackets fitted outside the mouth (Fig 10-18). Extraoral anchorage is usually intended to eliminate skeletal deformities, eg, to treat prognathism or in cases of maxillary atrophy.

The *headgear* is a device for extraoral anchorage in which a distinction is made between different directions of pull: cervical pull, horizontal pull, high pull, vertical pull, and frontal pull. It is an active device with fixed and removable components. There are three essential elements to a headgear: *(1)* head cap or neck pad with elastics for extraoral anchorage; *(2)* facebow for transferring forces (Fig 10-19); and *(3)* cemented bands with tubes to the maxillary molars, for intraoral application of force.

Headgear is used for the maxillary and mandibular dentition as well as the structures of the midface, with a dental and skeletal effect both in the distal movement of teeth or groups of teeth and in stabilizing molar anchorage in multiband treatment. It is also used for correcting inhibited sagittal development.

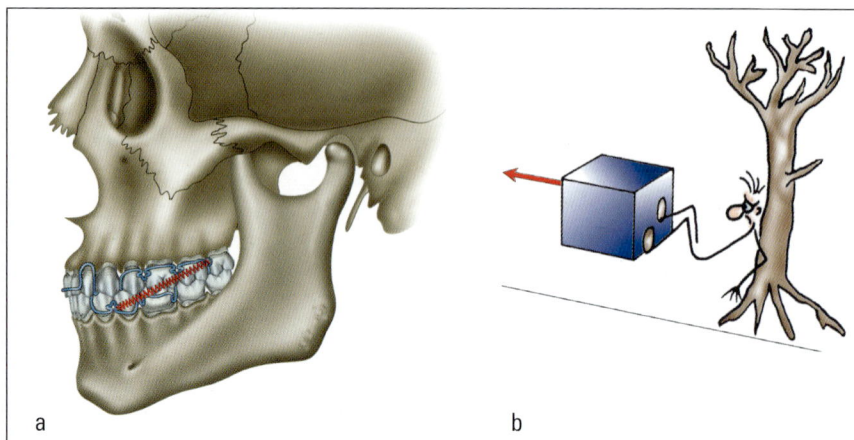

Fig 10-17 *(a and b)* Maxillomandibular distribution of forces arises due to maxillomandibular anchorage, eg, by an elastic between a mandibular and a maxillary appliance. In the allegorical depiction, the stick man braces himself against a tree to move the cube.

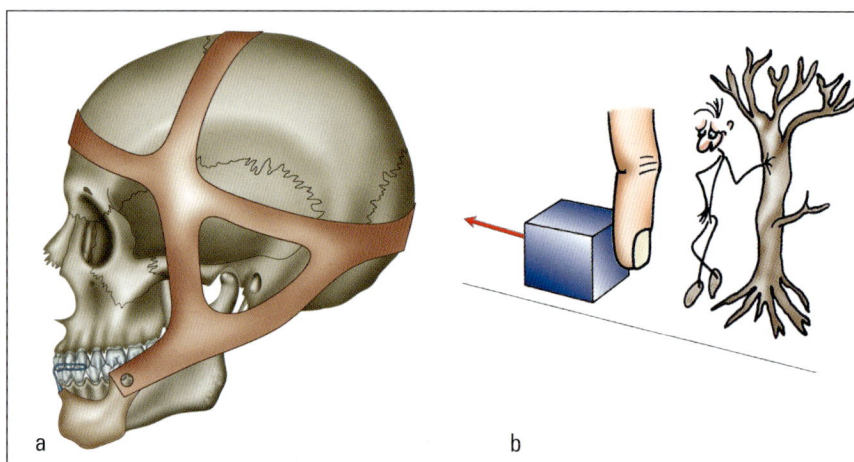

Fig 10-18 *(a and b)* Extraoral anchorage means distribution of forces between the appliance and the skull by bands or wire brackets, a chin cap, and neck bands. This makes it possible to move individual teeth or groups of teeth fitted with appliances. The allegorical view again illustrates the situation: While the stick man is busy directing matters, a force from outside pushes the cube in the desired direction.

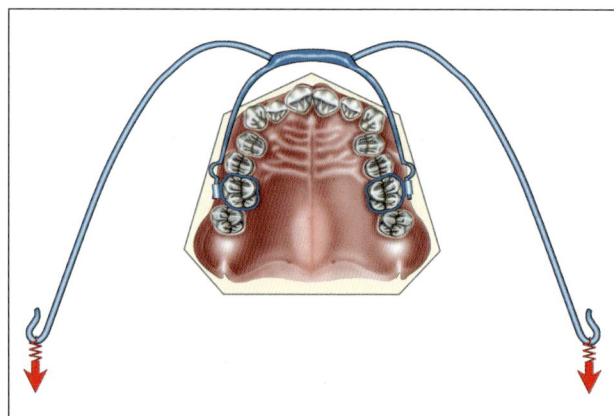

Fig 10-19 Extraoral anchorage involves a facebow for transferring forces on multiband appliances, plates, or functional orthodontic appliances. The facebow comprises an inner arch with a welded outer arch, which obtain their support on the head through a neck band or head cap. The illustration shows a standard facebow.

Classification of Orthodontic Appliances

Forms of dysgnathia can be treated with mechanically or functionally effective, active or passive, rigid or elastic appliances. In the case of extreme malpositions, surgical measures may become necessary prior to orthodontic treatment (eg, extraction to eliminate crowding). A fundamental distinction is made in orthodontic treatment devices between removable and fixed appliances.

Removable appliances are divided into three groups:

1. Active appliances only act in the maxilla or in the mandible.
2. Functional orthodontic appliances for simultaneous treatment of both jaws are passively acting appliances.
3. Retainers are used to secure the treatment outcome.

There are smooth crossovers between active and passive appliances because many have both active and passive design elements, and they are often used alternately.

Active appliances produce and transfer forces actively to the teeth, periodontium, areas of the jaw, and other parts of the masticatory system by means of springs, wire ligatures, screws, and elastics. These are plate or framework appliances and create their effect continuously or in fixed periods of wear.

Removable active appliances are used in the primary dentition as well as the mixed and permanent dentitions. In the primary dentition, reverse articulations (also known as *crossbites*) and individual malpositions can be corrected; in the mixed dentition, comprehensive functional orthodontic treatments are prepared, and in the permanent dentition they serve as retainers. They are fabricated by the dental technician on a working model according to the dentist's instructions and comprise the following components:

• Baseplate made of colored acrylic
• Retentive components made of hard wire to anchor the appliance

• Active components in the form of hard wire springs or double-thread screws

Passive appliances act on the teeth, periodontal tissues, alveolar process, jawbones, and TMJs with the functional forces of the masticatory, lingual, lip, and cheek muscles and influence these muscles directly by specifically stimulating, inhibiting, or re-educating them in their activity. Such appliances are functional orthodontic devices, usually removable and fitting loosely in the mouth; the fixed inclined plane is one exception.

Functional orthodontic appliances are based on the idea that form and function are directly dependent on each other. They manage without continuous application of forces and make use of forces within the biologic range of tolerance.

Functional orthodontic appliances are used in the mixed dentition to correct the position of the jaws in relation to each other. The activator as a typical functional orthodontic appliance is employed in the treatment of displaced occlusal position.

Crozat appliances are removable devices made of archwires that are soldered together and highly elastic. They act as both active and functional orthodontic treatment appliances.

Retainers stabilize corrected tooth positions and do not transfer any additional forces. Retainers can be designed as removable or fixed. A retainer is simply constructed and contains no active components, only retentive components.

Advantages of removable appliances include the following:

• They allow simple, safe treatment without causing any harm to the patient's health.
• No damage to the teeth occurs as a result of removing the appliance from the mouth to activate it.
• Problem-free cleaning allows for minimal caries attack.
• The treatment appliance is easy to remove.
• Targeted fluoridation of the teeth is possible.

Disadvantages of removable appliances include the following:

• Bodily tooth movements are not possible.
• The treatment outcome is dependent on patient compliance.

- Continuous, regular wearing periods are necessary.
- There may be poor wearing comfort and restriction of speech.

Fixed orthodontic appliances are intraoral band-arch appliances, inclined planes, and palatal expansion appliances.

Active Plate

Active orthodontic appliances include the removable, self-activating plates with which artificial, continuously applied orthodontic forces bring about changes in tooth or mandibular position by means of springs, screws, or elastics (Fig 10-20).

An *active plate* can expand dental arches in a transverse direction and stretch them in a sagittal direction. Individual tooth movements, such as tipping, rotation, and lateral displacement, can be achieved with them; reverse horizontal overlaps (also known as *overjets*) and locally limited reverse articulations can also be corrected with active plates. Malocclusions that are not limited to the alveolar region but have a skeletal origin cannot be readily treated with active plates.

Active plates are removable appliances fabricated by dental technicians. They generally have the following *advantages* over fixed appliances:

- Damage to the teeth can be avoided because patients are able to remove the appliance themselves if they experience pain.
- The action of orthodontic forces can be interrupted, and tissue structures adapt more quickly.
- Appliances and teeth can be cleaned more easily and more thoroughly.
- An appliance can be removed if a patient is troubled by the esthetic effect.

Disadvantages of removable active plates include the following:

- Wearing times can only be monitored with the patient's cooperation.
- Clumsy handling by the patient can damage the appliance.

- Mechanical effects of the retentive and active components can damage dental enamel.

The *elements of an active plate*—the baseplate, the retentive components, and the active components—perform various functions. To be able to carry out movements with active plates, the baseplate parts or retentive components must not inhibit tooth movement, which means that the direction and the magnitude of movement must be properly planned. Eruption movements of the teeth also must not be impeded by baseplate margins or bite planes.

The *baseplate* is a rigid acrylic plate that houses the retentive and active components and fits closely to the palate or the inside of the inferior alveolar ridge. It can be divided in a variety of ways, enabling the individual segments of the baseplate to be moved differently. The baseplate is fixed to the teeth with numerous clasps. The edge of the baseplate lies against the teeth below the tooth equator and extends into the interdental spaces. The baseplate may be lengthened or widened by means of anterior or posterior bite planes.

Posterior bite planes on the posterior tooth surfaces are used to inhibit vertical migration of the posterior teeth and block that of the anterior teeth (Fig 10-21), so that enforced occlusal positions (eg, reverse articulation of individual incisors) are corrected.

Posterior and anterior bite planes can be used to correct displacements of occlusal position as the mandible is guided into the intended position during biting. Joint changes can be stimulated, mandibular guidance being enforced with additional elastics.

The *action of the active plate* arises when the existing active components are activated between the segments of the baseplate. The baseplate margins exert pressure on the teeth and induce a change in the dental arch when the screws or Coffin springs are activated (Fig 10-22). Expansion, retraction, or extension of the dental arch can take place, depending on how the baseplate is divided and how the individual components are moved.

The *baseplate margin* can avoid individual teeth so that these teeth are excluded from the active effect of the plate. If the baseplate margin only avoids specific contact areas selectively, the

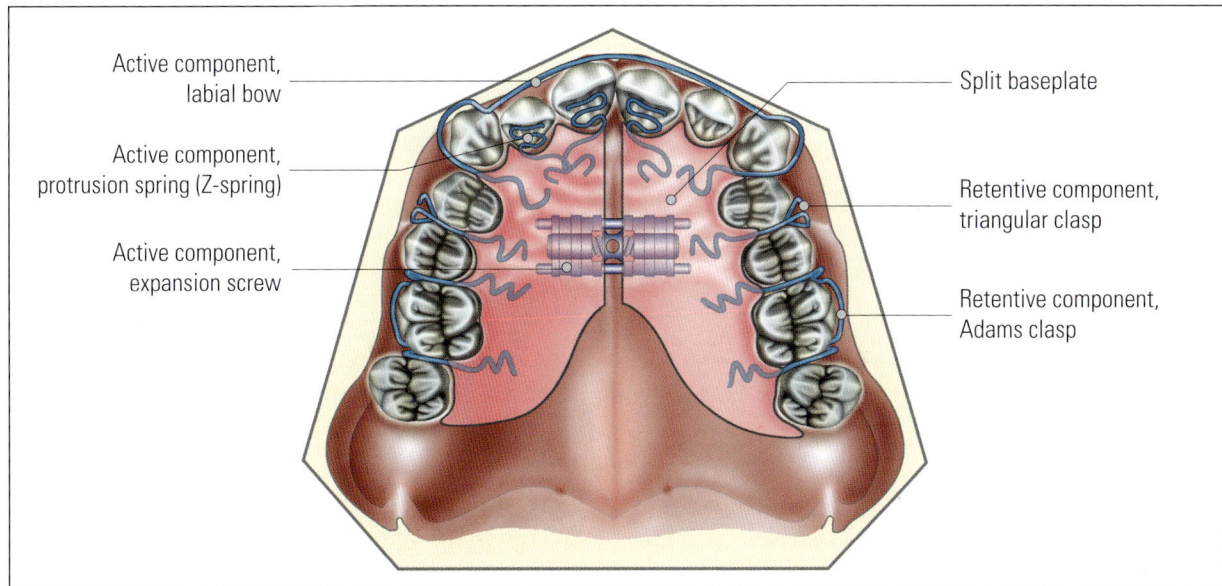

Fig 10-20 The active plate as a removable orthodontic appliance applies continuous artificial forces by means of springs, screws, and elastics. Based on the function, the different parts of the active plate are the baseplate, the retentive components, and the active components.

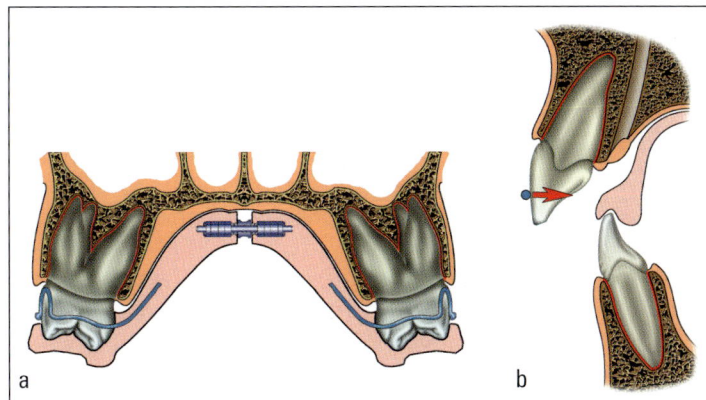

Active component, labial bow

Active component, protrusion spring (Z-spring)

Active component, expansion screw

Split baseplate

Retentive component, triangular clasp

Retentive component, Adams clasp

Fig 10-21 (a) Posterior occlusal planes in the posterior region inhibit vertical migration of the posterior teeth and block that of the anterior teeth, so that enforced occlusal positions (eg, reverse articulations) are corrected. (b) Antagonists can be restrained from the teeth being corrected by means of posterior occlusal planes.

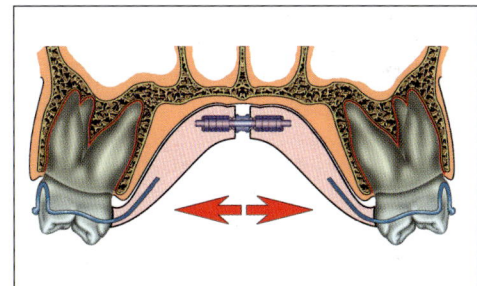

Fig 10-22 The action of an active plate arises as the baseplate margins exert a clamping effect between the teeth when the plate is inserted. Pressures on parts of the alveolar ridge and areas of compression and tension in the periodontal space develop equally, which in turn stimulates remodeling processes. A continuously exerted force may be generated if the expansion screw is regularly unscrewed by a fixed amount.

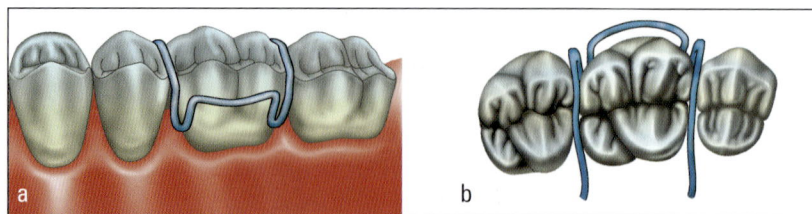

Fig 10-23 The Adams clasp (or crib) is used to anchor removable orthodontic applianc-es. Within the closed dentition, it can be guided into the interdental embrasure from the baseplate in a vestibular direction. Two U-loops have punctiform contact with the tooth in the undercut cervical area as they are placed obliquely at an angle to the tooth. The arms of the clasp must not interfere with occlusion. The height of the U-loops is deter-mined by the clinical crown, while the external width of the loop measures about 3 mm. The U-loop is fitted at such an angle to the tooth that punctiform contact is guaranteed.

rotation of an individual tooth may also be en-forced.

The clamping force applied when the appliance is inserted acts on the teeth. On insertion, the teeth tip and generate remodeling stimuli over ar-eas of tension and compression. As well as the re-modeling stimuli in the periodontal tissue, there is a compressive effect on the alveolar process, giving rise to changes in this area. In addition, the formation of new bone at the sutures may be initiated if tensile effects on this area exist. This leads to widening or extension of the palatal area.

Retentive components of an active plate

The clamping effect holds the active plate in the mouth until the teeth are tipped; once the remod-eling processes commence, the clamping effect subsides. Additional retentive components are therefore necessary. Spring components that per-form corrective functions cannot be used as re-tentive components. Because the spring force can only be as great as the normal clamping force of the baseplate, its effect will decline after the ap-pliance has been worn for a short period of time.

Retentive components are clasps whose spring action only starts once they are moved out of their resting position. They are guided into the under-cut areas of the teeth; they engage vestibularly, lie mainly pressure-free, and use the baseplate margin as their abutment. Retentive components may only be used indirectly for tooth movement when, fixed to the baseplate, they are moved

along with the baseplate. Retentive components have to participate in orthodontic tooth move-ments without loss of anchorage. After tooth movements have been achieved and after tooth growth, the position of the retentive components must be corrected. Retentive components are bent out of hard, round steel wire with a diameter of 0.5 to 0.7 mm. Thin wire is necessary because the retentive components are always guided in a vestibular direction over the closed dentition.

It is essential to ensure that retentive compo-nents exert no *regulating effects*. This is why the clasps only have punctiform contact with the teeth below the bulbous part of the tooth. If the clasps had linear contact, corrective treatment might ac-tivate orthodontic forces acting on the retaining teeth. With punctiform contacts, it is much easier to make a correction, especially when several teeth are incorporated with a closed wire band.

Four types of clasp (or crib) with different mod-ifications are used as retentive components: *(1)* Adams clasp, *(2)* eyelet or triangle (delta) clasp, *(3)* ball clasp, and *(4)* arrowhead clasp.

Other types of clasp are possible, and their val-ue depends on how well they fulfill their retaining function without being the source of uncontrolled orthodontic forces.

The *Adams clasp* enables the baseplate to be fixed to a single tooth, for which the maxillary posterior teeth are best suited. Mandibular poste-rior teeth are often still too short and hence have no undercut areas buccally. Therefore, the possi-bility of trimming the gingiva on the model un-til the necessary undercuts are exposed may be considered.

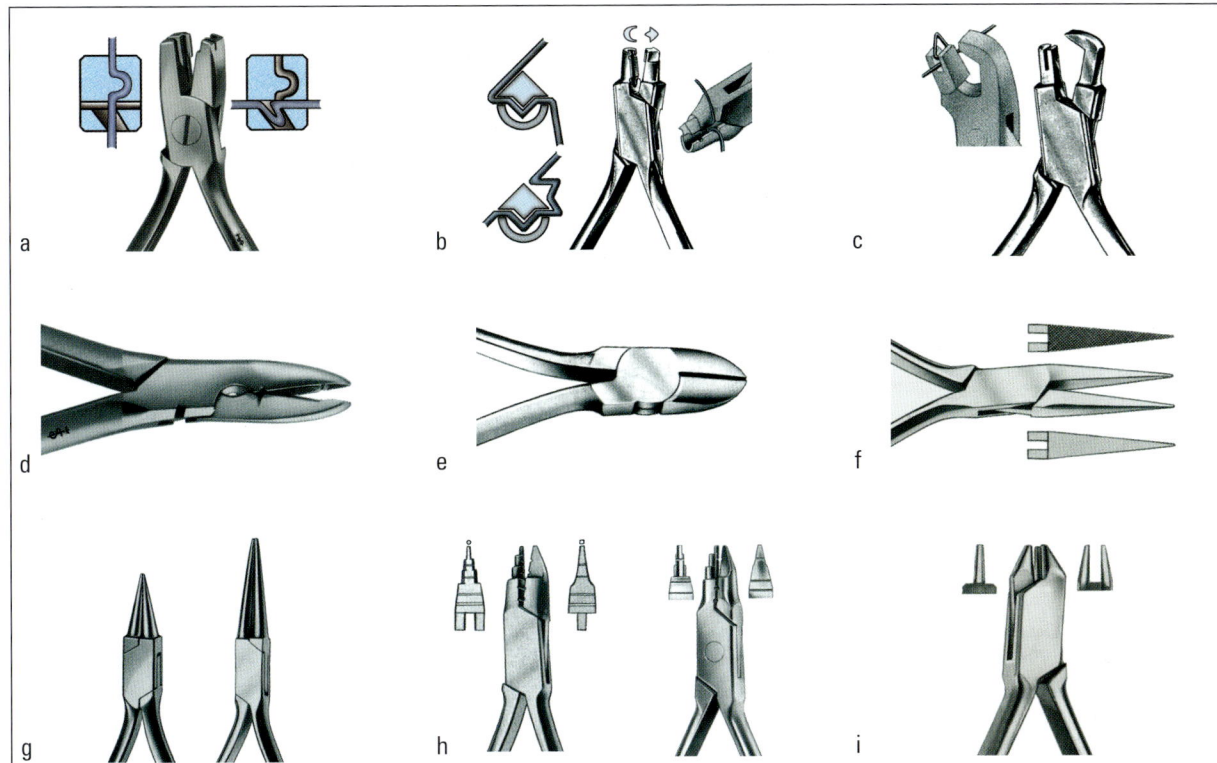

Fig 10-24 *(a)* Nance loop bending pliers for bending loop springs, loops, and Adams clasps (Aesculap). *(b)* Arrow-forming pliers, combination pliers for bending arrowhead clasps (Carl Martin). *(c)* Arrow clasp bending pliers for horizontal bending of the arrowhead to the dental arch (Carl Martin). *(d)* Waldsachs pliers have one hollowed-out jaw into which the other jaw fits (Aesculap). *(e)* Side-cutting pliers with cutters in a scissors arrangement to snip off wires. *(f)* Flat-nose pliers with or without serrated jaws for holding thin wires (Carl Martin). *(g)* Round pliers and round-nose pliers are suitable for bending loops and activating eyelets (Carl Martin). *(h)* Young loop bending pliers, universal pliers for bending different sizes of loops (Aesculap). *(i)* Three-prong pliers (Aderer pliers) have divided jaws into which one middle jaw engages.

The Adams clasp is a ***closed clasp*** with two U-shaped loops guided over the tooth at an acute angle (Fig 10-23). The tips of the loops (called the arrowhead) contact the tooth close to the interdental papillae in a buccal-approximal position. The buccal bar runs horizontally at a small distance from the tooth so that bending open or tightening the horizontal part can bring the loops closer together or move them further apart. If the U-loops are bent too acutely in relation to the tooth, the plate will be levered off. It is of primary importance, however, to avoid linear contact. Two crosspieces (known as "ears" or "arms") run interdentally over the dentition to the appliance baseplate, where they are anchored via relatively long retentive tails. The arms must not interfere with occlusion if the plate has no posterior occlusal planes.

The ***baseplate margin and Adams clasp*** engage the tooth on all sides; this means that bodily tooth movement can be initiated when the part of the baseplate with the Adams clasp is moved by a screw. So that the Adams clasp cannot bend out of shape, the parts extending transversally over the teeth can be reinforced by spikes.

An Adams clasp is fabricated from bent 0.7-mm spring hard wire or from semifinished parts. Flat-nose pliers and flat pointed pliers are required. (Figure 10-24 illustrates several types of wire-bending pliers and their specific indications.) First the length is transferred from the tooth to the horizontal buccal bar, and the ends of the wire are bent at right angles. The U-loops are then bent with the flat pointed pliers. The height corresponds to tooth height, and the maximum width is 3 mm.

The **U-loops** are bent at an angle of 45 degrees to the horizontal buccal bar, and the arms are guided interdentally over the dentition. The buccal bar must be adapted to the tooth contour. In the mandible, it will become necessary to place an occlusal rest on the middle of the tooth, starting from the lingual, so that the plate does not sink down to the floor of the mouth.

Triangle (or eyelet) clasps lie with the tip of their triangle or their eyelet curvature against the approximal area of two adjacent teeth, below the tooth equator but above the interdental papilla (Fig 10-25). They have only one arm running over the dentition. This type of clasp is bent out of 0.7-mm spring hard steel wire. The triangle is designed in accordance with the size and shape of the interdental space between the anchoring teeth. The triangle may be an equilateral triangle with a side length of 5 mm, while the eyelet, a modification of the triangle clasp, has a diameter of about 3 mm. The crosspiece of the clasp is laid over the dentition in the interdental embrasure and, with a retention arm, extends into the baseplate of the appliance. The relatively long crosspiece readily bends out of shape and therefore often has to be corrected, which damages the material. The clasps can break, be swallowed, or be aspirated into the trachea. In view of this notable disadvantage, arrowhead clasps tend to be preferred, or triangle clasps are only used temporarily.

The **difference in application** between eyelet and triangle clasps may be that triangle clasps extending into the interdental spaces could also be used as space maintainers, especially since the free triangular bracket can be activated for horizontal thrust. This jeopardizes the spring and clasp function because of the weak crosspiece. Eyelet clasps can be used as a technically simple retentive component.

The **ball clasp** is an eyelet clasp reduced to a ball (or droplet) in the actual area of retention (Fig 10-26). In the past, the ball used to be formed from a drop of solder at the end of the wire. Today it is used as a semifinished part and is made of 0.5- to 0.7-mm wire. The **ball** lies firmly in the interdental area, with the crosspiece guided over the dentition, and is sensitive to warping and can break after multiple corrections. To achieve an adequate length of spring arm, the crosspiece is lengthened in the vestibular direction, and the ball is placed in an arc in the interdental area of retention.

An **arrowhead clasp**, like an Adams clasp, has two arms that lie over the closed dentition (Fig 10-27). An arrow-shaped loop is formed, the arrowhead being bent toward the interdental retention area of two teeth. The long wire loops from the arms (as far as the arrow) run at a distance of about 1 mm from the gingiva and ensure that the arrowhead has a wide spring deflection.

The **arrowhead** contacts two teeth and can be worked with a certain pretension; the outer support is the edge of the baseplate. As the arrowhead contacts the tooth below its equator and in the process exerts some pressure, tooth growth is supported rather than impeded. This is reinforced by the fact that the arms do not run in the interdental embrasures of the anchoring teeth but at a distance from them in the approximal area of other teeth. Hence the arrowhead clasp can be used to a limited extent for single-tooth movement by shaping just half an arrowhead that only contacts one tooth and moves it.

Where a plate is normally anchored, two arrows are used in one **loop unit** per half jaw. If firmer retention is required, three arrows can be fitted into the interdental spaces as a loop unit for each half of the jaw. However, the longer the loop unit, the weaker the clasp structure will be.

An arrowhead clasp is bent out of 0.7-mm spring hard clasp wire; arrow-forming pliers and arrow clasp bending pliers are recommended for shaping the arrows according to a specific bending sequence.

Clasp forms taken from prosthodontics transfer uncontrolled forces due to linear contact, so they should not be used for orthodontic purposes.

The **C-clasp** (circumferential clasp) is a single-arm clasp made of 0.7-mm spring hard wire shaped into a small eyelet at the clasp tip. It runs from just above the gingival margin in a vestibular direction around the tooth.

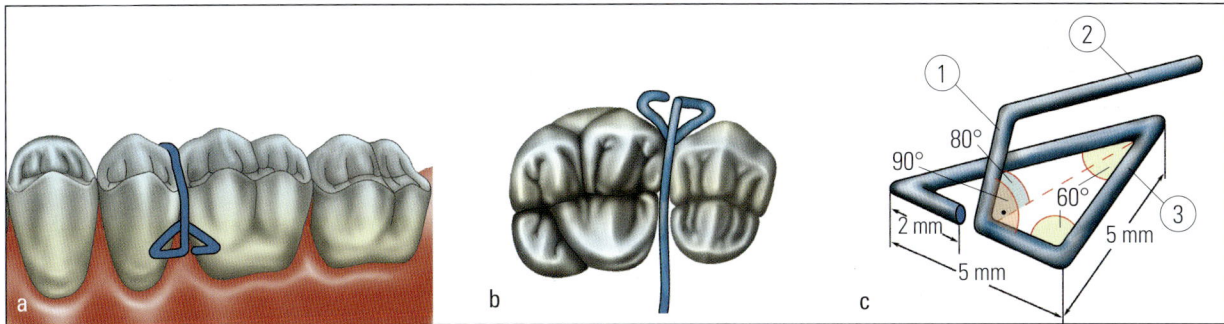

Fig 10-25 *(a to c)* The triangle clasp is a retentive component for the closed dentition. The tip of its triangle is aligned against the approximal area of two adjacent teeth so that punctiform contact arises below the tooth equator and above the gingival papilla. A distinction is made between a vertical piece *(1)* and a transverse piece *(2)*, which is guided over the dentition. The tip of the triangle *(3)* is bent at a 60-degree angle, as are the other angles of the triangle, producing an equilateral triangle with an edge length of about 5 mm. The vertical piece has to be bent at an angle of 80 degrees to the area of the triangle, but there is an angle of 90 degrees to the lateral part.

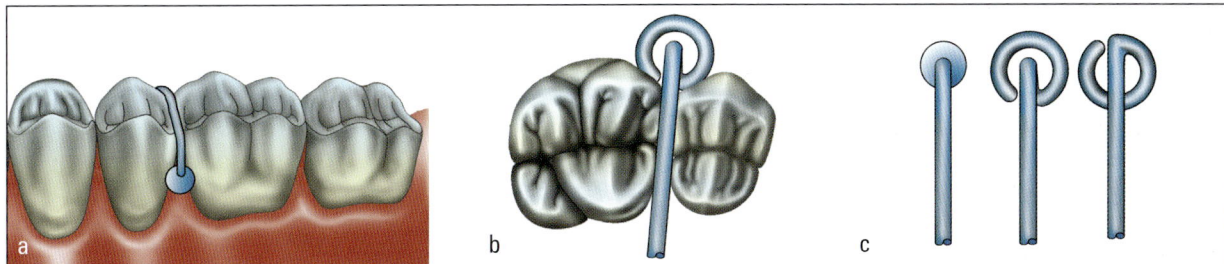

Fig 10-26 *(a to c)* The eyelet clasp is a modification of the triangle clasp. The open part of the eyelet and the eyelet extension contact in the approximal area of two adjacent teeth below the tooth equator but above the interdental papilla. Instead of an eyelet clasp, ball clasps also perform the retentive function. The eyelet of an eyelet clasp may be opened vestibularly so that punctiform contacts to the adjacent teeth arise within the curvature of the eyelet.

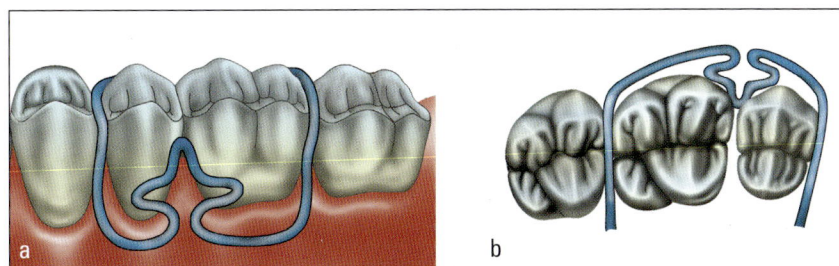

Fig 10-27 *(a and b)* The arrowhead clasp is one of the classic retentive components of orthodontics. Tooth movements can also be initiated with arrowhead clasps in a specific area of application. These clasps come in different wire thicknesses (0.5 to 0.7 mm), like Adams clasps, as semifinished parts. The crosspieces generally lie in the adjacent interdental embrasure, while the arrowhead shows between two teeth. The arrowhead is bent down to the approximal area. The loops of the vestibular sections can be activated so that the pressure of the arrowhead is variable.

Active components of an active plate

The continuous application of force by an active plate can be achieved by three mechanisms: *(1)* orthodontic screws, *(2)* spring components, or *(3)* elastics.

Orthodontic screws actively exert an effect on the teeth and dental arches via the baseplate margin. The screws currently available basically have the same structure and comprise the screw body, the screw spindle, and the guide pins (Fig 10-28). The screws are made from steel alloys resistant to conditions in the mouth; the screw body can be made of plastic or nonferrous metal alloys.

The *screw body* is divided, anchored in the acrylic of the appliance, and transfers the screw forces to the parts of the appliance. The screw spindle and the guide pins are fitted in parallel in the screw body. The screw body, spindle, and guide pins may be placed in a closed housing where the thread and guide tracks are captured in metal. However, screws are also available as skeletal finished parts where the thread and guide tracks lie in the acrylic of the appliance.

The *screw spindle* can have an opposing thread or a simple, one-sided thread. The screw with an opposing thread is used in reciprocal application of force, so that the split baseplate appliance transfers even, equal forces on both sides from the middle of the screw to the dental arches. The screw with a one-sided thread is used in stationary anchorage so that the large segment of the appliance transfers the force on one side to the segment being moved.

The *pitch* of the spindles is not equal in all screw designs but is between 0.64 and 0.90 mm for a rotation of 360 degrees. The overall expansion width, depending on the design and dimensions of a screw, is between 3 and 8 mm. If the spindle has an opposing thread, 360-degree rotation of the spindle achieves twice the pitch (expansion).

The *guide pins* are arranged parallel to the screw spindle in the screw body. As a result, the segments of the appliance are protected against twisting forces, and smooth running of the screw is guaranteed. In addition, it prevents the thread from winding back under stress.

The *mechanical effect* of the screws is based on clamping the appliance plate between the two segments of the dental arch being corrected. The clamping is made possible by the periodontal mobility of the teeth. The expansion of a plate by twisting the screw thread is matched to the width of the periodontal space to prevent any damage. On average, a child's periodontal space is 0.3 mm wide. A quarter turn of a screw with an overall thread pitch of 8.0 mm will narrow the periodontal space by 0.1 mm during reciprocal application of force.

The *pressure effect* achieved by the screw has to be so large that remodeling processes are initiated and remain continuously stimulated with a quarter turn per week. At the same time, the compressive forces must not stop blood circulation. Studies have proved the practicability of screws by comparing the degree of tooth loosening as a result of screws versus springs, showing that the screws caused markedly less tooth loosening.

Screws are classified according to their form and function. A distinction is made on the basis of the thread design and movement options:

- The *expansion screw* with two-sided thread is used for reciprocal application of force but also for selective application of force achieved by skillfully controlling the split between screw segments (Fig 10-29).
- The *sector screw* is used for moving individual sectors of the appliance during stationary application of force as a single-thread screw (Fig 10-30). As a tension (or lag) screw, it is screwed apart when incorporated, and the gap between the sectors is widened in keeping with the width of pull. If the screw is twisted together, the tensile effect enforces correction of the dental arch or single-tooth movement.
- The *telescopic screw* with a thread direction is used for single-tooth movement and made from acrylic or metal (Fig 10-31).
- The *swivel expansion screw* has two threads but no guide pins; instead it has a separate hinge that is fitted dorsally to the plate edge at the appliance gap. When the expansion screw is opened, the dental arch can be expanded in the anterior region, which is why the appliance plate should extend very far dorsally. The hinge may also be replaced by a wire.

Figures 10-32 to 10-36 show other varieties of orthodontic screws.

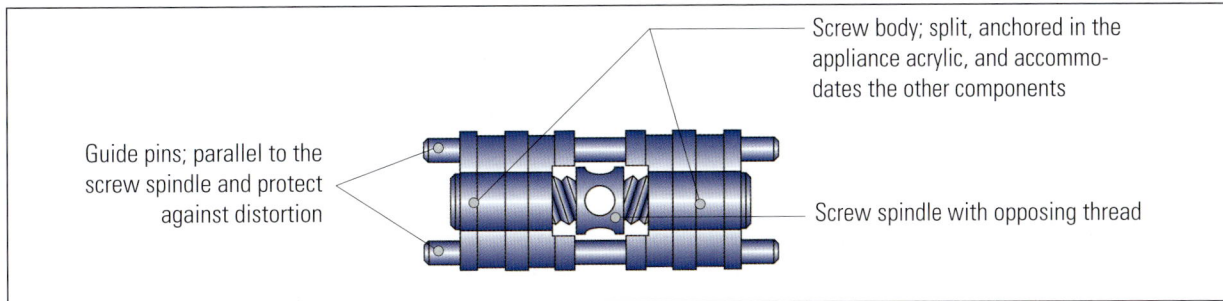

Guide pins; parallel to the screw spindle and protect against distortion

Screw body; split, anchored in the appliance acrylic, and accommodates the other components

Screw spindle with opposing thread

Fig 10-28 The expansion screw is an active component of an active plate; in principle it is broken down into the screw body, the screw spindle, and the guide pins.

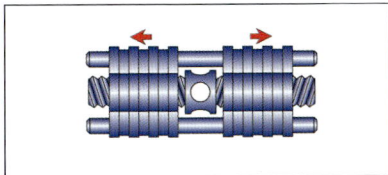

Fig 10-29 The expansion screw with two-sided thread is used for reciprocal as well as selective application of force.

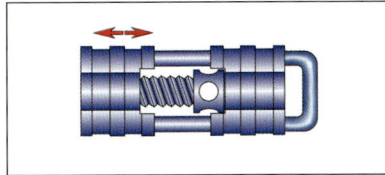

Fig 10-30 The sector screw with one-sided thread aids stationary application of force as a tension and expansion screw.

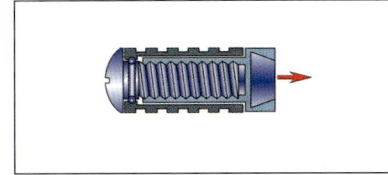

Fig 10-31 Telescopic screw with single thread for stationary application of force as a protrusion screw.

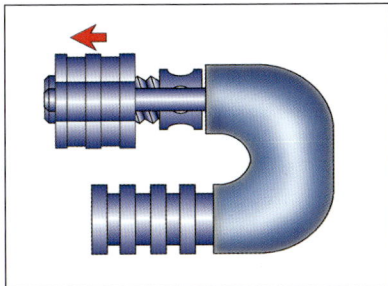

Fig 10-32 The prognathism activator screw is used with a double-plate for the mandible and the maxilla in the case of maxillomandibular anchorage.

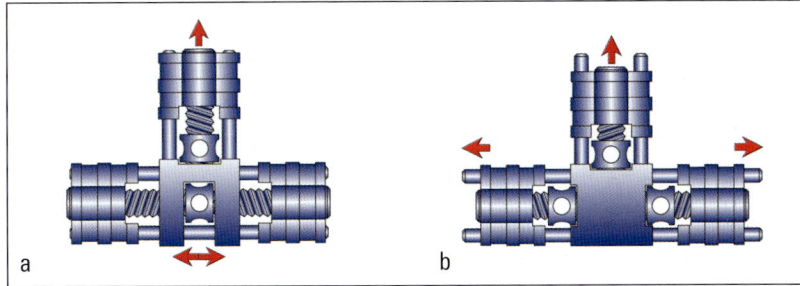

Fig 10-33 (a and b) The multisector screw by Bertoni for selective and reciprocal application of force comprises expansion screws arranged at 90-degree angles to each other. Alternately, protrusion and transverse thrust can be initiated with selective, stationary application of force when one screw segment at a time is adjusted.

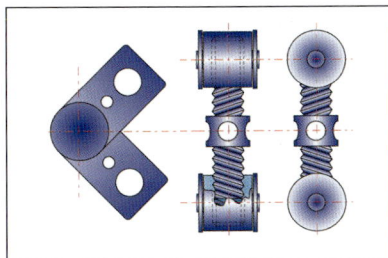

Fig 10-34 Fan expansion screw in two versions: The screw and hinge are separated (swivel expansion screw), and the screw and hinge are located together on one support.

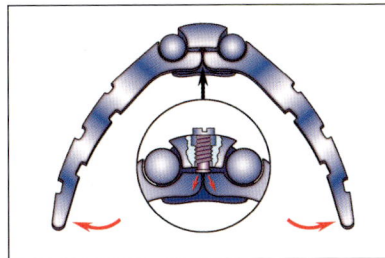

Fig 10-35 The posterior expansion screw is a fan-type expansion screw for distal expansion of the mandibular dental arch. The swivel arms are pushed apart with a screw in the housing block.

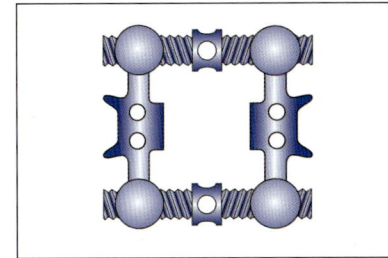

Fig 10-36 The double-fan screw involves two parallel spindles hinged with the screw bodies, each via two cylinders, for anterior, posterior, and transverse expansion.

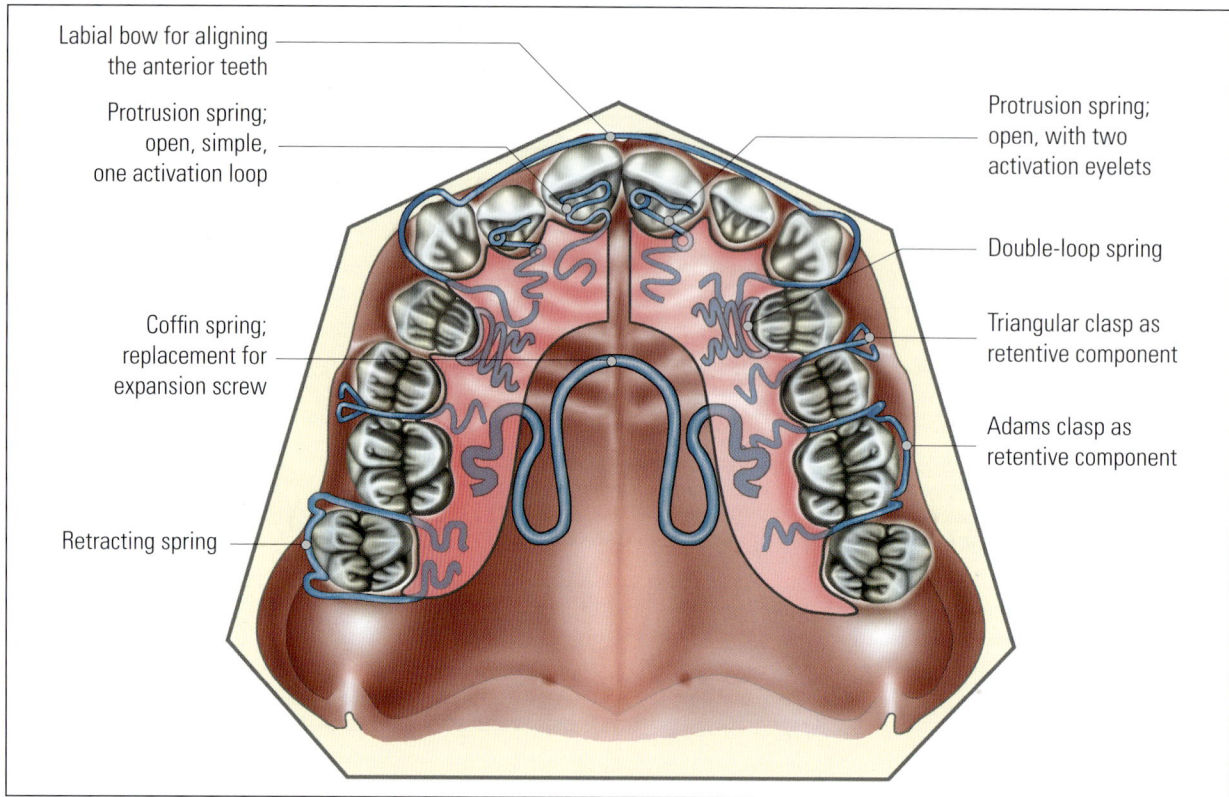

Fig 10-37 A wide variety of active components can be fitted to an active plate. Springs as active components for stationary application of force are highly variable in form and size. The shorter and thicker they are, the stiffer and stronger they are. The longer and thinner, the weaker they are, which means that widely varying forces can be applied.

Labial bow for aligning the anterior teeth

Protrusion spring; open, simple, one activation loop

Coffin spring; replacement for expansion screw

Retracting spring

Protrusion spring; open, with two activation eyelets

Double-loop spring

Triangular clasp as retentive component

Adams clasp as retentive component

Active spring components

Active spring components for tooth movement encircle the tooth in a linear fashion, exert spring pressure, and can be activated (Fig 10-37). The spring components of the active plate help to move sections of the dental arch or individual teeth.

The **mechanical effect** of spring components is different from that of screws. Screws exert a strong initial force that is tailored to the width of the periodontal space and is therefore biologically favorable. Springs are elastic and act with relatively weak but continuous pressure and with a thrust distance that is greater than the periodontal space. To exert effective pressure that will initiate remodeling processes, a specific spring force must be applied by a specific spring deflection. This means, however, that the continuously acting spring forces endanger the periodontal liga-

ment, and hence the appliances can only be worn on an hourly basis.

Furthermore, if the spring forces are applied in a punctiform fashion and lead to tipping of teeth, excessive pressure intensity can easily arise, which stops the blood flow in the periodontal ligament. Spring forces often lie within the third level of biologic intensity and can result in damage.

The **spring effect**, depending on function, is punctiform for tooth rotation or linear throughout the tooth width for protrusion or extrusion. The springs are generally covered in acrylic but exposed in the effective area on the tooth.

Short, thick springs are hard; long, thin springs are soft. Springs with punctiform contact will tip or rotate the tooth; spring loops with linear or flat contact may in some circumstances move the tooth in multipoint application of force.

When technicians are choosing or designing their own spring shapes, they should check what tooth movement is to be achieved by spring pressure. The position and form of the force being applied and the usable abutments must be borne in mind, as well as an unimpeded movement path for the tooth. It is also important to ensure that the retentive components of the appliance can be used for tooth movements as passive abutments or bodily clasps.

The *active components* of an active plate can be varied to match the task in hand and permit numerous movement possibilities. Depending on function, there are three *types of spring components*:

1. Springs as screw replacements
2. Springs for stationary application of force
3. Labial bows

Spring components as screw replacements are usually expansion springs. However, they may also be used as tension springs. In an omega shape, these are known as *Coffin springs* because they were being used as early as 1882 by S. H. Coffin. These Coffin springs take up less space than screws and allow variable movements of the appliance segments in different directions; ie, they can be used for any case that can be treated with screws. Their disadvantage is that patients cannot carry out activation themselves and the magnitude of force as a function of activation cannot be accurately measured. Continuous pressure in the third level of biologic intensity arises, which leads to damage.

A *Coffin spring* is bent out of 1.0- to 1.2-mm spring hard steel wire to form an 8- to 16-mm omega loop (Fig 10-38). It lies centrally in the maxilla and joins two sagittally sawn plate halves of an orthodontic monobloc or activator. Two small Coffin springs with 8-mm loop size opened up toward one another can be placed in a simple expansion plate to achieve torsional stiffness.

A Coffin spring can be activated at three places and offers the possibility of anterior, posterior, or total jaw widening. The larger the Coffin spring, the weaker the spring effect will be; the smaller the loop (or when two springs are mounted), the stronger the spring effect will be. The spring force cannot be measured as accurately as the expansion force of a screw.

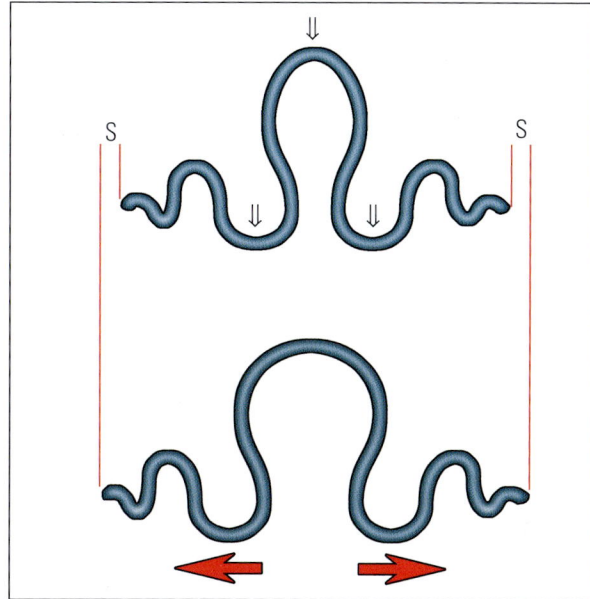

Fig 10-38 Springs can also be used as retentive components instead of screws. A Coffin spring made of 1.0-mm wire can achieve the same plate expansion as is possible with a screw. The omega-shaped loop is between 8 and 16 mm in size and can be activated at three points by the amount indicated by S.

A *Coffin plate* is an expansion plate whose edges lie palatally against the anterior and posterior teeth. It is sawn through in the middle, and the halves are pushed apart by a strong Coffin spring whose ends are fixed in the acrylic. By activation of the spring, the pressure can be evenly transferred to the alveolar processes or, if necessary, anteriorly increased.

Spring components for stationary force application

These active spring components act on individual teeth or groups of teeth. The spring forms can vary considerably in shape and size; differences can arise in terms of the effect and magnitude of force.

An *intermediate or interdental spring* for lateral, mesial, or distal tooth movements in the dental arch is bent out of spring hard round wire: 0.5 mm for anterior teeth, and up to 0.6 mm for canines and premolars. This kind of spring is basally let into the baseplate and can be activated;

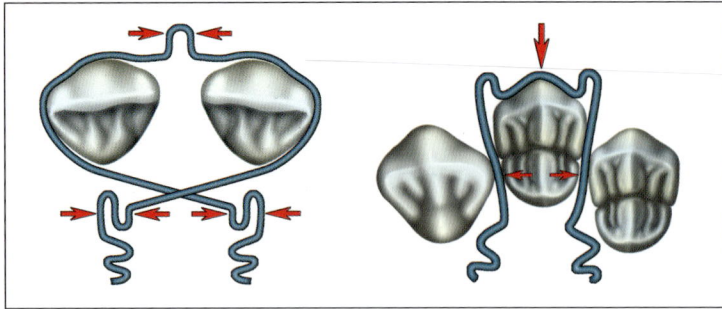

Fig 10-39 Retracting springs are used to pull the teeth back into the dental arch. Activation takes place at the vestibularly placed loops. With a closed outer spring, two teeth can be encircled so that they can be pushed together within the dental arch (eg, to close a diastema).

it is covered toward the tongue. It runs over the approximal surface in a vestibular direction; the springy part has an activation eyelet (loop or double loop). The end of the spring is bent round to form a loop and, coming from approximally, lies to a variable extent on the vestibular surface of the tooth being moved. When placed between two teeth in a closed form, it can be used to widen a gap, or it can be used with a U-shaped loop for readjusting or with crossed retentions for closing a diastema.

A *finger spring* is an interdentally acting intermediate spring for tooth movements in the sagittal and transverse directions that is fabricated from 0.6-mm spring hard wire. It has interdental/approximal contact with the tooth being moved and is referred to as an *interdental, intermediate, mesial,* or *distal spring*.

A *retracting spring* is an intermediate spring that fits closely to the tooth on the vestibular side and helps align individual teeth (Fig 10-39). The springy part runs in a U or V shape, is fitted with an activating eyelet (loop), and can be anchored in the body of the appliance or soldered to the labial bow.

Protrusion springs arising from an appliance plate are the most commonly used springs in orthodontics. They are open or closed, single-tail or double-tail spring loops that can be crossed over each other several times. The loops of 0.4- and 0.7-mm spring hard wire are used for single-tooth movement, tooth rotations, and movement of groups of teeth. *Frame loop, frame spring, paddle spring,* or *loop spring* are possible synonyms. The protrusion spring is let into the baseplate so that a basal guide fan is formed in the acrylic base in which the spring is free moving and can be acti-

vated. Activation is achieved as the loops are bent open at the bending points or the specially bent activation eyelets.

An *open protrusion spring*, in the form of a compressed S, has at least three activation loops running parallel to each other at a distance of 1 to 2 mm (Figs 10-40 and 10-41). The loop width corresponds to the mesiodistal width of the tooth being moved.

A *closed protrusion spring* is fabricated from 0.4- to 0.6-mm spring hard wire; both ends of the wire are firmly anchored in the acrylic base, making this spring less elastic (Fig 10-42). It can have one or two activation loops and run over all the anterior teeth and canines to act as a support to a labial bow.

Spring loops (guide loops) are classified as closed protrusion springs and can contact individual teeth, run over several teeth, or run over the whole of the anterior region (Fig 10-43). However, the position of force application in the coronal area is significant for tooth movement. Depending on the degree of tooth movement, it must be possible to activate the spring evenly throughout the movement path.

A *paddle spring* is a closed protrusion spring for single-tooth movement in which both ends of the wire are anchored in the acrylic base (Fig 10-44). It can be used for maxillary anterior teeth (but it tends to cause tipping) or for buccal movement of posterior teeth.

Elastics are mostly fitted between maxillary and mandibular appliance plates to correct a displacement of occlusal position. To treat a retrusive occlusion, a hook is mounted on the maxillary plate level with the canines and on the mandibular plate at the last molar. As a result,

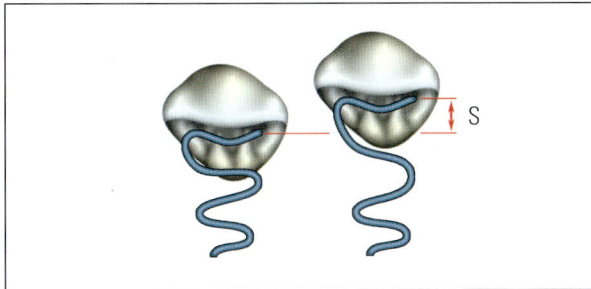

Fig 10-40 The simple open protrusion spring with an activation loop is relatively stiff and has only limited thrust distance (S).

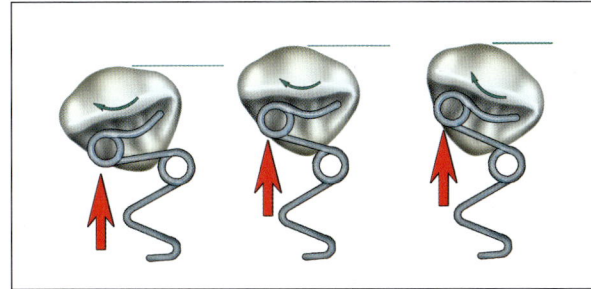

Fig 10-41 The open protrusion spring with two activation eyelets is relatively soft and allows differentiated direction of thrust.

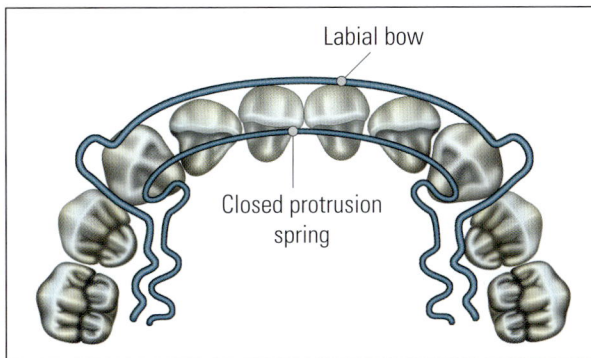

Fig 10-42 The closed protrusion spring made of 0.4- to 0.6-mm wire runs lingually over the incisors and canines and acts as the support for the labial bow; it can have one or two activation loops.

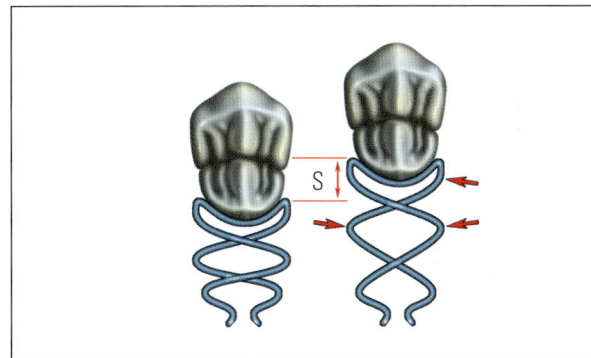

Fig 10-43 The spring loop (loop spring) with two activation arches allows gentle application of force and has wide freedom of movement (S). It should be classified as a closed protrusion spring and allows directed, controllable regulating thrust.

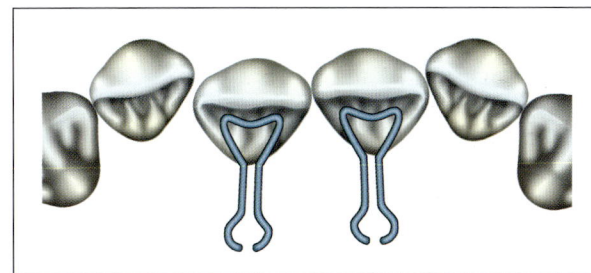

Fig 10-44 The paddle spring is a loop spring made of 0.4- to 0.6-mm spring hard wire for protrusion of anterior teeth; both ends of the wire lie in the appliance, and the paddle-shaped loop lies on the lingual surface of the anterior tooth.

the mandible is pulled forward. If prognathism is to be corrected, the hook arrangement in the maxilla and mandible is transposed to pull the mandible backward. The retentive components of the active plate have to be particularly numerous and secure when using elastics for correcting occlusal displacement. Elastics can also be used for rotation of twisted teeth. A circular wire or metal band is placed around a severely twisted tooth, to which a hook is fitted that does not impede rotation of the tooth. An elastic from this hook to the plate exerts a pull to rotate the tooth.

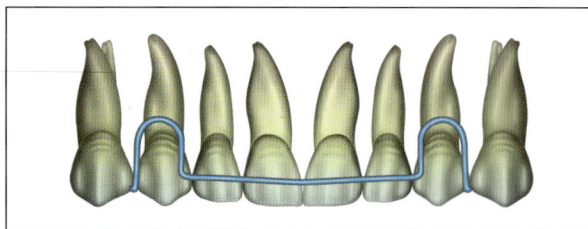

Fig 10-45 The labial bow is one of the activatable spring components. However, it can also take on a retentive function. It is used in both the maxilla and the mandible. The horizontal part of the labial bow runs along the incisal third of the incisors.

Labial bow

The labial bow is one of the most important activatable spring components of orthodontic appliances and is used in both the maxilla and the mandible (Fig 10-45). However, it can also take on a retentive function.

The ***labial bow*** is used as an active spring component for aligning the anterior teeth to create a harmonious dental arch or as a retentive component in distal movement of posterior teeth. As an active component, it can be placed against the incisors under tension for retrusion of the anterior teeth. It is also placed under tension when individual teeth are to be rotated, supplemented either by a protrusion spring to form an eccentric couple or the milled plate edge for punctiform placement. The effect of the labial bow under tension can be varied by positioning the plate edge and the bow at different heights in relation to the tooth so that this two-point application of force enforces eccentric tipping of the teeth. The labial bow can also lie against the anterior teeth without tension when the whole anterior section is moved by the split plate and when the position in relation to the plate edge is to remain fixed. When the anterior teeth protrude, the labial bow can also stick out to keep the lip away from the teeth and hence minimize lip pressure.

The following paragraphs describe the ***components*** of a labial bow.

The ***horizontal part*** is harmoniously curved to match the ideal dental arch form and at the incisors runs along the incisal third from the mesial third of one canine to the mesial third of the contralateral canine (Fig 10-46). To achieve a harmonious curvature, this section is bent with the fingers and not with pliers.

The horizontal part of the bow can be expanded by soldered springs for single-tooth movement (eg, by mesial and distal springs to close spaces between teeth). The labial bow may also be covered with plastic—as a passive retentive component—to fix the position of all the anterior teeth or individual incisors. This covering can also be applied at a later stage.

U-loops continue the harmonious curvature of the horizontal part. The U-loops are formed by bending the labial bow at the mesial third of the canines at right angles in a cervical direction. The loops protrude about 2 to 3 mm above the cervical margin. The loop width is roughly equivalent to two-thirds of the canine width because the distal limb of the loop must be bent approximately between the canine and the first premolar into the transverse part (Fig 10-47). The length of the U-loops is roughly equivalent to canine crown length. The loop serves to activate the labial bow and can help to correct the position of the canine.

A ***retraction loop*** is a loop in the distal limb of the U-loop that is guided over the labial surface of the canine at its equator (Figs 10-48 to 10-51). Thus, the U-loop can be exploited for movement of the canine by being shaped to form a loop guard.

A ***loop guard*** can also be shaped by placing the U-loop in a wavelike fashion over the labial surface. The whole labial bow can be guided wavelike over all the anterior teeth, where it acts as a lip bumper (see Fig 10-52).

The ***transverse part*** crosses the row of teeth and is bent into the appliance acrylic as a retentive component. The labial bow has the following features:

- The labial bow curvature must have a harmonious dental arch form.
- It runs along the incisal third of the incisors.
- The U-loops must bend at right angles at the mesial third of the canines.
- The limbs of the U-loop must run parallel and have the right height and width.

As an ***active anterior spring*** for retrusion of incisors, the labial bow is guided between the lateral incisor and the canines and is shaped from 0.6-mm wire. In this popular version, the movement of the labial bow takes place in harmonious shaping over the canine; a retraction loop is then

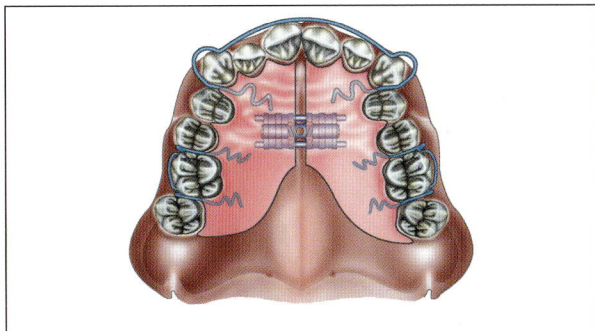

Fig 10-46 The curvature of the labial bow matches a harmonious dental arch curvature. The U-loops also continue the harmonious curvature over the canines.

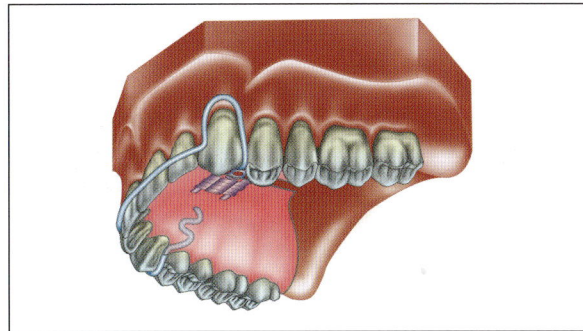

Fig 10-47 The U-loop of the labial bow starts approximally between the canine and the first premolar, runs 2 to 3 mm contact-free over the cervical margin of the canine, and has a width about two-thirds of the canine width.

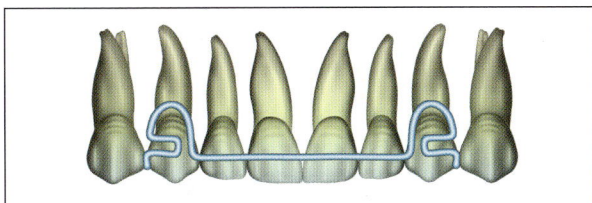

Fig 10-48 The distal limb of the U-loop can be bent into a retraction loop for the canine. The loop can be activated to guide the canine into the dental arch.

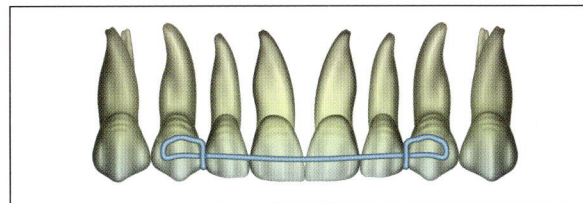

Fig 10-49 The retraction loop can also be placed mesially over the canine when the labial bow is guided interdentally between the lateral incisor and the canine from the baseplate.

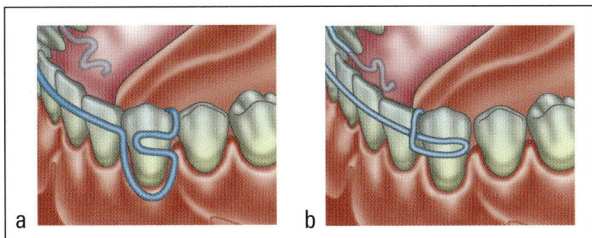

Fig 10-50 (a and b) Retraction loops for the mandible are shaped the same way as in the maxilla.

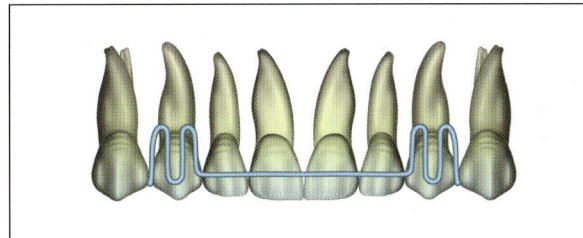

Fig 10-51 An activatable retraction loop is shaped like a double U. This can be used to realign a canine tipped out of the dental arch.

Fig 10-52 The labial bow can be guided over the anterior teeth of both jaws as a maxillomandibular bow. This lip bumper is intended to shield the anterior teeth from the lips.

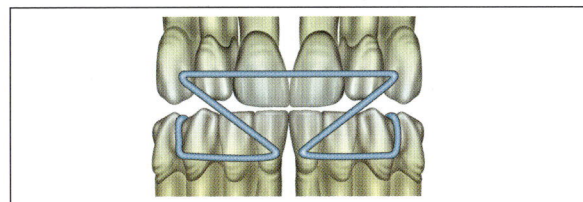

guided as far as the approximal area of the lateral incisor and canine, then the wire crosses over the transverse part. This produces an activatable loop guard for canine as well as incisor movement.

As a **maxillomandibular bow**, the labial bow made of 1.2-mm spring hard wire can be bent for maxillomandibular function (Fig 10-52). The wire formed of enlarged U-loops is guided from the maxilla to the mandibular anterior teeth.

Active plate designs

An active plate is also known as a **Schwarz plate** because A. M. Schwarz developed the plates into a system device, mainly used as retentive appliances. He transferred the typical retentive components to a simple expansion plate, including the arrowhead clasp he designed, and he fitted numerous active spring components for correcting defects of tooth position and the dental arch. Development of the two-thread expansion and tension screws furthered the design of the active plate.

The **basic form of active appliances** is the sagittally split plate, which is initially fitted with two simple Coffin springs and allows selective expansion of the anterior or posterior dental arch area. The highly variable design of the active plate—divided into several segments selectively movable against each other—greatly extends the range of uses so that nearly 90% of all anomalies of tooth position and dental arch can be corrected.

The effect of the appliances can be adapted very precisely to the particular case being treated by means of the **direction of cut** and variable division of segments, the use of several different screws, and omissions at the plate edge.

Division of the active plate into movable appliance segments follows three basic cut directions: *(1)* the sagittal split, *(2)* the transverse split, and *(3)* the Y-split, as well as combinations of these. Another possibility is a selective split for single-tooth movement, which leads to stationary application of forces.

Each of the tooth movements and dental arch corrections indicated by the different splits is possible in the opposite direction if opened screws are used with broadly worked division cuts. The screws are twisted together for orthodontic tooth movements. Once again, given movement thrusts on one side, the larger section of the dental arch is used as retention for stationary application of force.

For **anchorage** of the movable plate segments, the previously described retentive components and support spikes are fitted, while active spring components are attached for selective single-tooth movement. It is important to ensure that the appliances do not have too many components. It is always safer to carry out one correction at a time, using successive appliances for further correction.

The **sagittal split** is usually symmetric in the middle of the plate. The split is widened by means of the expansion screw, leading to bilateral expansion of the dental arch (Figs 10-53 to 10-55). As a rule, reciprocal application of force occurs. If the plate edge avoids a few teeth, these teeth will be excluded from the expansion. It is therefore possible to exclude all the anterior teeth from the expansion with a sagittally split plate. In fact, retrusion of the anterior teeth can be performed with a close-fitting labial bow at the same time as expansion of the posterior teeth because the bow is activated more and more during expansion of the plate.

The **transverse split** is made level with the canines and allows protrusive movement of the anterior teeth. At the same time, labially displaced canines can be pulled into the dental arch with retrusion springs. If the posterior plate segment is fixed to the posterior teeth, stationary forces are usually applied with a transverse split because the relatively immobile posterior teeth are only subliminally loaded in a labial direction during expansion of the dental arch (Fig 10-56).

The transverse split can also be used for selective expansion of sections of a dental arch or single-tooth movements. In the case of unilateral canine crowding with mesially migrated posterior teeth, the plate is divided on one side at the level of the canine and fitted with an expansion screw. By means of the screw force, the posterior teeth are moved distally and the canine is moved into the dental arch with a retraction loop from the labial bow. Even if individual teeth at the end of the dental arch have to be moved distally or mesially, a transverse split in the plate can be employed. Combined tension and expansion screws enable selective tooth movement via two transverse splits.

A **combination** of sagittal and transverse splits can be useful for unilateral dental arch expansion: An expansion screw is fitted in the sagittal split; directly in front of the screw, the split kinks transversally toward the dental arch that is to be expanded. The opposing dental arch and the anterior teeth offer stationary anchorage.

The **Y-split** is a practical combination of a sagittal and a transverse split, making it possible to apply combined (reciprocal and stationary) forces to three segments of an appliance (Figs 10-57 to 10-59). The typical Y-split has the sagittal cut run-

Fig 10-53 The effect of an expansion screw in an active plate with a sagittal split is reciprocal; ie, where the split is symmetric, the plate edges exert the same force on the dental arches. The plate edges press against the teeth but also against the alveolar ridges and palatal parts; these tissue areas are included in the expansion. The plate edges are shaped to omit any teeth that are to be excluded from the expansion.

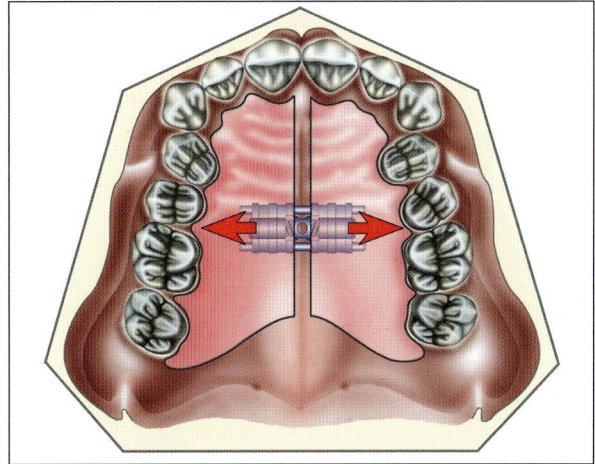

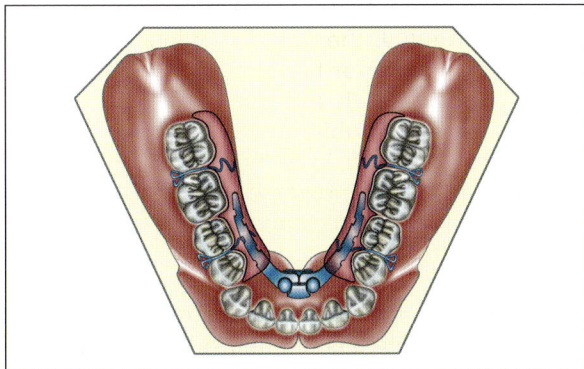

Fig 10-54 The posterior expansion screw is used in the mandible for distal expansion of the dental arch. The screw comprises a housing block, a split screw, the right and left pivot bearings, and the right and left swivel arms. The swivel arms can be swung apart via the split screw.

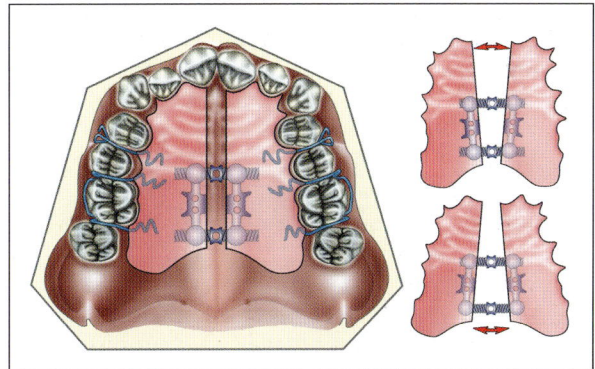

Fig 10-55 The double-fan screw comprises parallel spindles that are articulated with the screw bodies. This screw allows varying degrees of anterior, posterior, and transverse dental arch expansion.

Fig 10-56 Rather stationary force application is produced with an active plate that has a transverse split. Here the anterior dental arch is expanded, the plate body being supported against the posterior teeth.

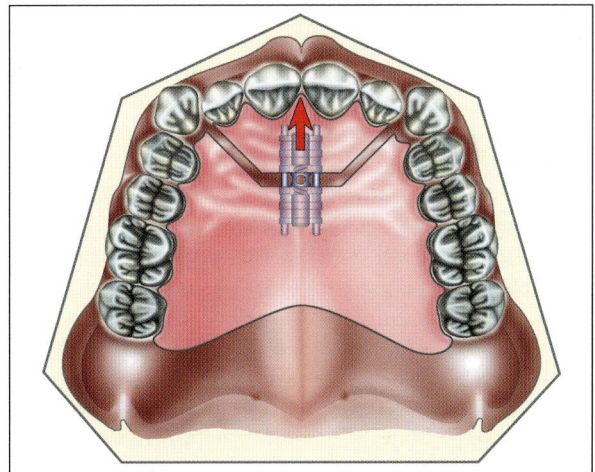

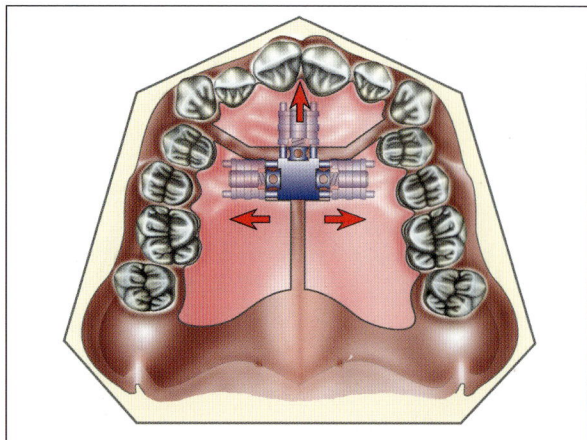

Fig 10-57 The Y-split of an active plate allows selective application of forces, depending on which screw spindle is activated. Thus, stationary force application can be produced by the posterior teeth for the anterior region, or the right segment of posterior teeth is expanded by means of the stationary anchorage at the front and on the left side.

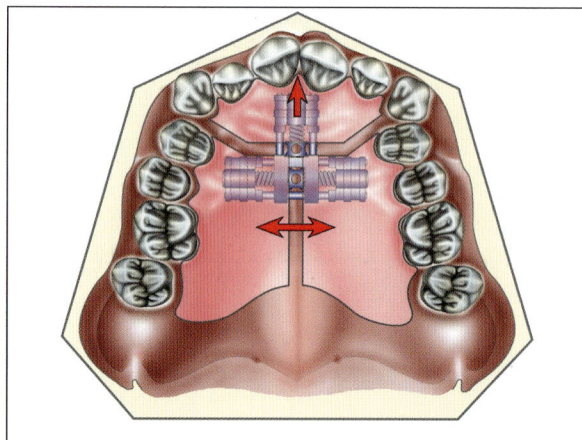

Fig 10-58 With this Y-split, stationary application of force can only be exerted on the anterior teeth, while only reciprocal force application for dental arch expansion can take place between the posterior segments of teeth.

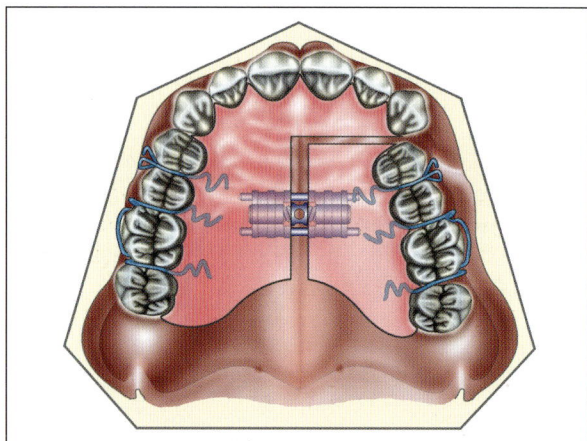

Fig 10-59 The combination of a sagittal split and a transverse split can be useful for one-sided dental arch expansion. An expansion screw is fitted in the sagittal split; directly in front of the screw, the split bends transversally as far as the dental arch that is to be expanded. The opposing dental arch segment and the anterior region offer stationary anchorage.

ning from the dorsal up to the middle of the plate, where it splits into two angled transverse cuts to the approximal areas between the lateral incisors and canines. Two expansion screws in the angled transverse cuts move the three segments against each other: If two expansion screws are opened to the same amount simultaneously, the anterior teeth move markedly in a labial direction and the posterior teeth move less markedly in the vestibular direction; the dental arch is slightly expanded.

Bilateral crowding can be corrected by moving the anterior region forward. Stationary applica-

tion of force can be achieved by selectively opening one screw, then the other; in the process, the posterior teeth are moved vestibularly as well as distally and on the side where the screw has been opened.

Selective single-tooth movement can be performed with a Y-split incorporating a sagittal cut that runs far forward and a transverse cut placed perpendicular to that. This will prevent expansion of the posterior region, while the posterior teeth move distally and labial anterior movement remains weakened.

Fig 10-60 Maxillomandibular anchorage with a double-plate for protrusion can be activated in a variety of ways: *(a)* A screw with a simple thread can be fitted between the maxillary and the mandibular plates. Here the maxillary incisor is to be pushed into the normal occlusal position. To achieve this, a labial bow loop is attached that is meant to shield the tooth from the upper lip. *(b)* In the same orthodontic case, the relative movement of the double-plate can be enforced via an inclined plane and an activatable loop spring.

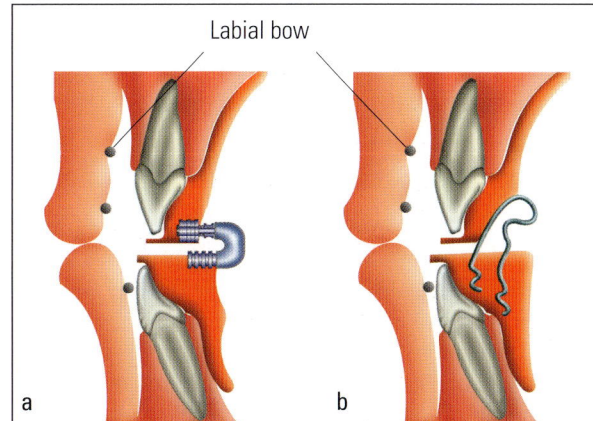

If even less ***movement of anterior teeth*** is planned, the Y-split is modified to block anchorage of the middle plate segment: Two sagittal cuts are made while a wide middle segment remains for the anterior teeth. The transverse cuts may run obliquely or vertically to the sagittal cut and hold the expansion screws. If one expansion screw then the other is moved alternately, ***stationary force application*** is possible with the anterior region remaining stationary as the posterior teeth are moved alternately distally and outward. A Y-split with a multisector screw for transverse and sagittal thrusts permits protrusive movement of the anterior teeth separate from expansion of the posterior region. Selective distal thrust of a posterior segment of teeth alternated with the opposite side can also be achieved with a multisector screw.

Double-plates

Active plates for treating positional anomalies can be fabricated in the maxilla and mandible and worn simultaneously to achieve the treatment objective. The dentitions are separated by occlusal guards so that the retentive components and active springs are not inadvertently activated and do not interlock or buckle during occluding. This offers the opportunity to join two appliances together for correcting an occlusal discrepancy. Elastics can be fitted to remedy a prognathic or retrognathic mandible. One appliance is firmly fixed in the maxilla, based on the principle of maxillomandibular anchorage, to correct the oc-

clusal discrepancy in the opposing jaw by traction (Fig 10-60).

Guide planes for protrusive or retrusive movement are placed horizontally when the appliances are moved against each other with a screw. One of the two plates has no fixed retentive components so that the mouth can be opened when the appliance is being worn.

Guide planes can be attached to the anterior region or placed in the posterior region. Anteriorly placed, they are held angled downward and backward for protrusive movement; if retrusive movement is to be achieved, they are worked so that they slope upward and forward. With the mouth closed, the appliances slide into the desired position as if on an inclined plane. If a spring loop is now incorporated into an appliance within the guide plane, it can be bent out in order to be activated, and the malposition is gradually guided back to a state of equilibrium. When correcting an occlusal anomaly, correction of the dental arch form is necessary if the opposing occlusion is not harmonious in the corrected position because the dental arch is too narrow or too wide for the new position. This is when a double-plate comprising active appliances proves very beneficial, because adjustment of the dental arch can be achieved during occlusal correction.

For practical purposes, occlusal records of the desired position are taken (forced occlusions); if that is not possible, the desired position is established by hand. The models are mounted in a fixator in the appropriate position.

Crozat Appliance

The appliances originally developed by George B. Crozat are a special form of orthodontic treatment appliance. The basic device, comprising lingually or palatally attached brackets made of heat-treatable 1.3-mm steel wire, can be extended with springs and hooks for elastics. The *Crozat appliance* controls growth forces during natural development of individual supportive tissues that are in the transitional stage during child facial development. The normal existing forces are directed into the "correct" path by gentle mechanical effects with a Crozat appliance; external forces applied are below-threshold stimuli and hence act through continuity.

The *treatment* is performed with extended appliances over prolonged periods of time and can last until the end of normal dentition growth. Treatment breaks are observed to allow growth reactions and analyze the state of the dentition for the next treatment phase. Alveolar bone growth is stimulated so that occlusal leveling can be performed and deep bites can be remedied. An esthetically and functionally satisfactory outcome is achieved, and neither tissue damage nor tooth loosening results from bone and root resorption.

The *advantages of a Crozat appliance* include the following:

• Moderate forces cause no tissue damage.
• Its slender frame facilitates self-cleaning.
• The appliance is esthetically acceptable.
• It has good wearing characteristics due to its slender frame.
• It causes virtually no speech restriction.
• It is easy to fabricate and handle.

The *disadvantages of a Crozat appliance* include the following:

• Late cases cannot be treated successfully.
• It requires a very long treatment period.
• The appliance is very susceptible to distortion.
• The patient's cooperation is required over long periods of time.

The *practicability of Crozat appliances* lies mainly in the support of sagittal and transverse den-

tal arch development. Single-tooth movement in a lingual or vestibular, mesial or distal direction as well as correction of tipping and rotation are possible with these appliances. It is even possible to eliminate occlusal discrepancies by means of maxillomandibular bracing with elastics.

Construction

Throughout the treatment period, the patient is always able to wear the same appliance because the appliance is a basic device that is extended or reduced in response to treatment progress. Furthermore, the appliance can be adapted to the enlarged, grown state of the dentition on a later model as it is bent to fit the new situation. Subsequent heat treatment removes stresses and strain hardening of the material so that the appliance regains adequate mechanical properties.

The basic appliance comprises the body wire and the retentive components in the posterior region; from there in a lingual direction lie two activatable wire arms directed mesially and in the maxilla two short bars directed buccally to the retentive components. These lingually and buccally placed extensions are attachment points for extending the appliance with bars, springs, and hooks. The lingual extensions can be activated and used for tooth movement. The individual components must be bent separately, then soldered together.

The *body wire* is formed by the transverse palatal bar in the maxilla (Fig 10-61) and by the lingual bar in the mandible (Fig 10-62). The body wire is shaped from 1.3-mm wire and runs from one retentive component (usually at the first molar) to the other half of the jaw. The wire must not touch the mucosa. The body wire is shaped to follow the normal course of a sublingual bar, which creates a 4-mm gap from the cervical margins without interfering with the floor of the mouth. It is soldered to the distolingual portions of the retentive components and can be activated for dental arch expansion by being bent open in the anterior curvature area. In the maxilla, the body wire runs transversally over the palatal vault and is fitted with an omega-shaped middle loop for activation. The middle loop is shaped to be large or small, depending on the degree of arch expansion. If the loop is bent open, spring force for lateral arch ex-

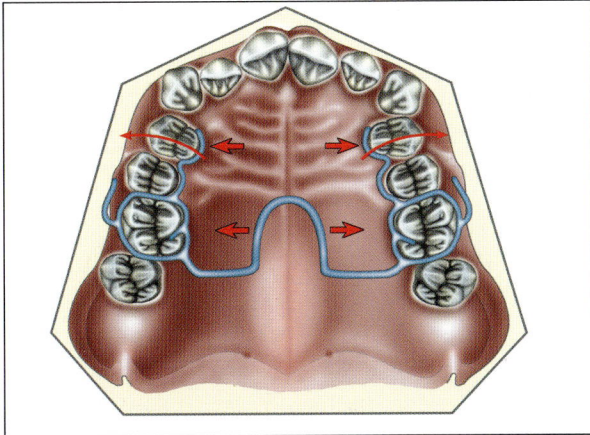

Fig 10-61 Crozat appliances for the maxilla are comprised of a body wire, an omega-shaped transverse bar that is soldered onto the retentive components. These retentive components are closed Jackson clasps around the first molars, from which the extension wires run lingually and buccally. The lingual arms contact both premolars, the buccal extension arm serving as the soldering point for additional elements.

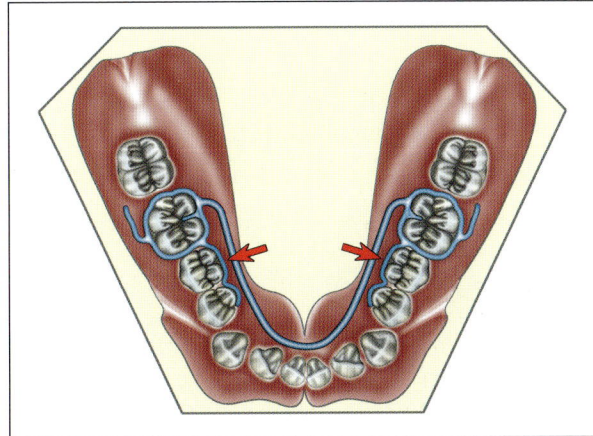

Fig 10-62 In the mandible, the body wire comprises the sublingual bar, which is also soldered to the Jackson clasps. The extension wires are again attached here. The lingual arms, as in the maxilla, bring about regulating thrust for the premolars, while the body wire is used for arch expansion.

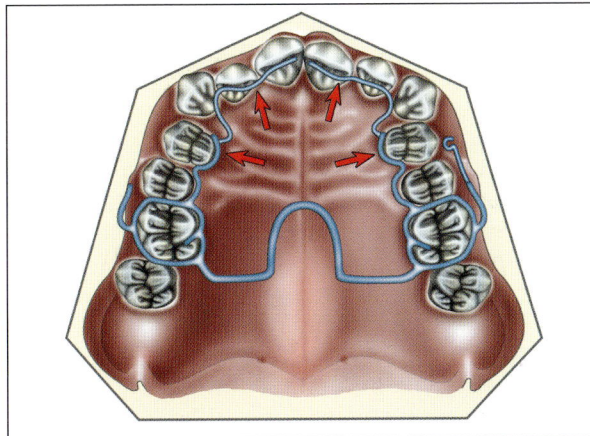

Fig 10-63 As auxiliary elements for the maxillary appliance, auxiliary spring arches can be attached lingually for moving the incisors. Buccal hooks can be soldered on and elastics fitted into these hooks for maxillomandibular anchorage.

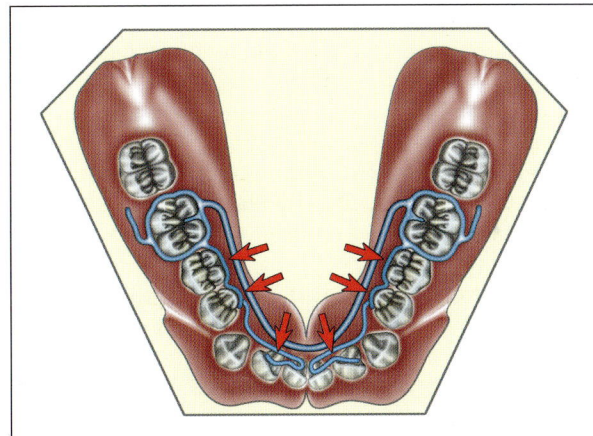

Fig 10-64 Lingual springs can also be attached in the mandible for adjusting the incisors. Activation loops for differentiated force application are fitted. The buccal extensions are bent distally to receive elastics from the maxillary appliance.

pansion arises. The maxillary wire also does not lie against the mucosa and is soldered distolingually with the retentive components.

Springs can be attached to the Crozat appliance to move the incisors (Figs 10-63 and 10-64).

The ***retentive components*** of the Crozat appliance are the ***Jackson clasps*** on the first molars (see Fig 10-61). This clasp is a closed wire loop made of 0.8-mm material that fits closely to the tooth on all sides (Fig 10-65). The Jackson clasp encircles the tooth bodily without itself having a clamping effect. Instead, four vertical clasp parts roughly parallel to each other lie in the mesial and distal interdental spaces and provide excellent control of the clasp. The clasp parts running vestibularly and lingually fit closely to the tooth hori-

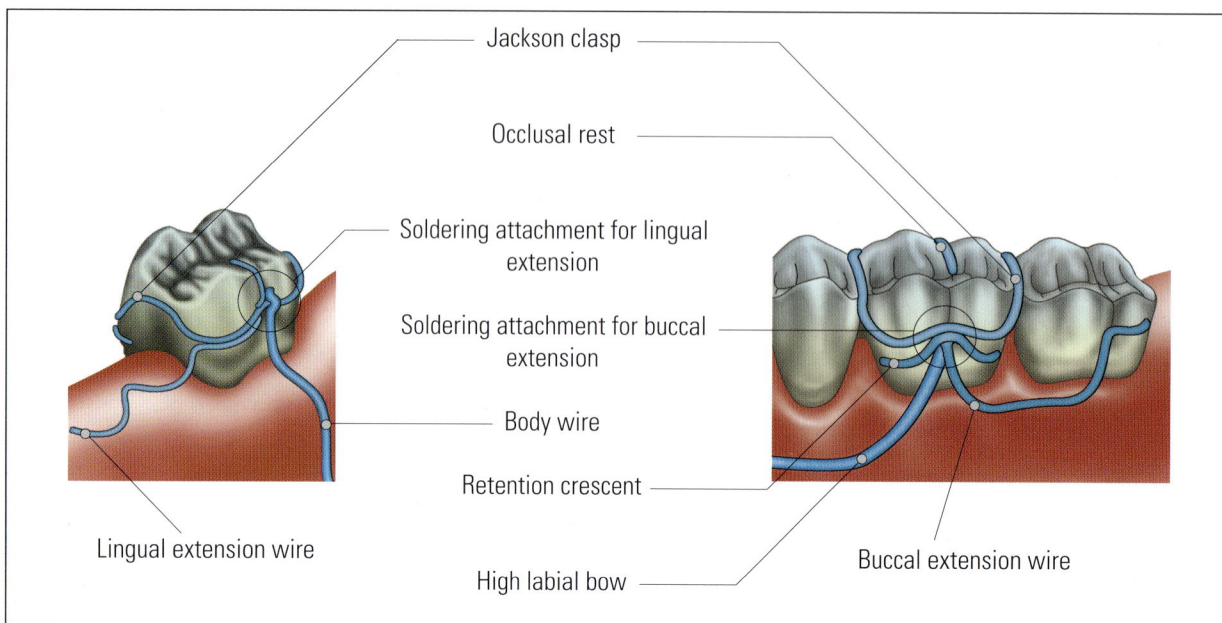

Fig 10-65 The Jackson clasp is a closed ring-shaped clasp. It is guided over the interdental embrasures and lies buccally and lingually at the tooth equator; it does not engage undercut areas, which is why a separate retention crescent is soldered on buccally. The soldering points for the individual components of the Crozat appliance are located on the retentive component. The individual parts are first bent, then fixed in position, then soldered at the specified points.

zontally. In the approximal area, the transverse parts of the clasp running from the lingual in a vestibular direction are fitted to the tooth without rest contact.

The functional supports of the clasp are the vertical wires at the four corners of the molars, which are known as *uprights* and fit as firmly as possible in the interdental spaces. The clasp has an occlusal rest to prevent it from slipping off in a cervical direction. This rest runs from the lingual in the central groove between the lingual cusps occlusally and is bent out of 1.0-mm wire profile and soldered.

The clasp effect of the Jackson clasp is produced with an additional crescent archwire. This crescent runs below the buccal part of the clasp and projects beyond the vertical part deep into the interdental spaces. The archwires are soldered to the buccal part in the middle.

Extension wires

The buccal and lingual extension wires are part of the basic Crozat appliance. Other additional el-

ements can be soldered to these wires without affecting the first solder. The lingual extension wires (lingual arms) take on guidance and corrective functions.

The lingual arms are made of 1.0-mm wire and run from the mesiolingual part of the clasp forward over the two premolars. They can lie directly against the premolar contours or only have punctiform contact with a tooth. A precisely fitted lingual arm takes on guidance functions, ensures positional stability, and may support lateral dental arch movements when the body wire is activated.

The buccal extension wires made from 1.3-mm round wire profile are mostly fitted in the maxilla and are soldered to the Jackson clasp. They serve as the soldering attachment for additional components and form right-angled short arches to the Jackson clasp without gingival contact.

The individual components are bent separately: First the Jackson clasp is bent with the rest and the crescent; then the body wire is bent, followed by the lingual and buccal extensions. These parts are fixed in the correct position on a second

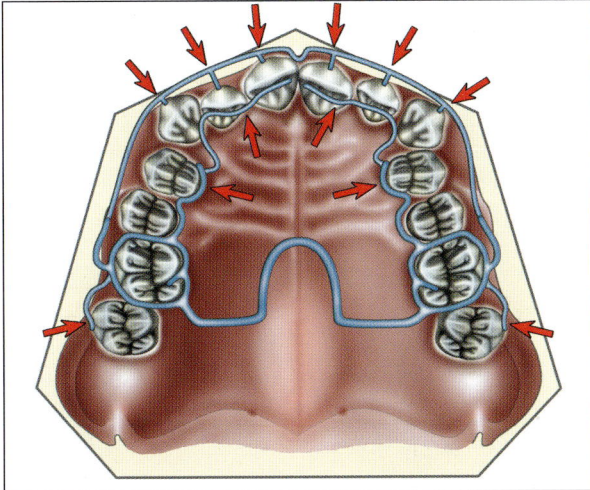

Fig 10-66 The Crozat appliance can be extended with a high labial bow. Vertical pins for adjusting the incisors come off this labial bow, which runs invisibly in the vestibular fornix. Highly differentiated adjustment is possible if lingual spring arches and labial bows are attached at the same time.

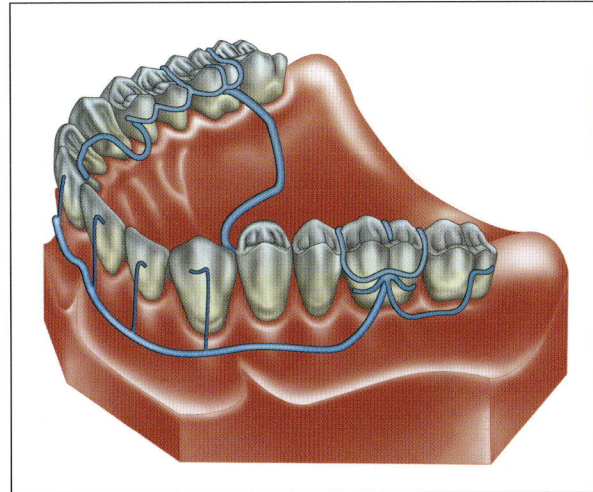

Fig 10-67 A vestibular view of the extended Crozat appliance shows the mechanism of action of the high labial bow, pins, and buccal extension. The buccal extension can be used for adjusting the second molars.

model made of soldering investment material and then soldered at the contact points. The soldering points are smoothed, and the appliance is polished. Stresses and strain hardening caused by finishing, polishing, and rebending are eliminated by heat treatment (annealing).

Additional elements for Crozat appliances include a high labial bow with pins, hooks and springs, as well as lingual auxiliary spring arches for movement of anterior teeth (Figs 10-66 and 10-67).

The **high labial bow** has a wire thickness of 1.3 mm and is soldered to the buccal extensions in the maxillary appliance. The bow runs outside the visible area in the vestibular space without touching the gingiva. The soldered pins (0.8 mm wide) extend from here to the labial surfaces of the teeth. At the level of the canines, hooks can be soldered on to receive elastics, which pull on the Jackson clasp at the hooks in the maxilla and are used for correcting occlusion. Hooks can also be attached to the high labial bow for elastics so that individual teeth can be rotated.

The lingual auxiliary spring arches are the counterparts to the high labial bow on the tongue side. They are bent out of 0.8-mm wire and fitted with additional activation loops. They are soldered to the existing lingual arms and run as far as the middle of the dental arch.

Treatment based on the Crozat approach involves several phases, for which the appliance has to be expanded and reworked. Each phase has different treatment goals, and the next phase is only started once the previous goal has been achieved.

Inclined Plane

The *inclined plane* is an appliance that fully implements the principle of functional orthodontics. It is only by biting together that the force is produced to trigger remodeling processes. This is a special acrylic appliance that is placed on the mandibular teeth and contacts only individual teeth in the opposing jaw. The force during biting is vectorially distributed to the inclined plane so that the tooth being corrected is pushed in a labial direction. The corrective forces arise intermittently and only at a magnitude that is within the physiologic range of tolerance.

The *indication for an inclined plane* is the adjustment of maxillary incisors that are lingually

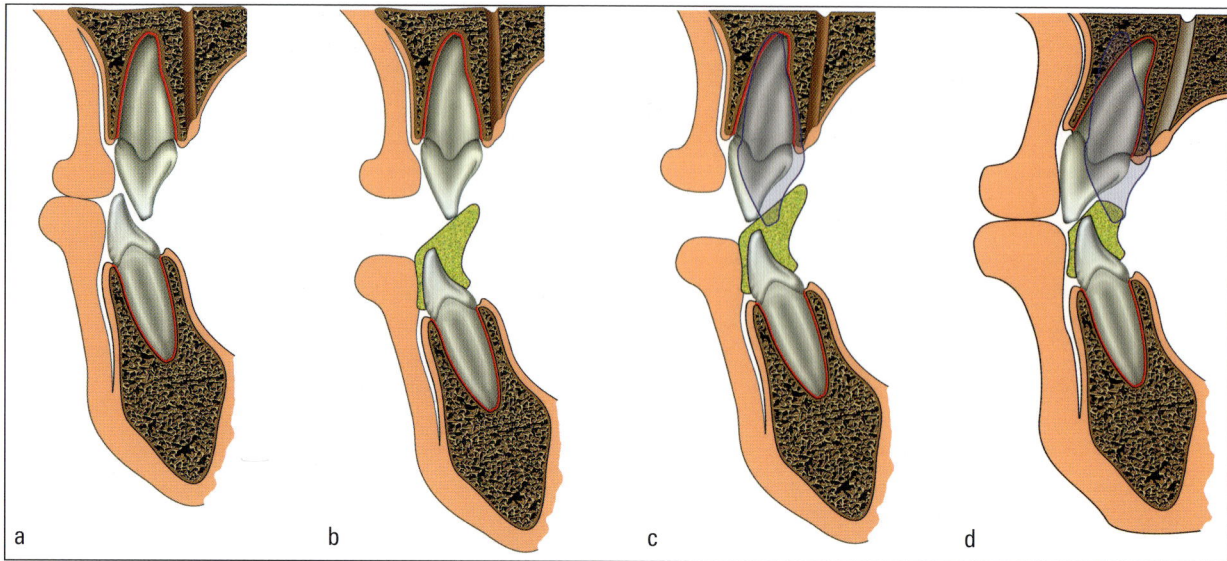

Fig 10-68 The principle of the inclined plane embodies the basic concept of an activator in a pure form, although the application of force is very crude. The inclined plane is used for moving individual teeth: *(a)* A maxillary incisor is inverted behind its mandibular antagonist. *(b)* An acrylic block is placed over the mandibular anterior teeth. A bite plane for the tooth being corrected is set at a very steep angle. When the patient bites down, a regulating thrust is exerted on the maxillary incisor. The steeper the inclined plane, the faster the adjustment takes place. *(c)* The inclined plane is reground to reflect the progress of the treatment. The mouth is able to close more and more as the orthodontic adjustment progresses. *(d)* Toward the end of the treatment (after about 6 weeks), the inclined plane is ground down as far as the incisal edges of the mandibular antagonists. The mouth is closed again.

tipped and caught behind the mandibular anterior teeth (Fig 10-68). To achieve stationary anchorage, the inclined plane at least embraces all four mandibular incisors without touching or irritating the gingiva.

Four incisors can be corrected effectively enough at the same time. During correction of the teeth, the periodontal tissues cannot be overloaded because the periodontium ensures that force is minimized in a reflex fashion.

If the distance to be spanned is very short, treatment success is quickly achieved. Therefore, correction of tooth position excluding antagonist contact is first undertaken with suitable active appliances, then adjustment is performed with an inclined plane within a very short treatment period.

A *reverse articulation of individual teeth* is often associated with crowding of teeth in that area. The teeth requiring correction overlap each other, and their movement is impeded. Therefore, the crowding must be rectified first.

Generally the inclined plane is firmly cemented. However, it can also be combined with a removable appliance that retrudes the mandibular teeth

at the same time. The mandibular incisors need to bridge one half and the maxillary teeth the other half of the distance being corrected. This involves a mandibular active plate with a tightened labial bow to which the inclined plane for the maxillary incisors is fitted.

For *retrusive movement*, the plate must be reduced behind the mandibular incisors. With the removable plate, the occlusal pressure is transmitted via the inclined plane to the maxillary teeth and also to the mandibular teeth to the same extent. To achieve stationary anchorage for the maxillary teeth and for the mandibular active components, the plate is anchored by the usual retentive components.

The *effect of the inclined plane* is dependent not only on the angle of inclination but also on the number of teeth being corrected, the distance to be bridged, and the freedom of direction of movement. If only one tooth has to be corrected, the entire occlusal force will act on its periodontium and stimulate remodeling. With an increasing number of teeth to be adjusted, the force is spread, and so is the tensile and compressive effect in the periodontal tissues of the involved teeth, until the force falls below a threshold and any orthodontic effect is lost.

The treatment period with an inclined plane should not be longer than 6 weeks because chewing activity is considerably restricted. The dentition must be kept out of antagonist contact so that only the tooth or teeth being corrected are loaded and repositioned. This results in lengthening of the unloaded teeth, which may lead to an anterior open bite. The steeper the inclined plane, the faster the adjustment is achieved.

Fabrication of an inclined plane takes place in the laboratory on models. However, it can also be modeled directly in the mouth. The entire mandibular dentition is enclosed in a block with a splint to ensure stationary distribution of forces and prevent lengthening at least of the mandibular incisors. The acrylic is pulled up for the width of the tooth being adjusted so that only the affected tooth is touched by the acrylic block when biting together and all the other teeth are kept out of contact.

The *acrylic bite plane* is placed at an angle of 45 degrees to the occlusal plane. In the mouth, the surface of the bite plane can then be ground into the optimum angle of inclination. In several consecutive sessions (about every 3 days), the bite plane is then ground off until the incisal edge of the mandibular incisor can be seen. The posterior teeth should have no contact during the treatment period; otherwise the inclined plane will not work.

Activators

The simple inclined plane as a fixed appliance or in conjunction with a removable mandibular plate is rarely used. However, all rigid functional orthodontic appliances operate on the principle of the inclined plane. The activator is the classic functional orthodontic appliance. This is a passive treatment appliance developed by V. Andresen and K. Häupl in the form of a double-plate that is used simultaneously for both jaws.

The *regulating effect* happens in all three planes of space: Dental arch expansion and narrowing, correction of misaligned individual teeth, and, most importantly, occlusal corrections can be successfully carried out. The appliance fits loosely in the mouth, is not fixed to the teeth, and only works when the teeth are brought together. The appliance impacts the teeth intermittently, and physiologic remodeling stimuli are supplied to the tissues.

The *effect of an activator* involves increasing the activity of muscles whose forces are suitable for remedying the malposition of teeth and occlusal anomalies. It works passively by the transfer of muscle stimuli from the masticatory, lingual, lip, and cheek musculature to the periodontal tissue, where it can trigger tissue remodeling. So that the appliance can bring the teeth together intermittently when the patient bites down, the two plates of the maxilla and the mandible have to be moved against each other. The jaws are no longer able to slide into a habitual terminal occlusion but are forced into a different, constructed position. For this purpose, the contact surfaces of the plates with the teeth can be milled out like inclined planes. The activator is first fitted with only a labial bow for the maxillary anterior teeth; spikes and guide wires can also be attached for transverse tooth movement (Figs 10-69 and 10-70).

The *passive appliance* comprises a reduced palatal plate. This merges into the mandibular plate, which in turn ends just before the floor of the mouth. The two plates are moved against each other in such a way that the lingual impression surfaces of the teeth lie in the proper position in relation to each other. A groove is created for the mandibular anterior teeth to bite into; the maxillary incisors do not contact the plate. A labial bow is provided for them. When the patient bites down, the mandible is pulled forward, the posterior teeth are blocked, and the maxillary anterior teeth contact the labial bow. Each individual tooth is now touched by the appliance in such a way that it tips in the desired direction. The maxillary and mandibular posterior teeth have plate contact only at the lingual surfaces, with the activator surfaces being inclined like an inclined plane to enforce tooth movement in the vestibular direction. The activator may additionally be shaped so that the inclined surfaces contact the maxillary posterior teeth not throughout the entire lingual surface but only in the mesiolingual segment, the intention being to stimulate distal movement of the posterior teeth.

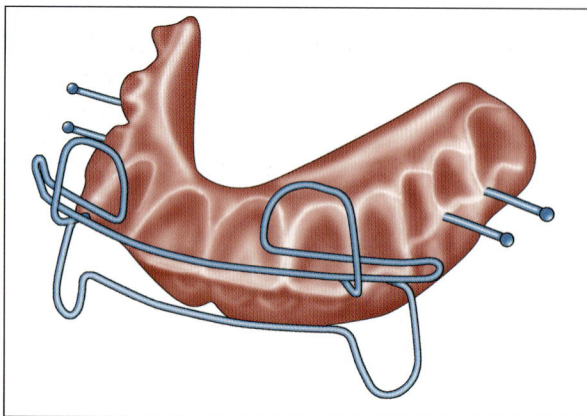

Fig 10-69 The activator comprises a double-plate for the maxilla and the mandible simultaneously, as well as labial wires, spikes, and guide wires, and it fits loosely in the mouth. The appliance does not become effective until the rows of teeth are brought together; the teeth impact each other intermittently, and the tissue receives physiologic remodeling stimuli. To achieve this, the two plates are moved against each other in a constructed occlusal position by the jaws.

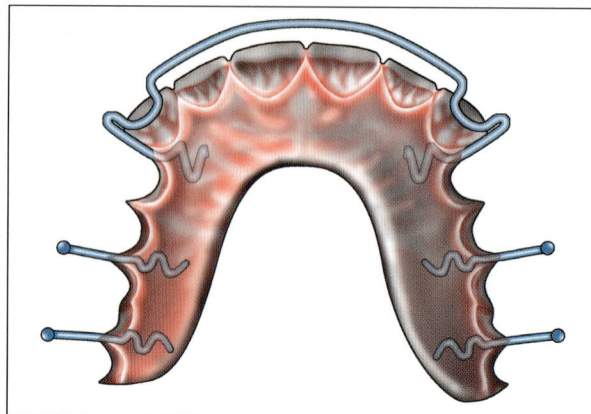

Fig 10-70 The mechanism of action of the activator involves ground inclined guide planes, as can be seen from this intaglio view. The forces for exerting pressure in this way arise through movements of the mandible during swallowing and breathing, tongue activities, and head movements during sleep. As well as reflex masticatory muscle activity, the functional interaction between the lip, cheek, and tongue muscles is gradually altered.

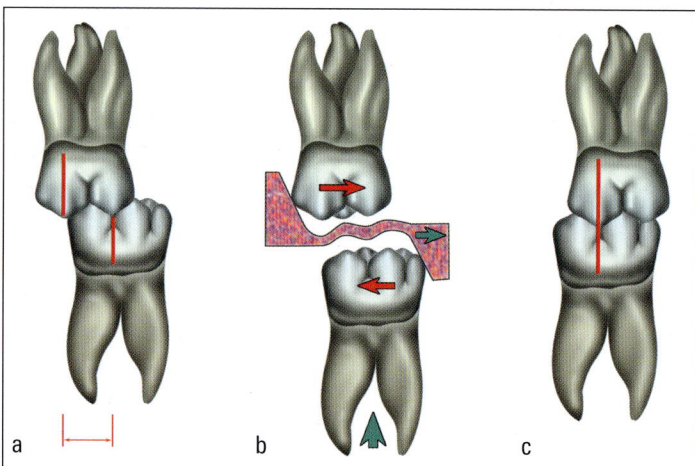

Fig 10-71 The regulating effect of an activator arises from an interaction between a mechanical effect and an increase in function or functional retraining of the neuromuscular system. For instance, if anomalies of tooth position or occlusal position (a) are to be remedied, the tooth guidance surfaces can be shaped on an appliance fitting loosely in the mouth so that a regulatory thrust is exerted on the teeth and parts of the jaws via inclined planes during reflex biting. A distal guidance surface is created for the mandibular tooth, which moves the tooth mesially and the appliance distally; the appliance presses the maxillary tooth distally with a mesial guidance surface (b). Extensive anomalies can be adjusted with this mechanism of action (c).

The occlusal surfaces of the posterior teeth are avoided so that vertical tooth movement is forced toward the occlusal plane. The mandibular anterior teeth are combined in a block by the interocclusal splint and thus held in their position. The maxillary incisors are retruded by the labial bow when the activator is palatally reduced. Biting together also pushes the labial bow against the maxillary anterior teeth and produces the impulse-type forces to stimulate reshaping of tissues.

The following *regulating thrusts* occur (Fig 10-71):

- Posterior dental arches are expanded.
- Maxillary posterior teeth move distally.
- Posterior alveolar processes are lengthened.
- Maxillary anterior teeth are retruded.
- The mandible is pulled forward.
- Joint changes and alveolar tissue changes are stimulated.

In this process, the **remodeling stimuli** arise not through continuous pressure but through the appliance being moved during muscle activity. The displacement of the mandible compared with the habitual resting position as a result of activator plates moved against each other is crucial because a regulating thrust occurs with every reflex movement of the mandible. Adjustment efforts can often be undertaken more quickly and more precisely with other orthodontic appliances but not as gently as with an activator. Sagittal occlusal correction is not accomplished as reliably with any other appliance or with such absolute simplicity as with this functional appliance.

Activator fabrication

First, two models are prepared on which the activator is to be fabricated from acrylic, and two duplicates are produced on which the activator is ground. A construction bite record is then fabricated to show the two models in relation to each other in the occlusal position that the activator is intended to enforce. The jaws lie in the construction bite just as they are meant to be positioned after the treatment. Isometric muscle contractions are produced by the construction bite when it goes 6 to 10 mm beyond the rest position in the vertical plane.

The following criteria apply to the **construction bite**:

• The **vertical distance** between the maxillary and mandibular dentition is so large that no antagonist contact occurs; the most favorable distance is 6 mm. However, if only a slight sagittal shift of occlusal position is required, a 10-mm opening will be more effective. This is because the force exerted when biting out of the blocked position should actually produce the physiologic stimuli.

• The **sagittal occlusal position** is intended to indicate the regular position, in which the first molars are the fixed points when the other teeth are missing or displaced in a mixed dentition. In disto-occlusion, protrusion by one premolar's width corresponds to TMJ tolerance. The protrusive position can generally be achieved without difficulty if the sagittal distance of the anterior teeth is sufficient. Where there is a deep vertical overlap, the anterior teeth are first brought into the edge-to-edge position.

• In **mesio-occlusion**, the mandible must be pushed into the rearmost position, which is possible by about 2 mm dorsally. For pronounced prognathism, it usually becomes necessary to keep the movement of the activator double-plates variable; ie, it must be possible to move them against each other with a screw in response to the progress of the adjustment.

• **Lateral adjustment** is performed by sliding the jaw midlines over each other. Where there are dental arch asymmetries, reverse articulation situations may arise, which also have to be re-adjusted by grinding on the activator. If necessary, unilateral dental arch constriction may be remedied by a swiveling activator wing.

In the **construction bite**, the working models are placed in the constructed relationship, and a wax squash bite is prepared. The construction bite taken on the model is tried in the patient's mouth, and then the models are placed in a fixator or a simple occluder with an occlusal height locking screw, with the hinge axis lying laterally next to the models. The oral cavity should be visible without any obstructions and accessible to working equipment. The models with the dorsal edges of the model base can also be lowered upright into plaster slurry, where they leave distinct impressions. Separator should be applied to the models so that they can be removed after the plaster has set. The plaster fixator is smoothed and shortened so that the models still have sufficiently secure guidance.

The **labial bow** is bent first. It contacts the maxillary incisors in the incisal third, incorporates the canine loop, is fed between the canine and the first premolar, and runs over the teeth in a palatal direction, where it is later anchored in acrylic. The canine loop can also be used for readjustment, depending on the progress of the treatment. The activator is then molded in wax: The double-plate fits closely to the palate and the alveolar process in the maxilla and mandible without restricting the floor of the mouth.

The **palatal plate** is reduced as far as possible. Therefore, the activator precisely covers the lingual surfaces of all the teeth as well as the occlusal surfaces of the posterior teeth and the mandibular anterior teeth. Basically, a wax splint covering the entire dentition is carved that reproduces the construction bite position.

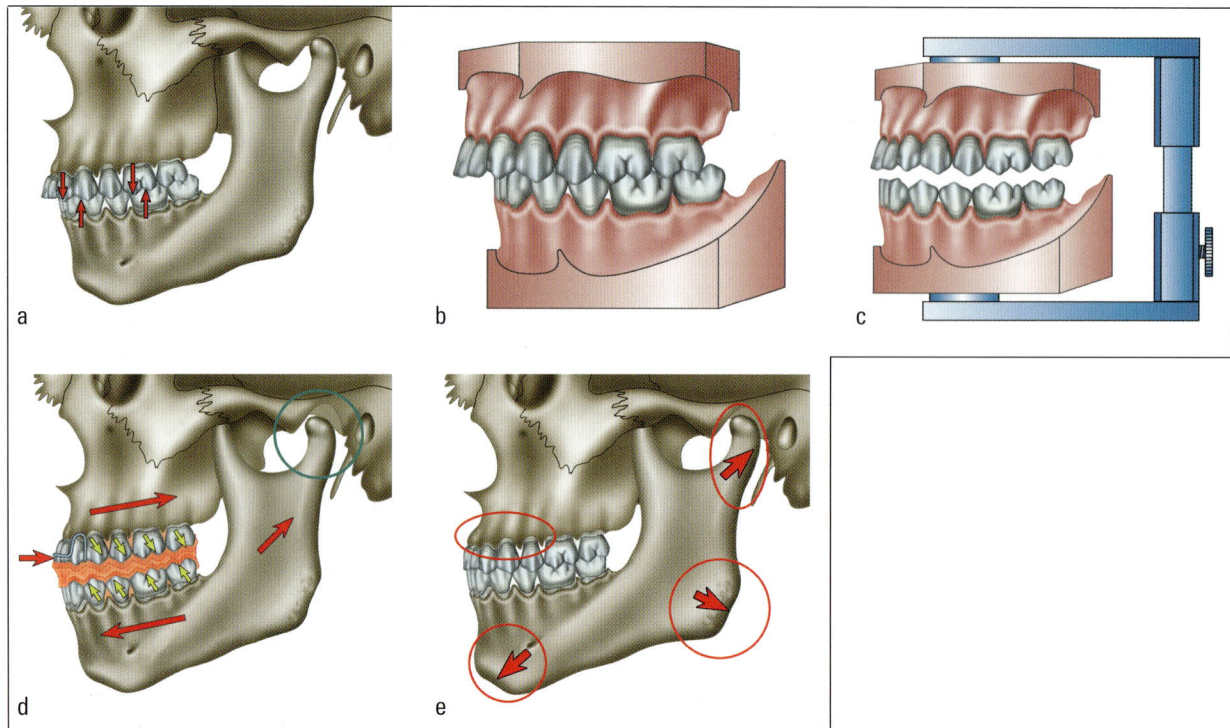

Fig 10-72 *(a)* Relatively reliable treatment of a distinct shift of occlusal position (here disto-occlusion) is possible with an activator. This requires a construction bite, which means the activator can become a function simulator. *(b)* The position of the jaws in relation to each other in reflexive terminal occlusion shows the shift of occlusal position as well as the prominence of the maxillary anterior teeth, which will also have to be corrected. *(c)* The jaws are placed in an eccentric mandibular position to each other, the construction bite. The vertical distance is about 4 to 10 mm, with the sagittal and lateral positioning corresponding to regular occlusion. *(d)* The physiologic remodeling stimuli arise because of reflex muscle activity when the mandible is brought into an eccentric position by the orthodontic appliance. As a result, growth stimuli occur in the distal direction in the maxilla and in the mesial direction in the mandible. *(e)* As well as the functional adaptive phenomena in the area of the alveolar processes of both jaws to correct intercuspation, changes occur in the TMJ (thickening of the condylar process), the angle of the jaw, and the chin.

A ***wax try-in*** can be carried out to check the position of the construction bite. However, the activator is generally fabricated immediately in acrylic. If the wax pattern can be accurately fabricated, which depends on the undercut situation and the shape of the teeth, the wax activator can be directly invested and completed in acrylic. Otherwise, the activator is invested on a model, usually that of the maxilla. Direct fabrication with self-curing acrylic, however, is the usual method. Once the activator is available in acrylic, it must be ground on the duplicate model.

Figure 10-72 illustrates the shift in occlusal position possible with an articulator, demonstrating the concept of the construction bite.

Grinding the activator

In addition to fabricating the construction bite, grinding is the most important measure in producing the appliance. Grinding ensures that all the intended tooth movements are possible. This working step is usually done by the dentist, but the experienced dental technician can carry out the basic grinding steps if a movement analysis has been discussed beforehand (ie, if it is decided which tooth is to be loaded or unloaded and how). The grinding is first done on the plaster model so that each grinding measure can be checked. Further grinding measures take place in follow-up sessions:

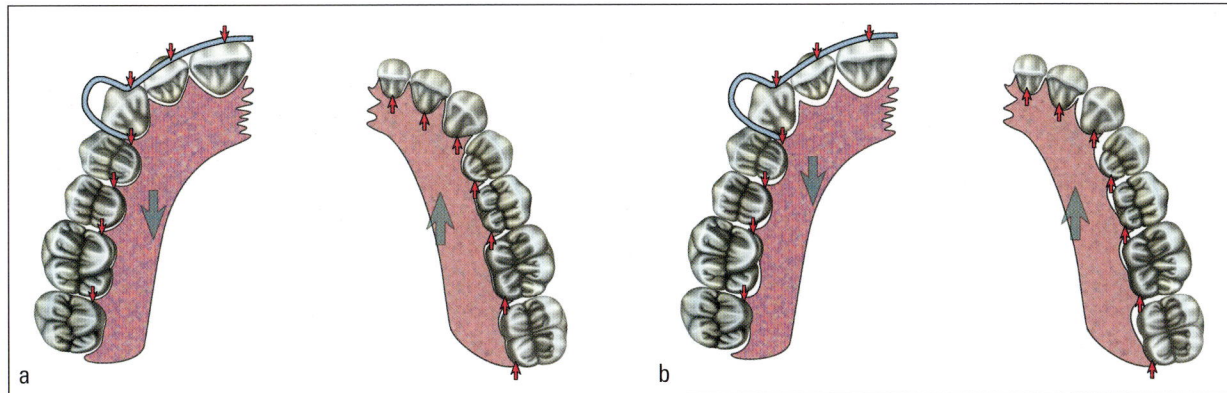

Fig 10-73 *(a)* Free grinding of the contact surfaces of the teeth in the direction of movement is unnecessary because the same effects occur even without free grinding. Grinding out guide depressions for the posterior teeth is in line with the idea of exposing the direction of movement of a tooth that is to be moved. Because the dental arches are to be shifted sagittally overall, only the vertical component is ground. *(b)* To compensate for residual gaps after extraction of a posterior tooth or if a group of posterior teeth is to be moved, the contact surfaces of the teeth are ground in such a way that a distally directed thrust occurs in the maxilla and a mesial thrust in the mandible. The palatal surfaces of the maxillary incisors are exposed if the anterior region is to be tipped inward.

1. ***Grinding on the posterior teeth*** starts as the chewing surfaces are exposed so that the activator margin contacts the posterior teeth only at the widest extent. The guidance surfaces should be ground steeply so that no acrylic gets in the way of a vertical movement of the posterior teeth if a deep bite is to be eliminated.

2. ***Free grinding of the contact surfaces*** on the maxillary teeth is done for distal movement so that only one mesiolingual contact remains. This free grinding of the guidance surfaces is not absolutely necessary, because the distal movement of the maxillary incisors will be enforced by the thrust from the activator, just as the mandibular incisors will be pushed mesially (Fig 10-73). It is debatable whether a preferred movement occurs if the guidance surfaces are freely ground separately for the maxillary and mandibular teeth.

3. ***Free grinding of the maxillary incisors*** for a possible retrusive movement is done by removing the acrylic palatally behind the incisors. The cervical margin and the alveolar process also must be uncovered in this area. Only the interocclusal splint for the mandibular anterior teeth is retained as a block. In the process, the interdental spaces and the cervical areas must also be exposed to prevent inflammation and too tight a fit.

4. ***Try-in and adjustment*** of the ground appliance is performed intraorally. The patient becomes familiar with the appliance, how to insert the appliance, and how to store it outside the mouth. It is also important to explain the mechanism of action of the appliance to the patient and to emphasize the regular wearing times and checkups.

The activator is generally worn at night; only at the start of the treatment should it be worn during the day for 2 or 3 hours (after lunch) so that the remodeling processes are maintained and not interrupted for long periods. Patients may also be instructed to do 5-minute pressing exercises twice a day.

The ***mechanism of action of the activator*** is mechanical, although no spring components or screws are used for support. The ground inclined guidance surfaces produce the intermittent loading and hence the areas of compression and tension in the periodontium.

The ***forces for this exertion of pressure*** arise due to mandibular movements when swallowing and breathing (mandibular movement synchronous with respiratory rate), tongue activity, and general head movements when sleeping.

The mandible is always forced into an eccentric position differing from the resting position, which

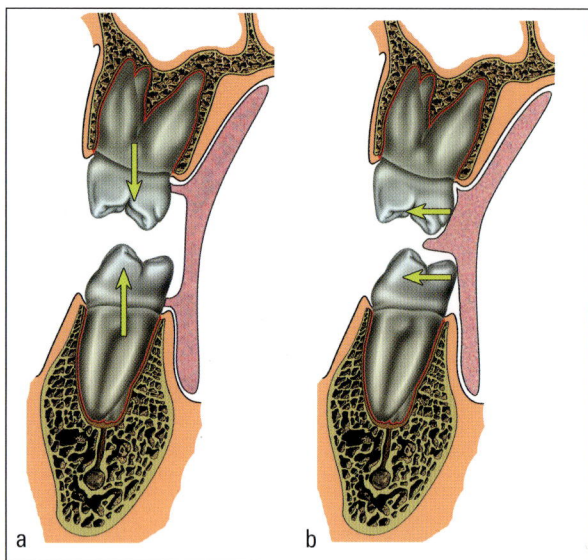

Fig 10-74 For an extrusive movement, the guide planes of the activator are ground out so that there is only one contact line below the tooth equator and the occlusal direction of movement remains clear (a). Dental arch expansion takes place via the tooth guide planes contoured as inclined planes; an occlusion rim remains occlusally (b).

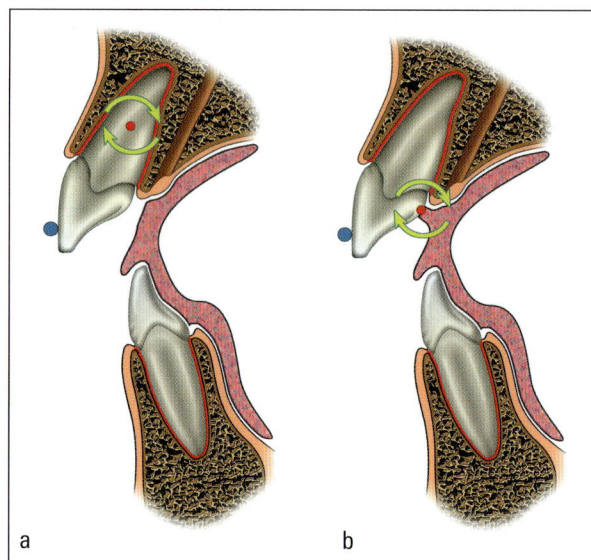

Fig 10-75 The incisors can be pushed back into the dental arch with the activatable labial bow. This involves single-point application of force if the activator stands freely lingually (a). Two-point application of forces exists if the activator margin contacts the incisor palatally and the activated labial bow tips the tooth inward. The activator edge is then the point of rotation (b).

means that forces are applied to the teeth via the activator and from there into the area of tissue remodeling. Excessive stresses are usually unlikely to occur because of the reflex coupling.

Masticatory muscle activity is altered by the activator as it initiates reflex biting movements. Unlike in deliberate biting, individual groups of teeth are only ever loaded by pressing exercises. In this respect, the activator differs from other appliances because it utilizes functional bodily forces and only to a small extent through deliberate biting. Although the forces are no different because the effect is the same in terms of tissue remodeling, this fact does relate to the property of the activator as a function stimulator. As well as reflex masticatory muscle activity, the functional interaction between lip and cheek muscles with the tongue musculature is gradually altered as well. The change in the position of the mandible relative to the maxilla and the altered tooth positions naturally have an impact on the musculature and its movement sequences.

Figures 10-74 and 10-75 illustrate the action of activators in the posterior and anterior teeth, respectively.

Activator designs

During the course of treatment with an activator, articular and periodontal tissue remodeling takes place slowly over the course of 2 or 3 years. The optimal activator effect happens during exfoliation; treatment should be finished after eruption of the maxillary second molars.

With ***slight reshaping***, suitable additional elements can be attached to the activator. Guide loops, spikes, and screw components for active appliances are used. These active components should be attached so that, like an activator, they only take effect when the mandible is pushed into the construction bite position by muscle activity. If malpositions of individual teeth or groups of teeth are to be corrected or if massive dental arch expansion needs to be carried out, there is the

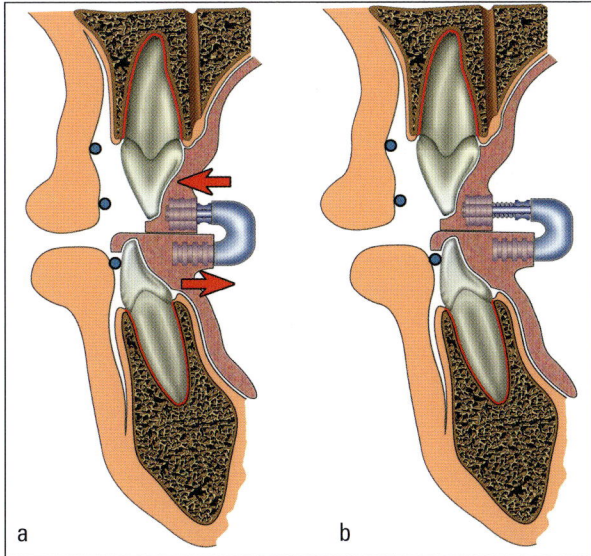

Fig 10-76 The bite-jumping (protrusive) double-plate comprises two separate plates for the maxillary and mandibular jaws, which are joined with a screw. The plate can be used for various correction procedures; here the inverted anterior region, combined with mesio-occlusion, is to be remedied. Fabrication with self-curing acrylics is relatively simple and straightforward if the plates are prepared separately and the guide planes are subsequently polymerized.

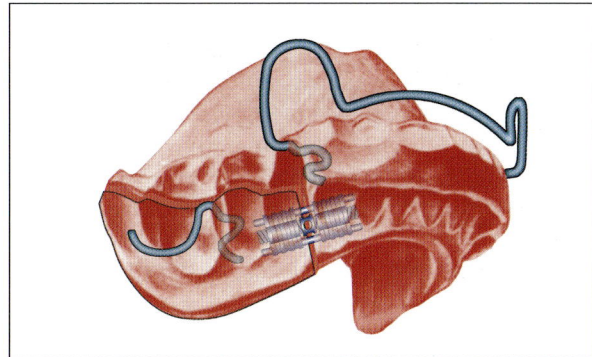

Fig 10-77 An activator fitted with an expansion screw is intended to move the mandibular incisors distally by a retrusive movement to eliminate a severely pronounced mesio-occlusion.

option of using active appliances before inserting the activator.

For **prognathism treatment** in which the mandible needs to be corrected over a greater distance than joint tolerance will allow, the activator can be separated horizontally in the area of the locked occlusion and fitted with an adjustment screw.

For this **occlusal correction**, the activator halves perforated in the region of the locked occlusion are pushed against each other in the sagittal direction so that the maxillary dental arch is brought forward and the mandibular arch backward. The posterior teeth in this region remain held in a splintlike fashion. In the anterior region, the mandibular plate part is milled lingually so that the lingual bow under tension presses the mandibular incisors lingually. The mandibular incisors must not be "nested" in a crowded state. A maxillary labial bow is additionally fitted and keeps the upper lip from lying closely against the maxillary incisors.

Protrusive (bite-jumping) and retrusive double-plates are two-part appliances that can be pushed against each other on a guide plane (Fig 10-76).

The retrusive or protrusive movement is produced with active appliances by different mechanisms: elastics, screws, activatable springs, and inclined guide planes. In the activator, the force for correcting an occlusal discrepancy must be applied by the masticatory muscles, which always want to pull the mandible into a habitual position. Two special screws are suitable for bite jumping or retrusive double-plates: (1) the prognathism screw and (2) the simple expansion screw. The screws are not used as on an active plate but are adjusted depending on the progress of the correction.

The **simple expansion screw** is placed with a sagittal direction of thrust at the dorsal edge of the maxillary plate. The screw section directed backward is held with an additional small plastic block from which two wire brackets run along the palate to the mandibular plate. If the expansion screw is now opened, the mandibular plate pushes in a distal direction (Fig 10-77). The advantage is that the tongue is not severely crowded (when a special prognathism screw is used, the tongue can be extremely crowded anteriorly). This is a screw whose movable part is bent over so that it extends downward into the mandibular plate.

Open bites can also be treated with an activator. The aim of the treatment must be to lengthen the anterior teeth and their alveolar processes while preventing further growth of the posterior teeth. The latter goal is achieved by interocclusal splints for the posterior teeth, while the anterior teeth are free-ground into the alveolar region. If lingual tipping of the anterior teeth is to be achieved, a rest can remain cervically while the labial bow lies tight to the tooth incisally. The direction of movement must be unimpeded, and there must be no anterior crowding. The activator with lateral interocclusal splints has another effect: When the mouth is closed, the mandible can be tipped around the interocclusal splint as the blocked incisors are approached and the condyles are lifted out of the fossae. Functional adaptation due to lengthening of the condyles and remodeling processes in the angles of the mandible are possible.

Several modifications of the activator are described in the literature as **maxillomandibular orthodontic appliances**. The following section provides brief descriptions of several different activators.

Brief outline of different activators

Monobloc activator

The **monobloc activator** is an appliance developed as an exercise device that embraces both jaws at once for correcting occlusal anomalies. It comprises an acrylic block for the maxilla and the mandible that is joined interocclusally (Fig 10-78).

In the **maxilla**, the greatly reduced acrylic base covers the palate in a horseshoe shape. The base is about 12 mm wide and flattens out. In the anterior region, the acrylic extends up to the incisal edges, and in the posterior region the occlusal surfaces are more than half covered.

In the **mandible**, the alveolar process is covered as far as the border of the floor of the mouth. Undercuts are blocked out. Anterior and posterior teeth are engaged as in the maxilla, with the occlusal surfaces two-thirds covered with an occlusal guard at least 3 mm thick.

The **labial bow** of the activator is used to retract the anterior teeth in the maxilla and is made of 0.9-mm spring hard wire. The transition of the labial bow into the acrylic block is kept free-moving to prevent fracture of the bow.

The monobloc activator can be used for widening the dental arches by means of a centrally positioned expansion screw. The sawn cut is placed sagittally in the middle.

Bimler appliance

This appliance (Bimler's "elastic occlusion former") differs considerably from a rigid form of activator. It is shaped from 0.9-mm strong steel wire. Only two thin acrylic plates lie palatally to the maxillary incisors, and a cap-shaped acrylic plate lies lingual to the mandibular anterior teeth (Fig 10-79). The palatal guide plates only fit closely to the maxillary incisors and anchor all the wire brackets. A **Coffin spring** links the two guide plates; the labial bow with a small buccinator loop is passed between the canines and first premolars. Lastly, a wire bracket as a replacement for a mandibular plate extends to the mandibular incisors, which it contacts below their equators. This wire then runs back down between the canines and first premolars over the dentition labially into the acrylic caps. Two wire brackets extend from the cap lingually behind the anterior teeth. The wire loops are guided differently depending on the aim of the treatment.

The **stimulating body** of this elastic occlusion-shaping appliance induces involuntary muscle reactions. Transverse mandibular movements are exploited for widening the dental arch, while vertical movements help to stretch the arch. The appliance is worn day and night for a quick outcome because it does not interfere with speech. It has to be adjusted in line with treatment progress, which is very difficult given the complicated wire bracket guidance.

Klammt's elastic open activator

The open activator is a maxillomandibular appliance comprising two lingual, lateral acrylic bodies that are joined by a transverse expansion screw or by a palatal bar (Fig 10-80).

The **standard appliance** comprises the lateral acrylic bodies, a palatal bar or a transverse screw,

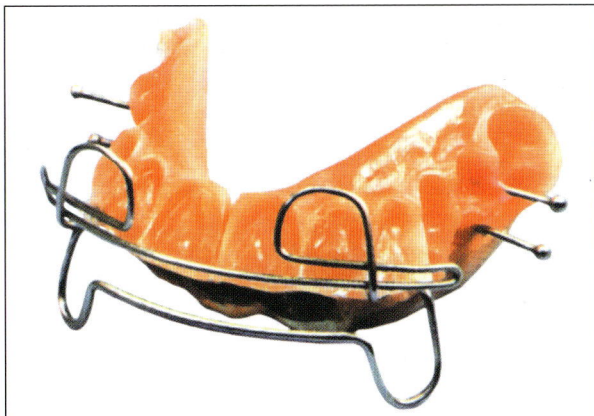

Fig 10-78 The monobloc activator fits loosely in the mouth as a double-plate for the maxilla and the mandible simultaneously. When the rows of teeth are brought together, the appliance impacts intermittently on the teeth and supplies physiologic remodeling stimuli to the tissues. So that the appliance can intermittently strike the teeth during biting, the two plates are in an eccentric position and the contact surfaces on the teeth are milled out like inclined planes.

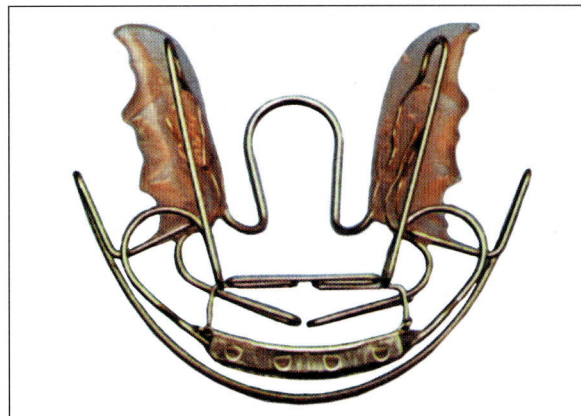

Fig 10-79 The Bimler appliance is a maxillomandibular elastic appliance made of 0.9-mm steel wire in which two thin acrylic plates fit closely to the posterior teeth and a cap-shaped acrylic plate lies against the mandibular anterior teeth. All the wire brackets are anchored in the lingual guide plates. The elastic appliance, as a stimulating body, induces involuntary muscle reactions. In addition to functioning as an early treatment appliance and retainer, this appliance is differentiated into three types that can be further subdivided according to tooth position and fitted with a variety of components.

labial bows paired for the maxilla and the mandible (with possible lip bumpers), and intraoral guide wires.

The *acrylic bodies* extend from the canine to the last posterior tooth; guide planes can be worked in, while the occlusal surfaces remain clear. The palatal bar made of 1.2-mm hard steel wire joins the two acrylic bodies. The palatal bar must not contact the mucosa or impede the tongue.

The *labial bows* made of 0.9-mm hard steel wire are passed between the canines and first premolars in a vestibular direction; they are formed into loops distally over the premolars and run over the anterior teeth. This means the labial bows take on the following *functions*:

- Shaping the dental arch from the incisors through to the premolars
- Controlling lip tone to shape the ideal dental arch
- Shielding the posterior teeth from the cheeks
- Vestibular guidance of the erupting canines and premolars

The *intraoral guide wires* made from 0.9-mm hard steel wire lie against the lingual surfaces of the incisors in pairs.

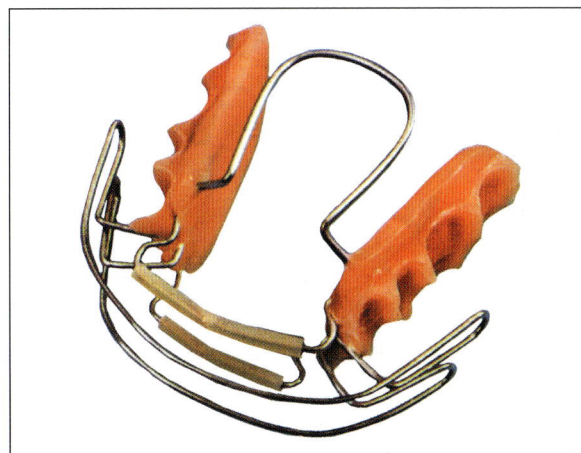

Fig 10-80 Klammt's elastic open activator is a maxillomandibular device comprising two reduced acrylic blocks (to avoid crowding the tongue) that lie against the posterior teeth and are joined by a Coffin spring (elastic appliance), a palatal bar, or an expansion screw (rigid appliance). The appliance carries two modified labial bows (top and bottom) to which lip bumpers may be fitted to hold back the lips. Guide loops are fitted intraorally for the anterior teeth; support spikes on the molars may be provided.

The **lip bumpers** can replace the labial bows in the maxilla or mandible and lie deep in the vestibular fornix.

Balters bionator

This is a functional orthodontic appliance made of a greatly reduced double-plate to which a widened labial bow and a palatally displaced "tongue bar" are attached (Fig 10-81a). It preferentially activates the vestibular musculature (lip closure) and the tongue (correct position and contact with the palate), which is the purpose of the lip bar with two buccinator loops and the tongue bar. It is indicated for shifting and leveling the occlusion and for correcting forms of dysgnathia arising from malfunctioning due to anomalies of the tongue and lip posture.

The **labial bow** (lip bar) lies at the level of the maxillary anterior teeth, bends down at the canines to the mandible, and is passed along the posterior teeth as a long buccinator loop. It then runs between the canines and premolars over the dentition into the acrylic of the appliance. It is shaped out of 0.9-mm hard steel wire and guided at a small distance from the tooth surfaces.

The **tongue bar**, like a tightened Coffin spring, runs dorsally over the palate; the 1.2-mm-thick wire is 1 mm away from the mucosa. This is intended to re-educate tongue activity.

The **acrylic plate** is very slender and mainly comprises a narrow mandibular base. The acrylic reaches the mandibular anterior teeth and, to provide better support for the appliance, is passed up to the occlusal surfaces of the posterior teeth.

The slender **basic appliance** can be worn all day long without restricting speech and achieves a quick result. It can be used as a distal activator (type 1) (Figs 10-81b and 10-81c).

The **shield appliance** (type 2) has an acrylic body that runs over the anterior palatal area in the frontal part of the maxilla (Figs 10-81d and 10-81e). Individual labial or buccal shields can be prepared for the vestibule. The shield appliance is used in an open bite and stops the tongue from sliding between the anterior teeth.

The **reverse appliance** (type 3) as a prognathism activator relates to the maximum retrusive position (Figs 10-81f and 10-81g). Compared with the basic appliance, its lip bar runs along the mandibular anterior teeth, and the lingual bar loop is bent forward. The lingual plate of the acrylic body runs over the incisal edges of the maxillary anterior teeth and contacts the palatal surfaces of the maxillary posterior teeth.

Fränkel functional regulator

The functional regulator is designed to alter the muscular function of the oral vestibule as the two buccal shields and lip pads keep development-inhibiting influences of the cheek, lip, and chin muscles away from the jaw and the shaping force of the tongue is fully exploited. The function regulator is indicated for defects of alveolar development such as mandibular retrognathia, deep bite, and prognathism.

The functional regulator is a reduced vestibular plate by which the acrylic part lies in the vestibule. Acrylic buccal shields vestibularly cover those parts of the dentition and alveolar ridge that are to be redeveloped.

Two wire brackets run vestibularly from the **buccal shields**: one as a labial bow in the maxilla and the other with two sublabial pads in the lower part of the vestibular fornix. The labial bow and sublabial pads push the mucosa from the alveolar bone and stimulate sagittal redevelopment of the apical bony base. To achieve this, the pads lie deep in the vestibular fornix at a distance from the alveolar ridge.

A **palatal loop** is bent in the maxilla as well as a guide loop for correcting the maxillary anterior teeth. In addition, clasplike wire loops can be used for single-tooth displacement. In the mandible, a guide loop also runs behind the anterior teeth.

Three types of functional regulator have been designed:

- **Type 1** comprises lateral shields, from which the maxillary labial bow and the mandibular wire bracket for the pads originate. In addition, there are two canine loops, one palatal bar, and a lingual bow with U-loops. Protrusive positions of the anterior teeth can be eliminated and dental arch expansion carried out.
- **Type 2** is used for correcting a disto-occlusion. The wire loops for the maxillary anterior teeth are intended to achieve retrusion. Additional wire loops for single-tooth movements can be fitted.

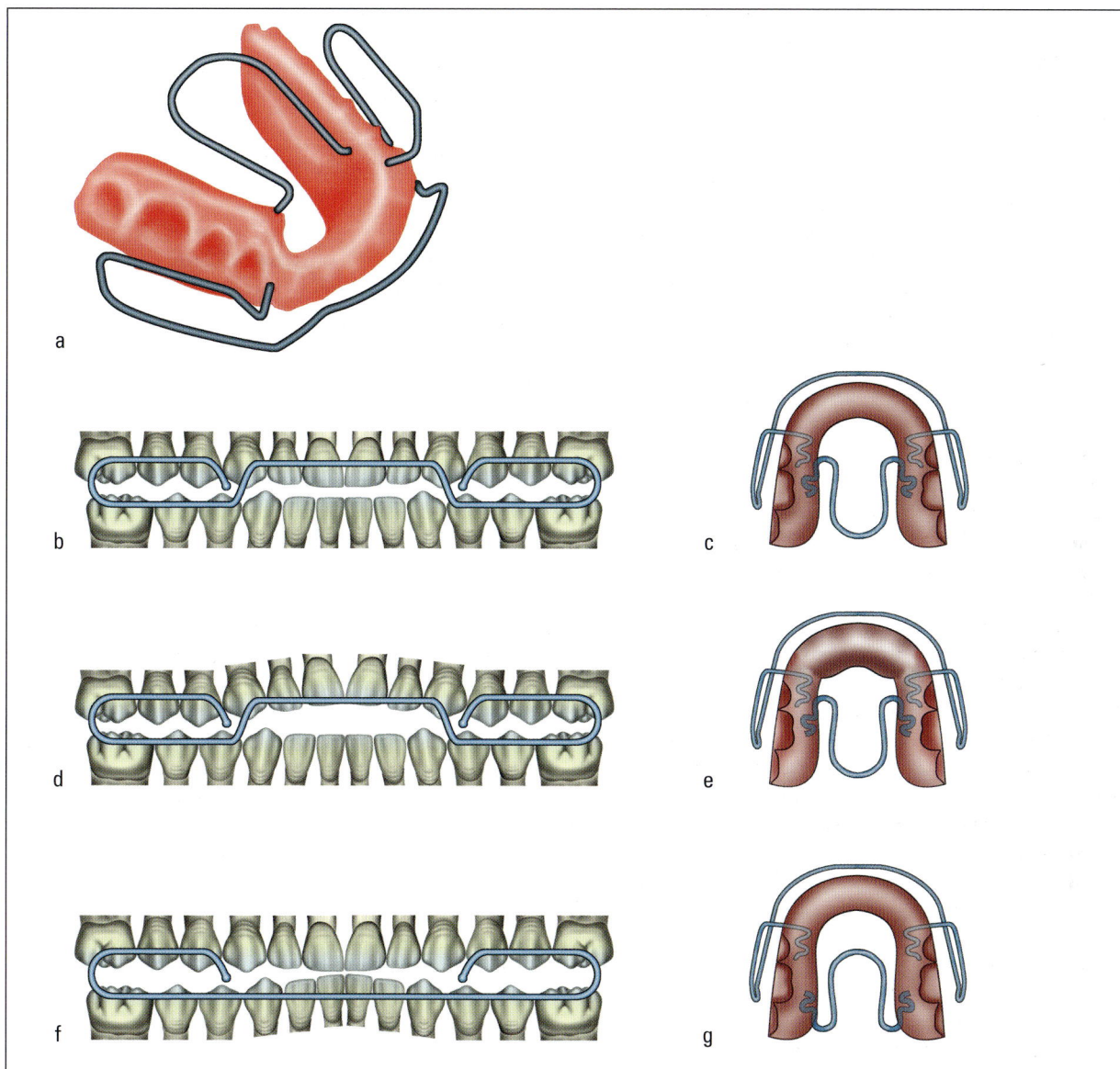

Fig 10-81 *(a)* Balters bionator is a passive appliance in the form of a reduced double-plate with widened labial bow and palatally placed lingual bar. The labial bow lies in the anterior region, bends down at the maxillary canines toward the mandible, and is passed along the posterior teeth as a long buccinator loop. Three types are identified for different treatment procedures. *(b and c)* The distal activator (type 1) is the basic appliance for regulating the occlusal position. An appropriate construction bite is required for this purpose. The lingual bar runs dorsally over the palate to stimulate the function of the tongue in relation to the lips and cheeks. *(d and e)* The shield appliance (type 2) is used to correct open bites. The acrylic body in the anterior region of the maxilla is guided over the anterior part of the palate, and labial or buccal shields can be prepared for the oral vestibule. The aim is to prevent the tongue from sliding between the anterior teeth. *(f and g)* The reverse bionator (type 3) is used for correcting prognathism. The lip bar runs along the mandibular anterior teeth, and the lingual bar loop is bent forward. The construction bite shows an extreme mandibular position.

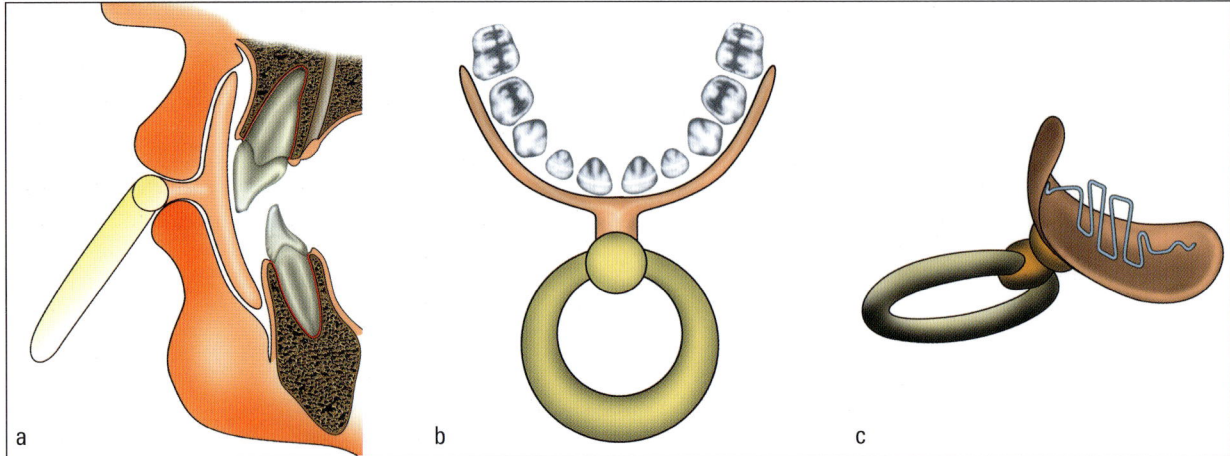

Fig 10-82 *(a)* The oral screen is usually supplied ready-made. It lies against the maxillary incisors as soon as the lips are closed and prevents further mouth breathing. It is suitable for early treatment of open bites. *(b)* The oral screen seen from above shows how the buccal muscles are held back so that tongue pressure can exert a possible effect of dental arch expansion. *(c)* The oral screen can be fitted with a lingual shield to prevent the tongue from pushing between the teeth. It can be used to treat open bites and cases of disto-occlusion.

• ***Type 3*** is used as a prognathism activator; lip pads are fitted in the maxilla, and the labial bow passes along the mandibular anterior teeth. A palatal bow in the maxilla is supplemented by a tight protrusion bar for stretching the maxillary anterior region.

Myofunctional therapy

Myofunctional therapy involves appliances for orofacial muscle exercises to repattern the activity of the masticatory, tongue, lip, and cheek muscles and re-educate them in order to correct anomalies of tooth and occlusal position. Functional orthodontic appliances for this therapeutic approach include oral screens.

Oral screens (vestibular screens) are simple appliances for increasing muscle activity by muscle exercises and tongue training for both the primary and the mixed dentition (Fig 10-82). Treatment with oral screens is a simple form of treatment. They can be used to:

• Carry out transverse development and shaping of the dental arches
• Eliminate harmful habits (habitual mouth breathing, finger sucking, lip biting, lip sucking)
• Eliminate disto-occlusion, open bites, and positional anomalies of the anterior teeth

The ***mechanism of action of oral screens*** consists of an active effect (myofunctional training) and a passive effect (pressure difference). The oral screen lying passively in the mouth shields against harmful influences of the cheek and lip muscles, allowing tongue pressure to have a dominant effect. The exercises with the oral screen have to be done several times a day to activate the right muscles.

During exercises, the patient tightly encloses the oral screen and pulls it out of the mouth against the resistance of the muscles. A distinct "plop" should be heard as this is done. Habitual mouth breathers are asked to switch to nasal breathing as the lips enclose the oral screen.

Stockfisch's kinetor is an appliance in the form of a double-cone activator block with lingual, elastic tube supports that press against the alveolar processes and the teeth during occluding and stimulate masticatory movements in all three planes of space, simultaneously stimulating the cheek muscles. It is used for jaw compression, protrusion with spaces and crowding, anterior crowding, deep vertical overlap, prognathism, and open bite. Expansion screws in the maxilla and mandible are used for this purpose. The kinetor is fabricated from ready-made parts, including four plastic parts to receive the exchangeable vestibular tubes, single tubes for raising the occlusion, and triple tubes for lowering the occlusion.

The **tooth positioner made from silicone** or other polymers helps to improve occlusion and intercuspation after multiband therapy or treatment with removable appliances. The tooth positioner is not a retainer but an active appliance for fixing a new masticatory pattern and a new intercuspation, for 1.0- to 1.5-mm corrections of tooth position, for controlled relapse before the use of a retainer, for patients who grind or clench, and for skeletal stabilization after maxillofacial surgery. The positioner is an appliance for eventual fine adjustment of the mandible into the centric position. This requires skull- and joint-related registration and fabrication in an articulator.

A diagnostic setup is first produced for **fabrication of a tooth positioner**. A setup is a saw-cut model in which all the teeth to be corrected are fitted with thin brass pins. The pins provide sufficient retention to the model teeth in the sagittal plane but allow changes of position in the vertical plane and rotation of the sawn-out model teeth.

The teeth in the setup are placed in the desired position without the sagittal relationship of the teeth being lost. In the correct position, all the teeth are fixed with adhesive wax and checked in the articulator via lateral movements. The positioner is then fabricated from silicone, self-curing acrylic, or thermoplastic resin. It is molded like a thick squash bite that encases all the teeth up to about 2 mm above the gingival margin; in the buccal and lingual area, it is 2 to 3 mm thick, and the interocclusal block is also about 2 mm thick.

Fixed Orthodontic Appliances

Tooth movements with active spring components, which contact the tooth in a punctiform or linear fashion, are basically achieved by single-point and two-point application of force. Bodily tooth movement by multipoint application of force cannot be performed with removable active plates. Bodily tooth movements are only possible if the tooth is rigidly contained and this rigid mounting is pushed in the desired direction parallel to an additional guide.

Rigid mountings encompass the tooth to be moved with a broad steel band. A mounting is welded to this steel band. A guide splint can be incorporated into this mounting, with which the tooth is moved.

The **technique for fixed appliances** involves fixing prefabricated auxiliaries to the teeth to allow the forces to act on the teeth. These auxiliaries can be steel bands, which already have the necessary mountings or can be welded in the individual position. The outer surface of the bands has a high-glaze finish, and the inner surface is rough so that it can be cemented onto the teeth.

The prefabricated mountings are referred to as **brackets** and **tubes**. In addition, lingual cleats can be used, which are double hooks that are welded onto the lingual side of the band and can receive elastics. These auxiliary parts are welded onto the bands or, as is usually the case today, bonded or cemented directly onto the tooth surface.

The **active components** in this technique are spring hard stainless steel wires that are braided with a round or square cross section and have high elasticity. The wires are shaped into the ideal arch form that is to be achieved at the completion of treatment. The auxiliaries and wires are supplied ready-made; the bands can also be prepared by the practitioner. This means that it is possible to produce fixed appliances directly on the patient; they supplement or replace removable active plates in certain treatment situations. A brief outline of the operating principle is provided here so that dental technicians can undertake certain partial jobs involved in fabrication.

Modern **multiband appliances** are multipurpose fixed appliances that can be used to do the following:

- Eliminate tipping and crowding of individual teeth
- Translate teeth and groups of teeth mesially and distally
- Correct faulty positioning of individual teeth (eg, lifting partially or completely buried teeth into the dental arch)
- Shift teeth in parallel planes
- Eliminate dental arch deformations
- Balance occlusal discrepancies and differences in occlusal height

These are all anomalies of tooth position that can also be remedied with an active plate. However, fixed appliances are predominantly used in late cases or when an active plate cannot be worn.

The **effect of fixed appliances** is based on the elastic spring forces of wires and elastics as well as screw forces acting specifically on the teeth, periodontal tissues, alveolar processes, jawbones, and TMJs.

Advantages of fixed appliances

- Can be used universally.
- Almost any correction aimed at an ideal arch form can be performed.
- Treatment period is relatively short (even in severe cases) and clear and manageable for the patient.
- All the auxiliaries are prefabricated and can be placed directly in the patient by the dentist.
- Corrections can be made immediately and directly in follow-up appointments.
- Patient cooperation is not required to ensure compliance.
- No damage to the appliance due to improper handling by patients.
- Treatment program is direct with straightforward planning.

Disadvantages of fixed appliances

- The amount of force cannot be objectively monitored.
- The appliance acts continuously with no interruption.
- Tissue damage, such as root resorption and shortening of the alveolar ridges, is possible.
- Limited cleaning ability with an increased risk of caries.
- Frequent radiographic checks are necessary.
- Multiband appliances or bonded brackets have an adverse impact in the social context.

Multiband technique

The mechanism of action of fixed appliances is based on an archwire being fixed in the brackets under tension. When the archwire is relaxed, it pulls the teeth in the direction of relaxation. The arches are made of thin and highly flexible wire that bridges the distances between the individual brackets. If the archwires are too thick, the periodontium might be damaged; if the elasticity of the wire is exceeded, it could be permanently deformed and become ineffective.

The **principle of treatment** involves controlling the orthodontic movements of the teeth with increasingly strong wires and bringing the teeth into the desired ideal position. The intraoral archwire is activated or the next-stronger archwire is inserted.

Activation is achieved by specific bending of the inserted wire to bring about horizontal changes of position, vertical shifts of position, or rotation movements.

The **treatment phases** of multiband techniques relate to the changes of tooth position:

1. Leveling phase involves eliminating vertical and horizontal positional anomalies.
2. Guidance and contraction phase involves movements along the arch for space closure.
3. Idealization phase means aligning all the teeth in the ideal position.
4. Retention phase takes place over a prolonged period after the active treatment is completed.

The **direction of pull** and hence the direction of movement of the teeth is always toward an ideal dental arch because, when the archwire is relaxed after the treatment, it resumes the ideal form it had before being put under tension.

The **brackets** are the precisely fitting guide splints for the wires, similar to the components in slide attachments but with wider-fitting tolerances. These guide splints are formed as half-tubes for the round wires or as square slots for square wire (Figs 10-83 and 10-84).

The **positioning of brackets** on the vestibular surfaces of the teeth is done so that the guide splints are vertical to the tooth axis and at the height of the contact points. The brackets are attached so that they lie at the midlines of the teeth, almost at a single height and in line (Fig 10-85). Before the start of treatment, the teeth are in their shifted axes. Therefore, the brackets need to be related to the tooth axis, and the guide slot for the square archwire needs to be aligned with the contact points. At the completion of treatment, the brackets should lie in common alignment. Attaching the brackets is the most important aspect of using fixed orthodontic appliances because this

Fig 10-83 The fixation components are the basic building blocks of fixed band appliances. The brackets have a vertical slot with a defined slot width and depth. The bracket body sits on a base that is bonded to the tooth or soldered to a steel band. There are wings at the sides of the bracket that receive ligatures (fixing wires) or elastics.

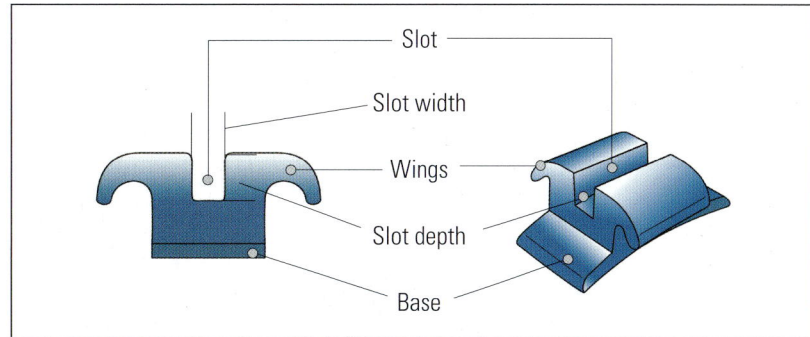

Slot
Slot width
Wings
Slot depth
Base

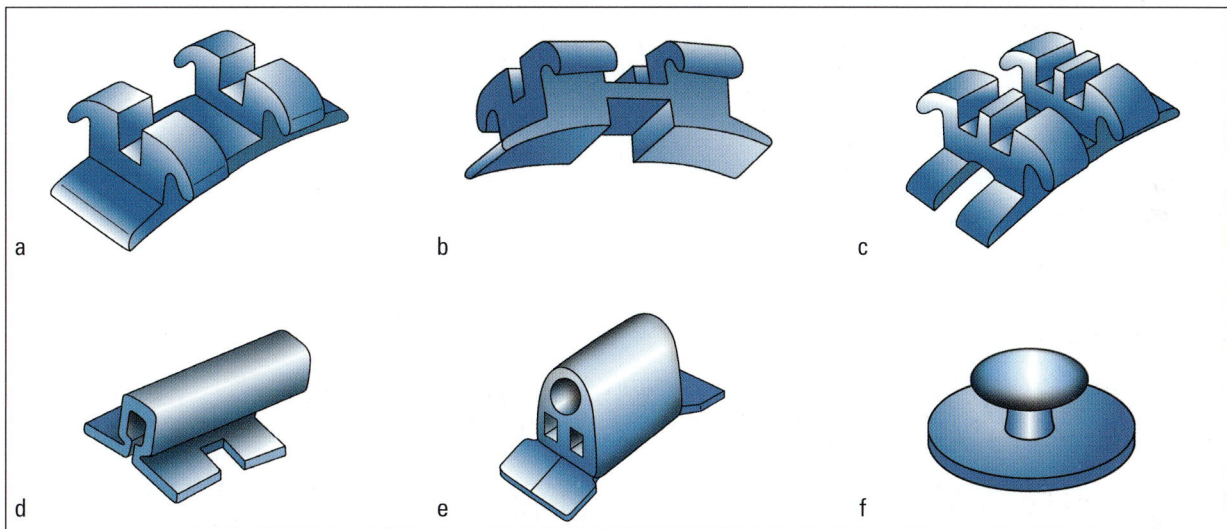

a
b
c
d
e
f

Fig 10-84 Various bracket designs are available. *(a)* Edgewise twin bracket for square bows. *(b)* A special design is the edgewise twin bracket with a vertical slot for additional components. *(c)* The special bracket with gingival and occlusal slots as well as slots close to the band is suitable for the edgewise and twin-wire technique. *(d and e)* The tubes receive the bow end and are usually fixed to the first molar. The tube width corresponds to the slot dimension of the brackets. As well as the simple tube, there are also combination tubes available for extraoral anchorage. *(f)* For the lingual surfaces of the teeth, there are additional lingual buttons for suspending elastics and ligatures.

Fig 10-85 The brackets should be mounted so that the middles of the slots lie on the midlines of the teeth, roughly at one height and in line with each other. Before the start of treatment, the teeth lie in the displaced axes. Therefore, it is necessary to relate the brackets to the tooth axis and the cusp height and to align the contact points using the slot for a square wire. At the end of treatment, the brackets should lie in common alignment.

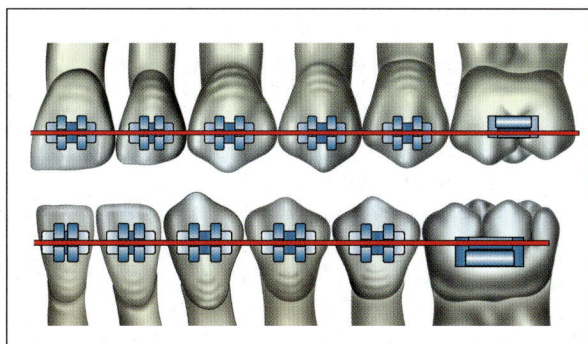

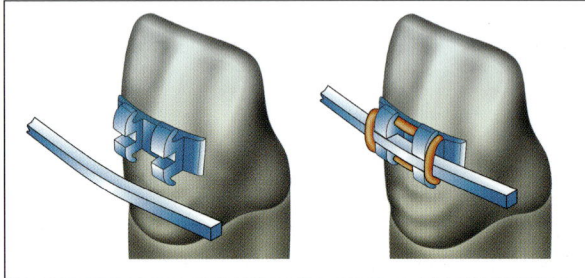

Fig 10-86 The bracket is bonded directly to the tooth enamel. An appropriately sized square archwire fits into the bracket and is anchored in the guide with small rubber loops. The square wire now pulls the tooth in the desired direction, depending on how the square archwire has been activated. A bodily movement is possible. The application of force on a tooth treated in this way corresponds to multipoint force application.

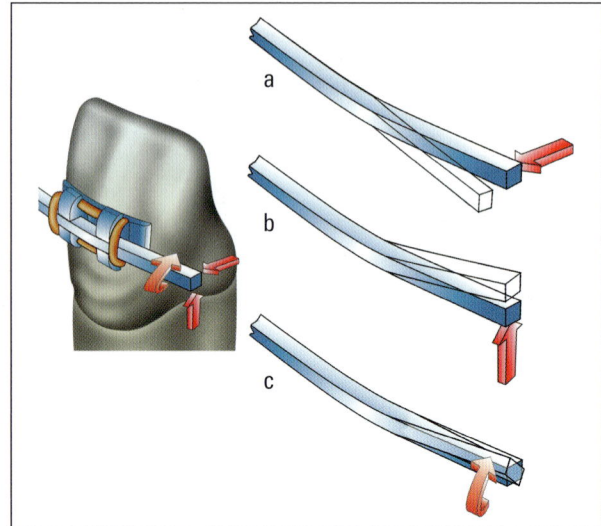

Fig 10-87 Bodily movement means that the tooth can be shifted in parallel as well as tipped and rotated. Three types of bends on the archwire are identified in relation to the reference planes: (a) first-order bend made in the horizontal plane; (b) second-order bend made in the vertical plane; (c) third-order bend made in the arch axis.

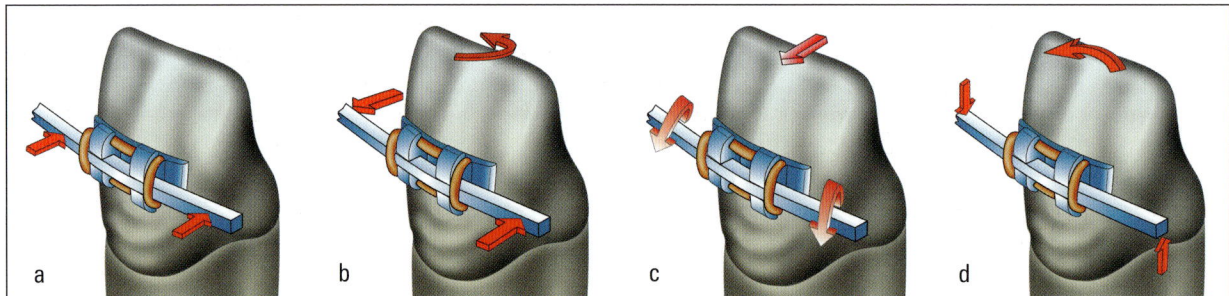

Fig 10-88 (a) When the wire is activated in the horizontal plane equally in one direction, the tooth is shifted in parallel. (b) If the wire is activated in the opposite direction, the tooth is rotated around its vertical axis. (c) Twisting the wire in the arch axis tips the tooth around this axis. (d) A second-order bend rotates the tooth around an axis in the horizontal plane.

determines the eventual tooth position. Single-tooth movements along the archwire or tipping parallel to it can also be carried out. If a space needs to be closed, the teeth to be corrected can be moved by elastics because the brackets are not only joined to the archwire but also linked to each other with elastics. The brackets and hence the teeth are pulled along the archwire.

Selective movement is possible when several anchor teeth are firmly fixed to the wire and the tooth being moved is flexibly connected to the wire. If a tipped tooth is to be aligned, a spring can be incorporated into the bracket and hooked onto the archwire under tension. Then the tooth being aligned is not connected directly to the archwire but indirectly via the spring.

Discrepancies of occlusal position can be remedied by elastics under maxillomandibular tension. If the elastics are stretched between individual antagonists, an open bite can also be

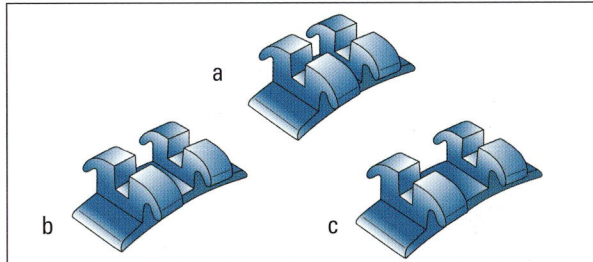

Fig 10-89 The edgewise twin brackets are available in narrow *(a)*, medium *(b)*, and wide *(c)* sizes to match the different tooth forms.

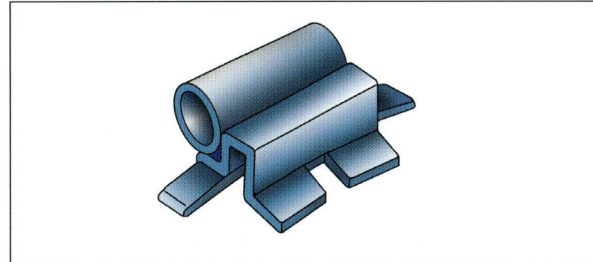

Fig 10-90 The combination tube is fitted with a tube for the edgewise arch and a tube for a facebow.

corrected. A tooth twisted in the dentition can be pulled into the normal position with elastics that are attached lingually to the tooth (via lingual cleats) then guided to the archwire.

The **palatal (or maxillary) expansion appliance** is a fixed active appliance comprising four orthodontic bands and an expansion screw that is cemented in place in the mouth. It rapidly pushes the halves of the maxilla apart within a few weeks and causes a fracture in the narrower area of the midpalatal suture. The aim is expansion in cases of a severely constricted maxilla with a unilateral or bilateral reverse articulation; at the same time, the nose is widened. In the process, the mucosal coverage of the oral and nasal cavity as well as the periosteal covering remain continuously intact. The fracture gap that is opened and kept open fully heals in about 6 months.

Figures 10-86 to 10-88 illustrate principles of the multiband technique.

Edgewise technique

The edgewise arch (square arch) technique is described here as the typical method of fixed orthodontic treatment. The edgewise technique involves working a square, spring hard archwire that is adapted to the desired width and form of the dental arch with special arch formers and is connected to the teeth with fixing components.

The **fixing components** are square brackets and tubes for fixing the ideal archwire (orthodontic ideal arch) (Figs 10-89 and 10-90). The standard edgewise bracket has a square, horizontal slot, but twin brackets with two adjacent slots can also be used. The brackets are matched to the different

tooth shapes in size, width, and base curvature. The fixation components can be fixed onto a cemented band or directly to the tooth by a direct bonding technique.

When **banding** teeth, the band must not damage the marginal border and tooth, which is achieved by good gingival and occlusal fit. The cement is used not only to fix the band but also for hygiene reasons because it fills the "gap" between tooth and band.

Acrylic, ceramic, or steel brackets are used in the **bonding technique**. Retention in the enamel is prepared by acid etching (eg, with phosphoric acid) of the teeth. The bracket is bonded to the etched tooth surface with a uniformly thin layer of adhesive.

In the **edgewise technique**, the archwires for each individual tooth are bent under tension: The edgewise (square) arch is first adapted to the ideal dental arch, then the wire is bent roughly into the position of the malpositioned tooth but only approximately. Once the wire is firmly attached to the tooth in the bracket, the tooth will be pulled in the direction of tension of the wire (Fig 10-91).

The **edgewise wire** does not sit fully in the bracket but is lifted out slightly. It is held in the bracket guide with small, taut elastomeric modules (like rubber bands). Forces now act on the tooth in two ways: the spring force of the tightened edgewise arch and the pulling force of the elastomeric modules. The forces act three-dimensionally on the tooth via the wire to correct the position of individual teeth, sections of the dental arch, or the entire dental arch.

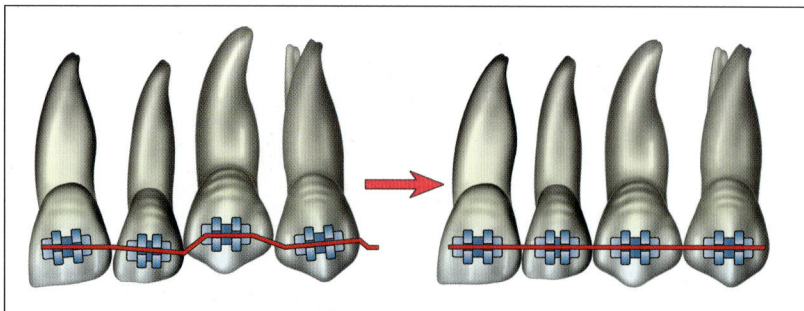

Fig 10-91 The edgewise arch is tightened in the activation areas and thus pulls each individual tooth in the desired direction; the force arises from pre-tension of the arch and at the same time from the bracing on each of the teeth involved. Treatment is completed when the edgewise arch takes on the harmonious dental arch form and the teeth are pulled into that position.

The **concept of the ideal arch** supposes that in an optimal masticatory system every tooth is correctly positioned in terms of anatomical contact points. Different prefabricated archwires are available for different individual sizes of dental arch. As well as narrow ones, there are wide versions for the maxilla and the mandible: ellipses, parabola, U-shaped, and V-shaped. Each archwire is divided into symmetric segments: anterior, canine, premolar, and molar segments. The placement of the fixing components is determined by this arrangement.

Fixing components can be **placed** in a variety of ways. Placement on the vestibular and the lingual surfaces of the teeth is possible.

The **bracket** is positioned in the middle on the dental crown while the horizontal bracket slot lies parallel to the incisal edge or the cusp tip so that, if the archwire were straight, the teeth would be in the regular position in relation to each other. The purpose of an edgewise approach is to guide the bracket position in the direction of the individual ideal arch with the orthodontic arches employed.

At the **start of treatment**, a highly elastic archwire is used to guide the teeth continuously in the desired direction; each new pair of archwire comes closer and closer to the ideal arch form. Each new archwire is stronger than the previous one and is prebent more precisely. The gradual alignment of the rows of teeth is characteristic of the edgewise technique. The archwire can be passively guided past individual teeth that are not to be incorporated into the ideal arch until a later stage.

There are various passive and active loops available as **special components** for individual correction of the position of single teeth in relation to the occlusal plane:

- Vertical loop for correction in the horizontal plane
- Horizontal loop for correction of extruded or intruded teeth
- Delta loop for correction of horizontal and vertical anomalies of posterior teeth
- Combination helix for correction in the vertical and horizontal planes for alignment and rotation
- Closing loops and bull loops for space closure in the mandible and maxilla

Figures 10-92 and 10-93 illustrate banded arches in the edgewise technique.

Multiband appliances

The **Begg technique** is an orthodontic technique with fixed appliances that uses special wires and brackets. The special types of bracket for this technique are called *Begg brackets*. Tipping as well as single-point contact can be achieved with these brackets. Tooth movements are enforced with light elastics. The archwire is fixed in the slots with lock pins.

The treatment takes place in three stages:

- **Stage 1:** The occlusion is opened, and the anterior teeth are placed in the edge-to-edge position; at the same time, crowding and tooth rotations are eliminated.
- **Stage 2:** If extraction therapy has taken place, the extraction spaces are closed.
- **Stage 3:** The tipped incisors and posterior teeth are aligned. Finally, fine adjustment of the teeth is carried out; the appliance is then removed.

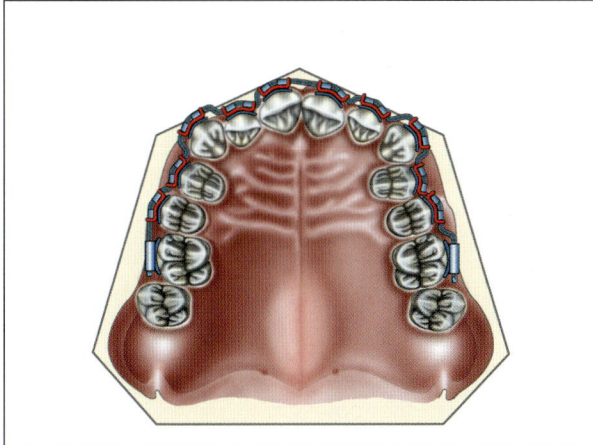

Fig 10-92 A fully banded jaw is shown here. The edgewise arch is preshaped on a model and given activation bends. The pre-tension of the arch must be checked and corrected in regular appointments. Depending on the progress of the treatment, new edgewise arches are shaped to replace the old ones.

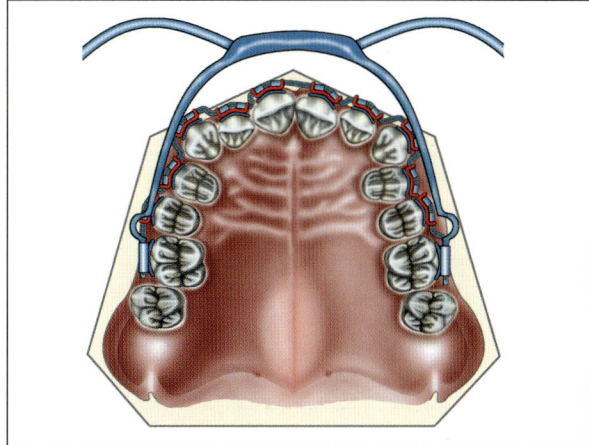

Fig 10-93 The banded jaw can be anchored extraorally with a facebow, either to fix the first molars or to achieve a shift of occlusal position.

Light wire technique denotes the use of fixed orthodontic appliances in which the outer arch of round highly elastic wire (0.3 to 0.45 mm) is fitted into the brackets on all the teeth. The force effect is minimized by guiding the wire into loops bent inward between the brackets. The arms of the bent-in loops run parallel at the same height before placement in the brackets. The basic shape of the arch corresponds to the intended ideal dental arch form. The archwire is inserted into the brackets under tension and fixed in place. It is anchored with horizontal tubes to the molars, which are also banded.

After fixation, the wire is under highly varied pre-tension for each tooth, depending on the defective position of the tooth concerned. In extreme positional anomalies, several archwires have to be individually shaped and inserted in successive treatment steps.

The *Ricketts technique* (bioprogressive technique) uses very thin and elastic wires that are gradually applied step by step to the banded teeth. The teeth are controlled with loop arches as far as possible and moved without frictional resistance.

The *twin arch technique* refers to the working of two archwires made of 0.25-mm wire that are guided into special brackets and tubes. The thin, spring hard wires exert only very weak spring forces. In addition, pressure and tension springs are used to tighten the wires.

The *bracket adhesive technique* refers to the multiband technique in which the orthodontic fixing components (brackets and tubes) are no longer fixed via bands but are directly bonded to the enamel pretreated with acid. An epoxy resin adhesive is used to bond brackets made of acrylic, porcelain, or metal to the enamel surface that has been conditioned with 40% phosphoric acid (H_3PO_4).

Direct bracket fixation requires no approximal separation of the teeth being banded. Only a few residual spaces remain after band removal, incompletely erupted teeth can be bonded, and better prevention of caries and gingivitis is ensured. Caries lesions are possible with the bracket adhesive technique in the marginal area around the brackets and in the interdental area, so intensive oral hygiene is required, with support from fluoridation measures.

Bonded brackets can be worked more quickly and more simply than bands. All individual tooth forms can be covered by a few standard bracket types, making extensive, costly band supports unnecessary. Vertical and horizontal placement of the brackets is far more difficult with the ad-

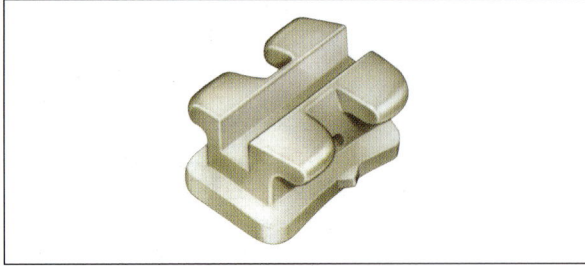

Fig 10-94 The standard brackets are supplied in tooth-colored acrylic for direct bracket fixation.

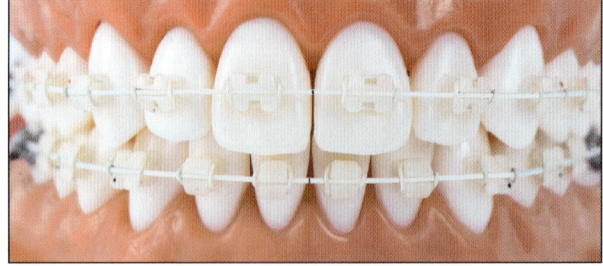

Fig 10-95 The tooth-colored brackets have high strength and high color stability; they are relatively unnoticeable in the mouth.

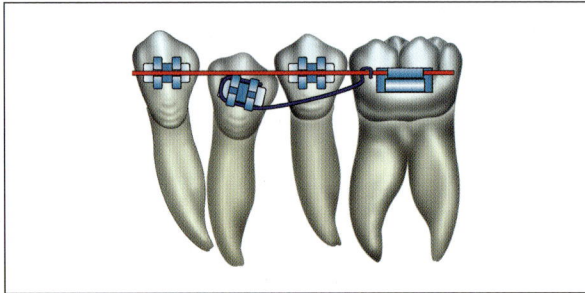

Fig 10-96 With additional wire components, the malposition of individual teeth can be corrected. Tipped teeth can be straightened with an uprighting spring until they can be integrated into the edgewise arch.

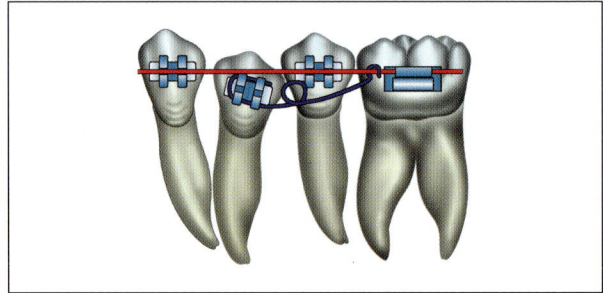

Fig 10-97 An uprighting spring can be fitted with a loop (activation eyelet). The spring can be inserted into the standard bracket and suspended in the edgewise arch.

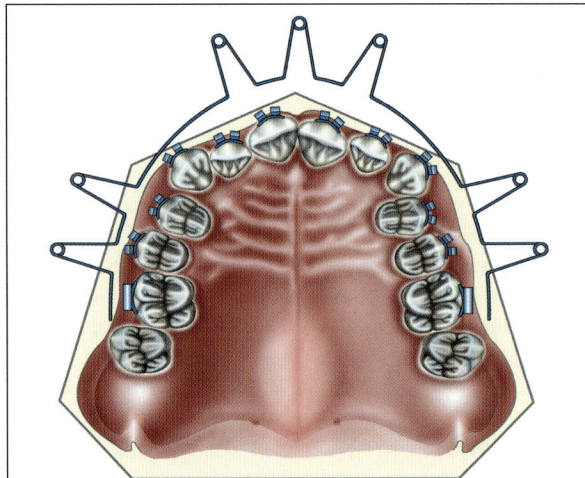

Fig 10-98 Instead of an edgewise arch, a relatively thin wire, as in the light wire technique, can be used. The round, highly elastic wire has the ideal dental arch form and several activation loops. The brackets are fixed to the teeth in the regular position.

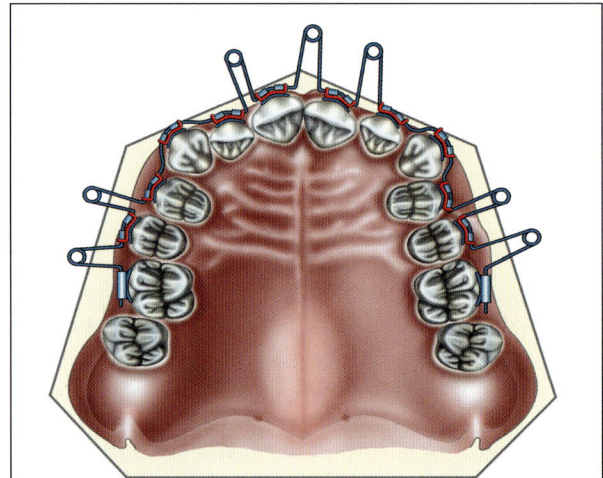

Fig 10-99 The wire is inserted under tension and fixed in the brackets. It now exerts continuous but very gentle force, which decreases gradually by the end of the treatment. The multipoint application of force is produced by the special form of bracket as a horizontal tube.

hesive technique. Bracket removal and subsequent enamel polishing are labor-intensive, and enamel chips or adhesive strands can appear in the enamel mantle.

High bond strength requires the acrylic to penetrate into the exposed microporosities of the conditioned enamel. The etched enamel surface must therefore have the following structure:

• Minimal, irreversible loss of height
• Rough, retentive microrelief with intraprismatic spaces
• Considerable enlargement of surface area for better wettability of the enamel

After etching, the dissolved residues of calcium crystals are removed from the enamel surface to achieve tight interlinking between the adhesive and the enamel.

Figures 10-94 to 10-99 illustrate various considerations of multiband appliances.

Lingual technique

Fixed appliances can be positioned lingually when the design of the lingual brackets is adapted to the oral conditions. The height of the brackets with adhesive base, bracket body, slots, and wings and the distance of the archwire from the tooth surface determine wearing comfort or can cause speech restriction or tongue irritation. The appliance must therefore have a very flat design.

In the *Incognito appliance system* from 3M Unitek, a computerized production process is used to customize and position the brackets for the individual patient. A precision silicone impression is first taken. The *silicone impression* must be completely bubble-free. Teeth and the whole gingival margin must be precisely recorded in the impression so that the tooth axes can be accurately defined.

Two dental stone models are prepared. In one model, the teeth are sawn out and set up in the ideal occlusal position intended at the end of treatment. This setup is then digitalized with a 3D scanner to produce a precise, virtual 3D model.

Based on this *virtual model*, a customized set of brackets for the individual patient is generated on the computer with special software. Appropriate bonding sites on the lingual surfaces are

first shaped, then the optimal positioning of the bracket bodies is determined. The individualized base of the bracket covers the greater part of the lingual surface with good accuracy of fit, which makes it much easier to carry out precise positioning and any rebonding that may be required.

After the *individual components* (base, bracket body, hook) have been precisely positioned on the screen, the rapid prototyping process takes place as the virtual brackets are converted into wax. Final completion can be done by precision casting with high-gold alloys. Thereafter, the correct dimensions of the slots for each bracket are checked by hand. The diameters of the arches and the slot sizes are perfectly harmonized with each other with variations of not more than 0.008 mm between slot and arch. Relative movements between the two parts—to the detriment of correction accuracy—are virtually ruled out.

The *finished gold brackets* are positioned and temporarily bonded onto the second dental stone model. From this situation of accurately positioned brackets, a silicone impression is taken in which the brackets are definitively fixed. The bonding surfaces of the brackets in the impression are pretreated for bonding to the tooth surfaces. The orthodontist can use this *silicone key* to fix all the brackets to the lingual surfaces with a special bonding agent in one operation. The brackets are then in the precise position that was predefined in the laboratory.

The *arch definition data* are generated at the same time as the virtual construction of the brackets and help to produce an arch sequence involving several archwires. The *course of the arch* is defined virtually on the computer and related to the position of the brackets. Highly complex bends result from the individual course of the arch, and these bends are made with a computer-controlled machine. The arch runs parallel and fits very closely to the tooth surfaces.

The *inserted wire* is shaped so that it pushes the teeth into the correct position during the course of treatment.

The *regulating thrusts* are performed by using elastics with the archwire. Insertion of the wires into the slots (ligation) is done with rubber link chains or wire ligatures that fix the wire very tightly in the slot. The regulating thrust arises from the differently sized archwires. The initial thermoelastic wires recover from their bending once they are at oral temperature and, in so doing, pull the tooth that is bodily clasped via the bracket.

These **superelastic arches** are used at the start of treatment to resolve malpositions. Later, non-superelastic (plastic deformable) arches are used that develop differing recovery forces due to different cross sections.

The **advantages of the Incognito appliance system** are the following:

• Accurate, arch-guided transfer of forces
• Adaptation of the brackets, even in cases of severe rotation and short clinical crowns
• Flexible, universal usability due to customized sets of brackets
• Esthetically highly advantageous

Figure 10-100 illustrates the production sequence for the Incognito appliance system.

Precision silicone impression.

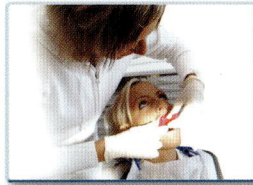

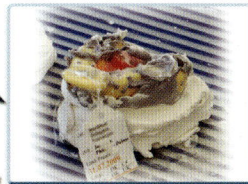

Model fabrication: two models made of dental stone.

A model is stripped down into dies and set up in a setup model.

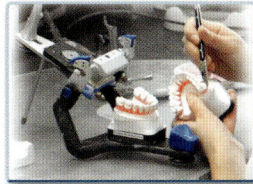

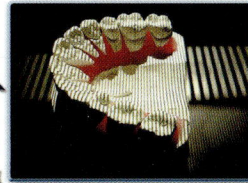

The setup model and second model are scanned.

The virtual model is checked, and tooth axes and bonding surfaces are defined on the computer.

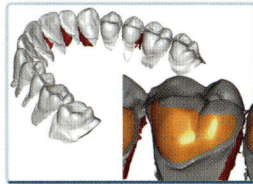

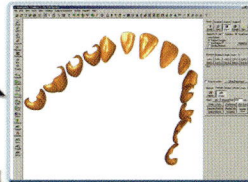

The lingual bonding surfaces are defined over the entire row of teeth.

Bracket bodies and hooks are precisely positioned, and the arch definition data are generated.

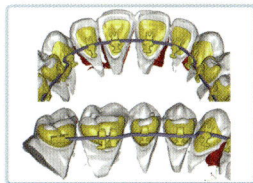

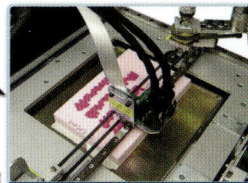

Virtual brackets are plotted in wax in a rapid prototyping process.

Brackets are fabricated in a casting technique with high-gold alloys.

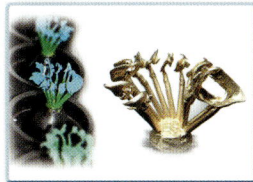

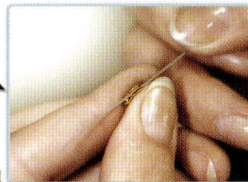

Quality control: slot width and depth are manually checked.

The brackets are fixed in their precise positions on the second model.

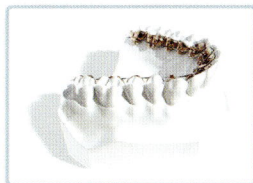

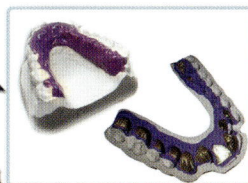

A transfer key is produced from silicone.

The arch sequences are curved with the computer-generated arch definition data.

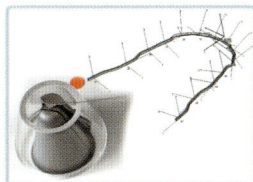

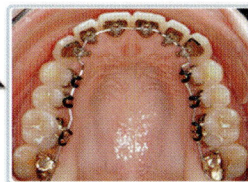

The brackets are bonded in a single working step with the transfer key, and the first archwire is inserted.

Fig 10-100 Production sequence for the Incognito appliance system. (Courtesy of 3M Unitek.)

Splint Therapy

Functional Disorders of the Orofacial System

The **orofacial system** includes the maxilla and the mandible with the sets of teeth, the masticatory muscles, the temporomandibular joints (TMJs), and the neuronal control with motor end plates. Functional diseases of this system develop as a result of multifactorial mechanisms. A functionally impaired masticatory system will display monotonous movement sequences, for instance, whereas variable movement patterns are seen in a healthy system (Fig 11-1).

Under certain circumstances, **functional disorders** may not cause any distinct symptoms in a patient and can only be identified by thorough investigation. If symptoms do occur, they frequently affect the muscles of mastication and the TMJs and are evident as tension, muscle and joint pains, jaw clicking, migraine-type headaches, and ringing in the ears (tinnitus). They can be divided into *myopathies* (muscular diseases) and *arthropathies* (joint diseases).

The purely **muscular diseases** range from dull muscle pain during mandibular movements to genuine tissue inflammation, muscle spasms through to changes in the muscle tissue (Fig 11-2). As well as physical illnesses, psychologic problems are a possible cause of muscular disorders.

The **physical causes** include occlusal discrepancies due to missing or displaced teeth, joint deformations and similar conditions, head or neck injuries, extremely wide mouth opening, or pathologic muscle tension due to postural abnormalities. Wrongly shaped chewing surfaces, wear facets in fillings, or prosthetic teeth indicate occlusal disorders that may induce muscular hyperactivity or parafunctional mandibular movements.

Psychologic problems caused by chronic stress lead to hyperactivity of the masticatory muscles and abnormal, enforced movement patterns (parafunctional habits). Such

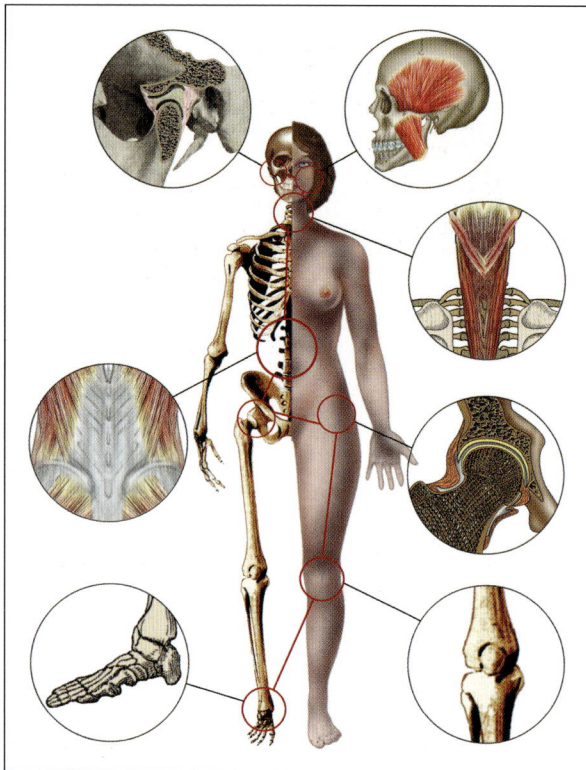

Fig 11-1 Functional disorders of the stomatognathic system (here a synonym for masticatory system) concern functional and structural disorders affecting the teeth, the TMJs, and the muscles of mastication. The terms *craniomandibular dysfunction* and *temporomandibular dysfunction* are used to refer to these functional disorders. The functions of the stomatognathic system are closely related to the functions of the cervical spine and the atlanto-occipital and atlantoaxial joints and can therefore be related to a diversity of symptoms, including diffuse toothache, tension in the jaw, mouth-opening problems, jaw clicking, tinnitus, facial pain, headache, pain at the back of the neck, tension headache, migraine, deafness, shoulder pain, lumbar pain, and spinal blockages. A connection with joint disorders in the hip, knee, and foot area is also suspected. In dentistry, this involves something of a paradigm shift: The entire masticatory system is no longer treated independently of the rest of the body, but close collaboration with orthopedists, osteopathic physicians, and physical therapists is sought.

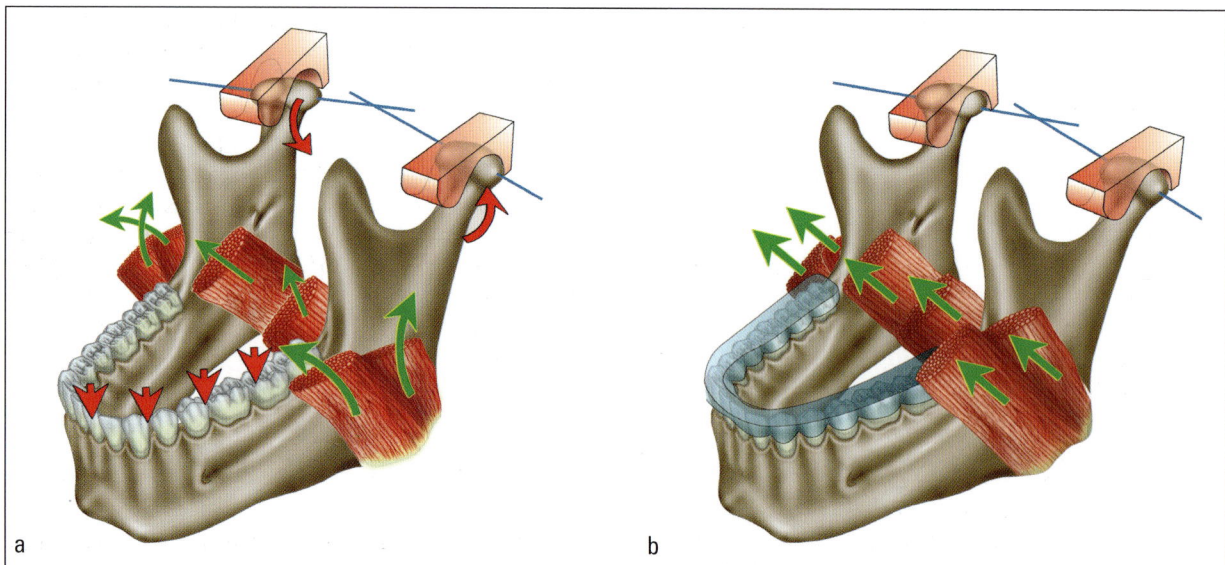

Fig 11-2 *(a)* Muscle incoordination results in faulty loading of the joints and a traumatic occlusion. *(b)* The aim of splint therapy is to restore the biostatics whereby the joints are unloaded as a result of balanced muscle function.

Fig 11-3 The histologic structural elements of a healthy TMJ are functionally harmonized parts that fit together: (1) mandibular fossa *(fossa mandibularis)*; (2) articular disc *(discus articularis)*; (3) joint capsule *(capsula articularis)*; (4) inferior joint space *(spatium articulare inferius)*; (5) condyle/mandibular head *(caput mandibulae)*. Functional disorders affect individual parts of the joint differently.

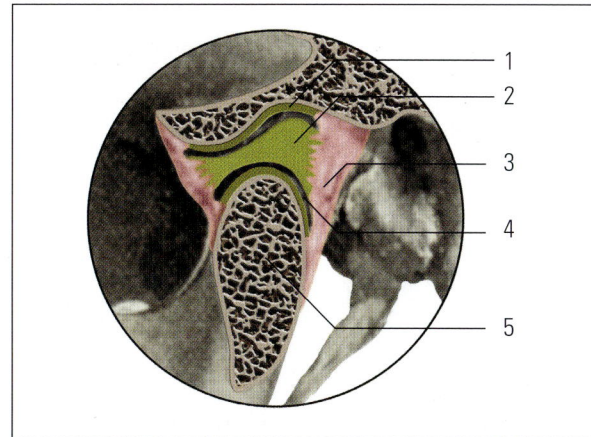

parafunctional activities always produce muscular problems, eg, grinding the teeth while asleep (bruxism). With bruxism, the force and duration of tooth contacts are prolonged; the muscles and periodontal tissues are overloaded; and tension headaches, joint pains, and muscle tension in the neck area can develop.

Physiologic tooth contacts (approximately 40 minutes a day) take place during chewing and swallowing, and the mean force level is 20 to 30 N, with peaks of up to 600 N. Periodontal tissues and masticatory muscles have long recovery periods in between. Loads of up to 950 N can arise from parafunctional masticatory movements such as grinding and gnashing of teeth.

Teeth grinding (bruxism or bruxing) refers to unconscious, rhythmic, compulsive, nonfunctional gnashing or clenching of the teeth by intermittent or persistent contractions of the masseter and temporal muscles, which is associated with grinding sounds.

Teeth grinding mostly happens at night during *REM* (rapid eye movement) sleep, but it can sometimes occur during the day, especially in stressful situations. A distinction is made between waking or daytime bruxism and sleep bruxism.

Disorders in the neurotransmitter system of the brain are considered to be *causes of teeth grinding*, which means bruxism is a centrally controlled and not a peripherally controlled disorder. Smoking, alcohol, illness, trauma, drug misuse, psychiatric disorders, and malocclusions favor this parafunctional activity. Stress or abnormally suppressed aggression as well as other psychologic factors have less influence than was previously thought to be the case.

Clenching as an apparently milder form of grinding, in which the teeth are only pressed onto each other and not rubbed against each other, is nearly as harmful. The abnormal masticatory forces during clenching and the transverse stresses during grinding lead to severe periodontal damage, considerable abrasion of the occlusal surfaces with wedge-shaped defects, and TMJ diseases and myopathies, muscle pains, or restricted movement of the masticatory muscles. Insomnia, sporadic headaches, and pains in the nape, back, neck, or shoulders arise.

These parafunctional movements can be treated and muscle tone normalized with what are known as *bruxism splints* or *muscle relaxation splints* in the form of occlusal guards. Splint therapy is intended to prevent damage to teeth, reduce grinding and clenching activities, and prevent sleep disturbances.

TMJ Diseases and Disorders

Diseases of the TMJs are mainly intra-articular disorders (Fig 11-3), with distinctions drawn between reversible microtrauma and irreversible macrotrauma and between congenital and acquired developmental disorders. Inflammatory microtraumas are joint noises (eg, clicking) occur-

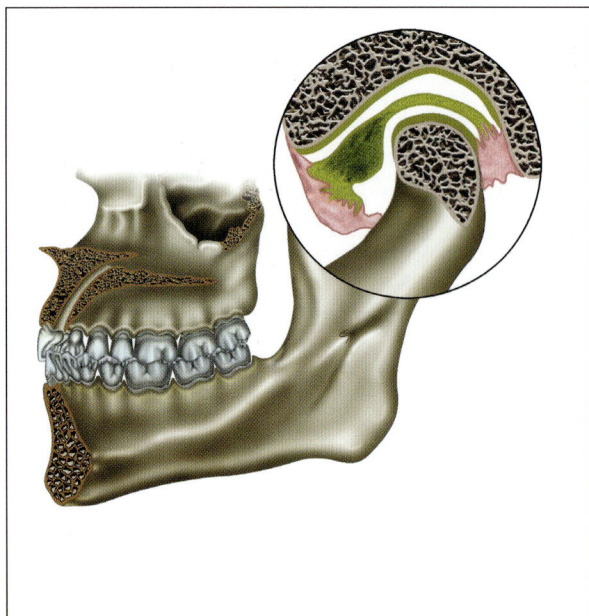

Fig 11-4 In anterior disc displacement, the disc lies anterior to the condyle while the mandible is in centric occlusion. It can be displaced centrally forward or laterally. Anterior displacement may remain constant during all mandibular movements so that all excursions of the mandible are associated with massive TMJ pain. However, when the disc slides into the correct condyle-disc relationship during mandibular movements, this is known as *disc displacement with reduction*.

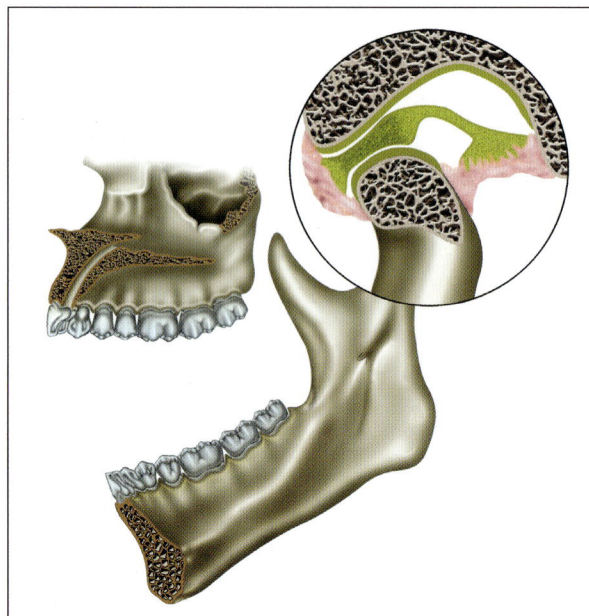

Fig 11-5 When the mouth is opened, the disc slides onto the condyle, which is accompanied by a distinct clicking or popping of the joint. At maximum mouth opening, the condyle-disc relationship corresponds to the normal position. If centric occlusion is resumed, the disc slides back in front of the condyle with a clicking or popping sound.

ring occasionally or constantly that result from rough joint surfaces caused by compression. If the compression is removed by means of a muscle relaxation splint (centric relation splint), the microtrauma is also eliminated.

Irreversible macrotraumas are partial or total, usually anterior displacements of the articular disc, with damage to the disc and to other joint structures, as well as massive joint changes (TMJ osteoarthritis; see Fig 11-6). In the case of partial or total anterior *disc displacement* (or *disc derangement*), the disc can be pushed back into its original position on opening (disc displacement with reduction), which is associated with a typical clicking or popping sound. Disc derangements and the associated displacement of the condyles are often caused by tooth loss, or the absence of individual support areas, and by occlusal disorders.

In this condition, the **articular disc** is displaced forward; ie, the disc lies anterior to the condyle when the mouth is closed (Fig 11-4). When the

mouth is opened, the disc slides onto the condyle (reduction of the disc), which is associated with a distinct clicking or popping of the joint. On maximum mouth opening, the condyle, disc, and fossa lie in the correct positions in relation to each other; once the mouth is closed, the disc slides forward again (disc prolapse) with distinct clicking (Fig 11-5). This opening and closing movement can be painful, but this functional disorder usually follows a pain-free course.

In **anterior disc displacement without reduction**, the disc remains anterior to the condyle throughout the entire opening and closing movement. In this case, the disc has sustained degenerative changes. Distinct pain occurs in the joint area during mandibular movement, and the mouth-opening movement is restricted.

Anterior disc displacement is treated with splints for repositioning the mandible. As a result, the disc is brought into a normal or improved position.

Fig 11-6 TMJ osteoarthritis. *(a)* Chronic traumatization of the TMJ (eg, due to bruxism) can affect the disc and the cartilage on the articulating surface. The disc may be abraded and even perforated, while the cartilage may be fibrillated, chipped, or worn away to the bone. *(b)* One form of degenerative change to tissue parts involves fusion of disc tissue with the cartilage alongside physiologic wear.

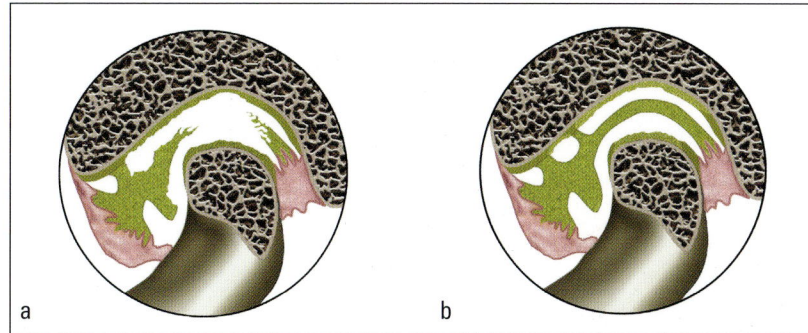

Degenerative changes (TMJ osteoarthritis) are apparent as extensive damage to articular soft tissues, such as massive wear of the joint cartilage, fibrillation of the bone at the condyles, and fibrillation of the disc, which may be perforated or completely abraded (Fig 11-6). As a result of these remodeling processes, mandibular movements are severely restricted, and stabbing pains occur in the joint area as well as rubbing joint noises. This is accompanied by functionally induced damage to the dental hard tissue, such as wear facets and wedge-shaped defects.

The *therapeutic measures* for functional disorders of the masticatory system are performed with occlusal guards, which change the occlusal conditions so that the TMJ symptoms are eliminated as well as the occlusal anomalies. Reorientation involving interaction of the occlusal pattern, muscles, joints, and nerves then ensues.

Splints produce physiologic, psychologic, and biomechanical effects as they:

- Stabilize the relationship between condyle and disc
- Remove occlusal interferences
- Relieve periodontal tissues (or implants)
- Diminish activities of the masticatory muscles
- Unload the TMJs
- Reduce tooth abrasion

They alter the vertical and anterior position of the mandible and the relationship of the condyle to the disc by repatterning the *neuromuscular habit*. Muscle pains, headaches, and subjective hearing problems can be eliminated in the process. Incorporating canine guidance into the splints keeps the posterior teeth apart during mandibular excursions. Movements out of centric occlusion lead to antagonist canine contact and disocclusion of the posterior teeth. The canine guidance produced by splints actually reduces contractile muscle activity considerably, which applies to chewing movements, teeth grinding, and eccentric clenching.

As muscle activity diminishes, the TMJ clicking during laterotrusive and protrusive excursions is reduced because the joints are relieved with less muscle contraction.

Splint Therapy for Functional Disorders

Splint therapy, as a biomechanical form of treatment, is used for a variety of functional disorders of the masticatory system. The treatment is carried out with occlusal splints and is indicated for:

- Myofascial pain in the TMJ area
- Acute TMJ inflammation
- Arthritic or rheumatic changes to the TMJ
- Parafunctional habits, such as nocturnal grinding and clenching of teeth
- Tinnitus, migraine, and tension headaches
- Vertical increase of occlusion and gnathologic occlusal changes
- Pre-prosthetic therapeutic measures

The terms *night guard, occlusal splint, occlusal plane, occlusion rim, occlusal splint,* and *stabili-*

Table 11-1   Summary of occlusal splints and intraoral appliances

Classification	Indications	Design
Reflex splints Stabilization splints Bruxism splints Anterior occlusal splints 	Interrupt parafunctional movement patterns Eliminate neuromuscular disorders Reduce muscle activity Achieve centric capability Stabilize the occlusion Treat bruxism Reduce periodontal loading and tooth abrasion	Firm elastic vacuum-formed sheets: • 1 to 2 mm thick • For the maxilla and the mandible • No occlusal guidance Acrylic splints with punctiform premature contact Prefabricated plastic sheets with capillary-linked cushions of water
Centric relation splints Michigan splint 	Restore the centric condylar position Neuromuscular relaxation for painful, tense muscles Create a pain-free joint position in TMJ osteoarthritis Treat advanced periodontitis Eliminate occlusal interferences	Hard acrylic splint for the maxilla covers all the teeth Flat occlusal surface for simultaneous occlusal contact of the mandibular occluding cusps Raises the occlusion by a maximum of 3 mm Canine guidance planes in the form of inclined planes for vertical opening in protrusive and lateral excursions
Eccentric splints Repositioning splints Distraction splints Interceptors 	Create the physiologic condyle-disc relationship Treat partial and total anterior disc displacement with and without reduction Eliminate joint clicking and TMJ pains Relieve compressed joints Stretch the muscles, ligaments, joint capsule, and neck of the joint	Acrylic splint for the maxilla and the mandible: • Areas into which the teeth bite if the occlusal depth is large • Anterior mandibular positioning and minimal occlusal raising • Wearing mode in the mandible Distraction splint/pivot splint: • Vacuum-formed splint for the maxilla with punctiform premature contact in the molar region (interceptor)
Special forms Hinge splints Aligners Retainers Mouthguards Miniplast splints	Treat obstructive sleep apnea Keep the upper airways clear Orthodontic treatment Fix the final tooth position Protect against injury in contact sports Various other minor treatments	Vacuum-formed sheets with tight fit for the maxilla and the mandible, connected with rods or screws to pull the mandible forward Series of stiff elastic vacuum-formed sheets fabricated according to constructed tooth position Stiff vacuum-formed sheets with approximately 10-mm-thick cushion Stiff or elastic vacuum-formed sheets for universal applications

zation splint are used as synonyms to describe the splints in splint therapy. There has been no systematic classification of these devices, so the collective term *occlusal splint* is used here. Occlusal splints can be classified differently based on their biomechanical effect, occlusal dimensions, and placement (whether in the maxilla or the mandible) as well as the materials used for their fabrication.

Occlusal splints are removable appliances for temporary use that are worn in the maxilla or the mandible. With these intraoral appliances, a new intercuspation position is created within the physiologic centric position of the mandible, and the occlusal relationships between the two dental arches are altered.

Night guards are transparent acrylic occlusion rims for the jaws that are worn at night. They are designed almost flat and have only a few depressions into which the opposing teeth occlude. Because acrylic is softer than teeth, the teeth no longer abrade each other but the guard instead. In addition, the TMJ is unloaded and relieved by a splint.

In addition to myoarthropathies (functional disorders of the muscle and joint complex), malocclusions, and occlusal anomalies, snoring and obstructive sleep apnea can be treated using **night guards.**

With splint therapy, there is **no splinting** such as that produced by elastic retentive components on partial dentures. Instead, splints separate the usual occlusion (decoupling the existing intercuspation) so that unloading of overloaded teeth, the muscles of mastication, and the TMJs can occur and faulty occlusal conditions can be corrected. Based on this definition, a *splint* becomes a therapeutic occlusal guide plate.

Occlusal changes due to elongation must not arise, which is why the splints cover all the teeth and support them antagonistically. These removable splints or guards are simple to fabricate and easy to handle. However, they have an adverse esthetic impact, may impede speech, and will encourage the accumulation of plaque, caries, and gingivitis.

Splints can be made of rigid or flexible acrylic or metal; they are either fixed with clasps or engage the undercuts of the teeth. A mouthguard (or mouth protector), covering the maxillary and mandibular teeth equally, is made from flexible material and is mainly worn for contact sports.

Materials are chosen on the basis of the desired function of the splinting and the properties of the materials:

• Transparent, hard, tough, and torsion-resistant acrylics for universal use
• Light-cured, translucent, or milky composites for occlusal buildups
• Flexible, transparent polyurethane
• Translucent, elastic thermoplastic material
• Thermoplastic acrylate in different grades of hardness and elasticity
• Elastic silicone materials in three grades of hardness and with good recovery properties
• Gold alloys and chrome-cobalt alloys

Classification of occlusal splints according to their biomechanical effect produces four groups (Table 11-1):

1. **Reflex splints** to interrupt parafunctional habits (eg, bruxism splints)
2. **Centric relation splints** to restore the centric condylar position (eg, Michigan splint)
3. **Eccentric splints** to treat disc displacements (eg, repositioning splints, distraction splints)
4. **Special forms** for a variety of therapeutic approaches

Reflex Splints

Joint diseases caused by disorders in dentition closure or stress-induced parafunctions can be treated with reflex splints, which interrupt the imprinted, pathologic movement pattern. This is done by raising the occlusal position and reducing muscle activity with a *bruxism splint* (see Fig 11-7). Neuromuscular diseases originating from psychologic stress and parafunctions can be treated with this kind of reflex splint. These are also used for acute joint pains as immediate treatment as well as for pretreatment prior to centric relation splints (to achieve centric capability).

Relaxation/myorelaxation splints are applied in cases of muscular dysfunction, underdevelopment, and functional atrophy in individual muscle

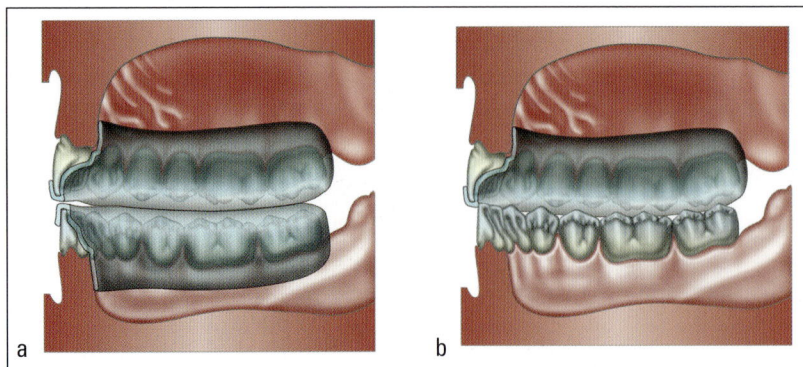

Fig 11-7 The simplest reflex splint is a smooth vacuum-formed sheet that raises the occlusion by a maximum of 2 mm. There is no occlusal guidance, so that relaxed joint play movements can be performed. Splints can be fabricated for the maxilla and the mandible *(a)* or for the maxilla alone *(b)*. These simple appliances can also be employed as bruxism splints.

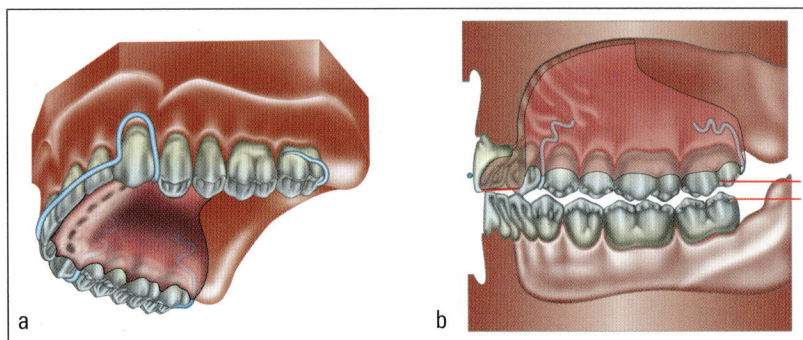

Fig 11-8 *(a and b)* The Hawley plate is an occlusal splint that is fitted with a labial bow and two molar clasps. A bite plane for the mandibular anterior teeth blocks the occlusion so that muscle relaxation can occur. This appliance is designed for temporary use for a maximum of 2 weeks.

segments. This involves seeking a pain-free mandibular position that serves as an interim stage of treatment.

Suitable *reflex splints* include smooth appliances made of 1.0- to 1.5-mm-thick, hard or soft vacuum-formed sheets that are pulled over the teeth and fabricated for the maxilla or the mandible without occlusal guidance (Fig 11-7), as well as splints made of self-curing acrylic that have punctiform premature contact (interceptors).

The *Hawley appliance* is a bite plane for the maxilla that is fitted with a flat palatal occlusal plateau for the mandibular incisors. This is intended to increase the vertical dimension and achieve disocclusion of the posterior teeth. The appliance lies lingually close to the teeth and is retained with a labial bow and two wire clasps on the molars (Fig 11-8). Incisal edges and occlusal surfaces are not covered.

The *labial bow* supports the maxillary anterior teeth. The horizontal bite plane is so wide that slight excursive movements are possible. To treat muscular hyperactivity, the appliance is inserted

for about 1 to 2 weeks to normalize muscle tone. As the muscles lengthen, a slight change in the condylar position is achieved and occlusal interferences are eliminated; overstimulation of the muscles can be reduced. Because the posterior teeth are not supported occlusally, they may overerupt, which is why the wearing time is limited to a maximum of 2 weeks.

The *Sved appliance* has the same function as the Hawley appliance and a similar form. It comprises a maxillary palatal plate that is held with two molar clasps (Fig 11-9). Instead of the labial bow, the plate is guided over the incisal edges of the maxillary anterior teeth to protect them against uncontrolled thrust. The bite plane is just as wide but sloped slightly lingually. The appliance is simple to fabricate and can also be inserted easily as it engages over the incisal edges of the maxillary anterior teeth.

A *splint with three-point support* is a Sved appliance with additional occlusal surfaces in the dorsal molar region. The purpose is to force eruption of the premolars. The plate wraps around the

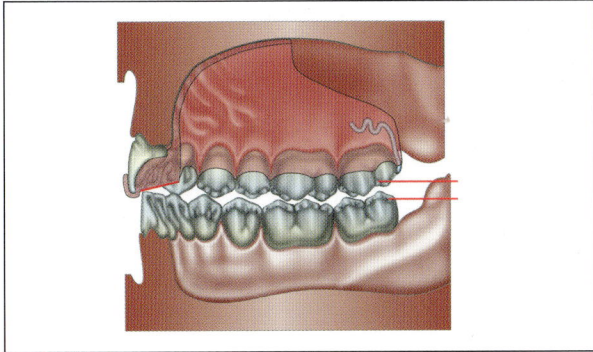

Fig 11-9 The Sved appliance, like the Hawley appliance, is a palatal plate with a bite plane for the mandibular anterior teeth used for temporary vertical opening to normalize muscle tone. Instead of the labial bow, an anterior wrapover of plastic serves to stabilize the maxillary anterior teeth. The bite plane is sloped lingually.

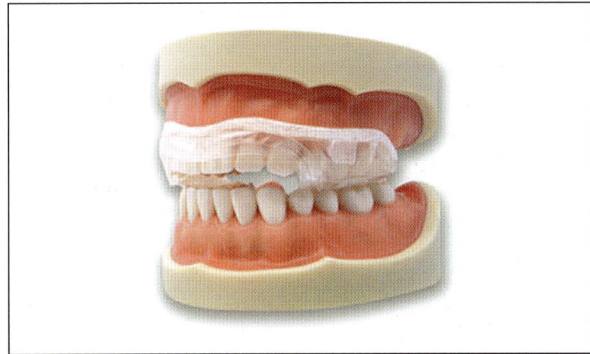

Fig 11-10 The Aqualizer can be worn in the maxilla concealed below the upper lip. The two liquid pads are positioned between the posterior teeth. The patient bites evenly on both pads, which improves the fit. When the Aqualizer is correctly seated, the patient will adopt the most agreeable occlusal position. The vertical opening should measure 1 to 2 mm. The Aqualizer can be worn during the day and also while asleep for a maximum of 8 hours per day. It is not a long-term splint and should be cleaned every day under water with a little dishwashing liquid. (Courtesy of Aqualizer.)

maxillary anterior teeth and the last molars, is held with wire clasps, and has an anterior occlusal plane as a sliding surface for the mandibular anterior teeth.

Anterior occlusal splints for temporary insertion (ie, a few hours) can be used to relax the muscles (eg, prior to intensive registration of relations) by eliminating occlusal interferences. These occlusal splints made of self-curing acrylic can be fabricated directly in the patient's mouth.

The **Aqualizer** is a prefabricated reflex splint filled with distilled water. This ready-made plastic sheet has water cushions on both sides acting as occlusal surfaces (Fig 11-10). Based on the principle of communicating vessels, whereby any homogenous liquid will always balance to the same level despite the shape or volume of the container, masticatory pressure is balanced with this appliance: Defective one-sided contact is prevented, and the TMJ is unloaded. The Aqualizer is an immediate splint that withstands even strong masticatory forces. The splint is made of a nylon sheet in the form of two occlusal pads filled with water, which are linked together by thin capillaries. All tooth contacts are cushioned by the water pads. The Aqualizer is available in two sizes and adapts to the dental arch on wearing.

Reflex splints are suitable neither as a preprosthetic measure where occlusal anomalies already exist nor as a means of producing the physiologic condylar position. They are also unsuitable for treating degenerative TMJ changes.

Centric Relation Splints

Centric relation splints (or simply *centric splints*) initiate self-centering of the condyles in the fossae, as established via a centric record. With the physiologic (relieved) joint position, neuromuscular relaxation is achieved, a pain-free therapeutic position is created in the case of intra-articular disorders, or pretreatment is undertaken for extensive occlusal correction (eg, in an abraded dentition).

Centric relation denotes the physiologic condylar position, a joint-related occlusal situation in which both condyles lie pressure-free in the centric position in the articular fossae. This position can be contrasted with maximal intercuspation. Therefore, the centric position of the condyles must be registered and transferred to an articulator to fabricate a centric relation splint.

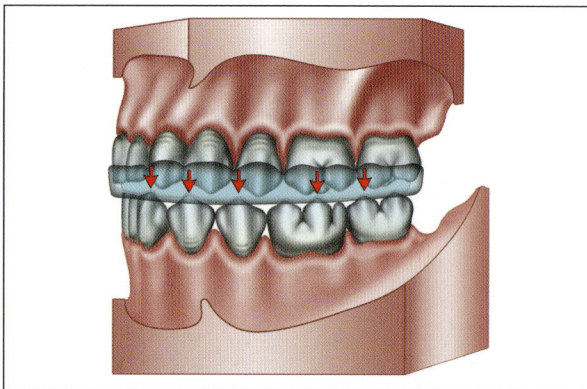

Fig 11-11 The centric relation splint is produced with a vertical opening that lies within the interarch distance. In the planned, physiologic, centric position, occlusal stops are ground for the mandibular occluding cusps. Pronounced canine-incisor guidance guides the mandible out of the opening movement into centric relation; during excursive movements, this canine-incisor guidance lifts the mandibular posterior teeth out of occlusion. Centric relation splints can be used as pretreatment for complex corrections of occlusal position.

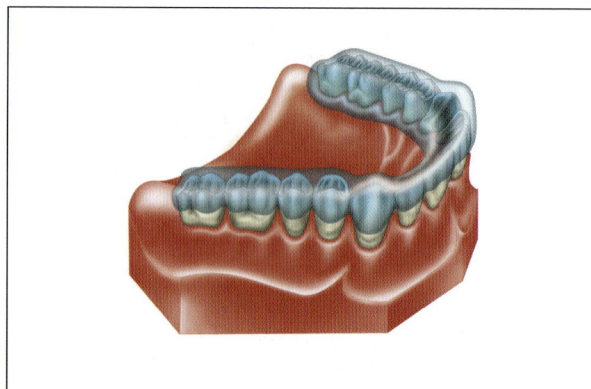

Fig 11-12 The stabilization splint wraps around the teeth in a vestibular direction as far as the equators of the teeth and leaves a generous amount of space from the palatal area. The occlusal surfaces are smooth without indentation marks for the posterior teeth. The canine-incisor guidance has a guide plane lingually with extensive freedom of movement in centric relation.

Cranium-related transfer of the maxillary model takes place in an articulator, in which the patient's movement parameters (eg, condylar path inclination, Bennett angle) can be set. For the interocclusal record registration, the patient's nerves and muscles must be relaxed; ie, the patient must be capable of achieving the centric position. This neuromuscular relaxation can be produced by prior treatment with reflex splints.

Variable *types of centric relation splints* are identified, as reflected in the following terms:

- Occlusion rim and relaxation plate
- Equilibration splint
- Michigan splint
- Stabilization splint
- Occlusion-raising splint

Vertical opening is produced with the *centric relation splint*, where the antagonists are positioned in punctiform, flat, but stable centric stops. The occlusal height lies within the interarch distance, and the horizontal relation is ground in the form of occlusal depressions for the active cusp tips (Fig 11-11). The grinding must be constantly adapted to the changing jaw relations.

In *protrusive and laterotrusive excursions*, the posterior teeth must be lifted out of occlusal contact, which is achieved with anterior canine guidance. The centric relation splints are fabricated for the maxilla and extended onto the palatal area to ensure sufficient stability. A centric relation splint can also be made into a prosthetic splint with artificial teeth for temporary replacement of support areas. In total tooth loss, centric relation splints are used to try out increases in occlusal height or removal of functional disorders.

The splint can be carved in wax and converted into acrylic or produced with self-curing or light-curing acrylics. After insertion of a centric relation splint, the centric contacts are ground until the contacts remain stable on the splint; aftercare is needed to grind off interfering contacts. The splint is worn all night and during the day as often as possible. Once the symptoms have subsided, the splint can be withdrawn after a few weeks' wear.

A *stabilization splint* is regarded as the standard appliance among centric relation splints and is used for painful, tense muscles; in cases of TMJ arthritis for relieving the joint structures; as a preprosthetic therapeutic aid; as well as in cases of advanced periodontitis. It is mainly worn at night,

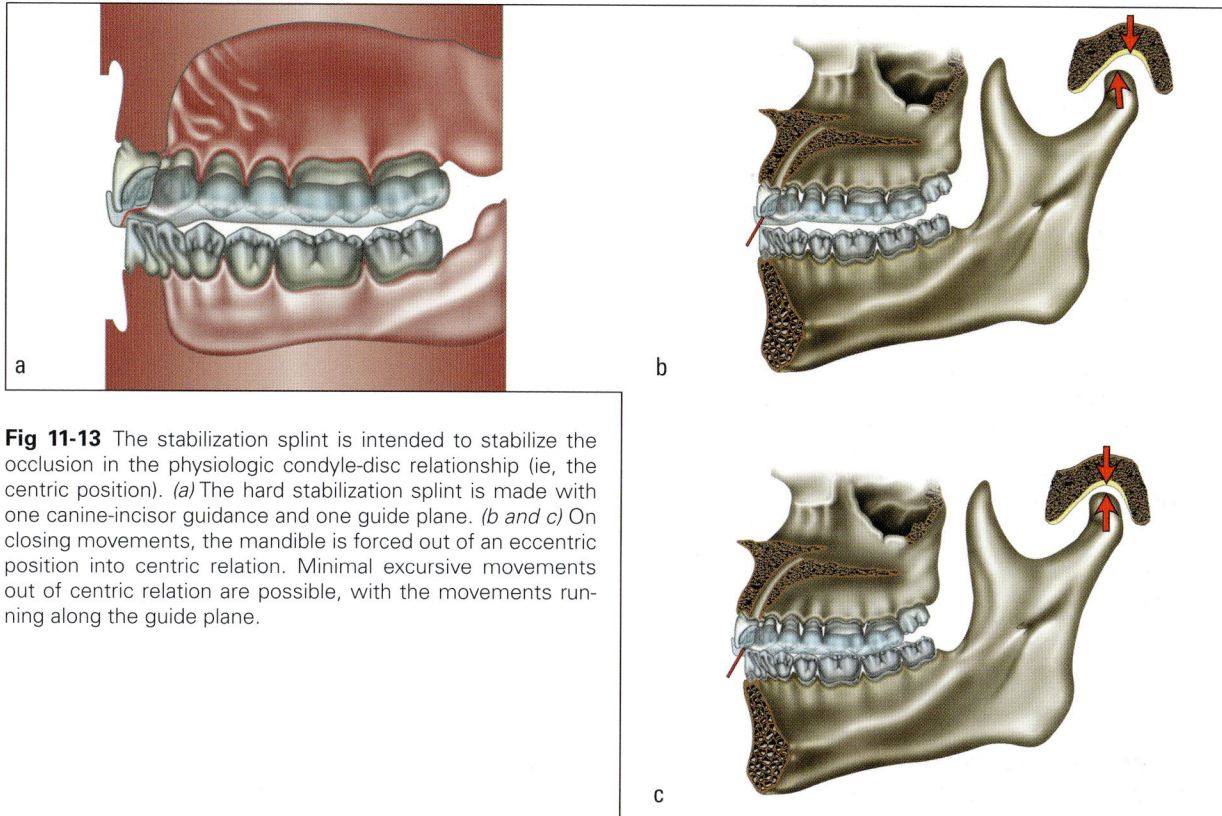

Fig 11-13 The stabilization splint is intended to stabilize the occlusion in the physiologic condyle-disc relationship (ie, the centric position). *(a)* The hard stabilization splint is made with one canine-incisor guidance and one guide plane. *(b and c)* On closing movements, the mandible is forced out of an eccentric position into centric relation. Minimal excursive movements out of centric relation are possible, with the movements running along the guide plane.

and wear is gradually reduced as the symptoms diminish.

The splint is fabricated from hard acrylic for the maxilla, covering all the teeth and keeping the occlusal surfaces flat. The acrylic wraps around the teeth to just above their equators (Fig 11-12). Guide planes for the anterior and posterior teeth can be incorporated to enforce canine guidance or canine-incisor guidance for the protrusive and lateral movements of the mandible (Fig 11-13).

Fabrication of the splint is performed on precisely mounted models (wax centric relation record, facebow) so that grinding can be done in the articulator. The splint can be carved in wax, invested, and fabricated by a hot-pressing process. On the maxillary model, the profile of the splint border is marked approximately 1 to 2 mm cervically below the tooth equators; a minimum distance of 1 mm to the marginal periodontium must be maintained. In the anterior region, the splint border projects only 1 mm beyond the incisal edge; the palate is avoided in a U shape. An occlusal elevation of approximately 2 to 3 mm is performed to ensure the minimum material thickness occlusally.

Michigan splint

The *Michigan splint* was developed in the 1950s at the University of Michigan. It is a hard, transparent acrylic splint that covers all the maxillary teeth and has flat, occlusal centric stops for the mandibular teeth so that, on jaw closure, there are even and simultaneous occlusal contacts of the mandibular teeth on the splint surface. This centric relation splint can be fabricated in an adjustable articulator and is fitted with a canine guidance that has a sufficiently steep inclination to prevent both working and nonworking contacts as well as anterior guidance contacts.

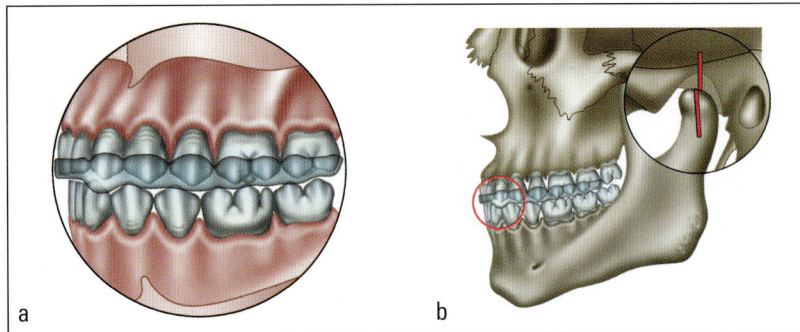

Fig 11-14 *(a and b)* A Michigan splint raises the occlusion in the centric position by about 2 mm; the condyle rotates out of the hinge position as far as the physiologic rest position at the maximum. All the posterior teeth contact the flat splint. The mandibular canines have freedom of movement out of centric occlusion on a canine guide plane. This is known as *freedom in centric occlusion*.

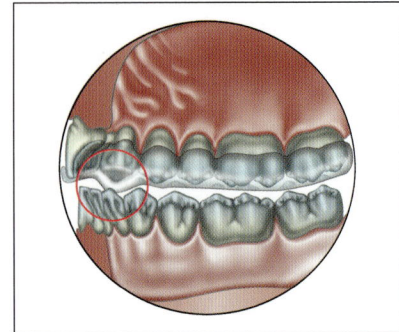

Fig 11-15 During movements out of centric occlusion beyond freedom in centric occlusion, the dentitions disocclude because the mandibular canine slips obliquely downward and forward on the steep canine guide plane and forces the dental arches apart.

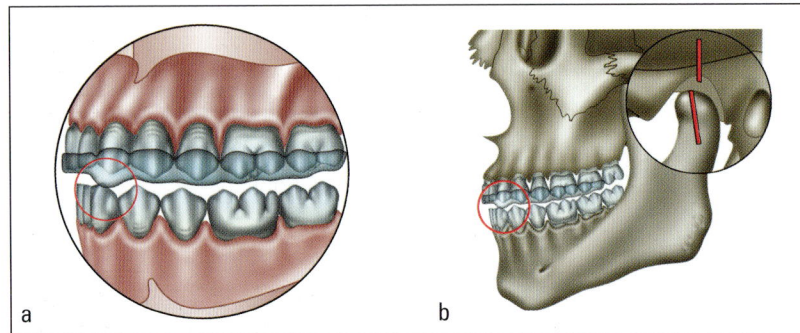

Fig 11-16 *(a and b)* The sloping canine guide plane is ground toward the movement of the mandible. During lateroprotrusive movements, slight mouth opening is enforced with the condyle rotating around its hinge axis.

The ***canine guidance*** of approximately 1 to 2 mm permits only minimal lateral or protrusive movements under full occlusal contact of the lateral splint surface before disocclusion occurs. These minimal movements are referred to as *freedom in centric occlusion*, and they have to be individually determined and worked into the canine guidance. The degree of freedom of movement permitted by the canine guidance must be adapted to different occlusal positions:

• Centric occlusion
• Habitual occlusion
• Occlusal position when swallowing
• Occlusal position when sleeping

Incisor guidance such that the splint disoccludes must not be present.

The Michigan splint in its basic form is hence a ***stabilizing centric relation splint*** with a defined occlusal elevation of 2 to 3 mm, canine guidance, and freedom of movement in the centric position (freedom in centric occlusion). It is used to treat malocclusions, to manage diseases of the muscles of mastication and pathologic TMJ changes (myoarthropathies), and to control bruxism. Figures 11-14 to 11-18 illustrate the actions and functions of the Michigan splint.

Because ***changes of mandibular position*** influence the neuromuscular system, especially the length of the muscles, muscle activity is markedly reduced by the use of a Michigan splint. A positive effect of the Michigan splint can be accurately demonstrated; ie, the splint therapy works even though the mechanisms of action cannot be clearly verified. There is hence something of

Fig 11-17 *(a)* In the centric position, the mandibular anterior teeth contact the splint evenly. Premature contacts upon gently guided mandibular closure must be ground back. *(b)* The canine guidance must be reground so that uniform sliding contact of the mandibular canine arises with all excursive movements and all the other teeth disocclude.

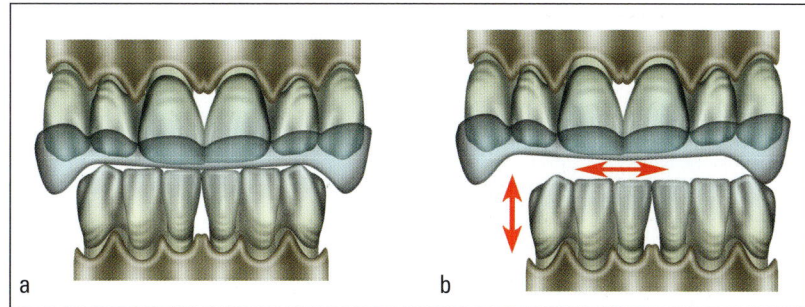

Fig 11-18 *(a to c)* The canine guide plane is ground toward freedom in centric occlusion. During these joint play movements, the occluding cusps of the mandibular posterior teeth should remain in sliding contact on the flat splint. The canine guide plane is shaped so steeply that the dentitions immediately disocclude when freedom in centric occlusion is left.

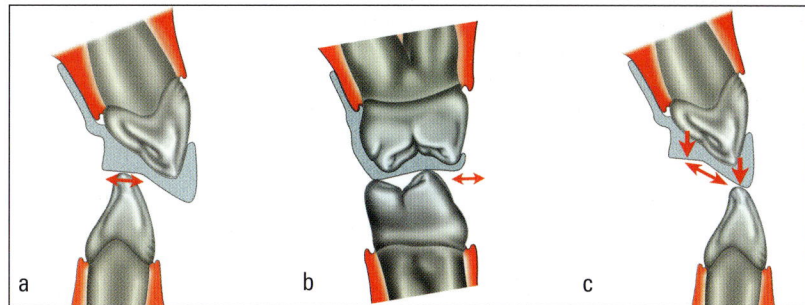

a placebo effect. The beneficial effect is based on the following conscious perceptions:

- It compensates for occlusal anomalies.
- It allows unloaded joint positioning.
- It counteracts bruxism and clenching.
- It prevents pathologic occlusal positions.

To **_fabricate the Michigan splint_**, the models are mounted in the articulator in the centric occlusal position with a facebow record. Joint values should be individually set, and the occlusal height and inclination of the incisal guide plate should be adjusted as follows:

- The vertical opening is arranged so that an interocclusal distance of 1 to 2 mm is present in terminal occlusion and in protrusive movements.
- The inclination of the incisal guidance is set up to allow border movements within the canine guidance.
- The height of the canine guidance should be designed so that all parts of the dentition disocclude in the edge-to-edge situation of the canines.

The splint in the maxilla is then carved in wax:

- The palatal border makes contact with the area of the palatal ruga, and the vestibular margin extends slightly above the tooth equators so that the splint can later be firmly clasped. After fabrication, it must be firmly seated without additional retentive components.
- Occlusally, a flat bite plane is created until only the buccal occluding cusps touch the splint. The bite plane follows the sagittal and transverse occlusal curves.
- The sloping canine guide plane is built up, and the movement paths of laterotrusion and protrusion are established on freedom in centric occlusion so that continuous contact of the canine guidance can ensue and until disocclusion of the posterior teeth occurs.

The splint is then fabricated in transparent thermoplastic polymer, the maxillary model is rearticulated, and the splint is reground in the articulator. The final grinding is done by the dentist. The Michigan splint must have an absolutely stable seating; it cannot rock. A splint that is not seated in a stable position must be remade.

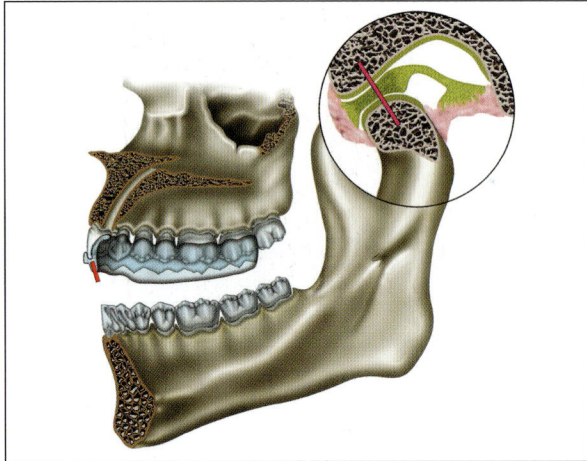

Fig 11-19 During an opening movement, an anteriorly displaced disc will slip onto the condyle with clicking noises and assume a correct condyle-disc relationship. This correct relationship of condyle to disc is to be fixed with an eccentric splint applied to a distinct protrusive position.

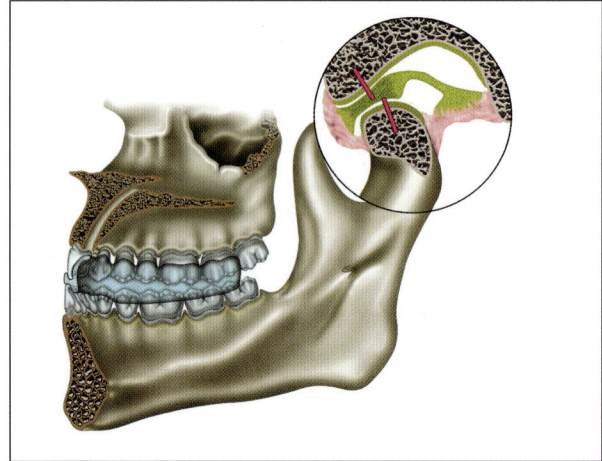

Fig 11-20 The splint must have a distinct anterior canine guidance and a large occlusal depth in the posterior region to maintain the eccentric position on mandibular closure. The splint is constantly reground during the treatment period until the normal terminal occlusion position is reached again.

Eccentric Splints

Repositioning splints and distraction (decompression) splints may be described as types of "eccentric splint" (ie, out of centric relation).

The ***repositioning splint*** can be used to bring the mandible into an anterior position in order to bring a partially or totally displaced articular disc into its physiologic position and create a click-free and painless situation. The aim is to restore a normal condyle-disc relationship through this temporary anterior displacement of the mandible.

Anterior displacement of the maxilla of not more than 1.0 to 1.5 mm by the splint is therapeutically successful. In a case of disc dislocation, the connective tissue suspending the disc is stretched or damaged, making it difficult to securely fix the condyle-disc relationship in the new occlusal position. This means that a relapse (recurrence) can happen after completion of treatment even in favorable conditions.

Repositioning splints are reground constantly during the wearing period to bring the mandible gradually out of the protrusive position back in a dorsal direction and the condyle back into its normal anatomical position (Fig 11-19). At the end

of treatment, a stable occlusion must exist and anterior canine guidance must be either present or producible by prosthetic methods.

This method requires regular appointments to ensure that the occlusal contact relationships are not altered, eg, no posterior open bite develops. Once the acute symptoms have subsided, the treatment should be continued with stabilization splints. The physiologic condyle-disc relationship is usually restored more quickly with stabilization splints.

The ***repositioning splint*** must be worn continuously, even while eating. The wearing time extends to a minimum of 6 months, until the joint noises and symptoms have disappeared. To prevent a relapse, a retainer can be used to stabilize the therapeutic position.

The ***therapeutic position*** (in the case of a repositioned disc) must be measured and transferred to an articulator so that the splint can be fabricated in that position. A repositioning splint should be made for the maxilla because of the wearing mode, and the occlusal contacts should be worked into it. So that the new position is found and fixed without any problems, anterior canine guidance and a large occlusal depth must be created (Fig 11-20).

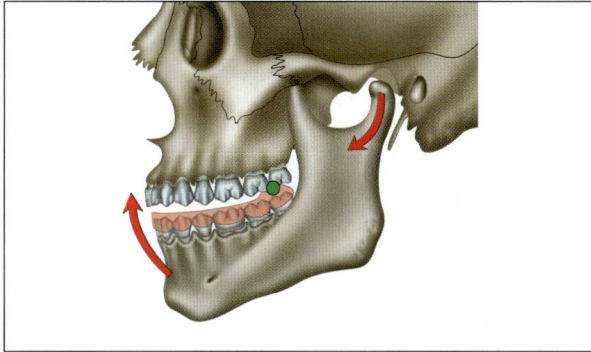

Fig 11-21 A center of rotation is fixed in the molar region with the pivot splint, the aim being to distract the condyles out of the joints and thereby relieve the joints.

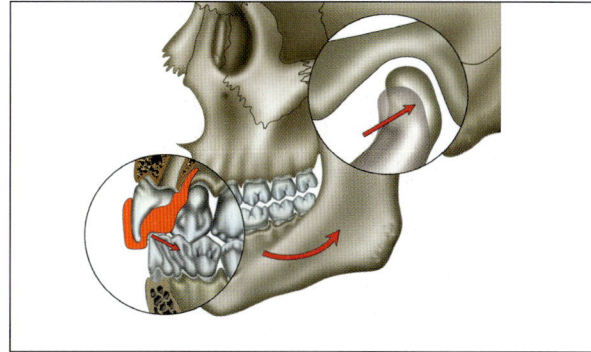

Fig 11-22 With an anterior jig, the aim is to achieve the best possible occlusal centric relation via three-point support from anterior and condylar points.

Fig 11-23 *(a and b)* An interceptor interrupts the parafunction of the musculature by raising the occlusal contacts through a vertical opening device in the posterior region, mainly positioned at the premolars. Once again, the TMJ is considerably relieved.

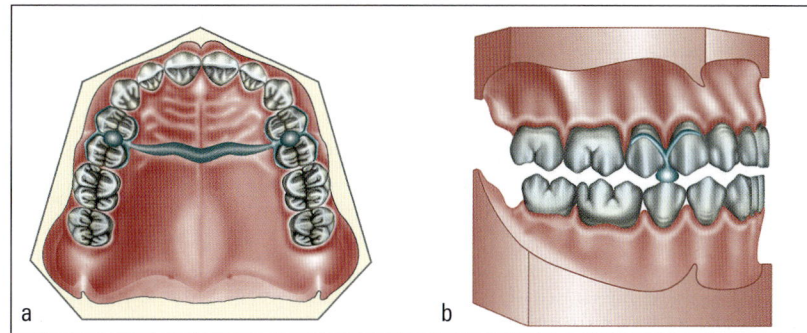

Repositioning splints are intended to ensure the centric mandibular position by means of uniform intercuspation where the teeth have numerous contacts with each other. Engagement in the contact pattern can thus be achieved without having to make any irreversible changes to the teeth.

A *distraction splint* (pivot splint, decompression splint) is the treatment method used to eliminate disc displacement without reduction or to relieve compressed TMJs by creating an artificial premature contact in the molar region (Fig 11-21). The TMJ is actually relieved when the condyle is pushed out of the fossa on biting together on the premature contact in the molars. As the joint is relieved, the joint capsules, muscles, and ligaments are stretched. To create the *artificial premature contact*, 0.3- to 0.9-mm-thick tin foil can be inserted into the condylar housing of the articulator so that the occlusion is raised in the dorsal area or the posterior teeth are blocked. The distraction splint is fabricated in this model position. The splint is worn as often as possible, until freedom from pain is achieved and unrestricted mouth opening is possible; this can take up to 6 months. The distraction splint with extreme distraction of 1 mm enables a displaced disc to be guided back, although with a risk of additional joint damage.

Partial splints can also be used to correct jaw relations.

The *anterior jig* offers incisal horizontal guidance to adjust the centric relation during prosthetic measures (Fig 11-22).

The *interceptor* is a clasp-retained palatal bar produced by model casting with bilateral ball-head or cylindric supports in the premolar region. It interrupts habitual parafunctions of the muscles of mastication by placing all the teeth out of contact (Fig 11-23).

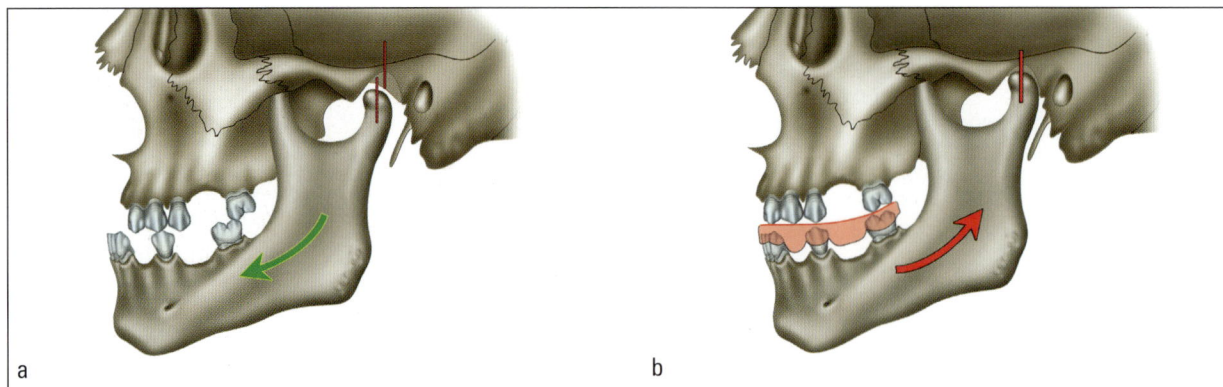

Fig 11-24 *(a)* One consequence of destruction of the dentition is displacement of the mandibular position with forced occlusal interlocking; the physiologic contact patterns are lost, and eccentric faulty contacts with tooth tipping ensue. The central position of the condyles in the fossa is shifted. *(b)* The faulty occlusion is raised by an occlusal splint; relaxation can occur, and unimpeded relieving movements can be performed. The occlusal splint initially has a flat surface without fixation of the occlusal position. The new mandibular relationship is established in a further treatment step.

Pre-prosthetic Treatment Measures

Progressive destruction of the masticatory system leads to functional disorders of the muscles, TMJs, and periodontal tissues. The vertical distances and horizontal relationships of the jaws are altered. The masticatory system adapts to the function that has been altered by loss of teeth or occlusal surfaces, but the malocclusions usually lead to hyperactivity of the muscles of mastication, which means that the normal neuromuscular program is disrupted. This results in neuromuscular coordination problems with avoidance or adaptive programs, giving rise to muscle diseases (myopathies) that also cause diseased change to the joint tissues.

Bruxism and *myoarthropathies* (muscle and joint diseases) are the clinical pictures that are triggered by impediments to occlusion.

A *definitive prosthetic treatment* can turn into treatment failure if the tissue parts do not have time to adjust to the newly reconstructed occlusal situation. *Pre-prosthetic splint therapy* aims to eliminate this disorder of neuromuscular coordination over a defined period of time and to carry out functional adaptation (Fig 11-24). In the process, the pain symptoms should be reduced and the impaired mandibular position should improve.

The following considerations apply to prosthetic structures:

- They may only be fabricated once there are no functional disorders of the masticatory system. Otherwise, functional therapeutic measures (regrinding, centric relation splints, long-term provisional restorations) need to be taken.
- They should be fabricated in a fully adjustable articulator; the models are adjusted with a joint-related facebow record.
- They should be realized with maximal intercuspation in centric relation of the mandible. If necessary, splint therapy should be initiated as a pre-prosthetic measure to establish the precise centric position.

The *objectives of splint therapy* as a pre-prosthetic measure are to correct the static and dynamic occlusal conditions in order to protect the teeth against progressive attrition; to change the condyle-disc relationship; to evenly distribute the forces acting occlusally; and to produce neurophysiologic effects that reduce the increased muscle activity.

A splint should interrupt pathologic reflex paths by using flat splint surfaces to eliminate the occlusal disturbances in the neuromuscular con-

Fig 11-25 *(a and b)* Occlusion-raising splints can be used in the mandible and have a distinct anterior canine guidance that can be ground based on the freedom in centric occlusion concept. The physiologic working length of the muscles of mastication can be restored by raising the teeth to the normal occlusal position.

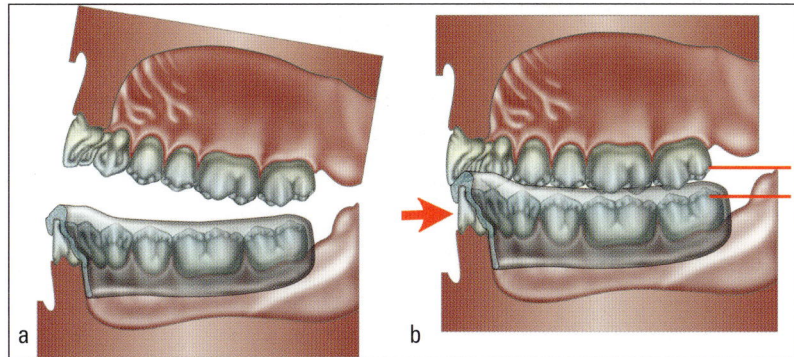

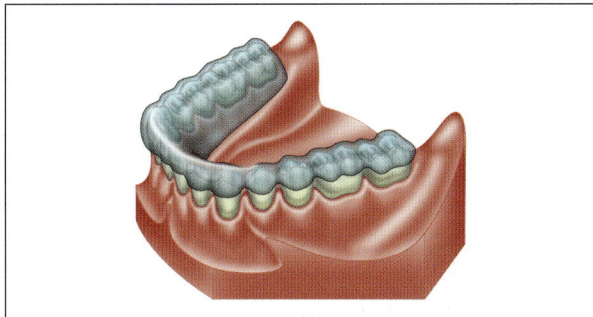

Fig 11-26 A fixation centric splint is a guide plane with anterior canine guidance that forces the mandible into the centric position. For the occluding cusps of the maxillary posterior teeth, contact areas are ground in centric relation. Freedom of movement is not provided for.

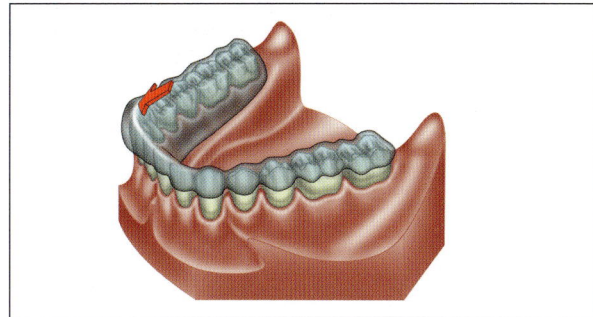

Fig 11-27 A masticatory muscle synchronizer has a tooth guide block intended to interrupt a parafunctional habit. Here a universally increased canine contact is built up, allowing the dental arches to disocclude when parafunctional laterotrusion is performed.

trol cycle of the masticatory system. Creation of the previous vertical distance eliminates sliding interferences and guides the musculature back to a normal functional sequence. If the enforced occlusal guidances are eliminated, muscular hyperactivity diminishes, the joints are relieved, and the pain symptoms of myoarthropathy disappear. The aim is therefore to restore the original occlusal position that will apply to the definitive restoration. The occlusal splints described in the following paragraphs are classified according to their pre-prosthetic treatment objective.

Occlusal splints are appliances with a flat surface for unimpeded relieving movements to treat a traumatic occlusion with eccentric faulty contacts due to tipping or migration of teeth and mandibular displacement. Decoding the faulty occlusion means that the centric relation of the condyles can be resumed, which is accomplished with retrusion splints.

Occlusion-raising splints can be used to increase a reduced vertical dimension resulting from posterior tooth loss or generalized abrasion (Fig 11-25). As the occlusal position is restored, the muscles of mastication regain their normal working length.

Fixation centric splints fix a specified intercuspation situation and are worn for a few months before definitive restoration work is started to establish an interference-free occlusion (Fig 11-26).

The ***masticatory muscle synchronizer*** is used for adapting the neuromuscular movement pattern, mainly in the mandible, as an occlusal splint with dominant anterior and canine guidance (Fig 11-27).

Occlusion rims are employed for orthodontic retrusion of the anterior teeth. They are mainly palatal plates with anterior occlusal platforms and a labial bar that are fixed to the maxillary molars with simple clasps.

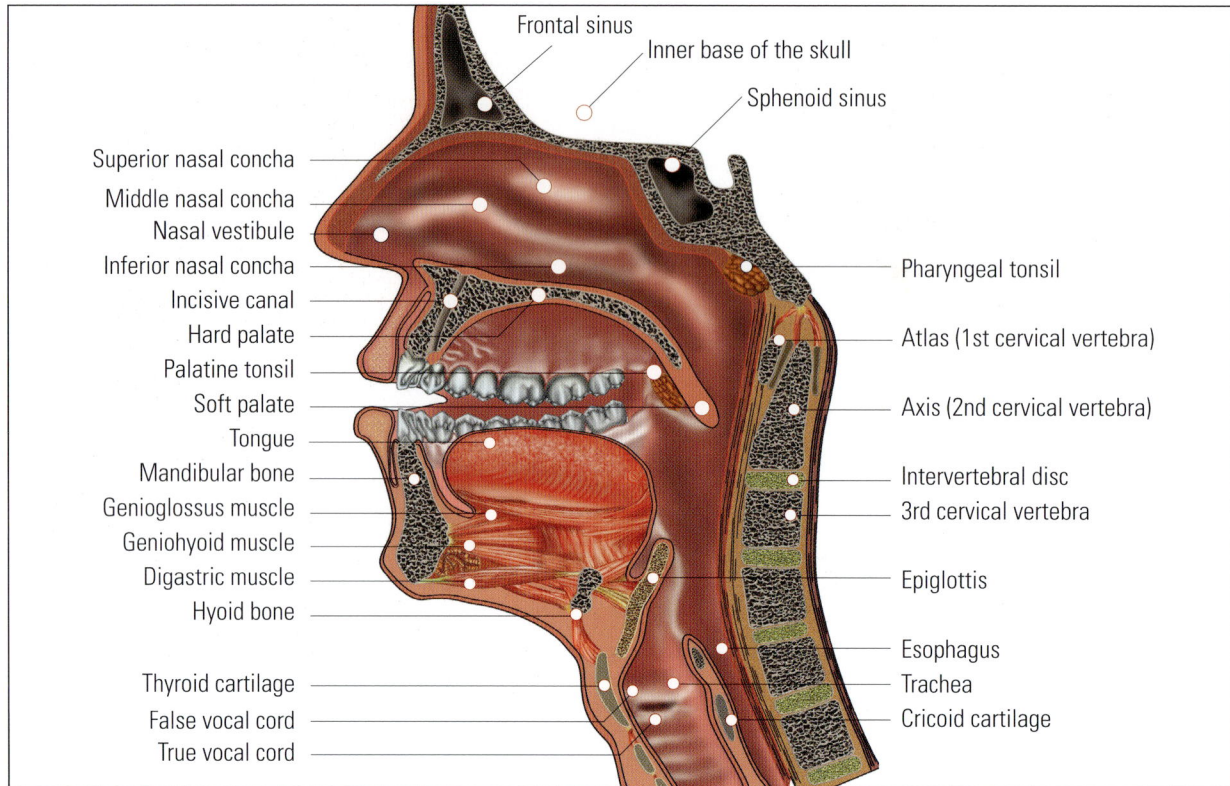

Fig 11-28 Median sagittal section through the pharynx and larynx shows the upper airways through the nasal cavity and the mouth. The area between the nasal cavity and the esophagus (gullet) about 10 to 12 cm in length is referred to as the *pharynx* (throat). The pharyngeal tonsils are located in the upper area of the pharynx (nasal part, *pars nasalis*); in a swollen state, they can constrict the upper airway. In the middle part of the pharynx (oral part, *pars oralis*), the palatine tonsils and the tongue can narrow the airway.

The **Shore plate** is a chewing pathway appliance for treating muscular dysfunction in a fully dentate dentition. The chewing pathway is shaped in plastic autopolymerizing acrylic resin onto the vacuum-formed splint.

Special Forms of Splint Therapy

Respiratory disorders with partial or complete displacement of the upper airways during sleep are associated with snoring noises that arise from vibration of the soft palate (Figs 11-28 and 11-29). Snoring is normally not harmful to health and does not require treatment. However, health may be impaired if respiratory arrest occurs for more than 10 seconds, despite breathing effort, because the upper airways are displaced. This arrest causes a decrease in oxygen saturation of the blood and triggers a waking reaction (Fig 11-30). Depending on the severity of this disorder, such respiratory arrest events followed by a waking reaction may occur between 5 and 40 times an hour (up to 100 times a night). The repeated waking reactions and interruption of sleeping phases cause increased drowsiness during the day. This condition is known as *obstructive sleep apnea* (OSA).

Snoring is a sign of this condition if it happens constantly and not sporadically. Sufferers are older, usually overweight adults. Abnormal anatomical proportions in the area of the upper airways may also be responsible for airway displacement, such as a long soft palate, an extended root of the

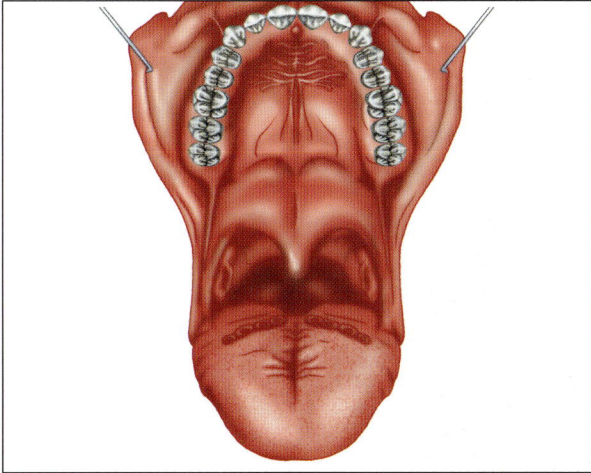

Fig 11-29 The upper airway crosses the passage from mouth to esophagus. During swallowing, the tongue presses the epiglottis shut so that no foreign bodies can get into the trachea. If the tongue falls backward during sleep, it can narrow the airway. The snoring noise arises when the soft palate is caused to vibrate.

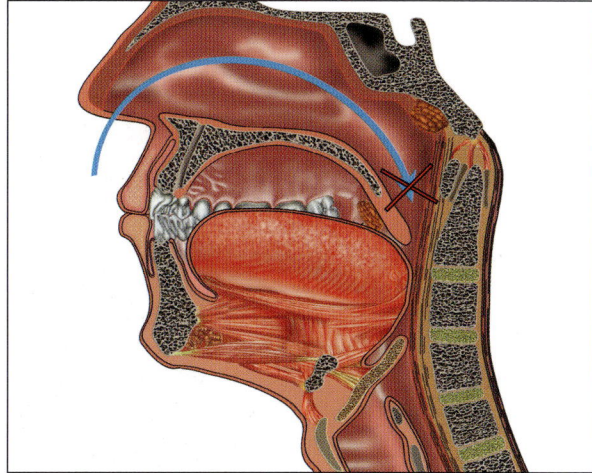

Fig 11-30 As the tongue presses against the soft palate and the airways are narrowed by the oropharynx, air has to be inhaled and exhaled with effort. The speed of flow increases in the narrowed air channel, but the flow of air is repeatedly interrupted. In the case of obstructive sleep apnea, respiratory arrest can occur several times and is accompanied by waking reactions. The upper airways can be kept clear and the snoring alleviated with an anti-snoring mouthpiece.

tongue, or a mandibular dental arch that is too narrow.

Treatment of particularly severe OSA cases involves positive pressure ventilation during sleep or surgical measures. Less severe cases can be treated with intraoral appliances that keep the upper airways open. These appliances include:

• Tongue retainers to pull the tongue forward
• Appliances to lift the soft palate
• Occlusal splints to pull the mandible forward

Tongue retainers are hollow bodies that encompass the tongue like a low-pressure chamber and hold it in an anterior position. As well as the body of the retainer, breathing tubes are attached. The retainer is fitted to the dentition and lies passively in the mouth.

Appliances to raise the soft palate are palatal plates fixed to the teeth with Adams clasps, and they carry a pelotte (a small, specially designed curved plate) on a spring loop. As a result, the soft palate is gently pressed upward, and snoring is prevented. The appliance is unsuitable for pa-

tients who exhibit a gag reflex to the appliance and is ineffective as a treatment method in OSA.

Anti-snoring mouthpieces are occlusion rims that pull the mandible downward and forward to widen the airways (Fig 11-31). The opening width and the protrusive position are determined individually and connected in a fixed-value device (mandibular protrusive splint). Split occlusion rims can also be fabricated with which the most effective protrusive position can gradually be found and adjusted.

An anti-snoring mouthpiece can be made in the form of two thick vacuum-formed sheets that are anchored to the teeth by a tight fit. They are connected via screws, linking arms (adjustable), or by a rigid acrylic block (fixed appliance). A rigid mouthpiece may also comprise a silicone block that holds the advanced mandibular position; it can be fabricated by the dentist directly in the mouth.

Aligners are transparent orthodontic splints, spring wires, or screws. Correction of tooth position is accomplished with a series of removable acrylic splints that initiate individual regulating thrusts. The initial orthodontic status is recorded three-dimensionally and developed in separate phases by computer-aided design technology, or even an analog technique, until the treatment objective is achieved. Individual splints to be worn for about 2 weeks are prepared in small correction steps. Orthodontic tooth movement occurs during this period, and the next modified splint is inserted until the projected treatment goal is attained. The splints are designed so that individual regulating thrusts are applied with defined force within the second level of biologic intensity and for a defined period of time. Different teeth or groups of teeth defined in the treatment plan are moved in each treatment phase. Therefore, long enough recovery phases for tissue adaptation are maintained before the next regulating thrust takes place.

Aligner splints are worn day and night, but they can be taken out to allow unimpeded eating and drinking as well as cleaning. They are transparent and therefore invisible, and they function without wires so that there is no rubbing on the teeth. The wearing characteristics are good, without long-term phonetic impairment. Wearers must maintain thorough oral hygiene.

The **Drum Miniplast splint** is a removable, universal occlusal splint that is made from a transparent 0.5- to 2-mm-thick vacuum-formed sheet for both the mandible and the maxilla. The term *Miniplast splint* can be regarded as a nonspecific synonym for a dental splint with a wide variety of treatment objectives.

Modified forms of the Miniplast splint can be described in relation to the specific application:

- A smooth, thick vacuum-formed splint that is not ground in is used as a **bruxism splint** to remove parafunctional movements.
- A thick vacuum-formed splint that is ground in centric occlusion aims to achieve a splinting effect and serves as a **relaxation splint** to reduce muscle tone.
- A thick **vacuum-formed splint reinforced with biting surfaces** that are based on a construction bite can compensate for faults of occlusal position.
- A thin, **elastic vacuum-formed splint** can be used as a carrier splint for a gel to bleach the teeth or can be coated with fluoride gel for fluoridation of the teeth.

- A thick, **stiff vacuum-formed splint** can be used to stabilize teeth loosened after trauma or gingival treatment (Fig 11-32).
- A **thick vacuum-formed splint** that encompasses both dentitions and is reinforced with elastic material acts as a **mouthguard** to protect against sports injuries.
- A **stiff vacuum-formed splint** that encompasses both arches and offers fixation can be used to stabilize the tooth position after an orthodontic measure; this splint can be interpreted as a **positioner or retainer**.

Retainers are used after an active orthodontic treatment phase to maintain the corrected tooth position until restructuring of the tissues affected by the orthodontic measures is completed. No teeth are moved any further in this treatment phase, which is known as the *retention phase* because it is intended to stop a return (recurrence or relapse) to the malposition of the teeth. If the retention period, which is almost as long as the active treatment period, is not adhered to, a relapse may occur and further treatment may become necessary. In extreme cases, lifelong retention will be required. After treatment with multiband appliances, the retention phase generally lasts longer. Retainers are rigid, thin, transparent acrylic plates that lie against the teeth lingually, are retained by an archwire running in the vestibular area, and permit unimpeded intercuspation. They should be worn all day; they do not interfere with phonetics and are almost invisible due to the clear plastic.

Lingual retainers or bonded retainers are fixed appliances that consist of a flexible wire that is fixed to the lingual surfaces by plastic adhesive. They are preferably inserted in the mandibular anterior region because the risk of relapse is greatest there. After treatment with removable appliances, the last appliance can be used as a retainer; none of the activatable parts (screws, springs, bars) are readjusted any further.

Mouthguards are intended to reduce injuries during contact and strength sports and are constructed or designed in keeping with the type of sport or the nature of the anticipated physical contact. The mouthguard can be fabricated in several layers; a hard base layer, extending over the whole palate and covering all the teeth occlusally, lies between two acrylic layers that remain soft

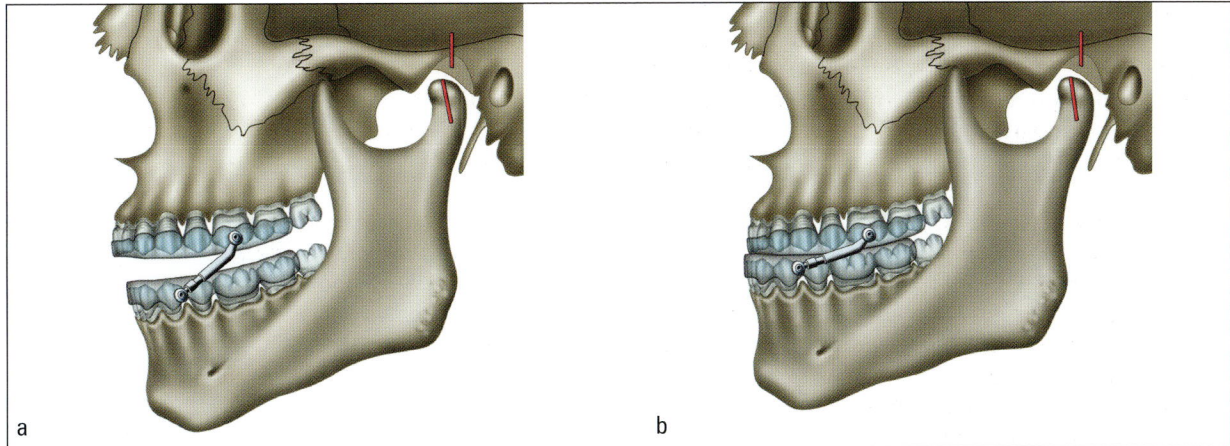

Fig 11-31 *(a)* The two parts of the anti-snoring mouthpiece are connected with an adjustable link. With the mouth open, the condyle slips downward and forward on the joint surface. *(b)* If the mouth is closed as far as the occlusal plane, the mandible with the floor of the mouth and tongue are pushed forward and the mandible remains slightly open. As a result, the upper airways are kept clear.

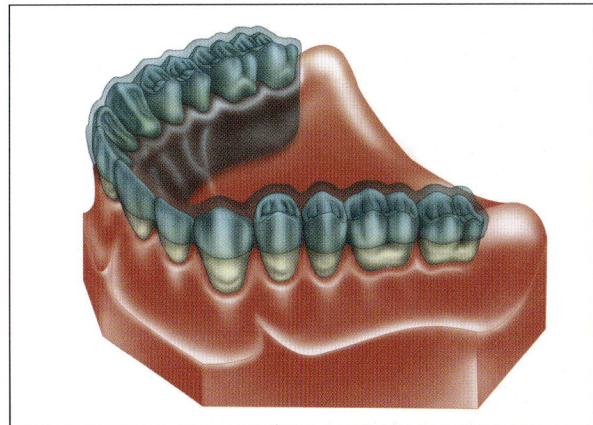

Fig 11-32 A Miniplast splint is a thermoplastically fabricated occlusal splint that can be used for traumatically loosened teeth. This universal occlusal plane for various therapeutic approaches encompasses all the maxillary teeth as far as the equators of the teeth and may partially extend onto the palatine vault. The areas of occlusion can be kept flat or fitted with selected occlusal indentations. As a centric relation splint, it can produce vertical opening within the physiologic rest distance of the jaws.

and fit closely to the teeth and jaws. The vestibular pad is applied to a thickness of 9 to 10 mm and extends into the vestibular fornices.

The term ***positioners*** denotes appliances that are made of elastic material and, where necessary, still allow fine correction of tooth position. After completion of treatment, the dental arch is sawn apart on the individual model, and the model teeth are placed in the ideal position. An elastic vacuum-formed splint is pulled onto this setup and represents this ideal position. The patient's teeth are gently pushed into the final position. After fine correction is performed with the positioner, a retainer is inserted that fixes the final tooth position.

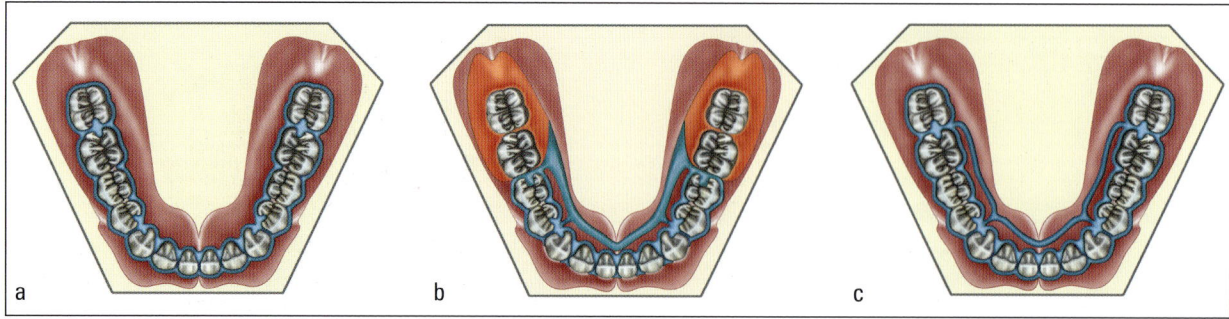

Fig 11-33 *(a)* The removable Elbrecht splint encloses the teeth lingually and vestibularly at the equators of the teeth. *(b)* A removable Elbrecht splint combined with a partial denture, the anterior teeth being grasped by cribs. *(c)* A removable Elbrecht splint with a sublingual bar for reinforcement.

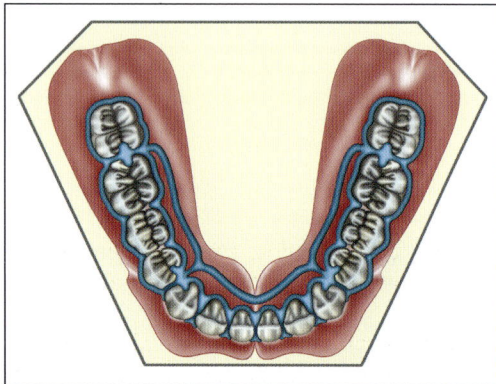

Fig 11-34 The crib splint with a sublingual bar to reinforce the splint. The cribs are guided interdentally in a vestibular direction.

Splint Therapy for Periodontal Treatment

Horizontal position is secured in clasp dentures by the rigid parts of cast clasps, such as clasp bodies, shoulders, and upper arms. They secure the denture against horizontal displacement and twisting and, in interaction with the rigid denture frames, evenly transfer masticatory pressure to other segments of the dental arch. They produce a splinting effect for the abutment teeth.

This **splinting effect** by clasp retention of periodontally compromised teeth can be exploited for therapeutic purposes when a dentition with spaces or wide sections of teeth is completely clasped together. Therefore, fixed or removable splints are fabricated to treat periodontally damaged dentitions with reduced loading capacity of individual teeth or groups of teeth or to stabilize dentitions with gaps.

Removable splints in the model-casting method as a continuous ring of clasps or in a cap shape are guided around the teeth and can be linked to a rigid unit by a large connector. They reduce horizontal and vertical movements of the splinted teeth without entirely preventing these movements.

Fixed splints comprise a soldered group of partial crowns that are anchored in the tooth by parallel grooves and parapulpal pins. Inlay splints are made up of mesio-occlusodistal inlays that are soldered together or joined with pin attachments. Fixed splinting components are periodontally hygienic and often esthetically more acceptable. However, they tend to provide local or complete blocking effects as they prevent both horizontal shifts and vertical movements of the clasped teeth. This gives rise to a block of resistance to all sagittally and transversally acting forces.

Partial dentures, which are used with rigid anchorage and support components, offer such blocks

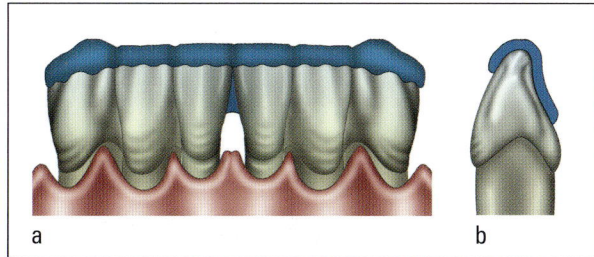

Fig 11-35 *(a and b)* The cap splint encloses the anterior teeth bodily above the equators of the teeth and covers the incisal edges.

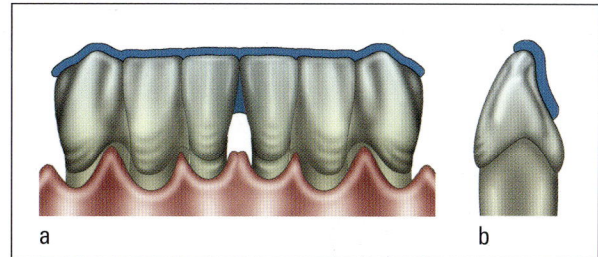

Fig 11-36 *(a and b)* The lingual splint covers the lingual surfaces of the teeth and is esthetically preferable to the cap splint.

of resistance. A primary blocking situation can be produced by bar connectors and a secondary blocking situation by telescope crowns and anchorage with attachments.

If a **splint is part of a denture** in the form of continuous reinforcement, the teeth and the denture form a functional unit that stabilizes the residual teeth, distributes masticatory pressure, and secures the horizontal position of the denture. Full reinforcement with alternating interdental insertion prostheses also delivers the desired splinting effects.

Splints can be fabricated without being integrated into a denture. The following paragraphs describe the different designs available.

The **Elbrecht splint** is a continuous bar produced by the model-casting method that is guided in a ring shape over the equator of each tooth (Fig 11-33); the splinting is stiffened by a large rigid connector (sublingual bar, reduced plate). The horizontal movements of the teeth are meant to be limited by this splinting so that the teeth are secured in their tooth bed. Because the splint also passes over the vestibular surfaces of the anterior teeth, it is esthetically disadvantageous and therefore is often modified into a crib splint.

In a **crib splint**, the continuous bar only runs on the lingual surfaces and engages in prepared niches on the incisal edges (Fig 11-34). The enclo-

sure and hence the splinting effect are limited in the process. The prepared incisal edges are at risk of caries.

The **cap splint** encloses the teeth incisally or on the masticatory surface with cast, accurately fitting caps (Fig 11-35). An excellent splinting effect is produced due to the good bodily grasp on the teeth. A cap splint is indicated if a sublingual bar cannot be placed because the floor of the mouth is high. Its disadvantages are the esthetic impression and the extensive coverage of the tooth surface, under which caries will develop if oral hygiene is poor.

The **lingual splint** covers the lingual surfaces of the teeth and has interdental cribs (Fig 11-36). It is indicated if the floor of the mouth is high, and it is esthetically better than a cap splint while producing the same splinting effects. Its disadvantages are again the extensive coverage with the risk of caries.

The **Weissenfluh splint** is a lingual splint that is suspended in the tooth with parallel pins. In addition, sleeves are cemented into parallel parapulpal drill holes in the lingual surfaces. The splinting effects and the esthetics are very good with this splint, but it is difficult to fabricate. Furthermore, there is also a risk of caries under the extensive coverage.

Index

Page numbers followed by "f" denote figures, and those followed by "t" denote tables.

A

Abducens nerve, 239f, 240
Abrasion
  description of, 76
  occlusal contacts, 148, 149f
  physiologic, 148
Accessory developmental groove, 95f, 96
Accessory nerve, 239f, 240
Acellular-afibrillar cementum, 52, 53f
Acellular-fibrillar cementum, 52, 53f
Activator
  Balters bionator, 342, 343f
  Bimler appliance, 340, 341f
  construction bite for, 335, 336f
  design of, 338–340
  expansion screw with, 339, 339f
  fabrication of, 335–336, 336f
  Fränkel functional regulator, 342, 344
  grinding of, 336–338, 337f–338f
  illustration of, 334f
  Klammt's elastic open, 340–342, 341f
  monobloc, 340, 341f
  open bite treated with, 340
  regulatory effect of, 333, 334f
  thrusts, 334f, 334–335
  wax try-in, 336
Active appliances, 309
Active plate
  actions of, 310, 311f
  active components of, 316, 317f
  design of, 324–327
  elements of, 310–312, 311f
  fixed appliances versus, 310
  function of, 310
  retentive components of, 312–315, 315f
  spring components of, 318–323, 318f–323f
Acute apical periodontitis, 287
Acute gingivitis, 285

Adams clasp, 312f, 312–313
Adrenal glands, 241f, 242
Adrenergic system, 240
Aging
  enamel affected by, 47
  facial expression muscles affected by, 229
Aligners, 362t, 375–376
Alveolar bone
  anatomy of, 57–59, 58f–59f
  composition of, 168, 169f
Alveolar foramina, 164, 165f
Alveolar jugae, 164, 165f, 170, 171f, 193, 195
Alveolar periodontium, 64f, 65
Alveolar processes, 59, 164, 165f
Alveolar ridge, 193
Alveolar septa, 164
Alveolar sockets, 20, 42f, 57f
Alveoli
  anatomy of, 167f
  maxillary, 164, 165f
  tooth position in, 62, 63f
Ameloblasts, 44, 45f, 47
Anaphase, 30, 30f
Anatomical crown, 20, 21f
Anatomical equator, 75, 75f
Anatomy
  definition of, 2
  directional, 5–8
  positional, 5–8
  subdivisions of, 3f
Anchorage, for force distribution, 306f–307f, 306–308
Angle characteristic, 72
Antagonists, 123, 123f, 139
Antagonists rule, 123, 123f
Anterior, 7
Anterior cranial fossa, 154
Anterior disc displacement, 360, 360f

Anterior fontanel, 156, 157f
Anterior jig, 371, 371f
Anterior nasal spine, 164, 165f
Anterior occlusal splints, 362t, 365
Anterior open bite, 127–128
Anterior reverse articulation, 129
Anterior teeth. See also Dentition; Teeth.
  activator effects on, 338f
  anatomy of, 21
  angle characteristic of, 73f
  canines. See Canine(s).
  definition of, 78
  incisal margin of, 72, 73f
  incisors. See Incisors.
  inclination of axes, 78, 78f, 87f, 93f
  intercuspation of, 124, 124f
  labial surfaces of, 78–79
  in occlusion, 230f
  position of, 135t
  primary, 111
  root characteristic of, 78, 79f
  successional, 114
  tipping of, 122, 122f
  vertical overlap with, 135t
  vestibular inclination of, 125
Anterior-supported occlusion, 214, 214f
Anti-snoring mouthpieces, 375, 376f
Apatite crystals, 36, 45–46
Apical, 7
Apical foramen, 6, 21, 21f, 55
Apical periodontium, 64f, 65–66
Apocrine glands, 186
Approximal, 7
Approximal contact points, 138, 138f
Approximal marginal ridges, 95
Approximal surfaces
  description of, 74, 75f
  mesial, 80, 82f
  of mandibular first molar, 109, 110f
  of mandibular first premolar, 99f, 100

of mandibular incisors, 84, 85f–86f
of mandibular second premolar, 101f, 102
of maxillary canines, 89f, 91
of maxillary first molar, 103f, 104, 105f
of maxillary first premolar, 96–97, 97f
of maxillary lateral incisor, 83f, 84
of maxillary second molar, 106f, 107
of maxillary second premolar, 97, 98f
Aqualizer, 365, 365f
Arch characteristic, 74
Arcon articulators, 249, 249f
Arrowhead clasp, 314, 315f
Arthritis, 181
Arthropathies, 357
Articular capsule, 180–181, 226f
Articular disc
  anatomy of, 178f, 180–181, 258
  displacement of, 360, 360f
Articular ligaments, 181, 182f
Articular tubercle, 177–179, 178f
Articulation surfaces, 148
Articulators
  anatomical values used, 250–251
  arcon, 249, 249f
  average-value. See Average-value articulators.
  classification of, 246–251
  components of, 245–246, 246f
  facebow technique, 266–267, 266f–267f, 271f
  fixed-value, 250, 251f
  fully adjustable, 258
  Gothic arch tracing, 264, 265f
  intercondylar distance of, 258, 259f
  jaw relation registration, 260–261, 261f–263f
  joint values, 272f, 272–273
  mounting models in, 267–271, 268f–271f
  nonarcon, 248, 248f
  reference planes for model adjustment, 246–247, 247f
  replication of joints and movements, 248–250
  system errors with, 258, 259f
Artificial replacement, 2
Atrophy, 2
Attached gingiva, 67
Attrition, 76
Auricle, 13f
Auriculo-infraorbital plane, 14
Auriculotemporal nerve, 244
Autonomic nervous system, 236, 240
Autonomic organs, 5

Average-value articulators
  definition of, 250, 252
  illustration of, 252f
  occlusal height in, 257, 257f
  occlusal plane in, 254f
  semi-adjustable, 253, 253f
  technique errors with, 254–257
Axon, 235

B

Balanced occlusion, 214–215, 215f
Balkwill angle, 118, 120f, 121, 252, 266
Ball clasp, 314, 315f
Ball-and-socket joint, 176, 177f
Balters bionator, 342, 343f
Basal, 7
Base of the skull, 154, 155f–157f
Basement membrane, 33f, 68
Begg brackets, 350
Begg technique, 350
Bennett angle, 211, 211f, 252, 272
Bennett movement, 209–212, 210f–211f, 258
Bennett side shift, 253, 253f
Bilateral reverse articulation, 131, 135t
Bimler appliance, 340, 341f
Biologic functional cycle, 8
Biologic intensity levels, 302–303, 303f
Bite plane. See Occlusal plane.
Body
  directional terms for, 7–8
  structure of, 3–5, 4f
Bonded brackets, 351
Bone
  alveolar, 57–59, 58f–59f
  composition of, 36
  constituents of, 37–38, 37f–38f, 44f
  development of, 36–37
  flat, 40
  form and function of, 38–40, 39f
  inorganic components of, 37
  irregular, 40
  long, 40, 40f
  membrane, 37
  organic components of, 37
  replacing, 37
  short, 40
  structure of, 36–37, 37f
Bone marrow, 36f, 38
Bonwill circle, 118, 118f
Bonwill triangle, 120, 120f, 252, 254, 258, 266

Bony palate, 166, 167f
Bony skull, 151, 152f
Bony substance, 36f, 38
Border movements, of mandible, 203–204, 203f–206f
Bracket adhesive technique, 351
Brackets, 346–348, 347f
Brain
  anatomy of, 236–238, 237f
  cranial nerves, 239f, 239–240
  segments of, 236–238, 237f
Brainstem, 238
Bruxism, 359, 372
Bruxism splints, 359, 362t
Buccal, 6, 7f
Buccal cavity, 192f, 193
Buccal cusps, 142f, 216
Buccal frena, 16, 17f, 18
Buccal frenulum, 192f, 193, 194
Buccal vestibular sulcus, 18
Buccinator muscle, 12, 16, 229f, 231f, 232
Bursae, 221

C

Calibration keys, 255–257, 256f
Camper facial angle, 14
Camper plane, 12f, 12–14, 119, 119f, 246, 247f, 252
Cancellous bone, 58, 58f
Cancellous tissue, 168
Canine(s)
  in alveolar bone, 59f
  definition of, 79
  description of, 21, 88
  mandibular, 22f, 91, 92f–93f
  maxillary, 22f, 88–91, 89f–90f, 93f
  occlusion of, 93f
Canine guidance, 79, 214, 214f, 368, 369f
Canine guidance ridge, 88
Canine-supported occlusion, 214, 214f
Cap splint, 379, 379f
Caput angulare, 233
Caput infraorbitale, 233
Caput zygomaticum, 233
Cardiac muscle, 218
Caries
  areas susceptible to, 276, 276f
  in dentin, 48
  description of, 283–285
  dietary factors, 284
  fluoride for prevention of, 290–291, 291f
  formation of, 283

lesion associated with, 283
prevention of, 290, 292
treatment of, 284–285
Carotid foramen, 155f
Cartilage, 40
Cartilaginous connective tissue. See
Fibrocartilage.
Cartilaginous joint, 175
Caudal, 8
C-clasp, 314
Cell(s)
as functional unit, 25–26
classification of, 26
cytoplasm of, 27f, 28
description of, 5
division of, 30–32
growth of, 25
illustration of, 27f
metabolism in, 25
microstructures of, 27f, 28–30
nucleus of, 26, 29f, 29–30
organelles of, 26, 27f
regulatory ability and reactivity of,
25
reproduction in, 25
Cell membrane, 26
Cell-poor cementum, 52
Cell-rich connective tissue, 34–35, 35f
Cellular-fibrillar cementum, 52, 53f
Cementoblasts, 52–53, 53f
Cementocyte, 53f
Cementoenamel junction, 67
Cementum
acellular-afibrillar, 52, 53f
acellular-fibrillar, 52, 53f
anatomy of, 42f, 51, 52f
cell-poor, 52
cellular-fibrillar, 52, 53f
collagen of, 52–53
composition of, 44, 44f
definition of, 51
formation of, 51–52, 53f
function of, 53
Central, 7
Central developmental groove, 95, 95f
Central fossa, 95f, 96
Centric occlusion, 203, 203f, 212, 213f,
215, 215f, 264, 272, 368
Centric records, 261, 272
Centric relation, 263f, 365
Centric relation splints
description of, 362t, 365
illustration of, 366f
Michigan splint. See Michigan
splint.

stabilization splint, 366–367,
366f–367f
types of, 366
Centric stops, 138, 140, 142f–143f,
216f
Centrosome, 27f, 28
Cephalometric planes, 12f–13f, 12–14
Cephalometry, 12
Cerebellum, 238
Cerebral gyri, 154
Cerebrum, 238
Cervical, 7
Cervical vertebra, 39f
Cheeks, 11–12
Chewing, 198
Chin, 12
Chin muscle, 229f, 233–234
Chlorhexidine, 289
Chondroblasts, 40
Christensen's phenomenon, 208f,
208–209
Chromatids, 30
Chromatin, 27f, 30
Chronic gingivitis, 285
Circumpulpal dentin, 51
Circumvallate papillae, 196–197,
196f–197f
Class II malocclusion, 127, 127f–128f
Class III malocclusion, 128f
Cleaning techniques, 289–291, 290f
Cleft lip, 277, 278f–279f
Cleft palate, 166, 277, 278f–279f
Clenching, 359
Clinical crown, 20, 21f
Closed dentition, 136–137
Coffin spring, 319, 319f, 340
Collagen, 52–53
Collum angle, 98, 99f
Columnar epithelium, 32, 33f
Compact substance, 36f, 38
Components, 146
Conditioned reflexes, 236
Condylar ball, 248
Condylar guidance, 206, 248
Condylar housings, 250
Condylar path, 179
Condylar paths, on fully adjustable
articulators, 272, 273f
Condylar process, 172, 172f
Condyle
anatomy of, 179f, 179–180
movement of, 206–207, 207f
Connective tissue
description of, 32, 34f–35f, 34–36
mucosal, 187

of marginal periodontium, 68, 69f
of periodontal ligament, 60
Contact areas, 139, 142f–143f
Contact points
approximal, 138, 138f
description of, 74, 75f, 138–149
function of, 138
Corona dentis, 6
Coronal, 7
Coronal pulp, 54f, 114
Coronal suture, 154, 157f
Coronoid process, 168, 171f, 174
Corpus callosum, 237f, 238
Cortex, 238
Cortical substance, 36f, 58
Cranial, 8
Cranial nerves, 239f, 239–240
Cranial sutures, 154, 156f–157f
Cranial vault
bones of, 156f–157f, 158, 159f
description of, 152f, 153
Cranium, 151, 152f
Crest line, 118
Crib splint, 378f, 379
Cribriform lamina, 58, 62
Cribriform plate, 168
Crista galli, 155f, 160
Cross line, 116, 117f
Crowding, 121f, 122, 134t, 326
Crown of tooth
anatomy of, 6, 20, 21f
defects of, 280–281
enamel covering of, 43
replacement of, 293
surfaces of, 71–74, 72f–73f
Crown-root angulation, 98, 99f
Crozat appliance
advantages and disadvantages of,
328
body wire of, 328–329, 329f
construction of, 328–330
description of, 309, 328
extension wires of, 330–331, 331f
high labial bow, 331, 331f
retentive components of, 329f,
329–330
springs attached to, 329, 329f
Crushing cusps, 94, 102
Cuboidal epithelium, 32, 33f
Curve of Spee, 126f, 127
Cusp(s), 94, 102
Cusp crest, 94
Cusp of Carabelli, 103f, 104, 107, 280
Cusp ridges, 94–95, 95f
Cusp slopes, 94, 95f

Cusp tip, 94, 94f
Cusp-fossa occlusion, 140
Cusp-fossa–marginal ridges
    occlusion, 140
Cytology, 2, 25
Cytoplasm, 27f, 28

D

Deciduous teeth, 20. *See also* Primary
    teeth.
Deep bite, 128–129, 133, 134t
Demastication, 76
Dendrites, 234f, 235
Dental, 18
Dental abrasion. *See* Abrasion.
Dental aplasia, 282
Dental arch
    asymmetry of, 299
    axis of symmetry, 118
    directional terms for, 6, 7f
    in horizontal plane, 115
    inhibited development of, 283
    length of, 116–117, 117f
    mandibular, 116, 298–299
    maxillary, 116, 116f, 298–299
    of primary dentition, 112, 112f
    positional terms for, 6, 7f
    vertical anterior, 125, 125f
    width of, 116, 117f
Dental floss, 290
Dental formulas, 22–23
Dental papilla, 42
Dental periosteum. *See* Periodontal
    ligament.
Dental pulp. *See* Pulp.
Dental services, 291–293, 292f
Dental technician, 293, 293f
Dental tissues
    anatomy of, 41, 42f
    classification of, 41
    development of, 41–43
    enamel. *See* Enamel.
Dentin
    anatomy of, 42f, 54f
    caries involvement in, 48
    cells involved in formation, 47–48
    characteristics of, 47–48
    circumpulpal, 51
    color of, 43
    composition of, 44, 44f
    formation of, 43, 49–51, 50f
    hypoplasia of, 280
    mantle, 51
    mineralization of, 51

odontoblast processes in, 48,
    48f–49f, 51, 54f
secondary, 48, 76
Dentinal tubules, 49, 49f
Dentinoenamel junction, 76
Dentinogenesis, 49–51, 50f
Dentition. *See also* Anterior teeth;
    Posterior teeth; Teeth; *specific
    teeth.*
closed, 136–137
form and function of, 115–118,
    116f–118f
in frontal plane, 129–133, 134t–135t
in horizontal plane, 118–123
permanent, 22, 112
primary, 20, 22–23, 112. *See also*
    Primary teeth.
in sagittal plane, 123f–128f, 123–129
temporary, 21
types of, 21–22
Denture-bearing areas
    in mandible, 193–195, 194f–195f
    in maxilla, 191–193, 192f
Dentures, 293
Depressor muscle of the angle of the
    mouth, 229f, 231f, 233
Depressor muscle of the lower lip,
    229f, 233
Dermis, 184, 184f
Dermoskeleton, 18
Desmodontium, 59. *See also*
    Periodontal ligament.
Developmental anomalies
    in jaw, 277–279
    in primary dentition, 278–279
    in teeth, 279–281, 281f
Diaphragm, 3
Diastema, 123
Diencephalon, 238
Digastric fossa, 170
Digastric muscle, 224f, 226, 227f
Direction, anatomical nomenclature
    for, 5–8
Disc displacement, 360, 360f
Dislocation, 181
Distal, 7, 7f
Distal approximal surface, 74
Disto-occlusion, 127, 127f, 134t
Distraction splint, 362t, 371, 371f
Disuse atrophy, 2
Dorsal, 7
Double-fan screw, 325f
Double-plates, 327, 339, 339f
Drum Miniplast splint, 376, 377f

Dynamic occlusion, 212, 214,
    214f–215f
Dysgnathia, 123, 131, 275

E

Eccentric occlusion, 214
Eccentric splints, 362t, 370–371,
    370f–371f
Edge-to-edge occlusion, 135t
Edgewise technique, 349–350,
    349f–350f
Elastic cartilage, 40
Elastic connective tissue, 36
Elastics, 320–321
Elbrecht splint, 378f, 379
Electric toothbrushes, 288–289
Electronic pantography, 264
Ellipsoidal joint, 176, 177f
Embryonic connective tissue, 35–36
Enamel
    aging effects on, 47
    anatomy of, 42f, 54f
    composition of, 44, 44f
    description of, 43–45
    erosion of, 285
    fluoridation of, 47
    formation of, 45–47
    functions of, 45
    mature, 44
    mineralization process of, 46
    in multicusped teeth, 47
    organic substance of, 44
    permeability of, 45
    posteruptive maturation of, 47
Enamel cap, 42f
Enamel cuticle, 44
Enamel epithelium, 42, 43f
Enamel hypoplasia, 279
Enamel matrix, 45
Enamel organ, 42
Enamel prisms, 45–46, 46f
Endocrine glands, 185, 241f, 242
Endoplasmic reticulum, 27f, 28
End-to-end occlusion, 135t
Epidermis, 184, 184f
Epiphyseal line, 36f
Epithelial root sheath, 43f, 47
Epithelial tissue, 32–34, 33f
Erosion, 285
Eruption, 112, 113f
Ethmoid bone, 152f, 155f, 160, 161f
Ethmoidal cells, 160
Ethmoidal crest, 165f
Eustachian tube, 192f, 193

Exfoliation of teeth, 20, 59
Exocrine glands, 185, 187f
Expansion screw, 316, 317f
External ear, 9
External enamel epithelium, 42, 43f
Extraoral anchorage, 307, 308f
Eyeballs, 10
Eyelids, 10, 11f

F

Face
  description of, 5
  features of, 9–12
  landmarks of, 10, 11f
  upper, 9
Facebow technique, 266–267,
    266f–267f, 271f
Facial bones, 152f, 153, 160, 161f
Facial clefts, 279
Facial expression muscles
  anatomy of, 229f
  description of, 228–229
  first antagonistic muscle pair,
    232–233
  second antagonistic muscle pair,
    233–234
Facial nerve, 239f, 240
False hyperdontia, 281, 282f
False hypodontia, 282
Fasciae, 221
Fauces, 14
Fédération Dentaire International
    tooth notation, 23, 24f
Fibroblasts, 55, 61
Fibrocartilage, 40
Fibrous connective tissue, 35f, 35–36
Fibrous joint, 175
Fibrous marginal zone, 189, 190f
Fibrous median zone, 189, 190f
Filiform papillae, 196, 196f–197f
Finger spring, 320
First cervical vertebra, 39f
Fischer angle, 273
Fixation centric splints, 373, 373f
Fixator, 250, 251f
Fixed orthodontic appliances
  advantages and disadvantages of,
    346
  brackets, 346–348, 347f
  description of, 310, 345–346
  edgewise technique, 349–350,
    349f–350f
  lingual technique, 353–354
  mechanism of action, 346

multiband, 345–353
  technique for, 345
Fixed splints, 378
Fixed-value articulator, 250, 251f
Flat bones, 40
Floor of the mouth, 14, 15f
Fluoride, 47, 290–291, 291f
Foliate papillae, 197
Follicle, 42, 59, 61
Fontanels, 154, 156, 157f
Force
  anchorage for distribution of,
    306–307, 306f–308f
  description of, 146–148
  transferring of, for tooth
    movements, 304–305, 305f
Form and function, 2, 71
Fornix, of lips, 10, 11f
Fränkel functional regulator, 342, 344
Frankfort horizontal plane, 14
Free alveolar border, 170, 171f–172f
Free gingiva, 67
Freeway space, 212, 213f
Frenulum of tongue, 194–196
Frontal, 8
Frontal bone, 152f, 156f–157f, 158,
    159f
Frontal nerve, 242
Frontal plane
  dentition in, 129–133, 134t–135t
  description of, 6, 6f
  mandibular border movements in,
    204
  tooth malposition in, 131–133,
    134t–135t
Frontal process, 164, 165f
Fully adjustable articulators, 258
Functional movements, 202
Functional orthodontics, 296, 297f
Fungiform papillae, 196, 196f–197f

G

Gag reflex, 16
Ganglia, 234
Ganglion cells, 234, 238
Gaps, 122–123
Generalized abrasion, 76
Genioglossus muscle, 198, 199f, 226f
Geniohyoid muscle, 224f, 226f–227f,
    228
Germ cells
  description of, 31
  tooth, 42, 43f
Germ teeth, 42, 43f

Gingiva
  attached, 67
  free, 67
Gingival, 7
Gingival epithelium, 68
Gingival sulcus
  anatomy of, 66f–67f, 67
  wound-healing process in, 68
Gingivitis, 276f, 277, 285, 286
Glabella, 13f
Glabella vertical, 14
Glands, 185–186, 187f
Glandular cells, 186
Glandular epithelium, 32, 33f
Glandular zone, 190, 190f
Glossopharyngeal nerve, 239f, 240
Gnathion, 13f
Golgi apparatus, 27f, 28
Gothic arch, 204, 205f
Gothic arch tracing, 264, 265f
Granulocytes, 34
Greater palatine canal, 158
Greater palatine foramen, 167f
Greater palatine process, 165f
Gustatory glands, 196, 197f

H

Habitual intercuspation, 212
Haderup system, 23
Hair, 185
Hand-guided occlusal registration,
    261
Hard palate, 14, 15f
Hard substances
  cementum. *See* Cementum.
  dentin. *See* Dentin.
  description of, 46–47
  elasticity of, 53
  enamel. *See* Enamel.
Harmonious occlusion, 212
Hertwig epithelial root sheath, 43f, 47
Haversian canals, 38
Hawley appliance, 364, 364f
Head
  anatomy of, 5
  cephalometric planes of, 12f–13f,
    12–14
  directional terms for, 7–8
Headgear, 307, 308f
Hinge joint, 176, 177f
Hinge splints, 362t
Hinge-axis orbital plane, 247, 247f
Histology, 2
Holocrine glands, 186

Horizontal abrasion, 76
Horizontal curvature characteristic, 72–74, 73f
Horizontal exfoliation of teeth, 20
Horizontal plane
  dentition in, 118–123
  mandibular border movements in, 204, 205f
  tooth malposition in, 121f–122f, 121–123
Hormones, 240–242, 241f
Human body. See Body.
Human face. See Face.
Hyaline cartilage, 40
Hyaloplasm, 28
Hydrostatic contact pressure, 68–69
Hydroxyapatite, 36, 44
Hyoglossus muscle, 198, 199f
Hyoid bone
  anatomy of, 160, 161f
  muscle groups of, 226–228, 227f
Hyperdontia, 281, 282f
Hyperplastic gingivitis, 285
Hypoglossal nerve, 239f, 240
Hypothalamus, 238

I

Incisal, 7
Incisal margin, 72, 73f
Incisal view
  of mandibular incisors, 84, 85f–86f
  of maxillary canines, 89f, 91
  of maxillary first molar, 103f
  of maxillary incisors, 80, 81f–83f, 84
Incisive bone, 14, 164
Incisive canal, 164, 165f
Incisive foramen, 14, 155f, 164, 167f
Incisive papilla, 14, 17f, 166, 190, 193
Incisive suture, 166, 167f
Incisors
  in alveolar bone, 59f
  description of, 21
  mandibular. See Mandibular incisors.
  maxillary. See Maxillary incisors.
  mesial tipping of, 122
Inclination of axes
  for mandibular canines, 93f
  for mandibular incisors, 87f
  for maxillary canines, 93f
  for maxillary incisors, 87f
Inclined plane, 331–333, 332f
Incognito appliance system, 353–354, 355f
Inferior alveolar nerve, 244

Inferior joint space, 178f, 180
Inferior labial frenulum, 194
Inferior nasal concha, 152f, 156f, 160, 161f
Infrahyoid muscle, 228
Infraorbital canal, 165f
Infraorbital nerve, 242–243
Infraorbital sulcus, 163, 165f
Infrazygomatic crest, 165f, 192f, 193
Interbrain, 238
Intercalated discs, 218
Intercellular space, 5
Interceptors, 362t, 371, 371f
Intercondylar distance, 258, 259f
Intercuspal position, 212
Intercuspation, 124, 124f, 134t, 212, 213f
Interdental brushes, 289, 290f
Interdental papilla, 74
Interdental space, 67, 74–75, 74f–75f
Interdental spring, 319–320
Interincisal angle, 78
Internal alveolar wall, 58
Internal enamel epithelium, 42–43, 43f
Interocclusal record, 261f, 272
Interphase, 31
Interpupillary line, 13f
Interradicular septa, 164, 167f
Interstitial abrasion, 76, 77f
Intraoral appliances, 362t
Irregular bones, 40
Islets of Langerhans, 242

J

Jackson clasps, 329–330, 330f
Jaw development
  anomalies of, 277–279
  inhibition in, 283
  normal, 277
Jaw relation registration, 260–261, 261f–263f
Jet irrigators, 289
Joint(s). See also specific joint.
  arthritis of, 181
  diseases of, 181, 183
  dislocation of, 181
  mobility of, 176, 177f
  sprain of, 181
  structure of, 175
  types of, 174–177
Joint bodies, 175, 176f
Joint capsule, 175, 176f, 178f, 181
Joint cartilage, 36f
Joint cavity, 175
Junctional epithelial cells, 68

Junctional epithelium, 68
Juncturae, 174, 175f

K

Klammt's elastic open activator, 340–342, 341f

L

Labial, 6, 7f
Labial bow, 322–323, 323f, 331, 364
Labial frenula, 16, 17f
Labial surface
  of anterior teeth, 78–79
  of maxillary canines, 89f
  of maxillary central incisor, 80, 81f
  of maxillary lateral incisor, 80
Labiomental groove, 10
Lacrimal bone, 152f, 156f–157f, 160, 161f
Lacrimal nerve, 242
Lambdoid suture, 154, 157f, 175f
Lamina externa, 151
Lamina interna, 151
Lateral, 8
Lateral fontanel, 156
Lateral forced guidance, 132
Lateral pterygoid muscle, 180, 224, 224f–225f
Lateral pterygoid nerve, 244
Laterodetrusion, 211
Lateroprotrusion, 211
Lateroretrusion, 211
Laterosurtrusion, 211
Laterotrusion, 211
Laterotrusive excursion, 366
Law of form and function, 2
Lesser palatine foramen, 167f
Leukocytes, 68
Levator muscle of the angle of the mouth, 229f, 231f, 233
Levator muscle of the upper lip, 229f, 231f, 233
Lingual, 7, 7f
Lingual cusps, 142f
Lingual frenum, 17f
Lingual nerve, 244
Lingual retainers, 376
Lingual splint, 379, 379f
Lingual surface
  description of, 74, 74f
  of mandibular first molar, 109, 110f
  of mandibular first premolar, 99f, 100
  of mandibular incisors, 84, 85f–86f

of mandibular second premolar, 101f, 102
of maxillary canines, 88, 89f
of maxillary first molar, 103f, 104, 105f
of maxillary first premolar, 96, 97f
of maxillary incisors, 79f, 80, 81f
of maxillary lateral incisor, 80, 83f, 84
of maxillary second molar, 106f, 107
of maxillary second premolar, 97, 98f
Lingual technique, for fixed orthodontic appliances, 353–354
Lingual tipping, 136, 137f
Lingula mandibulae, 174
Lips
  anatomy of, 10, 11f
  cleft, 277, 278f–279f
  muscles of, 11
Long bones, 40, 40f
Long centric, 215
Loose connective tissue, 35–36
Lower face, 9
Lower lip, 10, 11f
Lymph, 62
Lymphocytes, 34
Lysosome, 27f, 28

M

Macroscopic anatomy, 2
Macrotrauma, 360
Main developmental groove, 95, 95f
Malocclusion, 215
Mandible
  alveolar part of, 168, 170
  alveolar tubercle of, 195
  anatomy of, 17f, 152f, 156f–157f, 168–174, 169f, 171f–172f
  angle of, 172
  body of, 168, 170–171, 171f–172f
  centric stops in, 143f
  contact areas in, 142f
  denture-bearing areas in, 193–195, 194f–195f
  formation of, 59
  functional construction of, 168, 169f
  movements of. See Mandibular movement.
  rami of, 172–174, 173f–174f
  rotation axes of, 207f
  topography of, 170–171, 171f–172f
Mandibular branch, of trigeminal nerve, 244, 244f
Mandibular canal, 168, 169f

Mandibular canines, 91, 92f–93f
Mandibular dental arch
  form of, 116
  length of, 116, 298–299
Mandibular foramen, 172f, 174
Mandibular fossa, 155f, 177, 178f, 179
Mandibular incisal point, 119
Mandibular incisors
  anatomy of, 79
  central, 84, 85f
  inclination of axes, 87f
  lateral, 84, 86f
  maxillary incisors versus, 79
Mandibular molars
  anatomy of, 22f
  first, 109, 110f
  primary, 112
  roots of, 102
  second, 109, 110f
  third, 109
Mandibular movement
  Bennett movement, 209–212, 210f–211f, 258
  border movements, 203–204, 203f–206f
  guidance factors in, 206–209
  muscles of, 222–223, 223f
  overview of, 201–203
  tooth contacts during, 216f–217f, 216–218
Mandibular notch, 171f, 174
Mandibular premolars
  anatomy of, 22f
  first, 98–100, 99f
  maxillary premolars versus, 98
  second, 100–102, 101f
Mandibular protrusion, 129
Mandibular torus, 174
Mandibular tubercle, 18
Mantle dentin, 51
Marginal, 8
Marginal gingivitis, 285
Marginal periodontitis, 287
Marginal periodontium
  anatomy of, 42f
  connective tissue fiber structure of, 68, 69f
  definition of, 66
  gingival epithelium, 68
  gingival sulcus, 66f–67f, 67
  hydrostatic contact pressure of blood vessel system, 69
  illustration of, 64f
  junctional epithelium, 68
  prosthetic tooth replacement effects on, 70, 70f

structural elements of, 66f–67f, 67–70
surgical resection of, 303
tissue seal mechanisms in, 66–67
Masseter muscle, 224f–226f, 225, 231f
Masseteric nerve, 244
Masseteric tuberosities, 171f, 172
Masticatory, 7
Masticatory cycle, 202f, 203
Masticatory muscle synchronizer, 373
Masticatory muscles
  activator effects on, 338
  anatomy of, 224–225, 224f–226f
  description of, 222–223
Masticatory process, 202–203
Masticatory surface, 72
Masticatory system, 8, 10f
Mastoid fontanel, 157f
Mastoid process, 155f
Mature enamel, 44
Maxilla
  anatomy of, 17f, 152f, 156f–157f, 162–163, 162f–163f
  body of, 162
  centric stops in, 142f
  contact areas in, 143f
  denture-bearing area in, 191–193, 192f
  facial surface of, 162
  formation of, 59
  infratemporal surface of, 162–163
  mucosal covering in, 189–191
  nasal surface of, 163
  orbital surface of, 163
Maxillary branch, of trigeminal nerve, 242–244
Maxillary canines, 88–91, 89f–90f, 93f
Maxillary dental arch
  form of, 116, 116f
  length of, 116, 298–299
Maxillary hiatus, 163, 165f
Maxillary incisors
  anatomy of, 22f
  central, 80, 81f–82f
  inclination of axes, 87f
  lateral, 80, 83f, 84, 87f
  lingual surfaces of, 79f
  mandibular incisors versus, 79
  root of, 87f
Maxillary molars
  anatomy of, 22f
  first, 102–104, 103f, 105f, 111
  primary, 111
  second, 104, 106f, 107, 111
  third, 107, 107f–108f

Maxillary premolars
  anatomy of, 22f
  description of, 96
  first, 96–97, 97f
  mandibular premolars versus, 98
  second, 97, 98f
Maxillary processes, 163f, 164, 165f
Maxillary sinus, 163
Maxillary teeth
  anterior, 11
  inclination of, 129, 130f
Maxillary tuberosity, 17f, 18, 165f,
    167f, 190, 193
Maxillomandibular anchorage, 307,
    308f, 327f
Maxillomandibular bow, 323, 323f
Maximal intercuspation, 212, 213f
Medial pterygoid muscle, 224f–226f,
    225
Medial pterygoid nerve, 244
Median palatine raphe, 117f, 193
Median palatine suture, 14, 166, 167f
Median plane, 6, 6f
Medulla oblongata, 237f, 238–239
Medullary cavity, 36f
Meiosis, 31f, 31–32
Membrane bone, 37
Mental foramen, 170, 171f, 194
Mental spines, 170
Mental trigone, 170
Mental tubercles, 171f
Merocrine glands, 186
Mesial, 7, 7f
Mesial approximal surface
  description of, 74
  of maxillary canines, 88, 89f
  of maxillary first molar, 106f
  of maxillary first premolar, 97
  of maxillary incisors, 80, 82f
Mesial migration, of teeth, 300
Mesial tipping, 122
Mesio-occlusion, 128f, 129, 134t–135t
Metabolism, cellular, 25
Metaphase, 30, 30f
Metaplasm, 28
Michigan splint
  description of, 362t
  fabrication of, 369
  history of, 367
  illustration of, 368f
  muscle activity reductions using,
    368
Microscopic anatomy, 2
Midbrain, 238
Middle cranial fossa, 154
Midface, 9–10

Midface horizontal plane, 247, 247f
Miniplast splints, 362t
Mitochondrion, 27f, 28
Mitosis, 30f, 30–31
Model analysis, orthodontic, 297–299,
    298f–299f
Modiolus, 229f, 230, 231f
Molar(s)
  in alveolar bone, 59f
  description of, 21
  function of, 102
  mandibular. *See* Mandibular molars.
  maxillary. *See* Maxillary molars.
  occlusal contacts in, 143f
  primary, 112
  root apices of, 170
Molar triangle, 17f
Monobloc activator, 340, 341f
Mounting models, in articulator, 267–
    271, 268f–271f
Mouth
  angles of, 10
  floor of, 14, 15f
  nose and, distance between, 11
  orifice of, 10
Mouth breathing, open bite caused
    by, 133
Mouthguards, 362t, 376–377
Mucins, 186
Mucous membrane, 187–189, 188f
Multicellular organisms, 26
Multipoint force application, 304f, 305
Muscle
  anatomy of, 218–220
  as motor unit, 220–222
  cardiac, 218
  definition of, 218
  facial expression. *See* Facial
    expression muscles.
  hyoid bone, 226–228, 227f
  mandibular movement, 222–223,
    223f
  mouth-closing, 222–223
  shape of, 221, 221f
  skeletal, 220
  smooth, 218
  striated, 218–220
  structure of, 218, 219f
Muscle contractions, 220–221
Muscle power, 221
Muscle tone, 220
Myelin, 235
Myelin sheath, 235f
Mylohyoid line, 17f, 170, 172f, 194
Mylohyoid muscle, 14, 226f–227f, 228
Mylohyoid sulcus, 172f, 174

Myofibrils, 28, 219, 219f
Myofunctional therapy, 344f, 344–345
Myopathies, 357, 372
Myorelaxation splint, 363–364

N

Nasal, 8
Nasal bone, 152f, 156f–157f, 160, 161f
Nasion, 13f
Nasion vertical, 14
Nasociliary nerve, 242
Nasolabial sulcus, 10–11
Neck, 5
Neck (of tooth), 21
Nerve cells, 234f, 234–235
Nerve fibers, 235–236
Nerve tissue, 234–235
Nervous system
  autonomic, 236, 240
  hormonal control of, 240–242, 241f
  somatic, 236
Neurilemma, 235
Neurites, 234, 234f
Neurocytes, 234
Neuromuscular guidance, of
    mandibular movements, 206
Neuron, 234f, 235
Neurotransmitters, 235
Neutro-occlusion, 123–125, 124f, 127,
    131f, 134t
Night guards, 363
Nodes of Ranvier, 235
Nonarcon articulator, 248, 248f
Nonsupporting cusps, 94
Normal occlusion, 8
Nose, 11
Notation, for teeth, 22–23, 24f
Nuclear membrane, 27f, 29, 29f
Nucleolus, 27f, 29, 29f
Nucleus, 26, 29f, 29–30

O

Oblique line, 17f, 18, 170, 171f, 194
Obstructive sleep apnea, 374–375
Obturators, 166
Occipital, 8
Occipital bone, 152f, 155f, 157f, 158,
    159f
Occipital condyle, 155f
Occipital foramen, 155f, 158
Occipital lobe, 237f
Occipitomastoid suture, 157f
Occluder, 250, 251f
Occlusal, 7

Occlusal contacts
  abrasion of, 148, 149f
  anatomy of, 139f
  definition of, 138
  form and position of, 140–141,
    141f–143f
  forms of, 149f
  interlocking principle of, 139f
  punctiform, 141f, 144–148, 145f–147f
Occlusal field, 215
Occlusal interferences, 215
Occlusal plane, 119, 119f, 252, 310
Occlusal splints
  anterior, 365
  definition of, 363, 373
  reflex splints, 362t, 363–365,
    364f–365f
Occlusal surface
  description of, 72, 72f–73f
  of mandibular first molar, 109, 110f
  of mandibular first premolar, 99f,
    100
  of mandibular second premolar,
    101f, 102
  of maxillary first molar, 103f, 104
  of maxillary first premolar, 96, 97f
  of maxillary second molar, 106f, 107
  of maxillary second premolar, 97,
    98f
  of posterior teeth, 94f–95f, 94–96
Occlusion
  anterior teeth in, 230f
  anterior-supported, 214, 214f
  balanced, 214–215, 215f
  canine-supported, 214, 214f
  centric, 203, 203f, 212, 213f, 264,
    272, 368
  curves of, 125–127, 126f, 129–130,
    130f
  cusp-fossa, 140
  cusp-fossa–marginal ridges, 140
  definition of, 212
  disto-, 127, 127f, 134t
  dynamic, 212, 214, 214f–215f
  edge-to-edge, 135t
  end-to-end, 135t
  harmonious, 212
  mesio-, 128f, 129, 134t–135t
  neutro-, 123–125, 124f, 127, 131f,
    134t
  normal, 8
  posterior, 127, 127f
  prosthetic, 215
  sagittal curve of, 125–127, 126f
  static, 212
  transverse curve of, 129, 130f

Occlusion rims, 373
Occlusion-raising splints, 373, 373f
Oculomotor nerve, 239, 239f
Odontoblast(s)
  in dentin, 42, 43f, 48, 49f, 51, 54f
  in pulp, 55, 56f
Odontoblast processes, 48, 48f–49f,
  51, 54f
Odontogeny, 41
Olfactory nerve, 239, 239f
Omohyoid muscle, 228
Open bite
  activator for, 340
  anterior, 132f, 132–133
  in posterior segment, 133
Ophthalmic branch, of trigeminal
  nerve, 242
Optic canal, 158
Optic nerve, 239, 239f
Oral, 7, 7f
Oral aperture, line through, 13f
Oral cavity
  anatomy of, 14–16, 15f
  definition of, 14
Oral cavity proper, 14
Oral hygiene
  cleaning techniques, 289–291, 290f
  functions of, 287, 287f
  toothbrush for, 287–289, 288f
Oral screens, 344, 344f
Oral tipping, 122, 122f
Oral vestibule, 14, 16–18, 17f
Orbicularis muscle, 229f, 231f, 232
Orbital vertical, 14
Organ(s)
  definition of, 5
  formation of, 26
Organ systems, 5
Organism, 5
Orofacial system
  biologic functional cycle, 8
  components of, 8, 9f, 358f
  functional disorders of, 357–359,
    358f
  functions of, 9
  normal occlusion, 8
Oropharyngeal, 14
Orthodontic appliances
  activator. See Activator.
  active plate. See Active plate.
  classification of, 309–310, 310f
  Crozat. See Crozat appliance.
  description of, 296–297
  double-plates, 327
  inclined plane, 331–333, 332f

myofunctional therapy, 344f,
  344–345
Orthodontic screws, 316, 317f
Orthodontics
  definition of, 295
  functional, 296, 297f
  functions of, 295
  model analysis, 297–299, 298f–299f
  tooth displacement by, 297
Osseous joint, 175
Osteoarthritis, 181, 361f
Osteoblasts, 36–37
Oval foramen, 155f, 158
Overbite, 78
Overjet, 78, 310
Overlap, 78

P

Paddle spring, 320, 321f
Palatal, 7
Palatal expansion appliance, 349
Palatal raphe, 14
Palatal surface, 74
Palate
  anatomy of, 14–15, 15f
  cleft, 166, 277, 278f–279f
Palatine bone, 14, 152f, 155f, 160,
  161f, 167f
Palatine crest, 160
Palatine glands, 16, 189
Palatine mucous glands, 15
Palatine process, 164
Palatine rugae, 15, 17f
Palatine tonsils, 16, 196f
Palatine torus, 167f
Palpebral fissure, 10
Papillae, 196–197, 196f–197f
Paralingual area, 17f
Paraplasm, 28
Parasympathetic nervous system, 240
Parietal bone, 152f, 156f–157f, 158,
  159f
Parietal lobe, 237f
Parotid gland, 12, 188, 188f
Partial dentures, 378–379
Partial splints, 371
Passive appliances, 309
Pathologic disorders, 2
Pathology, 2
Pericranium, 153
Perikymata, 46, 46f
Periodontal diseases
  description of, 275–277, 276f
  factors associated with, 285

gingivitis, 276f, 277, 285, 286
periodontitis, 276f, 277, 285, 287
Periodontal ligament
anatomy of, 41, 42f
cells of, 61, 62f
connective tissue fibers of, 60–61, 60f–61f
fiber systems of, 61, 61f
nerve supply in, 63
tissue elements of, 60
tooth eruption and, 114
in tooth functioning, 63
Periodontal space
apical widening of, 65
description of, 55–56, 59–60
fibers in, 63, 65f
marginal widening of, 65
nerve fibers in, 63, 65f
Periodontal treatment, splint therapy for, 378–379, 379f
Periodontitis, 276f, 277, 285, 287
Periodontium
alveolar, 64f, 65
alveolar bone, 57–59, 58f–59f
apical, 65–66
blood supply to, 62, 62f
classification of, 64f–70f, 64–70
definition of, 56
functions of, 63–64
marginal. See Marginal periodontium.
structural elements of, 56f
syndesmosis, 55–56
Periodontosis, 287
Periosteal flap, 36f
Periosteum, 37
Peripheral, 8
Permanent dentition
definition of, 22, 112
eruption of, 112, 113f
Petrotympanic fissure, 181
Philtrum, 10
Physiologic abrasion, 148
Physiologic migration of teeth
description of, 300, 301f
mesial, 75, 138
Physiologic processes, 2
Physiologic rest position, 212, 213f
Physiologic tooth contacts, 359
Physiology, 2
Pineal gland, 237f, 241f, 242
Pit and fissure sealing, 291, 291f
Pituitary gland, 237f, 238, 241f, 242
Pivot joint, 177, 177f
Plane joint, 177, 177f
Plaque, 283, 283f

Pliers, 313, 313f
Pogonion, 13f
Pons, 237f
Pont's index, 116, 117f, 298
Position, anatomical nomenclature for, 5–8
Positioners, 377
Posselt's diagram, 204
Posterior, 8
Posterior cranial fossa, 154, 155f
Posterior expansion screw, 325f
Posterior fontanel, 157f
Posterior incisive muscle, 232
Posterior nasal spine, 17f, 167f
Posterior occlusal planes, 310, 311f
Posterior occlusion, 127, 127f
Posterior teeth. See also Dentition; Teeth.
activator effects on, 338f
anatomy of, 21
occlusal surfaces of, 94f–95f, 94–96
successional, 114
Posteruptive enamel maturation, 47
Pound line, 118, 118f
Premolar tangent, 120f, 121
Premolars
in alveolar bone, 59f
description of, 21, 96
mandibular. See Mandibular premolars.
maxillary. See Maxillary premolars.
occlusal contacts in, 143f
occlusal surface of, 73f
Primary dentition
damage to, 280
description of, 20, 22–23, 112
developmental anomalies in, 278–279
premature eruption of, 279
Primary teeth
anterior, 111
dental arch form of, 112, 112f
description of, 20, 22–23
eruption of, 112, 113f
germ cells of, 42
posterior, 112
pulp tissue of, 114
systematic extraction of, 282–283
vestibular view of, 111f
Prognathism, 128f, 129, 134t, 278, 339
Prophase, 30, 30f
Prosthetic equator, 75, 75f
Prosthetic occlusion, 215
Prosthetic tooth replacement, 70, 70f
Prosthion, 13f
Prosthodontics, 292f, 292–293

Protrusion springs, 320, 321f
Protrusive double-plates, 339, 339f
Protrusive excursion, 366
Pterygoid fovea, 172f, 174
Pterygoid processes, 158, 167f
Pterygoid tuberosities, 172, 172f
Pterygomandibular plicae, 192f, 193–194
Pterygomandibular raphe, 16, 17f, 18, 182f
Pterygopalatine nerve, 243–244
Pulp
age-related changes in, 55
anatomy of, 42f, 47, 53–55, 54f
coronal, 54f
functions of, 55
histologic elements of, 54f
irreversible damage to, from abrasion heat, 55
irritation to, 55
root, 54f
tissue composition, 55
Pulp cavity, 47, 53–55, 54f
Pulpitis, 276f, 277
Punctiform contacts, 141f, 144–148, 145f–147f

R

Rami, of mandible, 172–174, 173f–174f
Raphe-papillary transversal, 116
Reciprocal anchorage, 306, 306f
Red bone marrow, 38
Reduction division, 31
Reflex, 236
Reflex splints, 362t, 363–365, 364f–365f
Relaxation splint, 363–364
Remodeling processes
causes of, 297
in mesial migration, 300, 301f
in tooth movement, 300–302, 301f
Removable appliances, 309–310
Removable splints, 378
Replacing bone, 37
Repositioning splints, 362t, 370f, 370–371
Reproductive glands, 242
Respiratory disorders, splint therapy for, 374–377
Retainers, 309, 362t, 376
Reticular connective tissue, 35
Retracting spring, 320, 320f
Retroarticular process, 177, 178f
Retromolar trigone, 170–171, 172f

Retrusive double-plates, 339, 339f
Reverse articulation, 131, 135t
Reverse vertical overlap, 129
Ribosomes, 28
Rickets, open bite caused by, 133
Ricketts technique, 351
Ridge line, 118
Risorius muscle, 229f, 231f, 232
Root
  abnormal shapes of, 280, 281f
  description of, 6, 20, 21f
  of mandibular canines, 93f
  of mandibular second premolar, 100f
  of maxillary canines, 93f
  of maxillary central incisor, 80, 81f
  of maxillary incisors, 87f
  of maxillary posterior teeth, 108f
  of successional teeth, 113–114, 114f
Root apex, 21, 21f
Root canal, 47, 50f
Root characteristic, 78, 79f, 126f
Root pulp, 54f
Rotating condyle, 202
Rotation, 121–122, 122f, 135t
Rugae, palatine, 15

S

Saddle joint, 176, 177f
Sagittal, 8
Sagittal axis, 6, 6f
Sagittal Christensen's phenomenon, 208, 208f
Sagittal curve of occlusion, 125–127, 126f
Sagittal plane
  dentition in, 123f–128f, 123–129
  illustration of, 6, 6f
  mandibular border movements in, 204, 205f
  tooth malposition in, 127f–128f, 127–129, 134t
Sagittal protrusion, 128
Sagittal split, of active plate, 324, 325f–326f
Sagittal suture, 154, 157f
Saliva, 186
Salivary glands, 12, 186, 188, 188f–189f
Sarcoplasm, 218, 220
Schwann sheath, 235
Schwarz plate, 324
Secondary dentin, 48, 76
Sector screw, 316, 317f
Sella turcica, 155f

Sellar joint, 176, 177f
Semi-adjustable average-value articulators, 253, 253f
Sensory tissue, 32, 33f
Serous glands, 186
Sharpey fibers, 52–53, 53f, 56–58, 61f, 65, 168
Shearing cusps, 102, 135t
Sheath of Henle, 235
Shore plate, 374
Short bones, 40
Sialoliths, 186
Single-point force application, 304f, 305
Skeletal muscle, 220
Skeleton, 39f
Skin
  atrophy of, 185
  bacteria on, 185
  functions of, 183
  heat regulation functions of, 183
  irritation of, 185
  sensory function of, 183
  structure of, 184, 184f
Skin appendages, 184–185
Skin glands, 185
Skull, base of, 154, 155f–157f
Skull cap, 151
Smooth muscle, 218
Snoring, 374–375
Soft palate, 14, 15f, 16, 17f, 160
Soft tissue orbitale, 13f
Soft tissue porion, 13f
Somatic nervous system, 236
Somatic organs, 5
Spaces, 122, 134t
Specialist training, 1
Specialization, 1
Sphenofrontal suture, 154, 157f
Sphenoid bone, 18, 152f, 155f–157f, 158, 159f
Sphenoidal fontanel, 157f
Sphenomandibular ligament, 181, 182f, 226f
Spheroidal joint, 176, 177f
Spinal cord, 236
Spiralization, 30
Splints/splint therapy. *See also specific splint.*
  centric relation. *See* Centric relation splints.
  effects of, 361
  goals of, 358f
  indications for, 361
  intraoral appliances for, 362t
  materials used in, 363

objectives of, 372
occlusal splints, 362t
periodontal treatment using, 378–379, 379f
pre-prosthetic treatment measures, 372–374
respiratory disorders treated with, 374–377
special forms of, 374–377
Spongy bone, 58, 58f
Spongy substance, 36f, 38, 38f
Spring components, of active plate, 318–323, 318f–323f
Spring loops, 320, 321f
Squamous epithelium, 32, 33f
Squamous suture, 154, 157f
Stabilization splint, 361, 363, 366–367, 366f–367f
Static occlusion, 212
Stationary anchorage, 306–307, 307f
Stellate cells, 49
Stellate reticulum, 42–43
Stem fibers, 30
Stensen duct, 232
Sternohyoid muscle, 228
Sternothyroid muscle, 228
Stockfisch's kinetor, 344f, 344–345
Stratified epithelium, 33f, 34
Striated muscle, 218–220
Styloglossus muscle, 198, 199f
Stylohyoid muscle, 227f, 228
Styloid process, 182f
Stylomandibular ligament, 181, 182f
Subcutis, 184
Sublingual caruncles, 195
Sublingual fovea, 170, 172f
Sublingual gland, 14, 188, 189f
Submandibular fovea, 170, 172f
Submandibular gland, 14, 188–189, 189f
Subnasale, 13f
Successional teeth
  anterior, 114
  eruption of, 114
  germ teeth, 42
  posterior, 114
  root formation of, 113–114, 114f
Sucking, open bite caused by, 132–133
Sulcus brush, 290
Superior incisive muscle, 232
Superior joint space, 178f, 180
Superior labial frenulum, 192f, 193
Superior nasal concha, 160
Supernumerary teeth, 281

Supplemental developmental groove, 95f, 96
Supporting cusps, 94
Suprahyoid muscles, 226, 227f
Surface epithelium, 32, 33f
Sutures, cranial, 154, 156f–157f
Sved appliance, 364, 365f
Sweat glands, 185
Swivel expansion screw, 316, 317f
Symmetry plane, 6, 6f
Sympathetic nervous system, 240
Symphysis, 12, 168
Synapse, 235, 235f
Synarthroses, 56
Syndesmosis, 55–56
Synovial bursae, 176
Synovial fluid, 175
Synovial folds, 175
Synovial sheaths, 176

T

Taste, 197
Taste buds, 196–197, 197f
Teeth. See also Anterior teeth; Dentition; Posterior teeth; specific teeth.
  abnormal numbers of, 281–283, 282f
  anatomy of, 20–21, 21f, 41, 42f
  in animals, 18, 19f
  anterior, 21
  approximal surfaces of, 74, 75f
  contact points of, 74, 75f, 138–149
  crown of. See Crown of tooth.
  deciduous, 20. See also Primary teeth.
  developmental anomalies in, 279–281, 281f
  directional terms for, 6, 6f–7f
  eruption of, 112, 113f
  exfoliation of, 20
  form, formation, and function of, 18–20, 19f
  forms of. See Tooth forms.
  germ cells of, 42, 43f
  grinding of, 359
  layers of, 41, 42f
  lingual surfaces of, 74, 74f
  malposition of
    in frontal plane, 131–133, 134t–135t
    in horizontal plane, 121f–122f, 121–123
    in sagittal plane, 127f–128f, 127–129, 134t
  in mammals, 19f, 20
  mesial inclination of, 126f
  neck of, 21
  notation for, 22–23, 24f
  number of, 281
  occlusal surface of, 72, 72f–73f
  posterior, 21
  root of, 6, 20, 21f
  size of, 20
  space between, 122–123
  supernumerary, 281
  tipping movements on, 57
  vestibular surface of, 72, 72f, 74f
  word origin of, 18
Telescopic screw, 316, 317f
Telophase, 30, 30f
Temporal, 8
Temporal bone, 152f, 155f–157f, 158, 159f
Temporal muscle, 224, 224f–225f
Temporal nerve, 244
Temporary dentition, 21
Temporomandibular dysfunction, 358f
Temporomandibular joint
  anatomy of, 359f
  in animals, 180–181
  articular disc, 178f, 180–181, 258
  articular surface of, 179
  bony parts of, 177–179, 178f
  clenching of, 359
  connective tissue parts of, 178f, 179
  degenerative changes of, 361
  diseases and disorders of, 359f, 359–360
  joint capsule, 175, 176f, 178f, 181
  movement of, 201
  osteoarthritis of, 361f
Temporomandibular ligament, 181, 182f
Tendon sheaths, 176, 221
Tendons, 221
Terminal occlusion, 212
Thalamus, 238
Thymus gland, 241f, 242
Thyrohyoid muscle, 228
Thyroid gland, 241f, 242
Tight connective tissue, 36
Tipping
  lingual, 136, 137f
  mesial, 122
  oral, 122, 122f
  in sagittal direction, 136
  vestibular, 122, 122f, 136–137, 137f
Tissue
  bone. See Bone.
  classification of, 32–36
  connective, 32, 34f–35f, 34–36, 60
  definition of, 5
  dental. See Dental tissues.
  epithelial, 32–34, 33f
  muscle, 32
  nerve, 32
Tissue linkage, 137, 137f
Tongue
  description of, 195–196
  dorsum of, 196, 196f
  frenulum of, 194–196
  musculature of, 198, 199f
  papillae of, 196–197, 196f–197f
  root of, 196
Tongue retainers, 375
Tooth. See Teeth.
Tooth decay, 276, 283–285. See also Caries.
Tooth displacement, 122, 135t
Tooth forms
  characteristic features of, 71–74, 72f–74f
  description of, 76–77, 76f–77f
Tooth germs, 59
Tooth guidance, of mandibular movements, 206, 212–214, 213f. See also Occlusion.
Tooth inclination, of mandibular first premolar, 98, 99f
Tooth movements
  remodeling processes in, 300–302, 301f
  transferring forces in, 304–305, 305f
Tooth positioner, 345
Tooth replacement, 122
Toothbrushes, 287–289, 288f, 290f
Toothpastes, 289
Topographical anatomy, 2
Torus palatinus, 14, 17f
Trabeculae, 38
Tragion, 13f
Tragus, 13f
Trajectories, 153
Transfer RNA, 29
Translating condyle, 202
Transverse axis, 6, 6f
Transverse Christensen's phenomenon, 208f, 208–209
Transverse curve of occlusion, 129, 130f
Transverse palatine suture, 166, 167f
Transverse plane
  description of, 6, 6f
  tooth malposition in, 135t
Transverse split, of active plate, 324, 325f–326f

Traumatizing occlusion, 215
Triangle clasps, 314, 315f
Triangular ridges, 94
Trichion, 13f
Trigeminal nerve, 239f, 240, 242–244, 243f
Trochlear nerve, 239, 239f
True hyperdontia, 281, 282f
True hypodontia, 282
True joints, 174–175
Twin arch technique, 351
Two-point force application, 304f, 305
Tympanic tubercle, 178f, 179

U

U-loops, 322, 323f
Upper face, 9
Upper lip, 10, 11f
Uprights, 330
Uvula, 14, 15f

V

Vacuoles, 27f
Vagus nerve, 239f, 240
Velar clefts, 277
Velum palatinum, 16
Ventral, 8

Vertebrae, 39f
Vertical abrasion, 76
Vertical anterior dental arch, 125, 125f
Vertical axis, 6, 6f
Vertical curvature characteristic, 72
Vertical exfoliation of teeth, 20
Vestibular, 6, 7f
Vestibular fornices, 16, 17f, 191
Vestibular inclination of anterior teeth, 125, 129
Vestibular sulcus, 16, 18
Vestibular surface
  description of, 72, 72f, 74f
  of mandibular first molar, 109, 110f
  of mandibular first premolar, 98–100, 99f
  of mandibular incisors, 84, 85f–86f
  of mandibular second premolar, 101f, 102
  of maxillary canines, 88, 89f
  of maxillary first molar, 103f, 104, 105f
  of maxillary first premolar, 96, 97f
  of maxillary second molar, 106f, 107
  of maxillary second premolar, 97, 98f
Vestibular tipping, 122, 122f, 136–137, 137f
Vestibulocochlear nerve, 239f, 240

Vibrating line, 16, 17f, 190, 193
Viruses, 26
Visceral cranium, 152f
Volkmann canals, 38, 62
Vomer, 152f, 155f–156f, 160, 161f
von Korff fibers, 51

W

Wear facets, 76
Weissenfluh splint, 379
Wisdom tooth, 21

Y

Yellow bone marrow, 38
Y-split, of active plate, 324, 326f, 326–327

Z

Zsigmondy-Palmer system, 23, 24f
Zygomatic bone, 152f, 154, 155f–157f, 160, 161f
Zygomatic crest, 17f, 18
Zygomatic muscle, 229f, 231f, 233
Zygomatic nerve, 242
Zygomatic process, 164, 165f, 167f